GENERAL UROLOGY

7
Edition

GENERAL
UROLOGY

DONALD R. SMITH, MD

Professor of Urology and
Chairman of the Division of Urology
University of California School of Medicine
San Francisco

Consulting Urologist, San Francisco General Hospital
Consulting Surgeon (Urology)
Veterans Administration Hospital, San Francisco

Lange Medical Publications

LOS ALTOS, CALIFORNIA

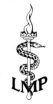

1972

A Concise Medical Library for Practitioner and Student

General Urology, 7th ed. $8.50

Current Diagnosis & Treatment (11th annual revision). Edited by M.A. Krupp and M.J. Chatton. 962 pp, *illus.*	1972
Current Pediatric Diagnosis & Treatment, 2nd ed. Edited by C.H. Kempe, H.K. Silver, and D. O'Brien. 1014 pp, *illus.*	1972
Review of Physiological Chemistry, 13th ed. H.A. Harper. 529 pp, *illus.*	1971
Review of Medical Physiology, 5th ed. W.F. Ganong. 573 pp, *illus.*	1971
Review of Medical Microbiology, 10th ed. E. Jawetz, J.L. Melnick, and E.A. Adelberg. 518 pp, *illus.*	1972
Review of Medical Pharmacology, 3rd ed. F.H. Meyers, E. Jawetz, and A. Goldfien. About 700 pp, *illus.*	1972
General Ophthalmology, 6th ed. D. Vaughan, T. Asbury, and R. Cook. 316 pp, *illus.*	1971
Correlative Neuroanatomy & Functional Neurology, 14th ed. J.G. Chusid. 453 pp, *illus.*	1970
Principles of Clinical Electrocardiography, 7th ed. M.J. Goldman. 400 pp, *illus.*	1970
Handbook of Psychiatry, 2nd ed. Edited by P. Solomon and V.D. Patch. 648 pp.	1971
Handbook of Surgery, 5th ed. Edited by J.L. Wilson. About 780 pp, *illus.*	1972
Handbook of Obstetrics & Gynecology, 4th ed. R.C. Benson. 774 pp, *illus.*	1971
Physician's Handbook, 16th ed. M.A. Krupp, N.J. Sweet, E. Jawetz, and E.G. Biglieri. 660 pp, *illus.*	1970
Handbook of Medical Treatment, 13th ed. Edited by M.J. Chatton. About 640 pp.	1972
Handbook of Pediatrics, 9th ed. H.K. Silver, C.H. Kempe, and H.B. Bruyn. 713 pp.	1971
Handbook of Poisoning: Diagnosis & Treatment, 7th ed. R.H. Dreisbach. 515 pp.	1971

Preface

This book was originally written for the medical student and for the medical practitioner who has not specialized in urology but whose practice requires a working familiarity with the diagnostic and therapeutic technics available for the management of genitourinary diseases and disorders. It has been a distinct pleasure to the author to find that residents in urology have also found the volume useful.

The thesis of the book is that although many urologic disorders produce few or no symptoms, the clues to their presence lie in careful history taking and physical examination and, above all, a personally performed study of the fresh, stained urinary sediment and utilization of the PSP renal function test, which also permits estimation of the amount of residual urine. In addition to excretory urograms, the need for voiding cystourethrograms has become increasingly apparent for demonstrating posterior urethral valves, congenital urethral stenosis in girls, and vesicoureteral reflux (the most common cause of acute and chronic pyelonephritis).

Throughout the book, new material has been added and emphases changed. The rather extensive bibliography has been brought up to date so that the reader can study any subject in depth.

I should like to reaffirm my gratitude to Dr. John A. Hutch for his advice and assistance in the preparation of the chapters on vesicoureteral reflux and the neurogenic bladder; to Dr. Marcus A. Krupp for his succinct summary of the problems of diagnosis of medical renal diseases; to Dr. Emil Tanagho for his excellent section on embryology; to Dr. Richards P. Lyon for his chapter on oliguria; to Dr. Rees B. Rees for his chapter on skin diseases of the external genitalia; and to Drs. Malcolm R. Powell and Jerome M. Weiss, whose chapter dealing with radioisotopic kidney studies remains unique in the urologic literature.

It is a pleasure to note that the Spanish translation of this book, published by El Manual Moderno of Mexico City, continues to receive wide acceptance in Central and South America. A German edition under the imprint of Urban & Schwarzenberg, published in 1968, has been well received. French, Greek, Portuguese, and Polish editions are now in preparation.

The author wishes to express his appreciation to his many urologic colleagues and former residents who have contributed valuable suggestions and criticisms over the years.

Donald R. Smith, MD

San Francisco, California
June, 1972

Table of Contents

1...

Anatomy of the Genitourinary Tract

Urology deals with diseases and disorders of the genitourinary tract in the male and of the urinary tract in the female. These systems are illustrated in Figs 1-1 and 1-2.

ADRENALS

Gross Appearance

A. Anatomy: Each kidney is capped by an adrenal gland, and both organs are enclosed within Gerota's (perirenal) fascia. Each adrenal weighs about 10 gm. The right adrenal is triangular in shape; the left is more rounded and crescentic. Each gland is composed of a cortex, chiefly influenced by the hypophysis, and a medulla derived from chromaffin tissue.

B. Relations: Fig 1-3 shows the relation of the adrenals to other organs. The right adrenal lies between the liver and the vena cava. The left gland lies close to the aorta and is covered on its lower surface by the pancreas; superiorly and laterally, it is related to the spleen.

Histology

The adrenal cortex is composed of 3 distinct layers: the outer zona glomerulosa, the middle zona fasciculata, and the inner zona reticularis. The medulla lies centrally and is made up of polyhedral cells containing eosinophilic granular cytoplasm. These chromaffin cells are accompanied by ganglion and small round cells.

Blood Supply

A. Arterial: Each adrenal receives 3 arteries: one from the inferior phrenic artery, another from the aorta, and the third from the renal artery.

B. Venous: The right adrenal blood is drained by a very short vein which empties into the vena cava; the left adrenal vein terminates in the left renal vein.

Lymphatics

The lymphatic vessels accompany the suprarenal vein and drain into the lumbar lymph nodes.

Ivemark, B., Ekström, T., & C. Lagergren: The vasculature of the developing and mature human adrenal gland. Acta pediat scandinav 56:601-6, 1967.

Johnstone, F. R. C.: The surgical anatomy of the adrenal glands with particular reference to the suprarenal vein. S Clin North America 44:1315-25, 1964.

KIDNEYS

Gross Appearance

A. Anatomy: The kidneys lie along the borders of the psoas muscles and are therefore obliquely placed. The position of the liver causes the right kidney to be lower than the left (Figs 1-3 and 1-4). The adult kidney weighs about 150 gm.

The kidneys are supported by the perirenal fat (which is enclosed in the perirenal fascia), the renal vascular pedicle, abdominal muscle tone, and the general bulk of the abdominal viscera. Variations in these factors permit variations in the degree of renal mobility. The average descent on inspiration or on assuming the upright position is 4-5 cm. Lack of mobility suggests abnormal fixation (eg, perinephritis), but extreme mobility is not necessarily pathologic.

On longitudinal section (Fig 1-5) the kidney is seen to be made up of an outer cortex, a central medulla, and the internal calyces and pelvis. The cortex is homogeneous in appearance. Portions of it project toward the pelvis between the papillae and fornices and are called the columns of Bertin. The medulla consists of numerous pyramids formed by the converging collecting renal tubules, which drain into the minor calyces.

B. Relations: Figs 1-3 and 1-4 show the relations of the kidneys to adjacent organs and

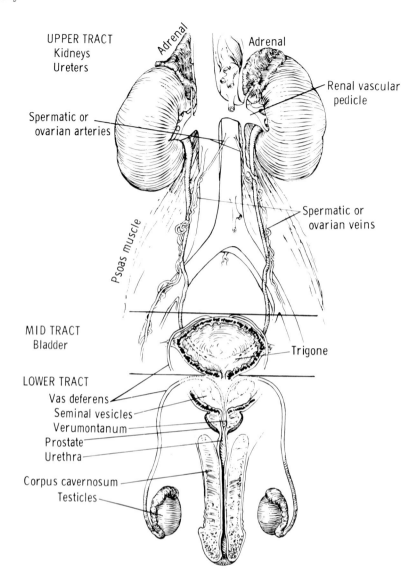

UPPER TRACT
Kidneys
Ureters

Adrenal

Adrenal

Renal vascular
pedicle

Spermatic or
ovarian arteries

Psoas muscle

Spermatic or
ovarian veins

MID TRACT
Bladder

Trigone

LOWER TRACT
Vas deferens
Seminal vesicles
Verumontanum
Prostate
Urethra
Corpus cavernosum
Testicles

Fig 1-1. Anatomy of the male genitourinary tract. The upper and mid tracts have urologic function only. The lower tract has both genital and urinary functions.

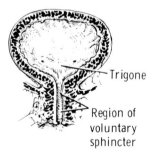

Trigone

Region of
voluntary
sphincter

Fig 1-2. Anatomy of the mid and lower tracts in the female.

structures. Their intimacy with intraperitoneal organs explains, in part, some of the gastro-intestinal symptoms which accompany genito-urinary disease.

Histology

A. Nephron: The functioning unit of the kidney is the nephron, which is composed of a tubule which has both secretory and excretory functions (Fig 1-5). The secretory portion is contained largely within the cortex and consists of a renal corpuscle and the secretory part of the renal tubule. The excretory portion of this duct lies in the medulla. The renal corpuscle is composed of the vascular glomerulus, which projects into Bowman's capsule, which, in turn, is continuous with the epithelium of the proximal convoluted tubule. The secretory portion of the renal tubule is made up of the proximal convoluted tubule, the loop of Henle, and the distal convoluted tubule.

The excretory portion of the nephron is the collecting tubule, which is continuous with the distal end of the ascending limb of the convoluted tubule. It empties its contents through the tip (papilla) of a pyramid into a minor calyx.

B. Supporting Tissue: The renal stroma is composed of loose connective tissue and contains blood vessels, capillaries, nerves, and lymphatics.

Blood Supply (See Figs 1-3 and 1-5.)

A. Arterial: Usually there is one renal artery, a branch of the aorta, which enters the hilum of the kidney between the pelvis, which normally lies posteriorly, and the renal vein. It may branch before it reaches the kidney, and 2 or more separate arteries may be noted. In duplication of the pelvis and ureter it is usual for each renal segment to have its own arterial supply.

This artery further divides into the interlobular arteries, which ascend in the columns of Bertin (between the pyramids) and then arch along the base of the pyramids (arcuate arteries). From these vessels smaller (afferent) branches pass to the glomeruli. From the glomerular tuft efferent arterioles pass to the tubules in the stroma.

B. Venous: The renal veins are paired with the arteries, but any of them will drain the entire kidney if the others are tied off.

Although the renal artery and vein are usually the sole blood vessels of the kidney, accessory renal vessels are common and may be of clinical importance if they are so placed as to compress the ureter, in which case hydronephrosis may result.

Lymphatics

The lymphatics of the kidney drain into the lumbar lymph nodes (Figs 17-1 and 17-2).

Barger, A. C., & J. A. Herd: The renal circulation. New England J Med **284**:482-90, 1971.

Black, D. A. K.: Renal rete mirabile. Lancet **2**:1141-51, 1965.

Castelli, W. A., & D. F. Huelke: The intrarenal vascular distribution in the human kidney. J Urol **102**:12-20, 1969.

Fetterman, G. H., & others: The growth and maturation of human glomeruli and proximal convolutions from term to adulthood. Pediatrics **35**:601-19, 1965.

Graves, F. T.: The arterial anatomy of the congenitally abnormal kidney. Brit J Surg **56**:533-41, 1969.

Layton, J. M.: The structure of the kidney from the gross to the molecular. J Urol **90**:502-15, 1963.

Mayerson, H. S.: The lymphatic system with particular reference to the kidney. Surg Gynec Obst **116**:259-72, 1963.

Osathanondh, V., & E. L. Potter: Development of human kidney shown by microdissection. IV. Development of tubular portions of nephrons. Arch Path **82**:391-402, 1966.

Roddie, I. C.: Modern views on physiology. XX. The kidney. Practitioner **205**:242-50, 1970.

Zamboni, L., & C. DeMartino: Embryogenesis of the human renal glomerulus. I. A histologic study. Arch Path **86**:279-91, 1968.

CALYCES, RENAL PELVIS, AND URETER

Gross Appearance

A. Anatomy:

1. Calyces - The tips of the minor calyces (4-12 in number) are indented by the projecting pyramids (Fig 1-5). These calyces unite to form 2 or 3 major calyces, which join the renal pelvis.

2. Renal pelvis - The pelvis may be entirely intrarenal or partly intrarenal and partly extrarenal. Inferomedially it tapers to form the ureter.

3. Ureter - The adult ureter is about 30 cm long, varying in direct relation to the height of the individual. It follows a rather smooth "S" curve. Areas of constriction are found (1) at the ureteropelvic junction, (2) where the ureter crosses over the iliac vessels, and (3) where it courses through the bladder wall.

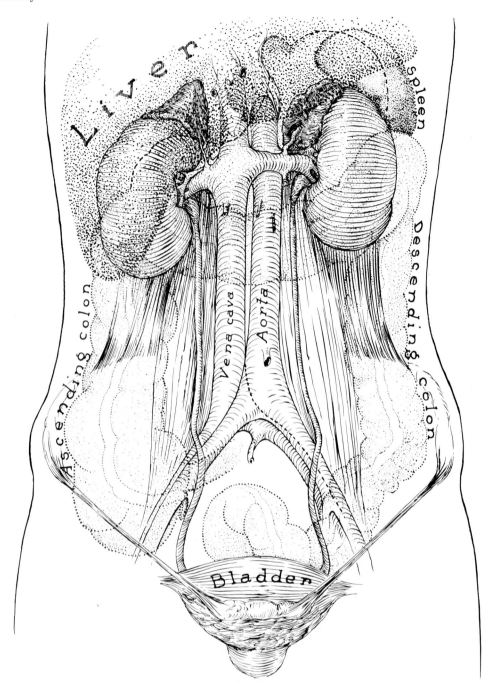

Fig 1-3. Relations of kidney, ureters, and bladder (anterior aspect).

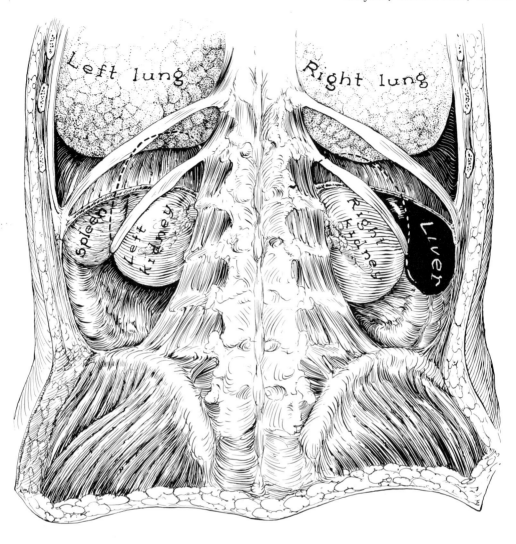

Fig 1-4. Relations of kidneys (posterior aspect).

B. Relations:

1. Calyces - The calyces are intrarenal and are intimately related to the renal parenchyma.

2. Renal pelvis - If the pelvis is partly extrarenal, it lies along the lateral border of the psoas muscle and on the quadratus lumborum muscle; the renal vascular pedicle is placed just anterior to it. The left renal pelvis lies at the level of the first or second lumbar vertebra; the right pelvis is a little lower.

3. Ureter - As followed from above downward, the ureters lie on the psoas muscles, pass medially to the sacroiliac joints, and then swing laterally near the ischial spines before passing medially to penetrate the base of the bladder (Fig 1-3). The uterine arteries are closely related to the juxtavesical portion of the ureters. The ureters are covered by the posterior peritoneum; their lowermost portions are closely attached to it, while the juxtavesical portions are embedded in vascular retroperitoneal fat.

As the vasa deferentia leave the prostate, they lie just medial to the ureters; just above the trigonal area the vasa pass anteriorly to the ureters on their way to the internal inguinal rings (Fig 1-6).

Histology (See Fig 1-5.)

The walls of the calyces, pelvis, and ureter are composed of transitional cell epithelium under which lies loose connective and elastic tissue (lamina propria). External to these are a mixture of spiral and longitudinal smooth muscle fibers. They are not arranged

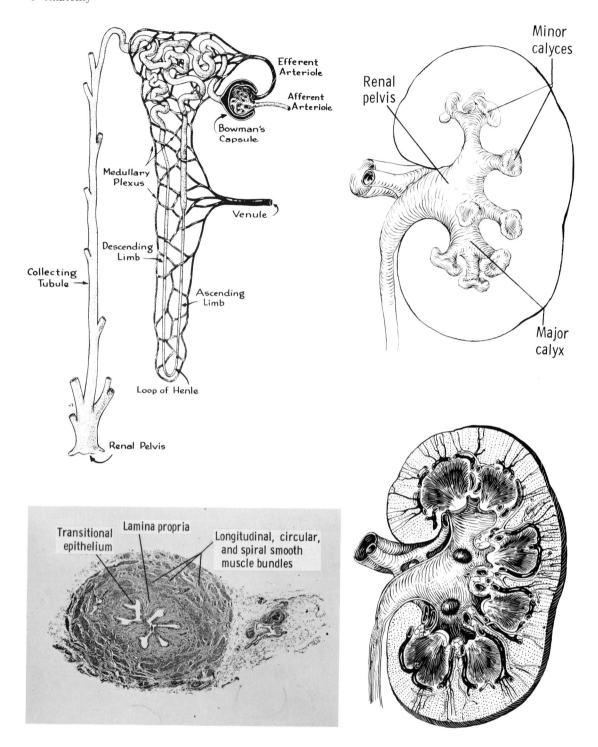

Fig 1-5. Anatomy and histology of the kidney and ureter. **Above left:** Diagram of the nephron and its blood supply. (Courtesy of Merck Sharp and Dohme: Seminar:9[3], 1947.) **Above right:** Renal calyces, pelvis, and ureter (posterior aspect). **Below left:** Histology of the ureter. The smooth muscle bundles are arranged in both a spiral and longitudinal manner. **Below right:** Longitudinal section of kidney showing calyces, pelvis, ureter, and renal blood supply (posterior aspect).

in definite layers. The outermost adventitial coat is composed of fibrous connective tissue.

Blood Supply

A. Arterial: The renal calyces, pelvis, and upper ureter derive their blood supply from the renal arteries; the midureter is fed by the internal spermatic (or ovarian) arteries. The lowermost portion of the ureter is served by branches from the common iliac, hypogastric, and vesical arteries.

B. Venous: The veins of the renal calyces, pelvis, and ureter are paired with the arteries.

Lymphatics

The lymphatics of the upper portion of the ureter as well as those from the pelvis and calyces enter the lumbar lymph nodes. The lymphatics of the midureter pass to the hypogastric and common iliac lymph nodes; the lower ureteral lymphatics empty into the vesical and hypogastric lymph nodes (Figs 17-1 and 17-2).

Cussen, L. J.: The structure of the normal human ureter in infancy and childhood. Invest Urol 5:179-94, 1967.

Sykes, D.: The morphology of renal lobulations and calyces, and their relationship to partial nephrectomy. Brit J Surg 51: 294-304, 1964.

BLADDER

Gross Appearance

The bladder is a hollow muscular organ which serves as a reservoir for urine. In women, its posterior wall and dome are invaginated by the uterus. The adult bladder has a capacity of 400-500 ml.

A. Anatomy: When empty, the adult bladder lies behind the symphysis pubis and is largely a pelvic organ. In infants and children it is situated higher. When it is full, it rises well above the symphysis and can readily be palpated or percussed. When overdistended, as with acute or chronic urinary retention, it may cause the lower abdomen to bulge visibly.

Extending from the dome of the bladder to the umbilicus is a fibrous cord, the medial umbilical ligament, which represents the obliterated urachus. The ureters enter the bladder postero-inferiorly in an oblique manner and at these points are placed about 2.5 cm apart (Fig 1-6). The orifices are situated at the extremities of the crescent-shaped interuteric ridge which forms the proximal border of the trigone. The trigone occupies the area between the ridge and the bladder neck.

The internal sphincter, or bladder neck, is not a true circular sphincter but a thickening formed by interlaced and converging muscle fibers of the detrusor as they pass distally to become the smooth musculature of the urethra.

B. Relations: In the male the bladder is related posteriorly to the seminal vesicles, vasa deferentia, ureters, and rectum (Figs 1-8 and 1-9). In the female the uterus and vagina are interposed between the bladder and rectum (Fig 1-10). The dome and posterior surfaces are covered by peritoneum; hence, in this area the bladder is closely related to the small intestine and the sigmoid colon. In both male and female the bladder is related to the posterior surface of the symphysis pubis, and, when distended, it is in contact with the lower abdominal wall.

Histology (See Fig 1-7.)

The mucosa of the bladder is composed of transitional epithelium. Beneath it is a well developed submucosal layer formed largely of connective and elastic tissues. External to the submucosa is the detrusor muscle, made up of a mixture of smooth muscle fibers which are arranged at random in a longitudinal, circular, and spiral manner.

Blood Supply

A. Arterial: The arterial supply to the bladder comes from the superior, middle, and inferior vesical arteries, which arise from the anterior trunk of the hypogastric artery. Smaller branches from the obturator and inferior gluteal arteries also reach this organ. In the female, the uterine and vaginal arteries also send branches to the bladder.

B. Venous: Surrounding the bladder is a rich plexus of veins which ultimately empties into the hypogastric veins.

Lymphatics

The lymphatics of the bladder drain into the vesical, external iliac, hypogastric, and common iliac lymph nodes (Figs 17-1 and 17-2).

Hodges, C.V.: Surgical anatomy of the urinary bladder and pelvic ureter. S Clin North America 44:1327-33, 1964.

Hutch, J.A.: The internal urinary sphincter: A double loop system. J Urol 105:375-83, 1971.

Tanagho, E.A., & D.R. Smith: The anatomy and function of the bladder neck. Brit J Urol 38:54-71, 1966.

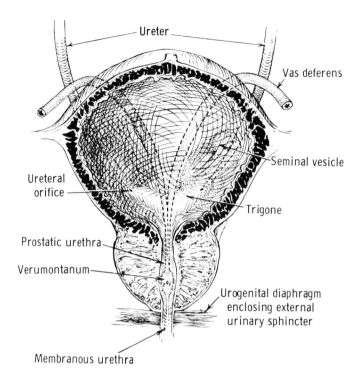

Fig 1-6. Anatomy and relations of the ureters, bladder, prostate, seminal vesicles, and vasa deferentia (anterior view).

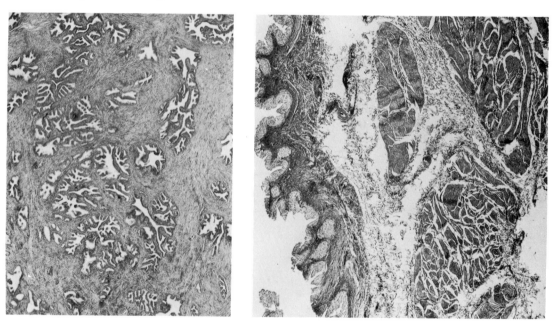

Fig 1-7. **Left:** Histology of the prostate. Epithelial glands embedded in a mixture of connective and elastic tissue and smooth muscle. **Right:** Histology of the bladder. The mucosa is transitional-cell in type and lies upon a well developed submucosal layer of connective tissue. The detrusor muscle is composed of interlacing longitudinal, circular, and spiral smooth muscle bundles.

Tanagho, E. A., & others: Observations in the dynamics of the bladder neck. Brit J Urol 38:72-84, 1966.

Hutch, J. A., & O. N. Rambo, Jr.: A study of the anatomy of the prostate, prostatic urethra and the urinary sphincter system. J Urol 104:443-53, 1970.

PROSTATE GLAND

Gross Appearance

A. Anatomy: The prostate is a fibro-muscular and glandular organ lying just inferior to the bladder (Figs 1-6 and 1-8). The normal prostate weighs about 20 gm and contains the posterior urethra, which is about 2.5 cm in length. It is supported anteriorly by the puboprostatic ligaments and inferiorly by the urogenital diaphragm (Fig 1-6). The prostate is perforated posteriorly by the ejaculatory ducts, which pass obliquely to empty through the verumontanum on the floor of the prostatic urethra just proximal to the striated external urinary sphincter.

B. Relations: The prostate gland lies behind the symphysis pubis. Closely applied to its posterosuperior surface are the vasa deferentia and seminal vesicles (Fig 1-8). Posteriorly it is separated from the rectum by the 2 layers of Denonvilliers' fascia, serosal rudiments of the pouch of Douglas which once extended to the urogenital diaphragm (Fig 1-9).

Histology (See Fig 1-7.)

The prostate consists of a thin fibrous (true) capsule enclosing the stroma, which is composed of connective and elastic tissues and smooth muscle fibers in which are embedded the epithelial glands. These glands drain into the major excretory ducts (about 25 in number), which open chiefly on the floor of the prostatic urethra. Just beneath the transitional epithelium of the prostatic urethra lie the periurethral glands.

Blood Supply

A. Arterial: The arterial supply to the prostate is derived from the inferior vesical, internal pudendal, and middle hemorrhoidal arteries.

B. Venous: The veins from the prostate drain into the periprostatic plexus, which has connections with the deep dorsal vein of the penis and the hypogastric veins.

Lymphatics

The lymphatics from the prostate drain into the hypogastric, sacral, vesical, and external iliac lymph nodes (Figs 17-1 and 17-2).

SEMINAL VESICLES

Gross Appearance

The seminal vesicles lie just cephalad to the prostate under the base of the bladder (Figs 1-8 and 1-9. They are about 6 cm long and quite soft. Each vesicle joins its corresponding vas deferens to form the ejaculatory duct. The ureters lie medially to each, and the rectum is contiguous with their posterior surfaces.

Histology

The mucous membrane is pseudostratified. The submucosa consists of dense connective tissue covered by a thin layer of muscle which in turn is encapsulated by connective tissue.

Blood Supply

The blood supply is similar to that of the prostate gland.

Lymphatics

The lymphatics of the seminal vesicles are those that serve the prostate (Figs 17-1 and 17-2).

SPERMATIC CORD

Gross Appearance

The 2 spermatic cords extend from the internal inguinal rings through the inguinal canals to the testicles (Fig 1-8). Each cord contains the vas deferens, the internal and external spermatic arteries, the artery of the vas, the venous pampiniform plexus (which forms the spermatic vein superiorly), lymph vessels, and nerves. All of the above are enclosed in investing layers of thin fascia. A few fibers of the cremaster muscle insert on the cords in the inguinal canal.

Histology

The fascia covering the cord is formed of loose connective tissue which supports arteries, veins, and lymphatics. The vas deferens is a small, thick-walled tube consisting of an internal mucosa and submucosa surrounded by 3 well defined layers of smooth muscle encased in a covering of fibrous tissue.

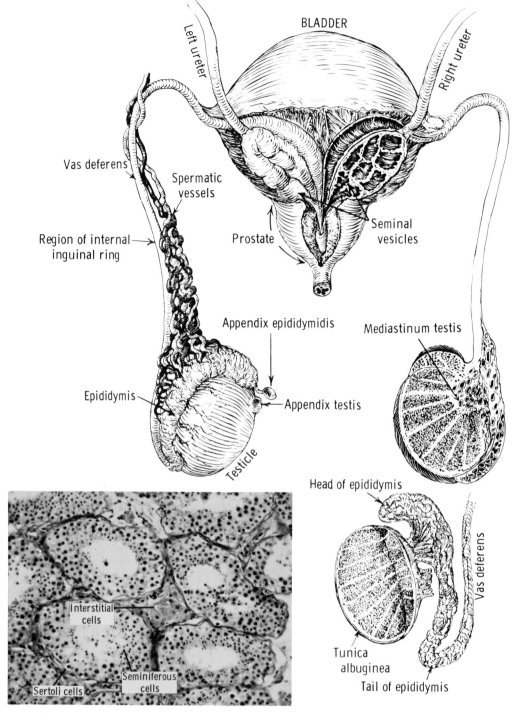

Fig 1-8. **Above:** Gross anatomy and relations of ureters, bladder, prostate, seminal vesicles, vasa deferentia, testes, and epididymides. **Below left:** Histology of the testis. Seminiferous tubules lined by supporting basement membrane for the Sertoli and spermatogenic cells. The latter are in various stages of development. **Below right:** Cross section of testis showing fibrous septa dividing organ into lobules.

Blood Supply

A. Arterial: The external spermatic artery, a branch of the inferior epigastric, supplies the fascial coverings of the cord. The internal spermatic artery passes through the cord on its way to the testis. The deferential artery is close to the vas.

B. Venous: The veins from the testis and the coverings of the spermatic cord form the pampiniform plexus, which, at the internal inguinal ring, unites to form the spermatic vein.

Lymphatics

The lymphatics from the spermatic cord empty into the external iliac lymph nodes (Figs 17-1 and 17-2).

Ahlberg, N. E., Bartley, O., & N. Chidekel: Right and left gonadal veins. An anatomical and statistical study. Acta radiol diag **4**: 593-601, 1966.

Bergman, L. L.: The regional anatomy of the inguinal canal. GP **26**:114-23, Oct 1962.

EPIDIDYMIS

Gross Appearance

A. Anatomy: The upper portion of the epididymis (globus major) is connected to the testis by numerous efferent ducts from the testis (Fig 1-8). The epididymis consists of a markedly coiled duct which, at its lower pole (globus minor), is continuous with the vas deferens. An appendix of the epididymis is often seen on its upper pole; this is a cystic body which sometimes is pedunculated but at other times is sessile.

B. Relations: The epididymis lies posterolaterally to the testis and is nearest to the testis at its upper pole. Its lower pole is connected to the testis by fibrous tissue. The vas lies posteromedial to the epididymis.

Histology

The epididymis is covered by serosa. The ducts in the upper pole of the epididymis are lined by columnar cells. The epithelium of the remainder is pseudostratified.

Blood Supply

A. Arterial: The arterial supply to the epididymis comes from the internal spermatic artery and the artery of the vas (deferential artery).

B. Venous: The venous blood drains into the pampiniform plexus, which becomes the spermatic vein.

Lymphatics

The lymphatics drain into the external iliac and hypogastric lymph nodes (Figs 17-1 and 17-2).

TESTIS

Gross Appearance

A. Anatomy: The average testicle measures about $4 \times 3 \times 2.5$ cm (Fig 1-8). It has a dense fascial covering called the tunica albuginea testis, which, posteriorly, is invaginated somewhat into the body of the testis to form the mediastinum testis. This fibrous mediastinum sends fibrous septa into the testis, thus separating it into about 250 lobules.

The testis is covered anteriorly and laterally by the visceral layer of the serous tunica vaginalis, which is continuous with the parietal layer that separates the testis from the scrotal wall.

At the upper pole of the testis is the appendix testis, a small pedunculated or sessile body which is similar in appearance to the appendix of the epididymis.

B. Relations: The testis is closely attached posterolaterally to the epididymis, particularly at its upper and lower poles.

Histology (See Fig 1-8.)

Each lobule contains 1-4 markedly convoluted seminiferous tubules, each of which is about 60 cm in length. These ducts converge at the mediastinum testis, where they connect with the efferent ducts which drain into the epididymis.

The seminiferous tubule has a basement membrane containing connective and elastic tissue. This supports the seminiferous cells, which are of 2 types: (1) Sertoli (supporting) cells, and (2) spermatogenic cells. The stroma between the seminiferous tubules contains connective tissue in which the interstitial Leydig cells are located.

Blood Supply

The blood supply to the testes is closely associated with that to the kidneys because of the common embryologic origin of the 2 organs.

A. Arterial: The arteries to the testes (internal spermatics) arise from the aorta just below the renal arteries and course through the spermatic cords to the testes, where they

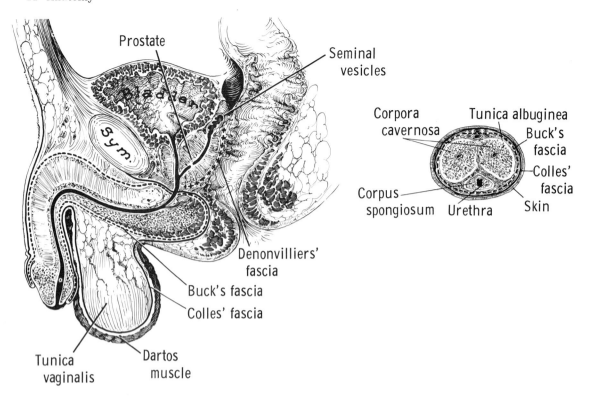

Fig 1-9. **Fascial planes of the lower genitourinary tract.** (After Wesson.) **Left:** Relations of bladder, prostate, seminal vesicles, penis, urethra, and scrotal contents. **Right:** Transverse section through penis. The paired upper structures are the corpora cavernosa. The single lower body surrounding the urethra is the corpus spongiosum.

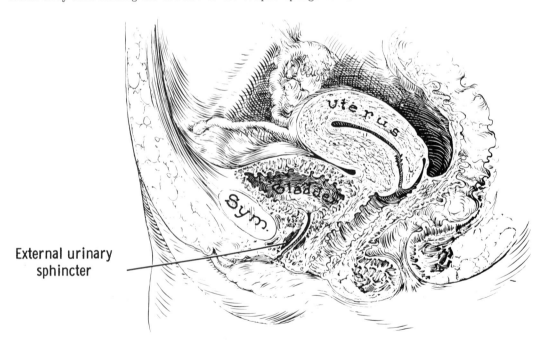

Fig 1-10. Anatomy and relations of the bladder, urethra, uterus and ovary, vagina, and rectum.

anastomose with the arteries of the vasa which branch off from the hypogastric artery.

B. Venous: The blood from the testis returns in the pampiniform plexus of the spermatic cord. At the internal inguinal ring the pampiniform plexus forms the spermatic vein.

The right spermatic vein enters the vena cava just below the right renal vein; the left spermatic vein empties into the left renal vein.

Lymphatics
The lymphatic vessels from the testes pass to the lumbar lymph nodes, which, in turn, are connected to the mediastinal nodes.

Busch, F.M., & E.S. Sayegh: Roentgenographic visualization of human testicular lymphatics: A preliminary report. J Urol 89:106-10, 1963.

SCROTUM

Gross Appearance
Beneath the corrugated skin of the scrotum lies the Dartos muscle. Deep to this are the 3 fascial layers derived from the abdominal wall at the time of testicular descent. Beneath these is the parietal layer of the tunica vaginalis.

The scrotum is divided into 2 sacs by a septum of connective tissue. The scrotum not only supports the testes but, by relaxation or contraction of its muscular layer, helps to regulate their environmental temperature.

Histology
The Dartos muscle, under the skin of the scrotum, is unstriated. The deeper layer is made up of connective tissue.

Blood Supply
A. Arterial: The arteries to the scrotum arise from the femoral, internal pudendal, and inferior epigastric arteries.

B. Venous: The veins are paired with the arteries.

Lymphatics
The lymphatics drain into the superficial inguinal and subinguinal lymph nodes (Figs 17-1 and 17-2).

PENIS AND MALE URETHRA

Gross Appearance
The penis is composed of 2 corpora cavernosa and the corpus spongiosum, which contains the urethra, whose diameter is 8-9 mm. These corpora are capped distally by the glans. Each corpus is enclosed in a fascial sheath (tunica albuginea), and all are surrounded by a thick fibrous envelope known as Buck's fascia. A covering of skin, devoid of fat, is loosely applied about these bodies. The prepuce forms a hood over the glans.

Beneath the skin of the penis (and scrotum) and extending from the base of the glans to the urogenital diaphragm is Colles' fascia, which is continuous with Scarpa's fascia of the lower abdominal wall (Fig 1-9).

The proximal ends of the corpora cavernosa are attached to the pelvic bones just anterior to the ischial tuberosities. Occupying a depression on their ventral surface in the midline is the corpus spongiosum, which is connected proximally to the under surface of the urogenital diaphragm through which emerges the membranous urethra. This portion of the corpus spongiosum is surrounded by the bulbocavernosus muscle. Its distal end expands to form the glans penis.

The suspensory ligament of the penis arises from the linea alba and symphysis pubis and inserts into the fascial covering of the corpora cavernosa.

Histology
A. Corpora and Glans Penis: The corpora cavernosa, the corpus spongiosum, and the glans penis are composed of septa of smooth muscle and erectile tissue which enclose vascular cavities.

B. Urethra: The epithelium of the urethra proximal to the glans is stratified or pseudostratified. The urethral mucosa which traverses the glans penis is formed of squamous epithelium. Proximal to this, the mucosa is transitional in type. Underneath the mucosa is the submucosa, which contains connective and elastic tissue and smooth muscle. In the submucosa are the numerous glands of Littré, whose ducts connect with the urethral lumen.

The urethra is surrounded by the vascular corpus spongiosum and the glans penis.

Blood Supply
A. Arterial: The penis and urethra are supplied by the internal pudendal arteries. Each artery divides into a profunda artery of the penis (which supplies the corpora cavernosa), a dorsal artery of the penis, and the bulbourethral artery. These latter branches

supply the corpus spongiosum, the glans penis, and the urethra.

B. Venous: The superficial dorsal vein lies external to Buck's fascia. The deep dorsal vein is placed beneath Buck's fascia and lies between the dorsal arteries. These veins connect with the pudendal plexus, which drains into the internal pudendal vein.

Lymphatics

Lymphatic drainage from the skin of the penis is to the superficial inguinal and sub-inguinal lymph nodes. The lymphatics from the glans penis pass to the subinguinal and external iliac nodes. The lymphatics from the deep urethra drain into the hypogastric and common iliac lymph nodes.

FEMALE URETHRA

The adult female urethra is about 3.5-4 cm long and 8 mm in diameter. It is slightly curved and lies beneath the symphysis pubis just anterior to the vagina.

The epithelial lining of the female urethra is squamous in its distal portion and pseudo-stratified or transitional in the remainder. The submucosa is made up of connective and elastic tissues and spongy venous spaces. Embedded in it are many periurethral glands, which are most numerous distally; the largest of these are the periurethral glands of Skene, which open on the floor of the urethra just inside the meatus.

External to the submucosa is a continuation of the inner and outer longitudinal smooth muscle layers of the bladder. These are surrounded by a sphincter of striated muscle in its middle third.

The arterial supply to the female urethra is derived from the inferior vesical, vaginal, and internal pudendal arteries. Blood from the urethra drains into the internal pudendal veins.

Lymphatic drainage from the external portion of the urethra is to the inguinal and subinguinal lymph nodes, and that from the deep urethra goes to the hypogastric lymph nodes (Figs 17-1 and 17-2).

Lindner, H.H., & S.E. Feldman: Surgical anatomy of the perineum. S Clin North America **42**:877-93, 1962.

Zacharin, R.F.: The anatomic supports of the female urethra. Obst Gynec **32**:754-9, 1968.

•   •   •

2...

Embryology of the Genitourinary System

Emil A. Tanagho, MD*

At birth, the genital and urinary systems are related only in the sense that they share certain common passages. Embryologically, however, they are intimately related. Because of the complex interrelationships of the embryonic phases of the 2 systems, they will be discussed here as 5 subdivisions: the nephric system, the vesicourethral unit, the gonads, the genital duct system, and the external genitalia.

THE NEPHRIC SYSTEM

The nephric system develops progressively as 3 distinct entities: pronephros, mesonephros, and metanephros.

Pronephros

This is the earliest nephric stage in man, and it corresponds to the mature structure of the most primitive vertebrate. It extends from the 4th to the 14th somites and consists of 6-10 pairs of tubules. These open into a pair of primary ducts, also formed at that same level, extend caudally, and eventually reach and open into the cloaca. The pronephros is a vestigial structure that disappears completely by the 4th week of embryonic life (Fig 2-1).

Mesonephros

The mature excretory organ of the higher fishes and amphibians corresponds to the embryonic mesonephros. It is the principal excretory organ during early embryonic life (4-8 weeks). It, too, gradually degenerates, although parts of its duct system become associated with the male reproductive organs. The mesonephric tubules develop from the intermediate mesoderm caudad to the pronephros shortly before pronephric degeneration. The mesonephric tubules differ from those of the pronephros in that they develop a cup-like outgrowth into which a knot of capillaries is pushed. This is called Bowman's capsule, and the tuft of capillaries is called a glomerulus. In their growth, the mesonephric tubules extend toward and establish a connection with the nearby primary nephric duct as it grows caudally to join the cloaca (Fig 2-1). This primary nephric duct is now called the mesonephric duct. After establishing their connection with the nephric duct, the primordial tubules elongate and become S-shaped. As the tubules elongate, a series of secondary branchings increases their surface exposure, thereby enhancing their capacity for interchanging material with the blood in adjacent capillaries. Leaving the glomerulus, the blood is carried by one or more efferent vessels that soon break up into a rich capillary plexus closely related to the mesonephric tubules. This is physiologically important. The mesonephros, which forms early in the 4th week, reaches its maximum size by the end of the second month.

Metanephros

The final phase of the development of the nephric system originates from both the intermediate mesoderm and the mesonephric duct. Development begins in the 5-6 mm embryo with a bud-like outgrowth from the mesonephric duct as it bends to join the cloaca. This ureteral bud grows cephalad and collects mesoderm from the nephrogenic cord of the intermediate mesoderm around its tip. This mesoderm with the metanephric cap moves, with the growing ureteral bud, more and more cephalad from its point of origin. During this cephalad migration, the metanephric cap becomes progressively larger and rapid internal differentiation takes place. Meanwhile, the cephalad end of the ureteral bud expands within the growing mass of metanephrogenic tissue to form the renal pelvis (Fig 2-1). Numerous outgrowths from the renal pelvic dilatation push radially into this growing mass and form into hollow ducts that branch and rebranch as

*Associate Professor of Urology, University of California School of Medicine, San Francisco.

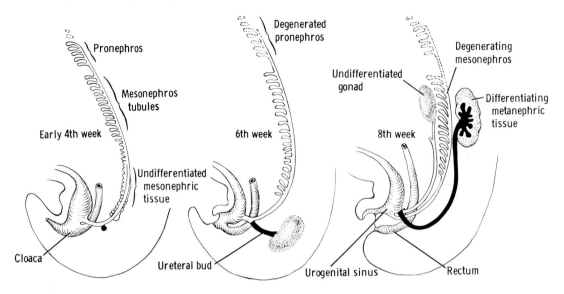

Fig 2-1. Schematic representation of the development of the nephric system. Only a few of the tubules of the pronephros are seen early in the 4th week, while the mesonephric tissue differentiates into mesonephric tubules that progressively join the mesonephric duct. The first sign of the ureteral bud from the mesonephric duct is seen. At 6 weeks, the pronephros has completely degenerated and the mesonephric tubules start to do so. The ureteral bud grows dorsocranially and has met the metanephrogenic cap. At the 8th week there is cranial migration of the differentiating metanephros. The cranial end of the ureteric bud expands and starts to show multiple successive outgrowths. (Adapted from several sources.)

they push their way toward the periphery. These form the primary collecting ducts of the kidney. Mesodermal cells become arranged in small vesicular masses that lie in close proximity to the blind end of the collecting ducts. Each of these vesicular masses will form a uriniferous tubule draining into the duct nearest to its point of origin. As the kidney grows, increasing numbers of tubules are formed in its peripheral zone. These vesicular masses develop a central cavity and become S-shaped. One end of the S coalesces with the terminal portion of the collecting tubules, resulting in a continuous canal. The proximal portion develops into the distal and proximal convoluted tubules and into Henle's loop; the distal end becomes the glomerulus and Bowman's capsule. At this stage, the undifferentiated mesoderm and the immature glomeruli are readily visible on microscopic examination (Fig 2-2). The glomeruli are fully developed by the 36th week or when the fetus weighs 2500 gm (Potter). The metanephros arises opposite the 28th somite (4th lumbar segment). At term, it has ascended to the level of the first lumbar or even the 12th thoracic vertebra. This ascent of the kidney is due not only to actual cephalad migration but to differential growth in the caudal part of the body as well. During the early period of

ascent (7th-9th weeks), the kidney slides up above the arterial bifurcation and rotates 90°. Its convex border is now directed laterally instead of dorsally. Further ascent proceeds more slowly until the kidney reaches its final position.

Certain features of these 3 phases of development must be emphasized. (1) The 3 successive units of the system develop from the intermediate mesoderm. (2) The tubules at all levels appear as independent primordia and only secondarily unite with the duct system. (3) The nephric duct is laid down as the duct of the pronephros and develops from the union of the ends of the anterior pronephric tubules. (4) This pronephric duct serves subsequently as the mesonephric duct and as such gives rise to the ureter. (5) The nephric duct reaches the cloaca by independent caudal growth. (6) The embryonic ureter is an outgrowth of the nephric duct; yet the kidney tubules differentiate from adjacent metanephric blastema.

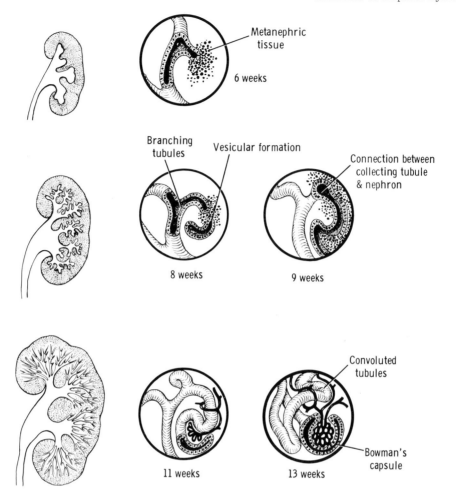

Fig 2-2. Progressive stages in the differentiation of the nephrons and their linkage with the branching collecting tubules. A small lump of metanephric tissue is associated with each terminal collecting tubule. These are then arranged in vesicular masses which later differentiate into a uriniferous tubule draining into the duct near which it arises. At one end, Bowman's capsule and the glomerulus differentiate, while the other end establishes communication with the nearby collecting tubules.

ANOMALIES OF THE NEPHRIC SYSTEM

Failure of the metanephros to ascend leads to **ectopic kidney.** An ectopic kidney may be on the proper side but low (simple ectopy) or on the opposite side (crossed ectopy) with or without fusion. Failure to rotate during ascent causes a **malrotated kidney.**

Fusion of the paired metanephric masses leads to various anomalies—most commonly **horseshoe kidney.**

The ureteral bud from the mesonephric duct may bifurcate, causing a **bifid ureter** at varying levels depending on the time of the bud's subdivision. An accessory ureteral bud may develop from the mesonephric duct, thereby forming a **duplicated ureter,** usually meeting the same metanephric mass. Rarely, each bud has a separate metanephric mass, resulting in **supernumerary kidneys.**

If the double ureteral buds are close together on the mesonephric duct, they will open near each other in the bladder. In this case, the main ureteral bud, which is the first to appear and the most caudal on the mesonephric ducts, will reach the bladder first. It will then start to move upward and laterally and will be followed later by the second accessory bud as it reaches the urogenital sinus. The main ureteral bud (now more cranial on the urogenital sinus) will drain the lower portion of the kidney. The 2 ureteral buds have reversed their relationship as they moved from the mesonephric duct to the urogenital sinus. This is why double ureters usually cross (Weigert-Meyer law). If the 2 ureteral buds are widely separated on the mesonephric duct, the accessory bud appears more proximal at the duct and will end in the bladder with an ectopic orifice lower than the normal one. This ectopic orifice could still be in the bladder close to its outlet, in the urethra, or even in the genital duct system (Fig 2-3). A single ureteral bud that arises higher than normal on the mesonephric duct can also end in a similar ectopic location.

Lack of development of a ureteral bud will result in a **solitary kidney** and a hemitrigone.

Ashley, D.J.B., & F.K. Mostofi: Renal agenesis and dysgenesis. J Urol **83**:211-30, 1960.

Cowinn, J.L., & B.W. Landry: Cystic diseases of the kidney in infants and children. Radiol Clin North America 6:191, 1968.

Murphy, W.K., Palubinskas, A.J., & D.R. Smith: Sponge kidney: Report of 7 cases. J Urol **85**:866-74, 1961.

Osathanondh, V., & E.L. Potter: Pathogenesis of polycystic kidneys. Type 4 due to urethral obstruction. Arch Path **77**:502-9, 1964.

Osathanondh, V., & E.L. Potter: Pathogenesis of polycystic kidneys. Survey of results of microdissection. Arch Path **77**: 510-2, 1964.

Persky, L., Izant, R., & R. Bolande: Renal dysplasia. J Urol **98**:431-5, 1967.

Traut, H.F.: The Structural Unit of the Human Kidney. Contribution to Embryology, No. 76, Carnegie Inst Pub No. 332, **15**: 103-20, 1923.

THE VESICOURETHRAL UNIT

The blind end of the hindgut caudad to the point of origin of the allantois expands to form the cloaca, which is separated from the outside by an ectodermal depression under the root of the tail. This depression is called the proctodeum, and a thin plate of tissue closing the hindgut is the cloacal membrane. At the 4 mm stage, starting at the cephalad portion of the cloaca where the allantois and gut meet, the cloaca progressively divides into 2 compartments by the caudad growth of a crescentic fold, the urorectal fold. The 2 limbs of the fold bulge into the lumen of the cloaca from either side, eventually meeting and fusing. The division of the cloaca into ventral (urogenital sinus) and dorsal (rectum) is completed during the 7th week. During the development of the urorectal septum, the cloacal membrane undergoes a reverse rotation so that the ectodermal surface is no longer directed toward the developing anterior abdominal wall but gradually faces caudally and slightly posteriorly. This growth change facilitates the subdivision of the cloaca and is brought about mainly by the development of the infra-umbilical portion of the anterior abdominal wall and by regression of the tail. The mesoderm that passes around the cloacal membrane to the caudal attachment of the umbilical cord proliferates and grows, forming a surface elevation, the genital tubercle. The further growth of this part of the abdominal wall progressively separates the umbilical cord from the genital tubercle. The division of the cloaca is completed before the cloacal membrane ruptures, and its 2 parts therefore open separately. The ventral part is the primitive urogenital sinus, which has the shape of an elongated cylinder and is continuous cranially with the allantois.

The urogenital sinus receives the mesonephric ducts. The caudad end of the mesonephric duct distal to the ureteral bud is progressively absorbed into the urogenital sinus. By the 7th week, both mesonephric duct and ureteral bud have independent opening sites. This will introduce an island of mesodermal tissue amid the surrounding endoderm of the urogenital sinus. As development progresses, the opening of the mesonephric duct (which will become the ejaculatory duct) migrates downward and medially. The opening of the ureteral bud (which will become the ureteral orifice) migrates upward and laterally. The absorbed mesoderm of the mesonephric duct expands with this migration to occupy the area limited by the final position of these tubes (Fig 2-3). This will later be differentiated as the trigonal structure, which is the only mesodermal inclusion in the endodermal vesicourethral unit.

The urogenital sinus can be divided into 2 main segments; the dividing line is the junction of the combined müllerian ducts with the urogenital sinus (Müller's tubercle), which is the most fixed reference point in the whole structure and which will be discussed below. The segments are as follows:

(1) The ventral and pelvic portion will form the bladder, part of the urethra in the male, and the whole urethra in the female. This portion receives the ureter.

(2) The urethral or phallic portion receives the mesonephric and the fused müllerian ducts.

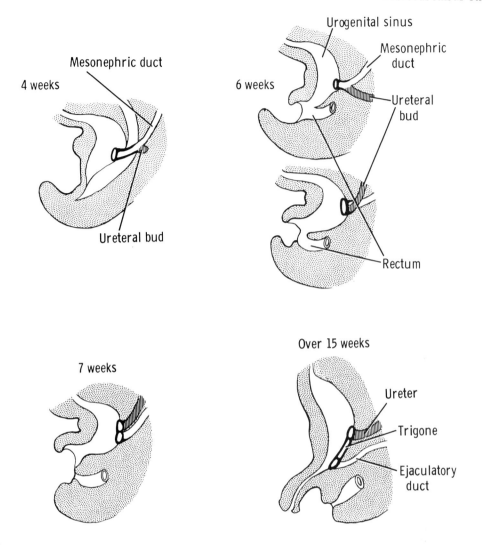

Fig 2-3. **The development of the ureteral bud from the mesonephric duct and their relationship to the urogenital sinus.** The ureteral bud appears at the 4th week. The mesonephric duct distal to this ureteral bud will be gradually absorbed into the urogenital sinus, resulting in separate endings for the ureter and the mesonephric duct. The mesonephric tissue that is incorporated into the urogenital sinus will expand and form the trigonal tissue.

This will be part of the urethra in the male and forms the lower 5th of the vagina and the vaginal vestibule in the female.

During the third month, the ventral part of the urogenital sinus starts to expand and forms an epithelial sac whose apex tapers into an elongated, narrowed urachus. The pelvic portion remains narrow and tubular, and this will form the whole urethra in the female and the supramontanal portion of the prostatic urethra in the male. The splanchnic mesoderm surrounding the ventral and pelvic portion of the urogenital sinus begins to differentiate into interlacing bands of smooth muscle fibers and an outer fibrous connective tissue coat. By the 12th week, the layers characteristic of the adult urethra and bladder are recognizable (Fig 2-4).

The part of the urogenital sinus caudad to the opening of the müllerian duct will form the vaginal vestibule and contribute to the lower 5th of the vagina in the female (Fig 2-5). In the male, it forms the inframontanal part of the prostatic urethra and the membranous urethra. The penile urethra is formed by the fusion of the urethral folds on the ventral surface of the genital tubercle. In the female,

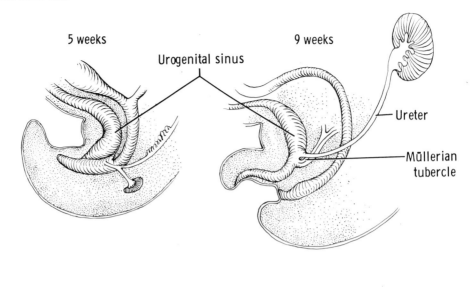

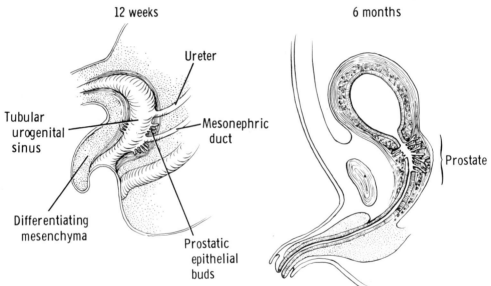

Fig 2-4. Differentiation of the urogenital sinus in the male. At the 5th week, the progressively growing urorectal septum is separating the urogenital sinus from the rectum. The former receives the mesonephric duct and the ureteral bud. It retains its tubular structure until the 12th week, when the surrounding mesenchyma starts to differentiate into muscle fibers around the whole structure. The prostatic gland develops as multiple epithelial outgrowths just above and below the mesonephric duct. During the third month the ventral part expands to form the bladder proper while the pelvic part remains narrow and tubular, forming part of the urethra. (Reproduced, with permission, from Tanagho and Smith: Mechanisms of urinary continence. I. Embryologic, anatomic, and pathologic considerations. J Urol **100**:640, 1969.)

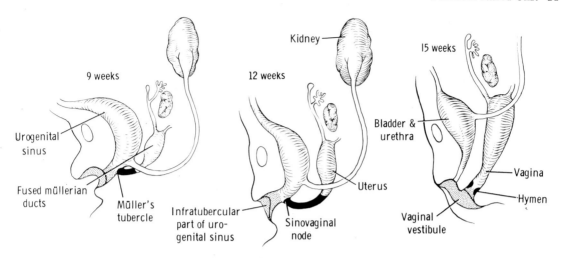

Fig 2-5. Differentiation of the urogenital sinus and the müllerian ducts in the female embryo. At 9 weeks the urogenital sinus receives the fused müllerian ducts at Müller's tubercle (sinovaginal node), which is solidly packed with cells. As the urogenital sinus distal to Müller's tubercle becomes wider and shallower (15 weeks), the urethra and fused müllerian duct will have separate openings. The distal part of the urogenital sinus will form the vaginal vestibule and the lower 5th of the vagina (shaded area), and that part above Müller's tubercle will form the urinary bladder and the entire female urethra. The fused müllerian ducts will form the uterus and the upper four-fifths of the vagina. The hymen is formed at the junction of the sinovaginal node and the urogenital sinus.

the urethral folds remain separate and form the labia minora. The glandular urethra in the male is formed by the canalization of the urethral plate. The bladder originally extends up to the umbilicus, where it is connected to the allantois that extends into the umbilical cord. The allantois usually is obliterated at the level of the umbilicus by the 15th week. The bladder then starts to descend by the 18th week. As it descends, its apex becomes stretched and narrowed and it pulls on the already obliterated allantois, now called the urachus. By the 20th week, the bladder is well separated from the umbilicus and the stretched urachus will become the middle umbilical ligament.

Begg, R.C.: The urachus, its anatomy, histology and development. J Anat 64:170-83, 1930.

Browne, D.: Some congenital deformities of the rectum, anus, vagina and urethra. (Hunterian Lecture). Ann Roy Coll Surgeons England 8:173-92, 1951.

Cullen, T.S.: Embryology, Anatomy and Diseases of the Umbilicus Together With Diseases of the Urachus. Saunders, 1916.

Dant, R.V., Emmett, J.L., & R.L.J. Kennedy: Congenital absence of abdominal muscles with urologic complications; report on a patient successfully treated. Proc Staff Mayo Clin 22:8-13, 1947.

Eagle, J.R., Jr., & G.S. Barrett: Congenital deficiency of abdominal musculature with associated genitourinary abnormalities: A syndrome. Report of nine cases. Pediatrics 6:721, 1950.

Hinman, F., Jr.: Surgical disorders of the bladder and umbilicus of urachal origin. Surg Gynec Obst 113:605-14, 1961.

Lattimer, J.K.: Congenital deficiency of the abdominal musculature and associated genitourinary anomalies: A report of 22 cases. J Urol 79:343-52, 1958.

Lowsley, O.O.: Persistent cloaca in the female: Report of two cases corrected by operation. J Urol 59:692-707, 1948.

Lowsley, O.S.: Congenital malformation of the posterior urethra. Ann Surg 60:733-41, 1914.

Ney, C., & R.M. Friedenberg: Radiographic findings in anomalies of the urachus. J Urol 99:288-91, 1968.

Stephens, F.D.: The female anus, perineum and vestibule: Embryogenesis and deformities. J Obstet Gynaec Brit Common 8:55-73, 1968.

Stephens, F.D.: Congenital Malformations of the Rectum, Anus and Genitourinary Tracts. Livingstone, 1963.

Wainstein, M.L., & L. Persky: Superior vesical fistula. An unusual form of exstrophy of the urinary bladder. Am J Surg 115:397-400, 1968.

THE PROSTATE

The prostate develops as a multiple solid outgrowth of the urethral epithelium both above and below the entrance of the mesonephric duct. These simple, tubular outgrowths begin to develop in 5 distinct groups at the end of the 11th week and are complete by the 16th week (112 mm). They branch and rebranch, ending in a complex ductal system that encounters the differentiating mesenchymal cells around this segment of the urogenital sinus. These mesenchymal cells start to develop around the tubules by the 16th week and become denser at the periphery to form the prostatic capsule. By the 22nd week, the muscular stroma is considerably developed and continues to progressively increase until birth.

From the 5 groups of epithelial buds, 5 lobes are eventually formed: anterior, posterior, median, and 2 lateral. Initially, these lobes are widely separated, but later they meet, with no definite septa dividing them. Tubules of each lobe do not intermingle with each other but simply lie side by side.

The anterior lobe tubules begin to develop simultaneously with those of the other lobes. Although in the early stages the anterior lobe tubules are large and show multiple branches, gradually they contract and lose most of these branches. They continue to shrink so that at birth they show no lumen and appear as small, solid, embryonic epithelial outgrowths. In contrast, the tubules of the posterior lobe are fewer in number, yet relatively larger, with extensive branching. These tubules, as they grow, extend posterior to the developing median and lateral lobes and form the posterior aspect of the gland, which may be felt rectally.

ANOMALIES OF THE VESICOURETHRAL UNIT

Failure of the cloaca to subdivide is rare and results in a **persistent cloaca**. Incomplete subdivision is more frequent, ending with **rectovesical, rectourethral, or rectovestibular fistulas** (usually with **imperforate anus** or **anal atresia**).

Failure of descent or incomplete descent of the bladder leads to a **urinary umbilical fistula (urethral fistula), urachal cyst,** or **urachal diverticulum,** depending on the stage and degree of maldescent.

Development of the genital primordia in an area more caudal than normal can result in formation of the corpora cavernosa just

caudad to the urogenital sinus outlet, with the urethral groove on its dorsal surface. This defect results in complete or incomplete **epispadias,** depending on its degree. A more extensive defect results in **vesical exstrophy.** Failure of fusion of urethral folds leads to various grades of **hypospadias.** This defect, due to its mechanism, never extends proximal to the bulbous urethra. This is in contrast to epispadias, which usually involves the entire urethra up to the internal meatus.

Amar, A. D., & J. A. Hutch: Anomalies of the ureter. Pages 98-164 in: Encyclopedia of Urology, Vol 7, Malformations. Springer-Verlag, 1968.

Chwalle, R.: The process of formation of cystic dilatations of the vesical end of the ureter and of diverticula at the ureteral ostium. Urol Cutan Rev 31:499-504, 1927.

Ericsson, N. O.: Ectopic ureterocele in infants and children. A clinical study. Acta chir scandinav Suppl 197, 1954.

Lenaghan, D.: Bifid ureters in children: An anatomical, physiological and clinical study. J Urol 87:808-17, 1962.

Meyer, R.: Normal and abnormal development of the ureter in the human embryo: A mechanistic consideration. Anat Record 96:355-71, 1946.

Randall, A., & E. W. Campbell: Anomalous relationship of the right ureter to the vena cava. J Urol 34:565-83, 1935.

Wershub, L. P., & T. J. Kirwin: Ureterocele, its etiology, pathogenesis and diagnosis. Am J Surg 88:317-27, 1954.

THE GONADS

Most of the structures which make up the embryonic genital system have been taken over from other systems, and their readaptation to genital function is a secondary and relatively late phase in their development. The early differentiation of such structures is therefore independent of sexuality. Furthermore, each embryo is at first morphologically bisexual, possessing all the necessary structures for either sex. The development of one set of sex primordia and the gradual involution of the other is determined by the sex type of the gonad.

The sexually undifferentiated gonad is a composite structure. Male and female potentials are represented by specific histologic elements (medulla and cortex) which have alternative roles in gonadogenesis. Normal differentiation involves the gradual predominance of one component.

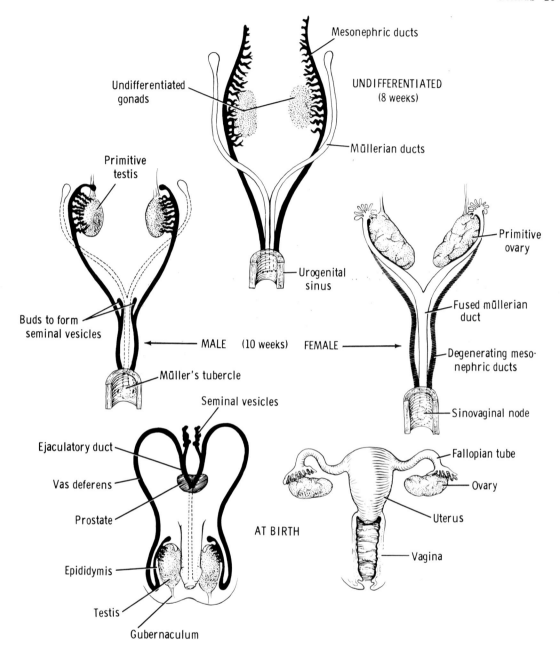

Fig 2-6. Transformation of the undifferentiated genital system into the definitive male and female systems.

The primitive sex glands make their appearance during the 5th and 6th weeks within a localized region of the thickening known as the urogenital ridge (this contains both the nephric and genital primordia). At the 6th week, the gonad consists of a superficial germinal epithelium and an internal blastema. The blastemal mass is mainly derived from proliferative ingrowth from the superficial epithelium that comes loose from its basement membrane.

During the 7th week, the gonad begins to assume the characteristics of a testis or ovary. Differentiation of the ovary usually occurs somewhat later than that of the testis.

If the gonad develops into a testis, the gland increases in size and shortens into a more compact organ while achieving a more caudal location. Its broad attachment to the mesonephros is converted into a gonadal mesentery known as the mesorchium. The cells of the germinal epithelium grow into the underlying mesenchyma and form cord-like masses. These are radially arranged and converge toward the mesorchium, where a dense portion of the blastemal mass is also emerging as the primoridum of the rete testis. A network of strands soon forms which is continuous with the testis cords. The latter also split into 3-4 daughter cords. These eventually become differentiated into the seminiferous tubules by which the spermatozoa are produced. The rete testis unites with the mesonephric components that will form the male genital ducts as discussed below (Fig 2-6).

If the gonad develops into an ovary, it (like the testis) gains a mesentery (mesovarium) and settles in a more caudal position. The internal blastema differentiates in the 9th week into a primary cortex beneath the germinal epithelium and a loose primary medulla. A compact cellular mass bulges from the medulla into the mesovarium and establishes the primitive rete ovarii. At 3-4 months of age, the internal cell mass becomes young ova. A new definitive cortex is formed from the germinal epithelium as well as from the blastema in the form of distinct cellular cords (Pflüger's tubes), and a permanent medulla is formed. The cortex differentiates into ovarian follicles containing ova.

Descent of the Gonads

A. The Testis: In addition to its early caudal migration, the testis later leaves the abdominal cavity and descends into the scrotum. By the third month of fetal life, the testis is located retroperitoneally in the false pelvis. A fibromuscular band (the gubernaculum) extends from the lower pole of the testis through the developing muscular layers of the anterior abdominal wall to terminate in the subcutaneous tissue of the scrotal swelling. The gubernaculum also has several other subsidiary strands that extend to adjacent regions. Just below the lower pole of the testis, the peritoneum herniates as a diverticulum along the anterior aspect of the gubernaculum, eventually reaching the scrotal sac through the anterior abdominal muscles (the processus vaginalis). The testis remains at the abdominal end of the inguinal canal until the 7th month. It then passes through the inguinal canal behind (but invaginating) the processus vaginalis (Fig 2-6). Normally, it reaches the scrotal sac by the end of the 8th month.

B. The Ovary: In addition to an early internal descent, the ovary becomes attached through the gubernaculum to the tissues of the genital fold and then attaches itself to the developing uterovaginal canal at its junction with the uterine tubes. This part of the gubernaculum between the ovary and uterus becomes the round ligament of the ovary; the part between the uterus and labia majora becomes the round ligament of the uterus. This prevents extra-abdominal descent, and the ovary enters the true pelvis. It eventually lies posterior to the uterine tubes on the superior surface of the urogenital mesentery, which has descended with the ovary and now forms the broad ligament. A small processus vaginalis forms and passes toward the labial swelling, but it is usually obliterated at full term.

GONADAL ANOMALIES

Lack of development of the gonads leads to **gonadal agenesis.** Incomplete development with arrest at a certain phase leads to **hypogenesis. Supernumerary gonads** are rare. The commonest anomaly involves descent of the gonads, especially the testis. Retention of the testis in the abdomen or arrest of its descent at any point along its natural pathway leads to **cryptorchidism,** which may be either unilateral or bilateral. If the testis does not follow the main gubernaculum structure but follows one of its subsidiary strands, it will end in an abnormal position, resulting in **ectopic testis.**

Failure of union between the rete testis and mesonephros results in a testis separate from the male genital ducts (the epididymis).

Burns, R. K.: Hormones and the Differentiation of Sex. In: Survey of Biological Progress, Vol 1. Academic Press, 1949.

Grossman, H., & S. D. G. Ririe: The incidence of urinary tract anomalies in cryptorchid boys. Am J Roentgenol 103:210-3, 1968.

Gruenwald, P.: The relation of the growing Müllerian duct to the Wolffian duct and its importance for the genesis of malformations. Anat Record 81:1-19, 1949.

Sugrue, D.: Male urogenital hypoplasia. Am J Surg 115:390-3, 1968.

THE GENITAL DUCT SYSTEM

Alongside the indifferent gonads, there are, early in embryonic life, 2 different yet closely related ducts. One is primarily a nephric duct (wolffian duct), yet it will also serve as a genital duct if the embryo develops into a male. The other (müllerian duct) is primarily a genital structure from the start.

Both ducts grow caudally to join the primitive urogenital sinus. The wolffian duct (known as the pronephric duct at the 4 mm stage) joins the ventral part of the cloaca, which will be the urogenital sinus. This duct gives rise to the ureteral bud close to its caudal end. The ureteral bud will grow cranially and meet metanephrogenic tissue. That part of each mesonephric duct caudad to the origin of the ureteric bud becomes absorbed into the wall of the primitive urogenital sinus so that the mesonephric duct and ureter open independently. This is achieved at the 15 mm stage (7th week). During this period, starting at the 10 mm stage, the müllerian ducts start to develop. They reach the urogenital sinus relatively late—at the 30 mm embryonic stage (9th week). This is the most constant and reliable point of reference in the whole system.

If the embryo develops into a male and the gonad starts to develop into a testis (17 mm, 7th week), the wolffian duct will start to differentiate into the male duct system, forming the epididymis, vas deferens, seminal vesicles, and ejaculatory ducts. At this time the müllerian duct proceeds toward its junction with the urogenital sinus and immediately starts to degenerate. It will only remain as a rudimentary structure.

If the embryo develops into a female and the gonad starts to differentiate into an ovary (22 mm, 8th week), the müllerian duct system forms the uterine (fallopian) tubes, uterus, and most of the vagina. The wolffian ducts, aside from their contribution to the urogenital sinus, remain rudimentary.

THE MALE DUCT SYSTEM

The Epididymis

Because of the proximity of the differentiating gonads and the nephric duct, some of the mesonephric tubules are retained as the efferent ductules and their lumens become continuous with those of the rete testis. These tubules, together with that part of the mesonephric duct into which they empty, will form the epididymis. Each coiled ductule makes a conical mass known as the lobule of the epididymis. The cranial end of the mesonephric duct becomes highly convoluted, completing the formation of the epididymis. Here there is a direct inclusion of a nephric structure into the genital system. Additional mesonephric tubules, both cephalad and caudad to those that were included in the formation of the epididymis, will remain as rudimentary structures, ie, the appendix of the epididymis and the paradidymis.

Vas Deferens, Seminal Vesicles, and Ejaculatory Ducts

The mesonephric duct caudad to that portion forming the epididymis will form the vas deferens. Shortly before this duct joins the urethra (urogenital sinus), a localized dilatation (ampulla) develops and the saccular convoluted structure that will form the seminal vesicle is evaginated from its wall. The mesonephric duct between the origin of the seminal vesicle and the urethra will form the ejaculatory duct. The whole mesonephric duct now achieves its characteristic thick investment of smooth muscle with a narrow lumen along most of its length.

Both above and below the point of entrance of the mesonephric duct into the urethra, multiple outgrowths of urethral epithelium mark the beginning of the development of the prostate. As these epithelial buds grow, they meet the developing muscular fibers around the urogenital sinus, and some of these fibers become entangled in the branching tubules of the growing prostate and become incorporated into it, forming its muscular stroma (Fig 2-6).

THE FEMALE DUCT SYSTEM

The müllerian ducts, which are a paired system, are seen alongside the mesonephric duct. It is not known whether they arise directly from the mesonephric ducts or separately as an invagination of the coelomic epithelium into the parenchyma lateral to the cranial extremity of the mesonephric duct, but the latter theory is favored. The müllerian duct develops and runs lateral to the mesonephric duct. Its opening with the coelomic cavity persists as the peritoneal ostium of the uterine tube (later it develops fimbria). The other end grows caudally as a solid tip and then crosses in front of the mesonephric duct at the caudad extremity of the mesonephros. It continues its growth in a caudomedial direction until it meets and fuses with the müllerian duct of the opposite side. The fusion is partial at first, so there is a temporary septum between the

Table 2-1. Male and female homologous structures.

Embryonic Structure	Male	Female
Mesonephric duct	Epididymis Vas deferens and seminal vesicles Ejaculatory ducts Appendix epididymidis Ureter, renal pelvis, etc Trigonal structure	Duct of epoophoron Gartner's duct Vesicular appendage Ureter, renal pelvis, etc Trigonal structure
Müllerian duct	Appendix testis Prostatic utericle	Fallopian tubes Uterus Vagina (upper 4/5)
Müller's tubercle	Verumontanum	Hymen (site of)
Sinovaginal bulb from urogenital sinus	Part of prostatic utricle	Lower 5th of vagina
Junction of sinovaginal bulb and urogenital sinus	Disappears normally (remnants probably form prostatic valves)	Hymen
Urogenital sinus Ventral and pelvic part	Urinary bladder (except the trigone) Supramontanal part of prostatic urethra	Urinary bladder (except the trigone) Whole urethra
Phallic or urethral portion	Inframontanal part of prostatic urethra Membranous urethra	Vaginal vestibule
Genital tubercle	Penis	Clitoris
Urethral folds	Penile urethra	Labia minora
Genital swellings	Scrotum	Labia majora
Gubernaculum	Gubernaculum testis	Ligament of ovary Round ligament of uterus
Genital glands	Testis	Ovary
Germinal cords	Seminiferous tubules	Pflüger's tube

2 lumens. This later disappears, leaving one cavity that will form the ureterovaginal canal. The potential lumen of the vaginal canal is completely packed with cells. The solid tip of this cord pushes the epithelium of the urogenital sinus outward, where it becomes Müller's tubercle (33 mm stage, 9th week). They actually fuse at the 63 mm stage (13th week), forming the sino-vaginal node, which receives a limited contribution from the urogenital sinus. (This contribution will form the lower 5th of the vagina.)

The urogenital sinus distal to Müller's tubercle, originally narrow and deep, shortens, widens, and opens to form the floor of the pudendal or vulval cleft. This results in separate openings for the vagina and urethra and also brings the vaginal orifice to its final position nearer the surface. At the same time, the vaginal segment increases appreciably in length. The vaginal vestibule is derived from the infratubercular segment of the urogenital sinus (in the male, the same segment will form the inframontanal part of the prostatic urethra and the membranous urethra). The labia minora are formed from the urethral folds (in the male they will form the pendulous urethra). The hymen is the remnant of the müllerian tubercle. The lower 5th of the vagina is derived from the contribution of the urogenital sinus with the sino-vaginal node. The remainder of the vagina and the uterus are formed from the lower fused third of the müllerian ducts. The fallopian tubes are the cephalad two-thirds of the müllerian ducts (Fig 2-6).

ANOMALIES OF THE GONADAL DUCT SYSTEM

Nonunion of the rete restis and the efferent ductules can occur and, if bilateral, lead to **azoospermia and sterility.** Failure of the müllerian ducts to approximate or incomplete fusion can lead to various degrees of **duplication** in the genital ducts. **Congenital absence** of one or both uterine tubes or of the uterus or vagina occurs rarely.

Arrested development of the infratubercular segment of the urogenital sinus leads to its persistence with the urethra and vagina having a common duct to the outside (**urogenital sinus**).

THE EXTERNAL GENITALIA

During the 8th week, external sex differentiation begins to occur. Not until 3 months, however, do the progressively developing external genitalia attain characteristics that can be recognized as distinctively male or female. During the indifferent stage of sexual development, 3 small protuberances appear on the external aspect of the cloacal membrane. In front is the genital tubercle and on either side of the membrane are the genital swellings.

By the breakdown of the urogenital membrane (17 mm, 7th week) the primitive urogenital sinus achieves a separate opening on the undersurface of the genital tubercle.

MALE EXTERNAL GENITALIA

The urogenital sinus opening extends on the ventral aspect of the genital tubercle as the urethral groove. The primitive urogenital orifice and the urethral groove are bounded on either side by the urethral folds. The genital tubercle becomes elongated to form the phallus. The corpora cavernosa are indicated in the 7th week as paired mesenchymal columns within the shaft of the penis. By the 10th week, the urethral folds start to fuse from the urogenital sinus orifice toward the tip of the phallus. At the 14th week, the fusion is complete and results in the formation of the penile urethra. The corpus spongiosum results from the differentiation of the mesenchymal masses around the formed penile urethra.

The glans penis becomes defined by the development of a circular coronary sulcus around the distal part of the phallus. The urethral groove and the fusing folds do not extend beyond the coronary sulcus. The glandular urethra is developed by the canalization of an ectodermal epithelial cord that has grown through the glans. This canalization progresses and reaches and communicates with the distal end of the previously formed penile urethra. During the third month, a fold of skin at the base of the glans begins growing distally and, 2 months later, surrounds the glans. This forms the prepuce. Meanwhile, the genital swellings shift caudally and are recognizable as scrotal swellings. They meet and fuse, resulting in the formation of the scrotum, with 2 compartments partially separated by a median septum and a median raphe, indicating their line of fusion.

FEMALE EXTERNAL GENITALIA

Until the 8th week, the appearance of the female external genitalia closely resembles that of the male except that the urethral groove is shorter. The genital tubercle, which becomes bent caudally and lags in development, becomes the clitoris. As in the male (though on a minor scale), mesenchymal columns differentiate into corpora cavernosa and a coronary sulcus identifies the glans clitoridis. The most caudal part of the urogenital sinus shortens and widens, forming the vaginal vestibule. The urethral folds do not fuse but remain separate as the labia minora. The genital swellings meet in front of the anus, forming the posterior commissure, while the swellings as a whole enlarge and remain separated on either side of the vestibule and form the labia majora.

ANOMALIES OF
THE EXTERNAL GENITALIA

Absence or duplication of the penis or clitoris is very rare. More commonly, the penis remains rudimentary or the clitoris may show hypertrophy. These may be seen alone or, more frequently, in association with **pseudohermaphrodism.** Concealed penis and transposition of penis and scrotum are relatively rare anomalies.

Failure or incomplete fusion of the urethral folds results in **hypospadias** (see above). Penile development is also anomalous in cases of **epispadias and exstrophy** (see above).

•   •   •

General References

Allan, F.D.: Essentials of Human Embryology. Oxford Univ Press, 1960.

Arey, L.B.: Developmental Anatomy; A Textbook and Laboratory Manual of Embryology, 6th ed. Saunders, 1954.

Blechschmidt, E.: The Stages of Human Development Before Birth; An Introduction to Human Embryology. Saunders, 1961.

Frazer, J.E.S., & J.S. Baxter: Manual of Embryology; the Development of the Human Body, 3rd ed. Williams & Wilkins, 1953.

Keith, A.: Human Embryology and Morphology, 6th ed. Williams & Wilkins, 1948.

Kjellberg, S.R., Ericsson, N.O., & U. Rudhe: The Lower Urinary Tract in Childhood: Some Correlated Clinical and Roentgenologic Observations. Year Book, 1957.

Patten, B.M.: Human Embryology, 2nd ed. Blakiston, 1953.

3...

Symptoms of Disorders
of the Genitourinary Tract

In the work-up of any patient the history is of paramount importance; this is particularly true in urology. It will be necessary to discuss here only those urologic symptoms which are apt to be brought to the physician's attention by the patient. It is important not only to know whether the disease is acute or chronic, but also whether it is recurrent, since recurring symptoms may represent acute exacerbations of chronic disease.

SYSTEMIC MANIFESTATIONS

Symptoms of fever, weight loss, and malaise should be sought. The presence of fever associated with other symptoms of urinary tract infection may be helpful in evaluating the site of the infection. Simple acute cystitis is essentially an afebrile disease. Acute pyelonephritis or prostatitis is apt to cause high temperatures (to 104° F), often accompanied by violent chills. Infants and children suffering from acute pyelonephritis may have high temperatures without other localizing symptoms or signs. Such a clinical picture, therefore, requires bacteriologic study of the urine without exception.

A history of unexplained attacks of fever occurring even years before may have been due to an otherwise asymptomatic pyelonephritis. Renal carcinoma sometimes causes fever which may reach 102° F or more. The absence of fever does not by any means rule out renal infection, for it is the rule that chronic pyelonephritis does not cause fever.

Weight loss is to be expected in the advanced stages of cancer, but it may also be noticed when renal insufficiency from obstruction or infection supervenes.

General malaise may be noted with neoplasm, chronic pyelonephritis, or renal failure.

LOCAL AND REFERRED PAIN

Two types of pain have their origins in the genitourinary organs: local and referred. The latter is unusually common.

Local pain is felt in or in the region of the involved organ. Thus, the pain from a diseased kidney (T10-12, L1) is felt in the costovertebral angle and in the flank in the region of and below the 12th rib. Pain from an inflamed testicle is felt in the gonad itself.

Referred pain originates in a diseased organ but is felt at some distance from that organ. The ureteral colic (Fig 3-3) caused by a stone in the upper ureter may be associated with severe pain in the ipsilateral testicle; this is explained by the common innervation of these 2 structures (T11-12). A stone in the lower ureter may cause pain referred to the scrotal wall; in this instance, the testis itself is not hyperesthetic. The burning pain with voiding which accompanies acute cystitis is felt in the distal urethra in the female or in the glandular urethra in the male (S2-3).

Abnormalities of a urologic organ can also cause pain in any other organ (eg, gastrointestinal, gynecologic) that has a sensory nerve supply common to both (Fig 3-2).

Kidney Pain (See Fig 3-3.)

Typical renal pain is usually felt as a dull and constant ache in the costovertebral angle just lateral to the sacrospinalis muscle and just below the 12th rib. This pain often spreads along the subcostal area toward the umbilicus. It may be expected in those renal diseases which cause sudden distention of the renal capsule. Acute pyelonephritis (with its sudden edema) and acute ureteral obstruction (with its sudden renal back pressure) both cause this typical pain. It should be pointed out, however, that many urologic renal diseases are painless because their progression is so slow that sudden capsular distention does not occur. Such diseases include cancer, chronic pyelonephritis, staghorn calculus, tuberculosis, and hydronephrosis due to mild

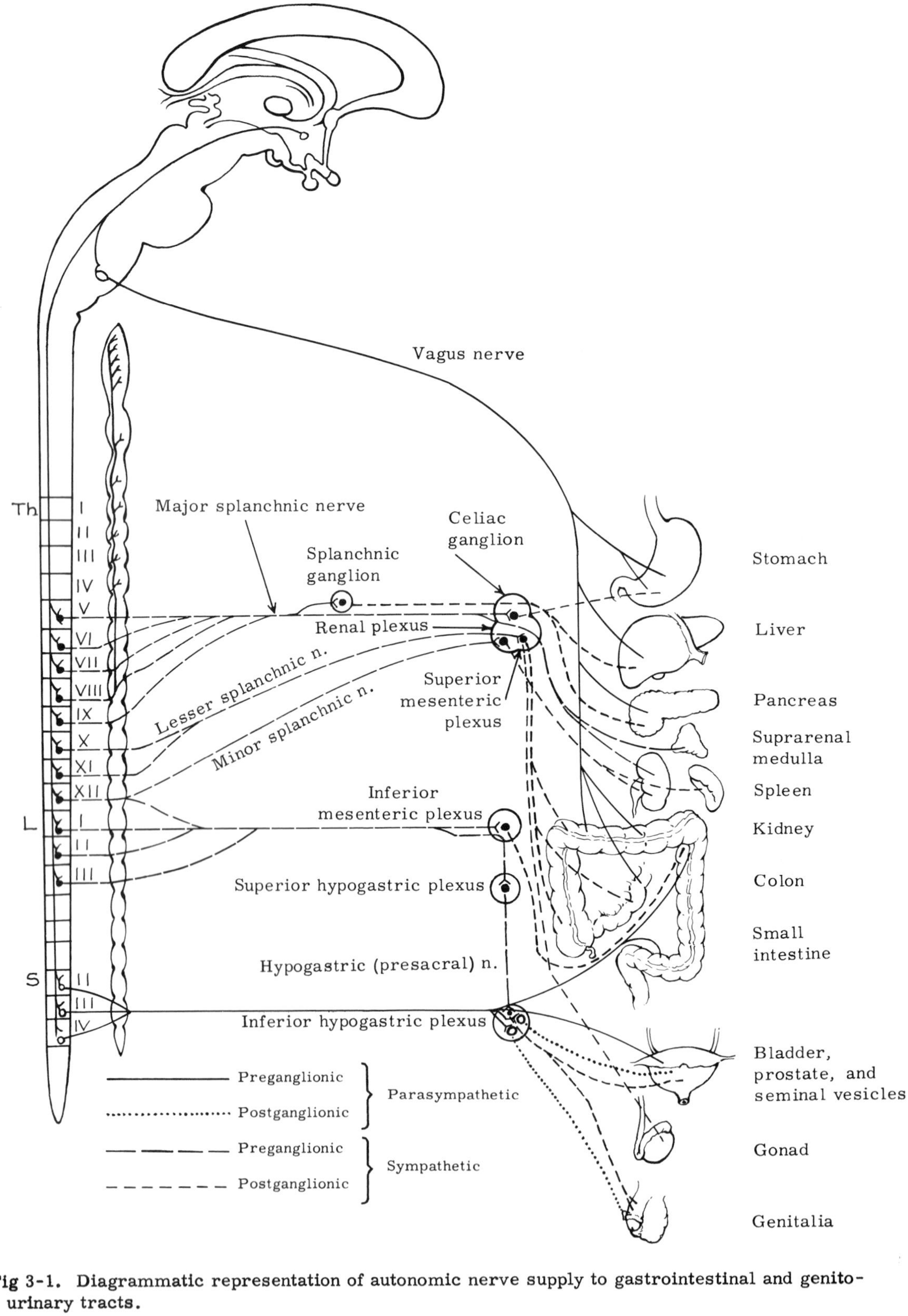

Fig 3-1. Diagrammatic representation of autonomic nerve supply to gastrointestinal and genito-urinary tracts.

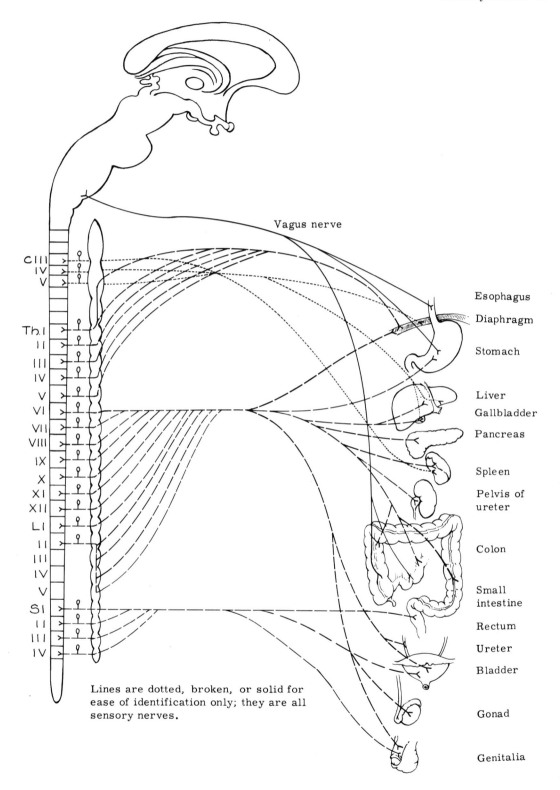

Fig 3-2. Diagrammatic representation of the sensory nerves of the gastrointestinal and genito-urinary tracts.

ureteral obstruction. Radiculitis commonly mimics renal pain.

Ureteral Pain (See Fig 3-3.)

Ureteral pain is typically stimulated by acute obstruction (passage of a stone or a blood clot). In this instance, there is back pain from capsular distention combined with severe colicky pain (due to renal pelvic and ureteral muscle spasm) that radiates from the costo-vertebral angle down toward the lower anterior abdominal quadrant, along the course of the ureter. In men it may also be felt in the bladder, scrotum, or testicle. In women it may radiate into the vulva. The severity and colicky nature of this pain are caused by the hyperperistalsis and spasm of this smooth muscle organ as it attempts to rid itself of a foreign body or to overcome obstruction.

The physician may be able to judge the position of a ureteral stone by the history of pain and the site of referral. If the stone is lodged in the upper ureter, the pain radiates to the testicle, since the nerve supply of this organ is similar to that of the kidney and upper ureter (T11-12). With stones in the midportion of the ureter on the right side, the pain is referred to McBurney's point and may therefore simulate appendicitis; on the left side, it may somewhat resemble diverticulitis or other diseases of the descending or sigmoid colon (T12, L1). As the stone approaches the bladder inflammation and edema of the ureteral orifice ensue, and symptoms of vesical irritability may occur. It is important to realize, however, that in mild ureteral obstruction, as seen in the congenital stenoses, there is usually no pain, either renal or ureteral.

Vesical Pain

The overdistended bladder of the patient in acute urinary retention will cause agonizing pain in the suprapubic area. Other than this, however, constant suprapubic pain not related to the act of urination is usually not of urologic origin. The relatively uncommon interstitial cystitis and vesical ulceration from tuberculosis may cause suprapubic discomfort when the

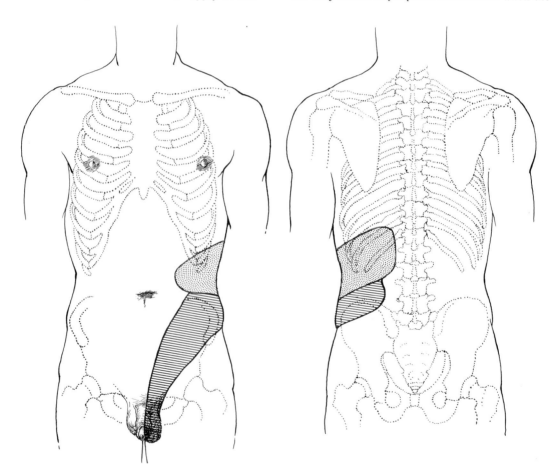

Fig 3-3. Referred pain from kidney (dotted areas) and ureter (shaded areas).

bladder becomes full, but this discomfort is usually relieved by urination.

The patient in chronic urinary retention due to bladder neck obstruction or to a neurogenic bladder may experience little or no suprapubic discomfort even though the bladder reaches the umbilicus.

The common cause of bladder pain is infection; the pain is usually not felt over the bladder but is referred to the distal urethra and is related to the act of urination. Terminal dysuria may be severe.

Prostatic Pain

Direct pain from the prostate gland is not common. Occasionally, when the prostate is inflamed, the patient may feel a vague discomfort or fulness in the perineal or rectal areas (S2-4). Lumbosacral backache is occasionally experienced as a referred pain from the prostate, but is not a common symptom of prostatitis. Inflammation of the gland may cause symptoms of cystitis.

Testicular Pain

Testicular pain due to trauma or infection is very severe and is felt locally, although there may be some radiation of the discomfort along the spermatic cord into the lower abdomen. It may involve the costovertebral area as well. Uninfected hydrocele and tumor of the testes do not commonly cause pain. A varicocele may cause a dull ache in the testicle that is increased after heavy exercise. At times the first symptom of an early indirect inguinal hernia may be testicular pain (referred). Pain from a stone in the upper ureter may be referred to the testicle.

Epididymal Pain

Acute infection of the epididymis is the only painful disease of this organ and is quite common. Some degree of neighborhood inflammatory reaction involves the adjacent testis as well, which further aggravates the discomfort. In the early stages of epididymitis, pain may first be felt in the groin or lower abdominal quadrant. (If on the right side, it may simulate appendicitis.) This may be a referred type of pain but can be secondary to associated inflammation of the vas deferens. The discomfort associated with epididymitis may reach the costal angle and may mimic ureteral stone.

Back and Leg Pain

Pain low in the back and radiating down one or both legs, especially when associated with symptoms of vesical neck obstruction, suggests metastases to the pelvic bones from cancer of the prostate.

Dowd, J.B.: Flank pain in nonurologic disease. M Clin North America 47:437-45, 1963.

GASTROINTESTINAL SYMPTOMS OF UROLOGIC DISEASES

Whether renal or ureteral disease is painful or not, gastrointestinal symptoms are often present. The patient with acute pyelonephritis will not only suffer from localized back pain, symptoms of vesical irritability, chills, and fever, but also from generalized abdominal pain and distention. The patient who is passing a stone down the ureter will have typical renal and ureteral colic and, usually, hematuria, and may experience severe nausea and vomiting as well as abdominal distention. However, the urinary symptoms so far overshadow the gastrointestinal symptoms that the latter are usually ignored. Inadvertent overdistention of the renal pelvis (eg, with opaque material in order to obtain adequate retrograde urograms) may cause the patient to become nauseated, to vomit, and to complain of cramp-like pain in the abdomen. This clinical experiment demonstrates the reno-intestinal reflex, which may lead to confusing symptomatology. In the very common "silent" urologic diseases, some degree of gastrointestinal symptomatology may be present which could mislead the clinician to seek the diagnosis in the intraperitoneal zone.

Cause of the Mimicry

A. Reno-intestinal Reflexes: These account for most of the confusion. They arise because of the common autonomic and sensory innervations of the 2 systems (Figs 3-1 and 3-2). Afferent stimuli from the renal capsule or musculature of the pelvis may, by reflex action, cause pylorospasm (symptoms of peptic ulcer) or other changes in tone of the smooth muscles of the enteric tract and its adnexa.

B. Organ Relationships: The right kidney is closely related to the hepatic flexure of the colon, the duodenum, the head of the pancreas, the common bile duct, the liver, and the gallbladder (Fig 1-3). The left kidney lies just behind the splenic flexure of the colon and is closely related to the stomach, pancreas, and spleen; inflammations or tumors in the retroperitoneum thus may extend into or displace intraperitoneal organs, causing them to produce symptoms.

C. Peritoneal Irritation: The anterior surfaces of the kidneys are covered by peritoneum. Renal inflammation, therefore, will cause peritoneal irritation, which leads to muscle rigidity and rebound tenderness.

The symptoms arising from chronic renal disease (eg, uninfected hydronephrosis, staghorn calculus, cancer, chronic pyelonephritis) may be entirely gastrointestinal and may simulate in every way the syndromes of peptic ulcer, gallbladder disease, appendicitis, or other less specific gastrointestinal complaints. If a thorough survey of the gastrointestinal tract fails to demonstrate suspected disease processes, the physician should give every consideration to study of the urinary tract.

Takacs, F.J.: The interrelationships of gastrointestinal and renal diseases. M Clin North America 50:507-14, 1966.

SYMPTOMS RELATED TO THE ACT OF URINATION

Many conditions cause symptoms of "cystitis." These include infections of the bladder, vesical inflammation due to chemical or x-ray radiation reactions, interstitial cystitis, prostatitis, senile urethritis, psychoneurosis, torsion or rupture of an ovarian cyst, and foreign bodies in the bladder. Often, however, the patient with chronic cystitis notices no symptoms of vesical irritability. In children following the taking of bubble baths, symptoms resembling cystitis may be noted secondary to the resulting urethritis.

Frequency, Nocturia, and Urgency
The normal capacity of the bladder is about 400 ml. Frequency may be caused by residual urine which decreases the functional capacity of the organ. When the mucosa, submucosa, and even the muscularis become inflamed (eg, infection, foreign body, stones, tumor), the capacity of the bladder decreases sharply. This decrease is due to 2 factors: the pain which results from even mild stretching of the bladder, and the loss of bladder elasticity which results from inflammatory edema. When the bladder is normal, urination can be delayed if circumstances require it, but this is not so in acute cystitis. Once the diminished bladder capacity is reached, any further distention may be agonizing, and the patient may actually urinate involuntarily if he does not void immediately. During very severe acute infections, the desire to urinate may be constant, and each voiding may produce only a few milliliters of urine. Day frequency without nocturia, and frequency lasting only a few hours (acute or chronic) suggest nervous tension.

Diseases that cause fibrosis of the bladder are accompanied by frequency of urination.

These include tuberculosis, interstitial cystitis, and bilharziasis. The presence of stones or foreign bodies causes vesical irritability, but secondary infection is usually the rule.

Nocturia is often a symptom of renal disease related to a decrease in the functioning renal parenchyma with loss of concentrating power. It commonly accompanies congestive heart failure and may be the earliest symptom noted. Nocturia may occur in the absence of disease by persons who drink excessive amounts of fluids in the late evening. Coffee and alcoholic beverages, because of their specific stimulating effects, often produce nocturia if consumed just before bedtime.

Burning Upon Urination
This is common in acute cystitis and prostatitis. In men, it is usually felt in the distal urethra just proximal to or in the glans. In women, it is ordinarily referred to the urethra. It is important to remember that it is rarely felt in the suprapubic area. This burning sensation occurs in association with the act of urination, although it may be more marked at the beginning, during, at the end, or occasionally after urination. It may be very severe. Vague pain in the urethra not associated with the act of voiding is usually not caused by urinary pathology. In men, it is apt to be a psychosomatic symptom; in women, however, it may occasionally be caused by chronic urethritis.

Enuresis
Strictly speaking, enuresis means bedwetting at night. It is physiologic during the first 2 or 3 years of life but becomes troublesome, particularly to parents, after that age. It may be functional or secondary to delayed neuromuscular maturation of the urethrovesical component, but it may present as a symptom of organic disease (eg, infection, distal urethral stenosis in girls, posterior urethral valves in boys, neurogenic bladder). If, however, pants wetting occurs also during the daytime or if there are other urinary symptoms, or if the enuresis persists beyond the age of 6 or 7 years, urologic investigation is essential. In adult life, enuresis may be replaced by nocturia, for which no organic basis can be found.

Symptoms of Prostatic Obstruction (See also pp 119, 272.)
A. Hesitancy and Straining: Hesitancy in initiating the urinary stream is one of the early symptoms of obstructions distal to the bladder. As the degree of obstruction increases, hesitancy is prolonged; the patient may have to strain in order to initiate urination.

B. Loss of Force and Decrease of Caliber of the Stream: Progressive loss of force and caliber of the urinary stream is noted as urethral resistance increases despite the generation of increased intravesical pressure.

C. Terminal Dribbling: This becomes more and more noticeable as obstruction progresses.

D. Acute Urinary Retention: Sudden inability to urinate may supervene. The patient experiences increasingly agonizing suprapubic pain associated with severe urgency. He may dribble only small amounts of urine.

E. Chronic Urinary Retention: This may cause little discomfort to the patient even though there is great hesitancy in starting the stream and marked reduction of its force and caliber. Constant dribbling of urine (paradoxical incontinence) may be experienced.

F. Interruption of the Urinary Stream: Interruption may be abrupt and accompanied by severe pain radiating down the urethra. This type of reaction strongly suggests the complication of vesical calculus.

G. Sense of Residual Urine: The patient often feels he still has urine in his bladder when he has finished urinating.

H. Recurring episodes of acute cystitis suggest the presence of residual urine.

Symptoms of Urethral Obstruction

In the male, the combination of a slow and bifurcated stream suggests urethral stricture. A slow, weak stream in the male infant or little boy is compatible with posterior urethral valves or congenital urethral stricture.

Little girls with or without urinary infection may have a slow, hesitant, or interrupted stream. This should suggest involuntary spasm of the periurethral striated musculature secondary to distal urethral stenosis (see p 385). Some women complain of constant impairment of urinary flow, in which case the possibility of urethral stricture should be investigated. Often, however, careful questioning will reveal that some voidings are slow while others are quite free. This is compatible with periodic periurethral muscle spasm on a psychogenic basis, or with urethritis.

Incontinence

There are many reasons for incontinence. The history often gives a clue to its cause.

A. True Incontinence: The patient may lose urine without warning; this may be a constant or periodic symptom. The more obvious causes include exstrophy of the bladder, epispadias, vesicovaginal fistula, and ectopic ureteral orifices. Injury to the urethral smooth muscle sphincters may occur during prostatectomy or childbirth. Congenital or acquired neurogenic diseases may lead to dysfunction of the bladder and incontinence.

B. Stress Incontinence: When slight weakness of the sphincteric mechanisms is present, urine may be lost in association with physical strain (ie, coughing, laughing, rising from a chair). This is common with cystocele and may occur with vesical neurogenic disease. The patient stays dry while lying in bed.

C. Urgency Incontinence: This type of urgency may be so precipitate and severe that there is involuntary loss of urine. Urgency incontinence not infrequently occurs with acute cystitis, particularly in women, for they seem to have relatively poor anatomic sphincters. Urgency incontinence is a common symptom of certain neurovesical diseases.

D. Paradoxical (Overflow or False) Incontinence: This is loss of urine due to chronic urinary retention or secondary to a flaccid bladder. The intravesical pressure finally equals the urethral resistance; urine then constantly dribbles forth.

Oliguria and Anuria

Oliguria and anuria may be caused by acute renal failure (due to shock or dehydration), fluid-ion imbalance, or bilateral ureteral obstruction.

Pneumaturia

The passage of gas in the urine almost always means that there is a fistula between the urinary tract and the bowel. This occurs most commonly in the bladder or urethra, but may be seen in the ureter or renal pelvis. Carcinoma of the sigmoid colon, diverticulitis with abscess formation, regional enteritis, and trauma cause most vesical fistulas. Congenital anomalies account for most urethral fistulas. Bacteria, by the process of fermentation, may rarely liberate gas.

Cloudy Urine

Patients often complain of cloudy urine, but it is most often cloudy merely because it is alkaline; this causes the precipitation of phosphate. Chyluria is a rare cause of cloudy urine. A properly performed urinalysis will reveal the cause of cloudiness.

Bloody Urine

Hematuria is a danger signal that cannot be ignored. It is important to know whether urination is painful or not, whether the hematuria is associated with symptoms of vesical irritability, and whether blood is seen in all or only a portion of the urinary stream. Some individuals will pass red urine after eating beets (particularly if they are anemic) or taking laxatives containing phenolphthalein, in which case the urine is translucent rather than opaque and contains no red cells. Because of the wide use of rhodamine B as a coloring agent in cookies, cakes, cold drinks, and fruit juices, children commonly pass red urine after the ingestion of these foods. This is the so-called Monday morning disorder. The hemoglobinuria seen in the hemolytic syndromes may also cause urine to be red.

A. Bloody Urine In Relation to Symptoms and Diseases: Hematuria associated with renal colic suggests ureteral stone, although a clot from a bleeding renal tumor can cause the same type of pain.

Hematuria is not uncommonly associated with nonspecific or tuberculous infection of the bladder. The bleeding is often terminal (bladder neck or prostate), although it may be present throughout urination (vesical or upper tract). Stone in the bladder often causes hematuria, but infection is usually present and there are symptoms of bladder neck obstruction, neurogenic bladder, or cystocele. When a tumor of the bladder ulcerates it is often complicated by infection and bleeding. Thus, symptoms of cystitis and hematuria are also compatible with neoplasm.

Dilated veins may develop at the bladder neck secondary to enlargement of the prostate. These may rupture when the patient strains to urinate.

Hematuria without other symptoms ("silent") must be regarded as a symptom of tumor of the bladder or kidney until proved otherwise. It is usually intermittent; bleeding may not recur for months. Complacency because the bleeding stops spontaneously must be condemned. Less common causes of silent hematuria are staghorn calculus, polycystic kidneys, solitary renal cyst, sickle cell disease, and hydronephrosis. Painless bleeding is common with acute glomerulonephritis. Recurrent bleeding is occasionally seen in children suffering from focal glomerulitis.

B. Time of Hematuria: Learning whether the hematuria is partial (initial, terminal) or total (present throughout urination) is often of help in placing the site of the bleeding. Initial hematuria suggests an anterior urethral lesion

(eg, urethritis, stricture, meatal stenosis in young boys). Terminal hematuria usually arises from the posterior urethra, bladder neck, or trigone. Among the common causes are posterior urethritis, and polyps and tumors of the vesical neck.

Total hematuria has its source at or above the bladder level (eg, stone, tumor, tuberculosis, nephritis).

Unusual Consequences of Micturition

Postmicturition syncope has been observed occasionally in men. Orthostatic hypotension and cardiac standstill have been observed in one patient. Psychomotor epilepsy and angina pectoris may be triggered by voiding.

Bennett, M.A., Heslop, R.W., & M.J. Meynell: Massive haematuria associated with sickle-cell trait. Brit MJ 1:677-9, 1967.

Bilinsky, R.J., Kandel, G.L., & S.F. Rabiner: Epsilon aminocaproic acid therapy of hematuria due to heterozygous sickle cell diseases. J Urol 102:93-5, 1969.

Davidson, A.I.G., & N.A. Matheson: Ovarian cysts and urinary symptoms. Brit J Surg 51:908-10, 1964.

Ferris, T.F., & others: Recurrent hematuria and focal nephritis. New England J Med 276:770-5, 1967.

Glasgow, E.F., Moncrieff, M.W., & R.H.R. White: Symptomless hematuria in childhood. Brit MJ 2:687-92, 1970.

Levin, S.: Red urine: The Monday morning disorder of children. Pediatrics 36:134-5, 1965.

Marshall, S.: The effect of bubble bath on the urinary tract. J Urol 93:112, 1965.

Morris, J.J., & H.D. McIntosh: Angina of micturition. Circulation 27:85-9, 1963.

Okamoto, K., Asechi, S., & K. Nagata: Distribution of chyluria and its treatment in Japan. Urologia Internat 17:241-56, 1964.

Redman, J.F., & J.E. Mobley: Sickle cell disease: Renal colic and microscopic hematuria. J Urol 100:594-5, 1968.

Silk, A.D.: Benign micturition syncope. California Med 111:355-6, 1969.

Zivin, I., & W. Rowley: Psychomotor epilepsy with micturition. Arch Int Med 113:8-13, 1964.

MANIFESTATIONS RELATED TO SEXUAL ORGANS

Symptoms

Many people suffer from genitourinary complaints on a purely psychologic or emotional basis. In others, organic symptoms may be increased in severity because of tension states. It is therefore important to seek clues which might give evidence of emotional stress.

In women, the relationship of the menses to ureteral pain or vesical complaints should be determined, although menstruation may exacerbate both organic and functional vesical and renal difficulties.

Many patients, particularly women, recognize that the state of their ''nerves'' has a direct effect on their symptoms. They often recognize that their ''cystitis'' or renal pain develops following a tension-producing or anxiety-producing episode in their personal or occupational environment.

A. Sex Difficulties in the Male: Men may complain directly of sexual difficulty. However, they are often so ashamed of loss of sexual power that they cannot admit it even to a physician. In such cases they come to him asking for ''prostate treatment,'' hoping that the physician will understand that they have sexual complaints and that they will be treated accordingly. The main sexual symptoms include impaired quality of erection, premature loss of erection, premature ejaculation, and even loss of desire. Since these symptoms are almost always psychologic in origin, this area must therefore be explored.

B. Sex Difficulties in the Female: Women suffering from the psychosomatic cystitis syndrome almost always admit to an unhappy sex life. They notice that frequency or pain often occurs at bedtime and on the day following the incomplete sexual act. Many of them recognize the inadequacy of their sexual experiences as one of the underlying causes of their urologic complaints; too frequently, however, the doctor either does not ask them pertinent questions or, if the patient volunteers this information, he ignores it.

In treating sex difficulties of suspected psychosomatic origin, the physician should explore pertinent facts concerning childhood, adolescence (sex education and experiences), marriage problems, and relationships with relatives, business associates, etc. Even if psychosomatic disease is strongly suspected before the history-taking has been completed, a thorough examination and laboratory survey must be done. Both psyche and soma may be involved, and the patient requires assurance that he is not suffering from organic disease. Although sexual interest and activity decline with advancing years, physically healthy men may continue to be sexually active into their eighth or ninth decades.

Objective Manifestations (See also Infertility, chapter 30.)

On occasion, a patient may have objective signs. The most common include urethral discharge, lesions of the skin, and scrotal, perineal, or abdominal masses.

Another symptom referable to the sex organs is that of bloody ejaculation. This is often associated with prostatitis, prostatic congestion, or hypertrophy of the mucosa of the seminal vesicles.

•　　•　　•

4...

Physical Examination of the Genitourinary Tract

The history will suggest whether a complete or partial examination is indicated. The symptom of urethral discharge probably does not require a thorough physical examination; on the other hand, painless hematuria would certainly require a careful examination of the genitourinary tract. The following is the urologic aspect of the physical examination of the patient.

EXAMINATION OF THE KIDNEYS

Inspection

On occasion a mass may be visible in the upper abdominal area which, if soft (eg, as in hydronephrosis), may be difficult to palpate. Fullness in the costovertebral angle may be consistent with malignancy (eg, neuroblastoma in children) or perinephric infection. The presence and persistence of indentations in the skin from lying on wrinkled sheets suggest edema of the skin secondary to perinephric abscess. If this is suspected, have the patient lie on a rough towel and observe for indentations.

Palpation of the Kidneys

The kidneys lie rather high under the diaphragm and lower ribs and are therefore well protected from injury. Because of the position of the liver, the right kidney is lower than the left. The kidneys are difficult to palpate in men because of the resistance of abdominal muscle tone and because the kidneys in men are more fixed than those of women and move only slightly with change of posture or respiration. On occasion the lower part of the right kidney may be felt, but the left kidney cannot usually be felt unless it is grossly enlarged or displaced.

The most successful method of renal palpation is carried out with the patient lying supine on a hard surface (Fig 4-1). The kidney is lifted by one hand in the costovertebral angle. On deep inspiration the kidney moves downward, and when it is lowest the other hand is pushed firmly and deeply beneath the costal margin in an effort to trap the kidney below that point. If this is successful the anterior hand can palpate the size, shape, and consistency of the organ as it slips back into its normal position.

The kidney can sometimes best be palpated with the patient sitting and the examiner standing behind him. At other times, if the patient is lying on his side, the uppermost kidney drops downward and medially, thereby making it more accessible to palpation.

An enlarged renal mass suggests compensatory hypertrophy (if the other kidney is absent or atrophic), hydronephrosis, tumor, cyst, or polycystic disease. A mass in this area, however, may be a retroperitoneal tumor, the spleen, a lesion of the bowel (eg, tumor, abscess), a lesion of the gallbladder or a pancreatic cyst. Tumors may have the consistency of normal tissue; they may also be nodular. Hydronephroses may be firm or soft. Polycystic kidneys are usually nodular.

An acutely infected kidney is tender, but this is difficult to elicit since marked muscle spasm is usually present. Since normal kidneys are often tender also, this sign is not always helpful.

Although renal pain may be diffusely felt in the back, tenderness is usually well localized just lateral to the sacrospinalis muscle and just below the 12th rib. This may be brought out by palpation or, more sharply, by fist percussion over that area.

Percussion of the Kidneys

At times a greatly enlarged kidney cannot be felt on palpation, particularly if it is soft. This can be true of hydronephrosis. Such masses, however, may be readily outlined by percussion, both anteriorly and posteriorly; this part of the examination should never be omitted. Percussion is of particular value in outlining an enlarging mass in the flank following renal trauma (progressive hemorrhage), where tenderness and muscle spasm prevent proper palpation.

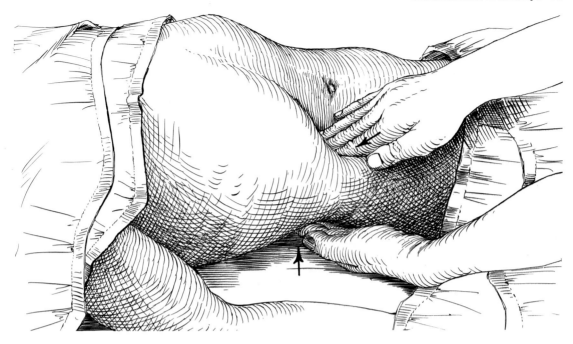

Fig 4-1. Method of palpation of the kidney. The posterior hand lifts the kidney upward. The anterior hand feels for the kidney. The patient then takes a deep breath; this causes the kidney to descend. As the patient inhales, the fingers of the anterior hand are plunged inward at the costal margin. If the kidney is mobile or enlarged, it can be felt between the 2 hands.

Transillumination

This maneuver may prove quite helpful in the child under 1 year of age who presents with a suprapubic or flank mass. A 2 or 3 cell flashlight with an opaque flange protruding beyond the lens is an adequate instrument. The flashlight is applied at right angles to the abdomen. The fiberoptic light cord, used to illuminate various optical instruments, is an excellent source of cold light. A dark room is required. A distended bladder or cystic mass will transilluminate; a solid mass will not. Flank masses may also be tested by applying the light posteriorly.

Differentiation of Renal and Radicular Pain

Radicular pain is commonly felt in the costovertebral and subcostal areas. It may spread along the course of the ureter as well and is the most common cause of so-called ''kidney'' pain. Every patient who complains of flank pain should be examined for evidence of nerve root irritation. The cause is often poor posture, arthritis, or intervertebral disk disease. Radicular pain may be noted as an aftermath of a flank incision. Pain experienced during the preeruptive phase of herpes zoster involving any of the segments between T11 and L2 may also simulate pain of renal origin.

Radiculitis usually causes hyperesthesia of the area of skin served by the irritated peripheral nerve. This hypersensitivity can be elicited by either pinching or pin-pricking the skin of the abdomen and flanks. Pressure exerted by the thumb over the facets, which are situated along the lateral edges of the vertebral bodies, will reveal local tenderness at the point of emergence of the involved peripheral nerve. This maneuver may reproduce the pain of which the patient complains.

Auscultation

Auscultation of the costovertebral areas and upper abdominal quadrants may reveal a systolic bruit which is often associated with stenosis or aneurysm of the renal artery. Bruits over the femoral arteries may be found in association with the Leriche syndrome, which may be a cause of impotence.

Arey, J. B.: Abdominal masses in infants and children. P Clin North America 10:665-91, 1963.

Bearn, J. G., & T. R. E. Pilkington: Organs palpable in the normal adult abdomen. Lancet 2:212-3, 1959.

Hand, M.: Radicular pain simulating urologic disease. J Urol 85:668-71, 1961.

Marshall, S., Lapp, M., & J.W. Schulte: Lesions of the pancreas mimicking renal disease. J Urol 93:41-5, 1965.

Mofenson, H.C., & J. Greensher: Transillumination of the abdomen in infants. Am J Dis Child 115:428-31, 1968.

Moser, R.J., & J.R. Caldwell: Abdominal murmurs, an aid in the diagnosis of renal artery disease in hypertension. Ann Int Med 56:471-83, 1962.

Museles, M., Gaudry, C.L., Jr., & W.M. Bason: Renal anomalies in the newborn found by deep palpation. Pediatrics 47:97-100, 1971.

EXAMINATION OF THE BLADDER

The bladder cannot be felt unless it is moderately distended. In the adult, if it is percussible, it contains at least 150 ml of urine. In acute or more commonly in chronic urinary retention, the bladder may reach (or even rise above) the umbilicus, in which case its outline may be seen and usually felt. (In chronic retention, where the bladder wall is flabby, the bladder may be difficult to palpate. In this instance, percussion is of great value.)

In the male infant or little boy, palpation of a hard mass deep in the center of the pelvis is compatible with a thickened hypertrophied bladder secondary to obstruction caused by posterior urethral valves.

A few instances have been reported wherein marked edema of the legs has developed secondary to compression of the iliac vessels by a distended bladder. Bimanual (abdominorectal or abdominovaginal) palpation may reveal the extent of a vesical neoplasm. To be successful it must be done under anesthesia.

Boyarsky, S., & J. Goldenberg: Detection of bladder distention by suprapubic percussion. New York J Med 62:1804-7, 1961.

Carlsson, E., & P. Garsten: Compression of the common iliac vessels by dilatation of the bladder. Acta radiol 53:449-53, 1960.

Stoutz, H.L.: Massive edema of lower extremities associated with overdistention of bladder. J Urol 86:503-4, 1961.

EXAMINATION OF THE EXTERNAL MALE GENITALIA

PENIS

Inspection

If the patient has not been circumcised, the foreskin should be retracted. This may reveal tumor or balanitis as the cause of a foul discharge. If retraction is not possible (ie, phimosis), surgical correction (dorsal slit or circumcision) is indicated.

The observation of a poor urinary stream is significant. In the newborn, neurogenic bladder or the presence of posterior urethral valves should be considered. In men, such a finding suggests urethral stricture or prostatic obstruction.

The scars of healed syphilis may be an important clue. An active ulcer requires bacteriologic or pathologic study (eg, syphilitic chancre, epithelioma). Superficial ulcers or vesicles are compatible with herpes; they are often interpreted by the patient as a venereal infection.

Meatal stenosis is a common cause of bloody spotting in the male infant. On rare occasions, it may be of such degree as to cause advanced bilateral hydronephrosis. It is easily corrected by meatotomy.

The position of the meatus should be noted. It may be located proximal to the tip of the glans on either the dorsum (epispadias) or the ventral surface (hypospadias). In either instance, there is apt to be abnormal curvature of the penis—dorsally with epispadias, ventrally with hypospadias. The urethral orifice is often stenotic.

Palpation

Palpation of the shaft may reveal a fibrous plaque involving the fascial covering of the corpora cavernosa. This is typical of Peyronie's disease. Tender areas of induration felt along the urethra may signify periurethritis secondary to urethral stricture.

Urethral Discharge

Urethral discharge is the most common complaint referable to the male sex organ. Gonococcal pus is usually profuse, thick, and yellow or gray-brown. Nonspecific discharges may be similar in appearance but are often thin, mucoid, and scanty. Although gonorrhea must be ruled out as the cause of a urethral discharge, a high percentage of such cases will be found to be nonspecific. Patients with urethral discharge should also be examined for other venereal diseases; double infection is not uncommon.

Bloody discharge should suggest the possibility of a foreign body in the urethra (male or female), urethral stricture, or neoplasm.

Urethral discharge must always be sought before the patient is asked to void.

SCROTUM

Infections and inflammations of the skin of the scrotum are not common. Small sebaceous cysts are occasionally seen. Malignant tumors are rare. The scrotum is bifid when midscrotal or perineal hypospadias is present.

Elephantiasis of the scrotum is caused by obstruction to lymphatic drainage. It is endemic in the tropics and is due to filariasis. Elephantiasis may result from radical resection of the lymph nodes of the inguinal and femoral areas, in which case the skin of the penis is also involved.

TESTIS

The testes should be carefully palpated with the fingers of both hands. A hard area in the testis proper must be regarded as a malignant tumor until proved otherwise. Transillumination of all scrotal masses should be a routine procedure. With the patient in a dark room, a strong flashlight is placed against the scrotal sac posteriorly. A hydrocele will cause the intrascrotal mass to glow red. Light will not be transmitted through a solid tumor. Tumors are often smooth but may be nodular. They seem abnormally heavy. A testis replaced by tumor or damaged by gumma is insensitive to pressure, and the usual sickening sensation is absent. About 10% of tumors are associated with a secondary hydrocele which may have to be aspirated before definitive palpation can be done.

The testis may be absent from the scrotum. This may represent transient (physiologic retractile testis) or true cryptorchism. Palpation of the groins may reveal the presence of the organ.

The atrophic testis (following postoperative orchiopexy, mumps orchitis, or torsion of the spermatic cord) is usually flabby and at times hypersensitive. Although spermatogenesis may be lost, androgen function is usually intact.

EPIDIDYMIS

The epididymis is sometimes rather closely attached to the posterior surface of the testis, and at other times it is quite free of it. The epididymis should be carefully palpated for size and induration. Induration means infection (primary tumors are exceedingly rare).

In the acute stage of epididymitis, the testis and epididymis are indistinguishable by palpation; the testicle and epididymis may be adherent to the scrotum, which is usually quite red. Tenderness is exquisite.

Chronic painless induration should suggest tuberculosis, although nonspecific chronic epididymitis is also a possibility. Other signs of tuberculosis of the genitourinary tract usually present include "sterile" pyuria, a thickened seminal vesicle, a nodular prostate, and "beading" of the vas deferens.

SPERMATIC CORD AND VAS DEFERENS

A swelling in the spermatic cord may be cystic (eg, hydrocele or hernia) or solid (eg, connective tissue tumor). The latter is rare. Lipoma in the investing fascia of the cord may simulate hernia. Diffuse swelling and induration of the cord is seen with filarial funiculitis.

Careful palpation of the vas deferens may reveal thickening (eg, chronic infection), fusiform enlargements (the "beading" caused by tuberculosis), or even its absence. The latter finding is of importance in the infertile male; it is rare.

TESTICULAR TUNICS AND ADNEXA

Hydroceles are usually cystic but on occasion are so tense that they simulate solid tumors. Transillumination makes the differential diagnosis. They may develop secondary to nonspecific acute or tuberculous epididymitis, trauma, or tumor of the testis. The last is a distinct possibility if hydrocele appears "spontaneously" between the ages of 18-35. It should be aspirated to permit careful palpation of underlying structures.

Hydrocele usually surrounds the testis completely. Cystic masses that are separate from but in the region of the upper pole of the testis are probably spermatoceles. Aspiration reveals the typical thin, milky fluid, which contains sperms.

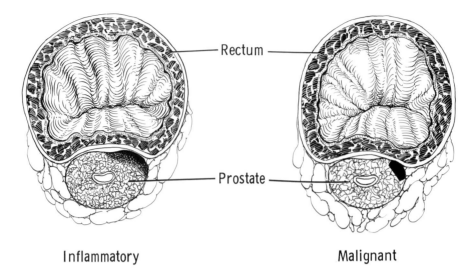

Inflammatory   Malignant

Fig 4-2. Differential diagnosis of prostatic nodules. Left: Inflammatory area is raised above the surface of the gland; induration decreases gradually at its periphery. **Right:** Cancerous nodule is not raised; there is an abrupt change in consistency at its edges.

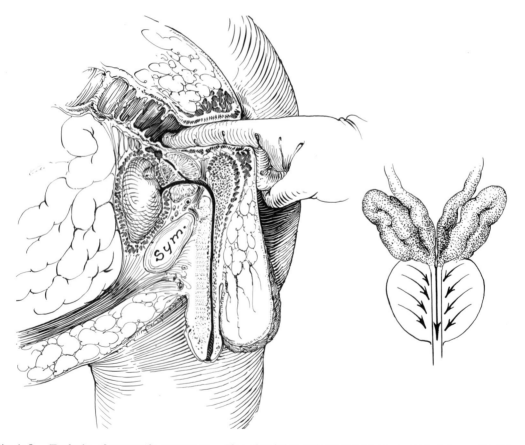

Fig 4-3. Technic of prostatic massage. The glandular substance is compressed from its lateral edges to the urethra, which lies in the center. (Drawing at right shows direction of pressure.) The seminal vesicles are then stripped from above downward.

VAGINAL EXAMINATION

Diseases of the female genital tract may secondarily involve the urinary organs, thereby making a thorough gynecologic examination essential. Commonly associated are urethrocystitis secondary to urethral diverticulitis or cervicitis, pyelonephritis during pregnancy, and ureteral obstruction from metastatic nodes or direct extension in cancer of the cervix.

Inspection

The urinary meatus may reveal a reddened, tender, friable lesion (urethral caruncle) or a reddened, everted posterior lip which is often seen with senile urethritis and vaginitis. Biopsy is indicated if a malignant tumor cannot be ruled out. Smears of discharges should be made. The diagnosis of senile vaginitis (and urethritis) is established by staining a smear of the vaginal epithelium with Lugol's solution. It should be examined immediately after rinsing because the brown dye in the cells quickly fades. Cells lacking glycogen (hypoestrogenism) do not take up the stain, whereas normal cells do.

Evidence of skenitis and bartholinitis may reveal the source of persistent urethritis or cystitis. The condition of the vaginal wall should be observed. Bacteriologic study of the secretions may be helpful. Urethrocele and cystocele may cause residual urine and lead to persistent infection of the bladder. A bulge in the anterior vaginal wall might represent a urethral diverticulum. The cervix should be visualized in order to note the presence of malignancy or infection. Biopsy or Papanicolaou preparations may be indicated.

Palpation

At times the urethra, the base of the bladder, and the lower ureters may be tender on palpation, but little can be deduced from this. Induration of the urethra or trigonal area or a mass involving either may be a clue to an existing neoplasm. A soft mass found in this area could be a urethral diverticulum. Pressure on such a lesion may cause pus to extrude from the urethra. A stone in the lower ureter may be palpable. Evidence of enlargement of the uterus (eg, pregnancy, myomas) or diseases or inflammations of the colon or adnexa may afford a clue to the cause of urinary symptoms (eg, compression of a ureter by a malignant ovarian tumor, endometriosis, or diverticulitis of sigmoid colon adherent to the bladder).

Carcinoma of the cervix may invade the base of the bladder, causing vesical irritability or hematuria; or its metastases to iliac lymph nodes may compress the ureters.

Rectal examination may afford further knowledge and is the obvious route of examination in children and virgins.

RECTAL EXAMINATION OF THE MALE

SPHINCTER AND LOWER RECTUM

The estimation of sphincter tone is of great importance. Laxity of the muscle strongly suggests similar changes in the urinary sphincters and detrusor and may be a clue to the diagnosis of neurogenic disease. In addition to the digital prostatic examination, the examiner should palpate the entire lower rectum and rule out stenosis, internal hemorrhoids, cryptitis, rectal fistulas, mucosal polyps, and rectal malignancies.

PROSTATE

Before the rectal examination is made, a specimen of urine for routine analysis should be collected. This is of the utmost importance, since prostatic massage (or even palpation at times) will force prostatic secretion into the posterior urethra. If this secretion contains pus, a specimen of urine voided after the rectal examination will be contaminated by it.

Size

The average prostate is about 4 cm in length and width. It is widest superiorly at the bladder neck. As the gland enlarges, the lateral sulci become relatively deeper and the median furrow becomes obliterated. The prostate may also elongate. It is necessary to realize that the clinical importance of prostatic hyperplasia is measured by the severity of symptoms and the amount of residual urine and not by the size of the gland. On rectal examination, the prostate may be of normal size and consistency in a patient with acute urinary retention.

Consistency

Normally, the consistency of the gland is similar to that of the contracted thenar eminence of the thumb (with the thumb completely opposed to the little finger). It is rather rubbery. It may be mushy if congested (due to lack of intercourse or to chronic infection with impaired drainage), indurated (due to chronic infection with or without calculi), or stony hard (due to advanced carcinoma).

The difficulty lies in differentiating firm areas in the prostate: fibrosis from nonspecific infection, granulomatous prostatitis, nodulation from tuberculosis, firm areas due to prostatic calculi or early cancer. Generally speaking, nodules caused by infection are raised above the surface of the gland. At their edges the induration gradually fades to the normal softness of surrounding tissue. In cancer, conversely, the suspious lesion is usually not raised; it is hard and has a sharp edge, ie, there is an abrupt change in consistency on the same plane. It tends to arise in the lateral sulcus.

Even the most experienced clinicians at times encounter trouble in this differentiation. In the absence of other signs of tuberculosis and in the absence of pus in the prostatic secretion, cancer is likely, particularly if an x-ray fails to show prostatic calculi (which are seen just behind or above the symphysis). Serum acid phosphatase determinations and radiographs of bones are of no help in diagnosing early carcinoma of the prostate.

Mobility

The mobility of the gland varies. Occasionally it has great mobility; at other times, very little. In advanced neoplasm it is fixed because of local extension through the capsule. The prostate should be routinely massaged in the adult and its secretion examined microscopically. It should not be massaged, however, in the presence of an acute urethral discharge, acute prostatitis, acute prostatocystitis, in men near the stage of complete urinary retention (because it may precipitate complete retention), or in men suffering from obvious cancer of the gland. Even in the absence of symptoms, massage is necessary, for prostatitis is commonly asymptomatic. Discovery of such silent disease and its eradication is important in preventing cystitis and epididymitis.

Technic of Massage

The patient should lean over the examining table so that his body is horizontal. His legs should be straight and his feet somewhat apart.

Methods of massage vary, but the basic maneuver is to press the gland substance firmly with the pad of the index finger in order to express secretion into the prostatic urethra. Start laterally and superiorly and massage toward the midline. A rolling motion of the finger is less traumatic to the rectal mucosa and prostate gland and is better tolerated by the patient. Finally, the seminal vesicles should be stripped from above downward and medially (Fig 4-3).

Copious amounts of secretion may be obtained from some prostate glands and little or none from others. This of course depends to some extent upon the vigor with which the massage is carried out. If no secretion is obtained, have the patient void even a few drops of urine; this will contain adequate secretion for examination. Microscopic examination of the secretion is done under low-power magnification. Normal secretion contains numerous lecithin bodies which are refractile, like red cells, but are much smaller than red cells. Only an occasional white cell is present. A few epithelial cells and, rarely, corpora amylacea are seen. Sperms may be present, but the absence of sperms is of no significance.

The presence of large numbers of pus cells is pathologic and makes the diagnosis of prostatitis. Stained smears are usually impractical. It is difficult to fix this material on the slide, and even when this is successful pyogenic bacteria are usually not found. Acid-fast organisms can often be found by appropriate staining methods.

On occasion it may be helpful to obtain cultures of prostatic secretion. After thorough cleansing of the glans and emptying of the bladder (to mechanically cleanse the urethra), massage is done. Drops of secretion are collected in a sterile tube of culture medium. Bacteriologic diagnosis is usually not helpful because antibiotic therapy is of little value in the treatment of chronic prostatitis.

SEMINAL VESICLES

Palpation of the seminal vesicles should be attempted. The vesicles are situated under the base of the bladder and diverge from below upward (Fig 1-9). Normal seminal vesicles are usually not palpable, but when they are overdistended they may feel quite cystic. In the presence of chronic infection (particularly tuberculosis) or in association with advanced carcinoma of the prostate, they may be markedly indurated. Stripping of the seminal vesicles should be done in association with prostatic massage, for the vesicles are usually infected when prostatitis is present. Primary tumors of the vesicles are very rare.

EXAMINATION OF LYMPH NODES
(See Figs 17-1 and 17-2.)

NEUROLOGIC EXAMINATION

Inguinal and Subinguinal Lymph Nodes

With inflammatory lesions of the skin of the penis and scrotum or vulva, the inguinal and subinguinal lymph nodes may be involved. Such diseases include chancroid, syphilitic chancre, lymphogranuloma venereum, and, on occasion, gonorrhea.

Malignancies (squamous cell carcinoma) involving the penis, glans, scrotal skin, or urethra in women metastasize to the inguinal and subinguinal nodes. Testicular tumors do not spread to these nodes unless they have invaded the scrotal skin or have been subjected to previous orchidopexy.

Other Lymph Nodes

Tumors of the testis and prostate may involve the left supraclavicular nodes. Cancer of the bladder and prostate typically metastasize to the hypogastric, external iliac, and preaortic nodes, although only occasionally are they so large as to be palpable. Masses near the midline in the upper abdomen in a young man should suggest cancer of the testis; the primary growth may be minute and completely hidden in the substance of what appears to be a normal testicle.

A careful neurologic survey may uncover sensory or motor impairment which will account for residual urine (neurogenic bladder) or incontinence. Since the bladder is innervated by the 2nd-4th sacral segments, much information can be gained by testing the sensation of the perianal skin, anal sphincter tone and by eliciting the Achilles tendon and bulbocavernosus reflexes. The bulbocavernosus reflex is normal if, with a finger in the rectum, the external anal sphincter and bulbocavernosus muscle can be felt to contract when the glans penis or clitoris is squeezed. If no contraction occurs, interruption of the sacral reflex arc (lower motor neuron lesion) is present.

Bors, E., & K.A. Blenn: Bulbocavernosus reflex. J Urol 82:128-30, 1959.

• • •

5...

Urologic Laboratory Examination

BLOOD COUNT

Erythrocytosis has been noted in association with 3-4% of urologic renal diseases, including carcinoma, hydronephrosis, and simple cyst. A number of instances have also been seen in association with uterine myomas and hepatoma. The erythropoietin level in the plasma is increased. Following definitive surgery, the erythropoietin level and the increased red cell count return to normal. If metastases later develop, erythrocytosis returns. (Note: Platelets, leukocytes, and other blood elements are usually not increased; the term "polycythemia" as applied to red blood cell count elevation in these disorders is a misnomer.)

Hypochromic anemia may occur in association with chronic pyelonephritis, uremia, and carcinoma.

EXAMINATION OF URETHRAL DISCHARGE IN THE MALE

A specimen of the discharge should be obtained before the patient voids. If discharge is absent at the time of examination, the urethra should be "milked" or the first portion of the voided urine can be collected and centrifuged. This sediment is similar to gross discharge.

The sediment or the actual discharge should be examined while wet. Trichomonads are seen as motile round bodies which are a little larger than pus cells. They may be cultured in a liquid liver or other suitable medium. The presence of lecithin bodies suggests that the discharge may be of prostatic origin. Pus and epithelial cells should be noted. If many epithelial cells are seen, chronic infection is probably present.

These secretions should also be stained. Methylene blue preparations permit clear observation of bacterial morphology. If cocci are present, Gram's stain (for gonococci) must be done.

EXAMINATION OF THE URINE

Urinalysis is without doubt the most important and the most poorly performed laboratory test in all medicine. There are 3 reasons for the inadequacy of so many urinalyses: (1) The urine is too often improperly collected, (2) it is not examined when fresh, and (3) examination of the sediment is frequently incomplete.

It is essential that the urine specimen be collected before the rectal examination is made. This guarantees that the urine will not be contaminated by infected prostatic secretion which may drain into the posterior urethra following this manipulation.

Proper Collection of Urine

In both men and women, the urethra harbors bacteria and a few pus cells. Any urine specimen voided into a single container will for this reason be contaminated by the normal urethral flora. This immediately clouds the interpretation of microscopic findings and often leads to the diagnosis of cystitis when the bladder urine actually contains no pus cells or bacteria. This applies particularly to women, in whom voiding causes urine to flow over the vulva and, at times, into the vagina.

A. Collecting Specimens From Men: Although "two-glass" and "three-glass" tests have been described, the simplest method of collecting urine from a man is to give him a clean glass and instruct him to start his stream into the toilet bowl or urinal. He should be instructed to retract a redundant foreskin. After the stream has thoroughly cleansed the urethra it should be directed into the glass (without interrupting the act of urination); before voiding has been completed, the glass should be removed. This affords a "midstream" (second glass) specimen which is as clean as that obtained by catheter.

B. Collecting Specimens From Women: Women should be placed in the lithotomy position. The labia are held apart. After the vulva has been cleansed, the patient is in-

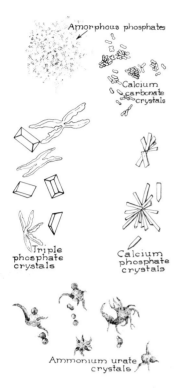

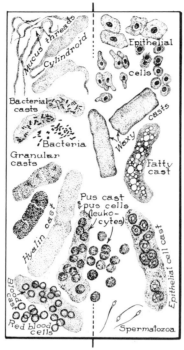

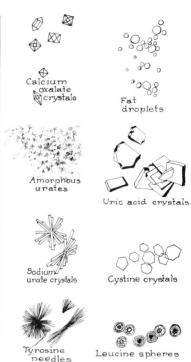

ALKALINE REACTION

Fig 5-1. Microscopic examination of urine sediment. (Redrawn after Todd and Sanford.)

ACID REACTION

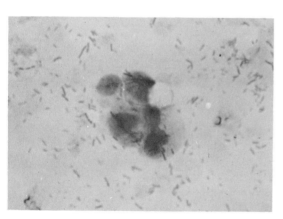

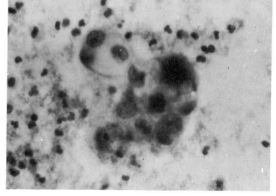

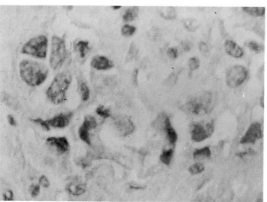

Fig 5-2. Urinary cytology. Above left: Triple-strength methylene blue stain of urinary sediment showing clumps of transitional cells with irregular and relatively large nuclei. Note presence of bacteria. **Above right:** Papanicolaou stain from same urinary sediment. Note similarity to methylene blue stain. **Left:** Biopsy of papillary vesical neoplasm from same patient. Clump of transitional cells in upper left hand corner is similar to those seen in urinary sediment.

structed to start voiding into a bowl held close to the vulva. The midportion of the stream should be collected in a sterile container.

Catheterization is also satisfactory and should not be avoided because of the fear of introducing infection with the catheter; the advantages of obtaining a "sterile" specimen far overshadow this slight risk, which may be further diminished by thorough irrigation of the bladder and the instillation of 30-60 ml of 1:5000 aqueous chlorhexidine solution or 0.5% neomycin. The passage of a catheter of moderate size (22 F) in women also permits exploration of the urethra and reveals stenosis, which may be the predisposing cause of the urinary infection.

C. Collecting Specimens From Children: If the boy or girl is old enough to cooperate, a midstream specimen can be collected as described above for men and women. The use of a plastic bag (after thorough antiseptic cleansing) for collection of urine in the neonate and infant is unsatisfactory from the bacteriologic standpoint. Davis and Chumley have shown that when little girls void in the supine position almost half of them reflux urine into the vagina. Boehm and Haynes, utilizing a technic which they term "midstream catch," report minimal bacterial contamination. After feed-

ing, and before the infant voids, the genital area is thoroughly cleansed with hexachlorophene detergent. The child is then held upside down (Fig 5-3). The spinal reflex of Perez is then elicited by stroking the back along the paravertebral muscles. Spontaneous voiding usually occurs within 5 minutes. The stream is directed into a sterile container.

One should not hesitate to catheterize little girls if other methods of urine collection fail. In similar circumstances, suprapubic aspiration may be considered in the male.

D. Stamey has stressed suprapubic vesical puncture as the ideal means of obtaining a truly sterile urine for bacteriologic analysis. It may be indicated in selected cases but hardly seems to lend itself to routine use.

Examination While Fresh

The "morning urine" is not an adequate urine specimen for routine examination of the urinary sediment. Even though the specific gravity of such a specimen is acceptable as a fairly dependable renal function test, the urinary sediment is abnormally altered after standing a few hours. Red cells break up and casts disintegrate as the urine becomes alkaline; bacteria, if not present in the fresh urine, enter the container and multiply rapidly. This can lead to the erroneous diagnosis of "urinary tract infection." Whether the physician is interested in the presence of red cells, casts, pus cells, or bacteria, a specimen that is not fresh is of little value. If urinalysis is to be dependable, the specimen must be collected properly and examined immediately.

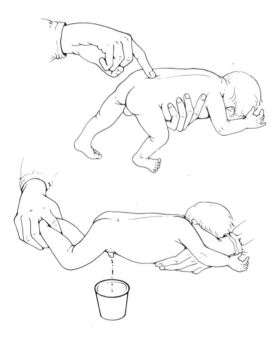

Fig 5-3. "Midstream catch" urine by the method of Boehm and Haynes. (Redrawn from Boehm, J.J., & J.L. Haynes: Bacteriology of "midstream catch" urines. Studies in newborn infants. Am J Dis Child 111:366, 1966.)

Microscopic Examination of Sediment After Centrifuging

The stained smear of urinary sediment, examined personally, is the most important step in urologic diagnosis and the best screening test for the presence or absence of infection. On occasion, although bacteria are seen on a stained smear, the cultures are returned as "negative." Since finding bacteria on a stained smear means that there are at least 10,000 organisms per ml, such a finding is pathognomonic of infection, and a negative culture in this instance should be ignored. A stained smear gives quick information so that immediate treatment can be instituted; a culture takes many hours to complete with loss of valuable time. Studies show that the correlation of stained smears with cultures is good. If the patient has symptoms compatible with urinary infection but pyuria and bacteriuria are absent, a culture should be obtained. This may negate the few errors encountered with the stained smear.

A. Wet Smear: This should be examined under low and medium power. White cells, red cells, crystals, and casts should be searched for, and the types of casts present should be noted (Fig 5-1). Squamous epithelial cells from the urethra and bladder neck are to be expected in the urine of the female; they are absent in men except in patients who are on estrogen therapy for cancer of the prostate. Trichomonads and yeast cells may also be seen.

B. Staining of the Sediment: Whether the wet smear reveals abnormalities or not, a stained smear must be examined. If pus cells appear to be present in a wet smear, staining of the sediment will aid in differentiating leukocytes and epithelial cells. The finding of transitional epithelial cells, singly or in clumps, strongly suggests vesical neoplasm (Fig 5-2). The stained smear will also identify the bacteria. This will allow the physician to select an antibiotic or chemotherapeutic agent immediately and on the basis of objective clinical information. Staining the urine when pus is present may also reveal that no bacteria can be seen. Such a "sterile" pyuria strongly suggests tuberculosis of the urinary tract. Death from renal tuberculosis may occur if the diagnosis is delayed, and late diagnosis is usually due to improperly performed urinalyses.

If no pus is found on the wet preparation, the sediment must still be stained, since about 30% of patients with chronic urinary tract infection have apyuric bacteriuria. One should not wait for the presence of pyuria or symptoms suggesting urinary tract diseases before considering such a possibility. This means that routine urinalysis in all patients, no matter what their symptoms, requires staining of the urinary sediment; until this has been done, urinary tract infection has not been ruled out.

1. For pyogenic organisms -

a. Triple-strength methylene blue is the stain of choice:

Methylene blue	1.5
Alcohol	30
N/10 potassium hydroxide	2
Distilled water, qs ad	120

Fix the sediment on the slide with heat. Take care to only **warm** the slide. Too much heat will distort the stained cells. Flood the slide with the dye for 10-20 seconds, then rinse and dry with heat. Do not blot since this is apt to remove the sediment. It is helpful to mark the slide through the area containing the stained sediment with a red wax pencil before the immersion oil is applied. This allows the microscopist to find the plane of the sediment with ease when the oil immersion lens is used. A cover slip is not necessary.

b. Gram's stain is of limited value in the study of urinary sediment. If rods are found, they are usually gram-negative; if cocci are found, they are usually gram-positive. Gram's stain has the disadvantage of repeated staining and washing, which may cause the sediment to be washed from the slide. It is useful in the identification of the gonococcus.

(1) Fix the sediment with heat.

(2) Stain with crystal violet for 1 minute.

(3) Wash in tap water.

(4) Stain with Lugol's solution for 1 minute.

(5) Wash in tap water.

(6) Decolorize with 95% alcohol or acetone-alcohol for 30 seconds or less.

(7) Wash in tap water.

(8) Stain with safranin for 30 seconds.

(9) Wash in tap water and dry with heat.

2. Acid-fast (Ziehl-Neelsen) stains should be done if a "sterile pyuria" is found or if urinary tuberculosis is suspected. The centrifuged sediment from 15 ml of urine discloses tubercle bacilli in half the cases. If a 24-hour urine specimen is centrifuged it will reveal tubercle bacilli in about 70-80%. The technic for Ziehl-Neelsen staining is as follows:

a. Stain heat-fixed smear with steaming Ziehl's carbolfuchsin for 5 minutes, or leave in cold stain for 24 hours. Cold Kinyoun carbolfuchsin acid-fast stain may be applied for 5 minutes.

b. Wash in tap water.

c. Decolorize with acid-alcohol until only a slight pink tinge remains.

d. Wash in tap water.

e. Counterstain with triple-strength methylene blue for 10-20 seconds.

f. Wash in tap water and dry with heat.

Cultures for Bacteria

A. Quantitative Cultures: Some type of quantitative estimation of the number of bacteria must be made; pour-plates and colony counts should be done. It is essential that the colony count be judged in the light of the specific gravity of the specimen. A count of 1000 organisms per ml in urine with a specific gravity of 1.002 is significant. A similar count in 1.030 urine might be compatible with urethral contamination. If urine which is not too dilute has been collected properly and plated immediately, a count of fewer than 1000 organisms per ml is compatible with urethral contamination. Only counts above 1000 organisms per ml should be considered significant. The acceptance of the popular concept that 100,000 organisms per ml is the "breaking point" between contamination and true infection causes many urinary tract infections to be missed. This high count allows for errors in collection of the urine and delays in transport to the laboratory. Quantitative cultures are also useful for preparing antibiotic sensitivity tests, which are helpful in the definitive treatment of infections.

Stamey and McLin and Tavel have described and evaluated simplified methods of quantitative urine culture applicable to office practice. The advantages of such office procedures are absolute control of the method of collection of urine by the physician and the opportunity for immediate plating. Few hospitals can compete with these technics, which make available a quantitative culture within hours. With such a method, a colony count of 1000 per ml is significant. Drug sensitivity disks can be placed on 1 plate, thus affording quick guidance in the choice of antibiotic.

B. Cultures for Tubercle Bacilli: If stained smears are negative for tubercle bacilli, cultures should be made. Even if the smears reveal acid-fast organisms, cultures should be done, since the finding of the bacteria in the stained sediment, although it is strong presumptive evidence, is not definitive proof of the presence of tuberculosis.

Guinea Pig Inoculation

This should be performed on all patients suspected of having tuberculosis of the urologic organs. Since it fulfills all of Koch's postulates, a positive guinea pig test is unequivocal evidence of tuberculous infection.

Other Tests of the Urine

A. Urinary pH: Normal kidneys contribute to the control of body pH by excreting urine in the pH ranges of 4.5 to about 7.5. The former figure is typical of diabetic acidosis. Readings above 7.5 mean that urea-splitting organisms are present. Despite a low blood pH, the urinary pH in renal tubular acidosis varies between 6.0 and 7.0.

B. Cytology: (See Fig 5-2.) Transitional cells shed from tumors of the urinary tract may be demonstrated either by the Papanicolaou technic or by methylene blue stain. The latter is as efficient as the former. Men do not shed epithelial cells unless they are taking estrogens, in which case squamous cells are seen. Women commonly shed squamous cells from the bladder neck and urethra. Both may pass small round transitional cells, however, if acute cystitis is present.

These stains correlate well with the presence of transitional cell neoplasms of the renal pelvis, ureter, or bladder but have not been too helpful in suggesting the presence of adenocarcinoma of the kidney.

C. Hormone Tests: In the presence of a testicular tumor, estimates of the amount of chorionic gonadotropin are of great importance in calculating the prognosis and may help to evaluate the presence or absence of metastases after the primary tumor has been removed. Determination of the amounts of 17-ketosteroids, pituitary gonadotropins, corticosteroids, and estrogens in the urine may be helpful in certain endocrine disorders, including infertility in the male.

D. The Sulkowitch test affords a rough estimate of the amount of calcium excreted in the urine. The patient should be instructed to refrain from drinking milk or eating cheese 3-4 days before the test is done. The Sulkowitch test is useful in uncovering hyperparathyroidism as a cause of urinary calculus formation. Sulkowitch reagent is made up according to the following formula:

Oxalic acid	2.5
Ammonium oxalate	2.5
Glacial acetic acid	5
Distilled water, qs ad	150

To 5 ml of urine, add 2 ml of Sulkowitch reagent. The amount of calcium is estimated by the speed of precipitation and the intensity of the cloud; it is graded from 0 to 4+.

Lack of reaction is compatible with hypoparathyroidism (it may be negative in acute pancreatitis), whereas a strongly positive test means hypercalciuria and suggests the presence of hypercalcemia. This test is indispensable in the study and management of patients suffering from urinary stone; it must, however, be correlated with the specific gravity of the urine.

E. Lactic Acid Dehydrogenase (LDH): This enzyme has been found to be significantly elevated in most potentially fatal medical renal diseases and chronic pyelonephritis. Increased levels are also observed in patients with cancer of the kidney, bladder, and prostate.

Amador, Dorfman, and Wacker have studied the urinary levels of LDH and alkaline phosphatase activities in the differential diagnosis of renal and other diseases (Table 5-1). The levels of both enzymes are normal in renal cyst, adrenocortical hyperplasia, benign prostatic hyperplasia, benign essential hypertension, and acute cystitis and pyelonephritis. Since the LDH test is rather nonspecific and since 75% of patients with an elevated level of the enzyme prove to have urinary infection, the simple test of urinalysis is usually definitive. Gault and Geggie have found this a poor diagnostic step.

Table 5-1. Urinary levels of LDH and alkaline phosphatases in disease states.

Diseases	Urinary Levels Of	
	LDH	Alkaline Phosphatase
Cancer of bladder Chronic pyelonephritis Sclerosing glomerulo- nephritis Malignant hypertension	↑	Normal
Cancer of kidney, pros- tate Adrenocortical adenoma and cancer Acute and chronic glo- merulonephritis (various types) Acute tubular necrosis	↑	↑

F. Vanilmandelic Acid (VMA): Vanilmandelic acid is the urinary metabolite of the catecholamines, including dopa, dopamine, norepinephrine, normetanephrine, and metanephrine. VMA levels are elevated in patients with pheochromocytoma, neuroblastoma, and ganglioneuroma. VMA determination is, therefore, a simple yet efficient screening test for these conditions. Estimation of the various catecholamines probably affords a little better diagnostic accuracy.

Summary

The stained smear of the sediment from a properly collected urine is all that is needed to diagnose most cases of urinary tract infection. Bacteriologic cultures may be required in patients who are acutely ill or in those who suffer from chronic or recurrent disease.

Abbott, G. D., & F. T. Shannon: How to aspirate urine suprapubically in infants and children. Clin Pediat 9:277-8, 1970.

Amador, E., Dorfman, L. E., & W. E. C. Wacker: Urinary alkaline phosphatase and LDH activities in the differential diagnosis of renal disease. Ann Int Med 62:30-40, 1965.

Boehm, J. J., & J. L. Haynes: Bacteriology of "midstream catch" urines. Studies in newborn infants. Am J Dis Child 111:366-9, 1966.

Bower, B. F., & G. S. Gordan: Hormonal effects of nonendocrine tumors. In: Annual Reviews of Medicine, Annual Reviews 16: 83-118, 1965.

Brody, L. H., Salladay, J. R., & K. Armbruster: Urinalysis and the urinary sediment. M Clin North America 55:243-66, 1971.

Budinger, J. M., & M. Cavallo: Detection of hematuria with a paperstrip indicator. Am J Clin Path 42:626-9, 1964.

Cohen, S. N., & E. H. Kass: A simple method for quantitative urine culture. New England J Med 277:176-80, 1967.

Davis, L. A., & W. F. Chumley: The frequency of vaginal reflux during micturition—its possible importance to the interpretation of urine cultures. Pediatrics 38:293-4, 1966.

Friedman, S. A., & J. L. Gladstone: The effects of hydration and bladder incubation time of urine colony counts. J Urol 105: 428-32, 1971.

Gault, M. H., & P. H. S. Geggie: Clinical significance of urinary LDH, alkaline phosphatase and other enzymes. Canad MAJ 101: 208-15, 1969.

Grabstald, H., & M. K. Schwartz: Urinary lactic dehydrogenase in genitourinary tract disease. JAMA 207:2062-6, 1969.

Lawson, J. S., & A. S. Hewstone: Microscopic appearance of urine in the neonatal period. Arch Dis Childhood 39:287-8, 1964.

McLin, P., & F. R. Tavel: Urine culture and direct sensitivity testing: A rapid simple method for use in the office. Clin Med 78: 16-21, Dec. 1971.

Northway, J. D.: Hematuria in children. J Pediat 78:381-96, 1971.

Park, C-H, & others: Reliability of positive exfoliative cytology study of the urine in urinary tract malignancy. J Urol 102:91-2, 1969.

Pryles, C. V., & B. Lustik: Laboratory diagnosis of urinary tract infection. P Clin North America 18:233-44, 1971.

Rehm, R. A., & A. Fishman: The value of the urine smear in detecting bacteriuria. J Urol 89:930-2, 1963.

Ritter, S., Spencer, H., & J. Smachson: The Sulkowitch and quantitative urine calcium excretion. J Lab Clin Med 56:314-20, 1960.

Rubin, M. I., & T. Baliah: Urinalysis and its clinical interpretation. P Clin North America 18:245-64, 1971.

Schulte, J. W., & others: A simple technic for recognizing abnormal epithelial cells in the urine. J Urol 89:615-25, 1963.

Stamey, T. A.: Office bacteriology. J Urol 97:926-34, 1967.

Sunderman, F. W., Jr.: Measurements of vanilmandelic acid for the diagnosis of pheochromocytoma and neuroblastoma. Am J Clin Path 42:481-97, 1964.

Tunnessen, W. W., Smith, C., & F. A. Oski: Beeturia: A sign of iron deficiency. Am J Dis Child 117:424-6, 1969.

Williams, C. M., & M. Greer: Homovanillic acid and vanilmandelic acid in diagnosis of neuroblastoma. JAMA 183:836-40, 1963.

RENAL FUNCTION TESTS

The kidneys have 3 primary functions: (1) the regulation of sodium chloride, potassium, and water (fluid and ion) balance, (2) the regulation of body pH, and (3) the excretion of the end products of metabolism

Proteinuria

The presence of proteinuria as measured by sulfosalicylic acid or indicator papers must be explained, although random tests may be misleading. Proteinuria must be correlated with the specific gravity of the specimen. A mere trace of protein in urine with a specific gravity of 1.004-1.010 is compatible with a significant 24-hour loss of protein in a patient with marked impairment of renal function, even uremia. Amounts of protein up to 100 mg/24 hours are normal.

Sulfosalicylic acid (but not Albustix®) gives a positive test for proteinuria in the presence of some radiopaque chemicals used in excretory urography.

Heavy proteinuria is seen in nephrosis and, at times, glomerulonephritis; but the clinical picture and other findings in the urinary sediment usually lead to the proper diagnosis. The heaviest proteinuria may be noted in children with high fever and severe dehydration and in orthostatic proteinuria. Proteinuria is not, therefore, necessarily pathognomonic of intrinsic renal disease.

Urine Specific Gravity

The specific gravity of the urine is a simple and significant test of renal function, although determination of osmolality may be more accurate. Normal kidneys in young persons can concentrate to 1.040; at age 40, to 1.036; at age 50, to 1.030. Thus, a specific gravity of 1.030 in a man 70 years old implies not only excellent renal function but also intense dehydration. With marked hydration, the specific gravity may fall to 1.000. Urine densities above 1.040 suggest that the specimen contains radiopaque fluid.

In the presence of diminishing renal function, there is progressive loss of concentrating power until 1.006-1.010 is reached. The power of dilution, however, tends to be maintained until renal damage is extreme. Even in uremia, although the concentrating power is limited to 1.010, dilution in the range of 1.002-1.004 may still be found. Therefore, a specific gravity of 1.004 in a random urine specimen does not guarantee adequate renal function. Oddly, the fixation point of specific gravity with advanced hydronephrosis is closer to 1.006, and even in this circumstance dilution may reach 1.002.

Urinary specific gravity rises as the radiopaque medium used in excretory urography is excreted. Total renal function may be estimated by subtracting the specific gravity of the preinjection specimen from the specific gravity of the urine voided any time up to 2 hours after the infusion. An increase of 0.025 units or more indicates good total renal function. Less than this implies impaired function. In the uremic patient, little change is observed.

The PSP (Phenol Red) Test (Also a measure of residual urine.)

The patient is instructed to void. Exactly 1 ml of phenosulfonphthalein (containing 6 mg of the dye) is then given intravenously with a tuberculin syringe (the ampule contains 1.2 ml). The patient should drink no more than 200 ml of water during each of the 2 subsequent half-hour periods. (Do not force fluids before or during the test, since excretion of PSP is not dependent upon urine flow. Furthermore, rapid vesical filling causes an obstructed bladder to lose tone, and the amount of residual urine is thereby increased.) Collect urine specimens one-half hour and, if excretion is less than 50%, 1 hour after the injection. Alkalinize with 5-10 ml of 10% NaOH to bring out the red color. Dilute the specimen with water to a volume of 1000 ml if the dye appears in good concentration. If the specimen is pale, dilute with only 250 ml or 500 ml, in which case the resulting percentage should be divided by 4 or 2, respectively. The percentage of dye recovered is measured by means of colorimetry. Collections beyond the first hour are of no value.

At times the urine may have a brownish hue; this usually occurs in "stagnant" (residual) urine. The azo dyes (eg, Pyridium®, Azogantrisin®, and Bromsulphalein®) interfere with accurate estimation of PSP excretion. Probenecid (Benemid®) depresses PSP excretion by 67% because it interferes with the transport of the dye.

If a catheter is in the bladder, it is necessary to irrigate it at the time of collection of each specimen because an indwelling catheter does not completely empty the bladder. The PSP excretion may be low if the test is done shortly after excretory urography, for both the radiopaque fluid and PSP compete for transport on protein molecules.

The average amount of dye normally recovered in the first half-hour specimen is 50-60%; the second specimen contains 10-15%. The normal total, then, for 1 hour is 60-75%. The normal PSP in children (infants excepted) is 5-10% higher than in the adult. An unusually high PSP in an adult is compatible with surgical or congenital absence of one kidney with compensatory hypertrophy of its mate.

Table 5-2. Examples of PSP excretion.

	I		II		III	
1/2 hour	25 ml	15%	30 ml	35%	25 ml	25%
1 hour	55 ml	25%	40 ml	25%	50 ml	25%
Totals	80 ml	40%	70 ml	60%	75 ml	50%

From such excretion curves the approximate amounts of residual urine can be estimated:

$$\frac{\text{Vol}^1\ (50 \text{ or } 60\ -\ \text{PSP}^1)}{\text{PSP}^1} = \text{Approximate amount of residual urine (in ml)}$$

Vol^1 = the volume of the first specimen.
PSP^1 = the percentage of PSP recovered in the first specimen.
"50 or 60" = the expected normal PSP excretion after 1/2 hour.
(The second half-hour does not enter into this calculation.)

The amount of residual urine in each of the above examples can therefore be calculated as follows:

$$\text{I} \qquad \frac{25\ (60\ -\ 15)}{15} = \frac{1125}{15} = \text{About 75 ml residual urine}$$

$$\text{II} \qquad \frac{30\ (60\ -\ 35)}{35} = \frac{750}{35} = \text{About 21 ml residual urine}$$

$$\text{III} \qquad \frac{25\ (60\ -\ 25)}{25} = \frac{875}{25} = \text{About 35 ml residual urine}$$

A "diaper" PSP test can be done on infants, even the newborn. The dye is given intramuscularly and the diaper is removed after 3 hours. It is placed in a graduate which is filled to the 1000 ml mark. The normal PSP in infants is 50% or more in 3 hours. Even at the age of 3 days, at least 30% will be excreted in 3 hours. In the presence of vesical outlet obstruction, bilateral renal damage, or vesicoureteral reflux, little of the dye may be recovered. Such a finding requires explanation.

The PSP test is a test of renal blood flow and tubular function. Since urologic renal diseases primarily affect the tubules, the test has obvious value as an index of the presence and extent of urologic renal damage. The test has the advantage of being simple, and in most cases it also affords a fairly accurate estimate of residual urine. If the urine specimen collected half an hour after the intravenous injection contains 50% or more of the dye, renal function is good and, if the urine volume is small (eg, 25-50 ml), there can be no significant residual urine. The test can therefore be stopped at that point, for nothing further can be learned from a second specimen. If the first specimen does not contain the normal amount of dye, a second specimen should be collected at the end of the second half-hour.

The presence of residual urine (vesical or bilateral ureterorenal) is suggested if a "flat" or "uphill" curve is obtained in association with (1) a fairly good total PSP in 1 hour, (2) a morning specific gravity of 1.024 or better, or (3) a normal serum creatinine. With increasing degrees of renal damage and in the absence of residual urine, the following PSP curves are to be expected in one hour: 40%—15%, 30%—10%, and 20%—10%. Even poorly functioning kidneys do not produce an "uphill" curve since 70% of the dye is cleared the first time around. When damage is severe, the total PSP is low and the curve "flat" (10%—10%, 5—5%, Trace—Trace).

The examples of PSP excretion in Table 5-2 therefore imply the presence of residual urine, for the curves are "flat" or nearly so, or "uphill."

When PSP curves are flat and their totals are low (eg, 20%—15%, 10%—10%, or 5%—5%), a serum creatinine should be obtained. If normal, a PSP of 50%—60% in the first half-hour can be assumed and the calculation of the amount of residual urine made. The same would be true if the specific gravity of the urine were 1.024 or higher. If there is doubt in the physician's mind, immediate catheterization should be performed and the PSP content of the retained urine added to that obtained during the test. This maneuver will show total PSP excretion and give an estimation of residual urine.

The use of the PSP test for estimation of total renal function and of residual urine, if present, makes it one of the most valuable routine office diagnostic procedures. It is a more useful test of renal function than measurement of nitrogen retention. It is inexpensive and affords real information in one-half hour, and it estimates degrees of renal damage before the uremic stage is reached. This test should be a routine laboratory procedure like the complete blood count and urinalysis. Since so many serious renal diseases are silent, the PSP test may occasionally pick up such a case. Many patients in uremia both feel and look well. A PSP of better than 30% in the first half-hour rules out uremia due to renal failure; only when it is 30% or less should tests for nitrogen retention be done.

In unilateral renal disease (eg, hydronephrosis), the specific gravity or concentration tests may show impairment because of the mixing of the urine from the good kidney with that from the diseased. The PSP, however, will usually be normal, because of the compensatory hypertrophy of the good kidney. In this instance, then, the PSP is a more dependable test of total renal function than concentrating power.

The same is true when residual urine is present in the bladder. A dilute urine retained in the bladder will lower the specific gravity of the concentrated fluid which is produced by dehydration, and the inference of renal impairment may be made. The PSP, however, will give a "flat" curve with a fairly normal total (eg, 25%—20%: total, 45%), which suggests the presence of residual urine.

For these reasons, concentration tests should be performed in conjunction with the PSP. This will help to prevent errors which might occur in the interpretation of the concentration test in certain urologic disorders.

Gault & Fox have described the 60-minute plasma PSP concentration as a test of renal function. One mg of PSP/kg body weight is given IV. The residual plasma level at 1 hour is estimated. A high level implies impaired renal function. This method is of value if the urine is bloody, but in other circumstances the routine PSP test or determination of the BUN and creatinine levels seems simpler.

Endogenous Creatinine Clearance

Although creatinine is filtered through the glomerulus and PSP is excreted by the tubules, these tests tend to parallel each other because most renal diseases involve both renal elements (Table 5-3). Thus, the creatinine clearance is roughly equal to twice the excretion of PSP in the first half-hour. The clearance of endogenous creatinine approximates the glomerular filtration rate (GFR) as measured by inulin. The normal values vary between 72-140 ml/min.

Blood Nitrogen Levels

In the face of bilateral ureteral or bladder neck obstruction, bilateral vesicoureteral reflux, shock, or heart failure, the flow of urine down the tubules is slowed. This allows over-reabsorption of urea nitrogen; creatinine is not so affected. Such a phenomenon is compatible with the counter-current theory of renal function. When the urinary tract is normal and unobstructed, the plasma urea-creatinine ratio is 10:1. When there is significant bilateral urinary stasis or diminished renal blood flow, the urea-creatinine ratio rises to 20-30:1. A similar pattern is seen when there is extravasation of urine into the peritoneal cavity. Thus, the combination of both serum BUN and creatinine determinations is of considerable diagnostic importance as a screening test.

In the adult the upper limits of normal are creatinine, 1.4 mg/100 ml; BUN, 15 mg/100 ml; and NPN, 35 mg/100 ml. Up to age 5 the normal creatinine is 0.8 mg/100 ml; BUN, 8 mg/100 ml; and NPN, 20 mg/100 ml.

Young children with advanced bilateral hydronephrosis may have a fixed specific gravity of 1.006 with a trace of protein and yet have a serum creatinine level within the normal range. A "diaper" PSP test will reveal the renal damage or suggest residual urine.

Serum Electrolytes   (See Inside back cover.)

The estimation of the concentration of serum electrolytes is important in patients with suspected fluid-ion imbalance or oliguria, hyperparathyroidism, hyperaldosteronism, and chronic renal failure.

Urine Chloride Concentration (Bedside Test of Scribner)

One of the prime functions of the kidneys is the regulation of body sodium chloride in relation to body water. In the face of sodium chloride excess, the kidneys can excrete up to 375 mEq/L of salt. With sodium chloride deprivation, normal kidneys can so efficiently withhold salt that its concentration in the urine falls to zero. As renal function fails, the specific gravity becomes fixed at 1.006-1.010 (stage of uremia); with further damage, the PSP excretion finally falls to a trace. The last measurable function that the kidneys lose

Table 5-3. Correlation of PSP test, serum creatinine, and creatinine clearance (no residual urine).

One-half Hour PSP	Specific Gravity	Serum Creatinine (mg/100 ml)	Creatinine Clearance (ml/min)
50 and higher	1015-1040	to 1.4 (normal)	100 and higher
30	1.010	1.7	60
20	1.010	2.0	40
10	1.010	2.4	20
5	1.010	3.4	10
0	1.010	4.0 and higher	5 or less

is sodium chloride regulation. In lower nephron nephrosis (acute tubular necrosis) the chloride concentration becomes fixed at 30-40 mEq/L. The only exception to this rule is the relatively rare incomplete tubular lesion in which the chloride concentration may be fixed at a point between 20-100 mEq/L.

It is obvious, then, that the estimation of the urine chloride is helpful in the treatment of fluid and electrolyte derangements and in the estimate of renal function. A urine chloride of 250 mEq/L implies good renal tubular function and sodium chloride excess. Similarly, a concentration of 1-2 mEq/L of chloride also implies adequate tubular function but sodium chloride depletion or retention (eg, heart failure).

When specific gravity becomes fixed, those mechanisms having to do with ammonia and bicarbonate substitution are sharply limited. Under these circumstances, the urine sodium concentration tends to equal the level of chloride in the urine unless the patient is receiving excess base (sodium lactate or bicarbonate).

Barsocchini, L. M., & D. R. Smith: Diaper phenolsulfonphthalein test in the newborn infant. J Urol 91:195-7, 1964.

Berliner, R. W., & C. M. Bennett: Concentration of urine in the mammalian kidney. Am J Med 42:777-89, 1967.

Dossetor, J. B.: Creatininemia versus uremia. The relative significance of blood urea nitrogen and serum creatinine concentrations in azotemia. Ann Int Med 65:1287-99, 1966.

Galambos, J. T., Herndon, E. G., Jr., & G. H. Reynolds: Specific-gravity determination, fact or fancy. New England J Med 270:506-8, 1964.

Gault, M. H., & I. Fox: The sixty-minute plasma phenolsulfonphthalein concentration as a test of renal function. Am J Clin Path 52:345-50, 1969.

Harrow, B. R., Sloane, J. A., & L. Salhanick: Clinical evaluation of renal function tests. J Urol 87:527-34, 1962.

Harrow, B. R., & J. A. Sloane: Value of concentration test in determining renal function. Postgrad Med 37:A48-55, 1965.

Lyon, R. P.: Hypogravic urine with uremia and normotension. J Urol 82:558-61, 1959.

Lyon, R. P.: Measurement of urine chloride as a test of renal function. J Urol 85:884-8, 1961.

Marshall, S.: A test of renal function: Excretion of contrast medium as measured by urinary specific gravity. Brit J Urol 36:519-23, 1964.

Newcombe, D. S., & A. S. Cohen: Uricosuric agents and phenolsulfonphthalein excretion. Arch Int Med 112:738-41, 1963.

Richardson, J. A., & P. E. Philbin: The one-hour creatinine clearance rate in healthy men. JAMA 216:987-90, 1971.

Scribner, B. H.: Bedside determination of chloride. Proc Staff Meet Mayo Clin 25:209-18, 1950.

Smith, D. R.: Estimation of the amount of residual urine by means of the phenosulfonphthalein test. J Urol 83:188-91, 1960.

Tjan, H. L., & others: Creatinine clearance in clinical medicine. California Med 98:121-8, 1963.

Undeman, R. D., VanBuren, H. C., & L. G. Raisz: Osmolar renal concentrating ability in healthy young men and hospitalized patients without renal disease. New England J Med 262:1306-9, 1960.

Young, J. D., Jr., de Mendonca, P. P., & D. Bendhack: A comparison of phenolsulfonphthalein excretion with the renal clearance of creatinine and PAH. Ann Surg 169:724-6, 1969.

•   •   •

6...

Diagnosis of Medical Renal Diseases

Marcus A. Krupp, MD*

The medical renal diseases are those that involve principally the parenchyma of the kidneys. Many of the symptoms and signs of urinary tract disease are common to both "medical" and "surgical" diseases of the kidneys and other urologic organs. Hematuria, proteinuria, pyuria, oliguria, polyuria, pain, renal insufficiency with azotemia, acidosis, anemia, electrolyte abnormalities, hypertension, headache, and ocular involvement may occur in a wide variety of disorders affecting any portion of the parenchyma of the kidney, its blood vessels, or the excretory tract.

Every effort must be made to rule out non-surgical disease of the urinary tract before resorting to diagnostic or therapeutic procedures which may prove to be unnecessary or dangerous.

A complete medical history and physical examination, a thorough examination of the urine, and blood chemistry examinations as indicated are essential initial steps in the work-up of any patient.

History

A. Family History: The family history may reveal disease of genetic origin, eg, tubular metabolic anomalies, polycystic kidneys, unusual types of nephritis, or vascular or coagulation defects which may be essential clues to the diagnosis.

B. Past History: The past history should cover infections, injuries, and exposure to toxic agents, anticoagulants or drugs which may produce toxic or sensitivity reactions, including blood dyscrasias. A history of diabetes, hypertensive disease, and collagen disease may be obtained. The inquiry must also be calculated to elicit symptoms of uremia, debilitation, and the vascular complications of chronic renal disease.

Physical Examination

One must look for such physical signs as pallor, edema, hypertension, retinopathy, and the stigmas of congenital disease (eg, enlarged kidneys with polycystic disease).

Urinalysis

Examination of the urine (see p 46) is the most essential single part of the investigation.

A. Proteinuria of any significant degree (++ to ++++) is suggestive of "medical" renal disease (parenchymal involvement). Proteinuria should be interpreted with consideration of the urine specific gravity, since a proteinuria of + in a dilute urine may indicate a significantly great protein loss. Formed elements present in the urine usually establish the diagnosis. Only after careful examination of the patient and suitable urine specimens, as well as analysis of the chemical constituents of the blood, is urography or cystoscopy justified.

1. "Pathologic" proteinurias - Significant proteinuria is present in glomerulonephritis, subacute or chronic nephritis, nephrotic syndrome, collagen disease, diabetic nephropathy, myeloma of the kidney, and polycystic kidney disease.

2. "Nonpathologic" proteinurias - When investigating causes one must be careful not to overlook mild cases of glomerulonephritis or other parenchymal disease.

a. "Physiologic" proteinuria - After vigorous exercise or protracted physical effort, protein, erythrocytes, casts, and tubule cells may appear transiently in the urine. Repeat examination of the urine after a period of rest usually resolves the problem.

b. Orthostatic proteinuria - Some persons have proteinuria when they are up and about, but not while recumbent. In any patient with proteinuria, the degree of proteinuria is always more pronounced when the patient is upright, and especially when he is active. Absence of proteinuria when the patient is supine during the period of urine formation confirms the diagnosis of orthostatic proteinuria.

---

*Clinical Professor of Medicine, Stanford University School of Medicine, Stanford, California; Director, Palo Alto Medical Research Foundation, Palo Alto, California.

B. Red Cell Casts: Although red cells in
the urine indicate extravasation of blood anywhere along the urinary tract, the occurrence
of red cells in casts proves the renal origin
of the bleeding. The erythrocytes forming
typical red cell casts are from the glomeruli
or the upper portions of the nephron.

C. Fatty casts and oval fat bodies (tubule
cells showing fatty changes) occur in degenerative diseases of the kidney (nephrosis, glomerulonephritis, collagen disease, amyloidosis,
and damage due to such toxins as mercury).

D. Other Findings: The presence of abnormal urinary chemical constituents indicative of
metabolic disorders involving the kidneys may
be the only evidence of such disease. These
include diabetes mellitus, renal glycosuria,
aminoacidurias (including cystinuria), oxaluria,
gout, hyperparathyroidism, hemoglobinuria,
and myoglobinuria.

Brody, L.H., & others: Urinalysis and the
urinary sediment. M Clin North America
55:243-66, 1971.
Lippman, R.W.: Urine and the Urinary Sediment; a Practical Manual and Atlas, 2nd ed.
Thomas, 1957.

GLOMERULONEPHRITIS

Following streptococcal infections (especially with type 12 hemolytic streptococci and
a few other strains), an autoimmune reaction
involving the kidney may occur. Evidence of
the renal lesion usually appears a few weeks
after the infection. Typical findings in the
acute stage are oliguria, hematuria, proteinuria, and evidence in the urine sediment of
glomerulitis (red cell casts) and of general
parenchymal involvement (tubule cells, leukocytes, and hyaline and granular casts). Headache, moderate edema, hypertension, and
mild azotemia are usually present. After the
acute phase has passed, a prolonged latent or
subclinical stage may be evidenced only by the
findings in the urine of protein, increased
numbers of erythrocytes and leukocytes, and
tubule epithelial cells and casts, some containing red cells and epithelial cells. The
degenerative or nephrotic stage is indistinguishable from other forms of the nephrotic
syndrome. The terminal stage is that of renal
insufficiency, in which traces of the latent or
nephrotic urine findings may still exist.

RENAL INVOLVEMENT
IN COLLAGEN DISEASES

The collagen diseases frequently produce
symptoms and signs of renal disease indistinguishable from acute or chronic glomerulonephritis, nephrosis, renal vein thrombosis,
and renal infarction. Although it may not be
accurate to classify all of these disorders as
collagen diseases, acute disseminated lupus
erythematosus, polyarteritis nodosa, sclero-
derma, dermatomyositis, and thrombotic
thrombocytopenic purpura have been implicated in producing a syndrome resembling glomerulonephritis. In about $1/3$ to $1/2$ of cases, the
urine sediment is diagnostic, containing red
blood cells and red blood cell casts; renal
tubule cells, including some filled with fat
droplets; and waxy and granular broad casts.
The presence of these formed elements is
indicative of active glomerular and tubular
disease with extensive focal destruction of
nephrons. The symptoms and signs of the
primary disease help to differentiate the form
of collagen disease present. When collagen
disease involves the kidneys, complete recovery or successful long-term amelioration of
the disease is not likely to occur.

NEPHROTIC SYNDROME

The nephrotic syndrome is characterized
by massive pitting edema, massive proteinuria, hypoalbuminemia, hypercholesterolemia,
and formed elements in the urine (fatty tubule
cells, fatty and waxy casts, and often red
cells). Azotemia is usually not marked.

Most cases of the nephrotic syndrome are
idiopathic and are associated with glomerular
lesions. The most common lesion is characterized by thickening of the basement membrane and distortion and fusion of the epithelial cell foot processes. Less commonly, the
glomeruli show proliferation of epithelial cells
and formation of crescents in Bowman's capsule.

The nephrotic syndrome may also appear
in the course of glomerulonephritis, collagen
disease involving the kidney (especially lupus
erythematosus), amyloidosis, following renal
vein thrombosis, following exposure to a specific allergen (eg, poison oak, bee venom),
or as a result of drug toxicity (eg, trimetha-
dione, mercury compounds).

Table 6-1. Common patterns of abnormal urine composition in disease.*

Disease	Specific Gravity	Protein†	Red Cells†	Casts†	Microscopic (Casts and Cells) and Other Findings
Normal	1.003-1.030	0 to trace (0-0.05 gm)	0 to occ	0 to occ	Hyaline casts (urine must be acid and fresh or preserved).
Diseases with high fevers	Increased	Trace or +	0	0 to few	Hyaline casts, tubule cells.
Congestive heart failure	High; varies with renal function.	1-2+	0 to +	+	Hyaline and granular casts.
Eclampsia	Increased	3-4+	0 to +	3-4+	Hyaline casts.
Diabetic coma	High	+	0	0 to +	Hyaline casts, glucose, ketone bodies.
Acute glomerulo-nephritis‡	Increased	2-4+	1-4+	2-4+	Blood, cellular, granular, hyaline casts; renal tubule epithelium.
Degenerative phase glomerulo-nephritis	Normal or increased	4+	1-2+	4+	Granular, waxy, hyaline, fatty casts; fatty tubule cells.
Terminal phase glomerulo-nephritis	Low, fixed	1-2+	Trace to +	1-3+	Granular, hyaline, fatty, broad casts.
Lipoid nephrosis	Very high	4+	0 to trace	4+	Hyaline, granular, fatty, waxy casts; fatty tubule cells.
Collagen diseases	Normal or decreased	1-4+	1-4+	1-4+	Blood, cellular, granular, hyaline, waxy, fatty, broad casts; fatty tubule cells.
Pyelonephritis	Normal or decreased	0 to +	0 to +	0 to +	Leukocyte and hyaline casts, pus cells, bacteria.
Benign hyper-tension (late)	Normal or low	0 to +	0 to trace	0 to +	Hyaline and granular casts.
Malignant hyper-tension	Low, fixed	1-2+	Trace to +	1-2+	Hyaline and granular casts.

*Modified from Krupp & others: Physician's Handbook, 16th ed. Lange, 1970.
†Quantities expressed in scale of 0-4+.
‡May be anuric, or have low, fixed specific gravity.

INTERCAPILLARY GLOMERULOSCLEROSIS

A complication of diabetes mellitus, this syndrome may resemble nephrosis or may appear as renal insufficiency. Urinalysis reveals proteinuria and the presence of formed elements, including hyaline and waxy casts, red cells, and tubule cells, some of which contain fatty droplets. Glycosuria may or may not be present when the blood glucose is elevated. Diabetic retinopathy is frequently present.

CYSTIC DISEASES OF THE KIDNEYS

Congenital structural anomalies of the kidney must always be considered in any patient with hypertension, pyelonephritis, or renal insufficiency.

Polycystic disease is familial and usually becomes manifest in early adult life. Hematuria, urinary tract infection, flank pain, and renal insufficiency with hypertension constitute the usual manifestations of the disease. Urography reveals the typical stretched calyceal system and renal enlargement (see p 334).

Cystic diseases of the renal medulla have been recognized with increasing frequency. Medullary cystic disease is familial and usually becomes symptomatic during adolescence with anemia, azotemia, acidosis, and hyperphosphatemia. Hypertension may occur. Another type of medullary cystic disease is sponge kidney. The disease is asymptomatic and is identified by the characteristic appearance of the urogram, which shows enlargement of the papillae and calyces and small cavities within the pyramids (see p 347).

METABOLIC RENAL DISEASES

In all cases of renal calculus and renal calcinosis, a careful search must be conducted for general metabolic disease.

CHRONIC RENAL INSUFFICIENCY

In addition to the disorders listed above, other relatively common diseases may present with renal insufficiency.

Essential Hypertension

Essential hypertension, especially "malignant hypertension," may produce arterial and arteriolar changes in the kidneys resulting in uremia. The terminal state is often indistinguishable from other causes of uremia, and the urine often contains moderate amounts of protein, red blood cells, epithelial and white cells, and casts (including broad and waxy casts). Even at postmortem examination, the kidney may be so damaged that the true nature of the disease cannot be determined.

Chronic Pyelonephritis

Chronic pyelonephritis may destroy so much of the kidney substance that all of the classical signs of renal insufficiency are present, which makes it extremely difficult to differentiate this disorder from other causes of advanced or terminal renal disease. The urine is often sterile at this stage of the disease; repeated cultures must be made to rule out infection. The urine may contain protein and formed elements present in other diseases producing renal failure. A recent or remote past history of urinary tract infection may be the only clue to the bacterial origin of the renal disease, but such a history is often lacking.

Multiple Myeloma

Multiple myeloma may first produce signs of renal failure because of extensive interstitial nephritis or because of amyloidosis. Other signs of myeloma establish the diagnosis: bone changes, anemia, hyperproteinemia (M protein occurring in the beta or gamma fractions), characteristic plasma cell displacement of the bone marrow, and Bence Jones protein in the urine. Bone pain and pathologic fractures often are present.

Caution: Excretory urograms are contraindicated in the presence of this disease; a number of deaths have been reported.

Analgesic Nephropathy

Associated with long term ingestion of phenacetin alone or in analgesic mixtures, serious damage to the kidney may occur with resultant renal insufficiency. Peritubular and perivascular inflammation accompany degenerative changes in tubule cells. Renal papillary necrosis extending into the medulla may involve many papillae. Hematuria, polyuria, renal colic, and evidence of renal insufficiency are common manifestations. Urograms show typical cavities and ring shadows of areas of destruction of papillae (see p 156).

•　　•　　•

General References

Black, D. A. K. (editor): Renal Disease, 2nd ed. Oxford Univ Press, 1967.

Bricker, N. S., & others: Renal function in chronic renal disease. Medicine **44**:263-88, 1965.

De Wardener, H. E.: The Kidney: An Outline of Normal and Abnormal Structure and Function. Little, Brown, 1961.

Earley, L. E., & others: Nephrotic syndrome. California Med **115**:23-41, Nov 1971. (Editorial by A. S. Relman: The nephrotic syndrome. California Med **115**:58-61, Dec 1971.)

Forster, R. P.: Kidney, water, and electrolytes. Ann Rev Physiol **27**:183-232, 1965.

Krupp, M. A.: Genitourinary Tract. Pp 477-504 in: Current Diagnosis & Treatment, 1972. Lange, 1972.

Lindheimer, M. D., & others: The kidney in pregnancy. New England J Med **283**:1095-7, 1970.

Milne, M. D. (editor): Management of renal failure. Brit M Bull 27:95-185, 1971.

Pitts, R. F.: Physiology of the Kidney and Body Fluids, 2nd ed. Year Book, 1968.

Smith, H. W.: The Kidney: Structure and Function in Health and Disease. Oxford Univ Press, 1952.

Strauss, M. B., & G. Welt (editors): Diseases of the Kidney, 2nd ed. Little, Brown, 1971.

Symposium on diseases of the kidney. M Clin North America 55:1-266, 1971.

Symposium on glomerulonephritis. Bull New York Acad Med 46:747-888, 1970.

Symposium on uremic toxins. Arch Int Med 126:773-910, 1970.

7...
Roentgenographic Examination of the Urinary Tract

PLAIN FILM OF ABDOMEN

A plain film of the abdomen, also called a KUB (kidney, ureter, and bladder), is a helpful step in the presumptive diagnosis of genitourinary disease (Figs 7-1 and 7-2). Since gastrointestinal and urologic diseases tend to mimic each other, it may be helpful in differential diagnosis as well.

Renal Shadows
A. Kidney Size: A plain film of the abdomen will usually show the renal outlines. They may be obscured, however, by bowel content, lack of perinephric fat, or a perinephric hematoma or abscess, which typically obliterates the renal shadow. This difficulty, however, may be overcome by tomography. Congenital absence of a kidney may be suggested. If both kidneys are unusually large, polycystic kidney disease, multiple myeloma, lymphoma, amyloid disease, or hydronephrosis may be present. If both are small, the end stage of glomerulonephritis or bilateral atrophic pyelonephritis must be considered. Unilateral enlargement should suggest renal tumor, cyst, or hydronephrosis, whereas a small kidney on one side is compatible with congenital hypoplasia, atrophic pyelonephritis, or an ischemic kidney. Normally, the left kidney is 0.5 cm longer than its mate. Discrepancy in the relative size of one kidney may imply renal ischemia.

B. Position: In 90% of cases, the right kidney is lower than the left, because of displacement by the liver. If a kidney appears to be abnormally displaced, a retroperitoneal tumor should be suspected (eg, adrenal tumor, pancreatic pseudocyst).

The axes of the kidneys are oblique to the spine; their lower poles are farther apart than their upper poles because they lie along the borders of the psoas muscles. If their axes are parallel to the spine (which means that the lower ends of the kidneys are lying on the psoas muscles), the possibility of "horseshoe" kidney should be considered.

C. Shape: The shape of the kidney should be studied. A lobulated edge might suggest polycystic kidney disease. An expansion of one pole of a kidney is compatible with tumor, cyst, or carbuncle.

Calcification
Because a plain film of the abdomen is 2-dimensional, it is practically impossible to make a positive diagnosis of stone in the urinary tract except in the instance of a staghorn calculus, which forms a perfect cast of the pelvis and calyces, thereby simulating a urogram. All one can usually say from study of a plain film is that there are opaque bodies in the region of the adrenal, kidney, ureter, bladder, or prostate. Oblique and lateral films, as well as visualization of the urinary tract with radiopaque fluids, are necessary in order to actually place the calcification in the respective organs.

Punctate calcification in the adrenals suggests tuberculous involvement (Fig 13-2) or neuroblastoma (Fig 20-3). Adrenal calcification follows spontaneous hemorrhage into the gland (Fig 7-14). Numerous small calcific bodies in the parenchyma of a kidney may suggest tuberculosis or medullary sponge kidney (Fig 21-9), although nephrocalcinosis (Fig 15-12) caused by primary or secondary hyperparathyroidism or hypercalciuria should be considered. About 7% of malignant renal tumors contain some calcification. Calcifications in the veins in the perivesical area (phleboliths) may simulate stone in the ureter, but as a rule they are perfectly round, often laminated and contain radiolucent centers. Calcified mesenteric lymph nodes may also resemble stone. Linear calcification lying to the left of the lumbar spine is compatible with aneurysm of the abdominal aorta. An aneurysm of the right renal artery (Fig 21-11) may be confused with a gallstone. Calcifications at the junction of the hypogastric and iliac arteries are often seen just below the sacroiliac joints and may therefore be confused with ureteral stones. A stone in the appendix may occasionally be confused with stone in the ureter. Radiopaque gallstones may overlie the kidney, but an oblique or lateral film will

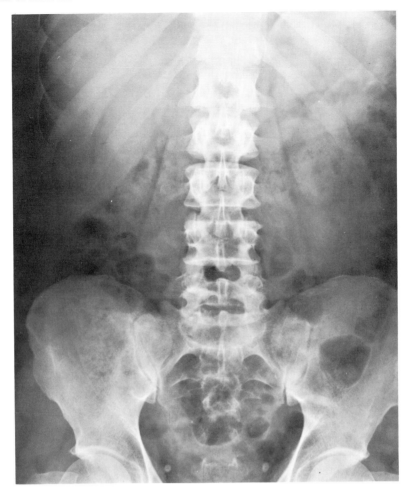

Fig 7-1. Normal plain film of abdomen. Bones are normal, psoas shadows well demarcated, renal shadows normal. The bladder contains some urine. Two phleboliths are seen in the region of the lower ureters and bladder.

demonstrate that the opacity is anterior to the kidney. Uterine fibroids and, occasionally, diseased ovaries may undergo pathologic calcification. Moles on the skin and swallowed pills or foreign bodies may be radiopaque. The wall of an adrenal or renal cyst may contain calcium.

Psoas Shadows

The psoas muscles usually stand out sharply. If one is obliterated and the kidney shadow on that side is absent, and if there is scoliosis of the spine with its concavity on the side of the defect, perinephric or paranephric abscess or hematoma is a possibility.

Bone Shadows

Survey of the bones may reveal arthritic change, which may suggest that what was thought to be kidney pain is really caused by

radiculitis. Gross spina bifida may be noted; the sacrum may be absent. Such findings would suggest the presence of neurogenic bladder (Fig 7-17). Metastases should also be sought. If osteoblastic, they almost certainly arise from the prostate; if osteolytic, the common primary sites are in the breast, thyroid, lung, and kidney.

Gastrointestinal Shadows

A plain film, by demonstrating gas in the small bowel, may lead to the diagnosis of bowel obstruction, although the initial impression may have been disease of the urinary tract. Gas under the diaphragm with the patient in an upright posture makes the diagnosis of a ruptured viscus (eg, perforated peptic ulcer). A large renal mass may displace all intestinal gas from that area (Fig 7-2).

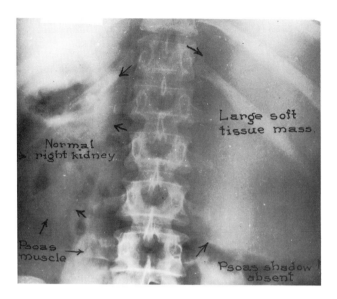

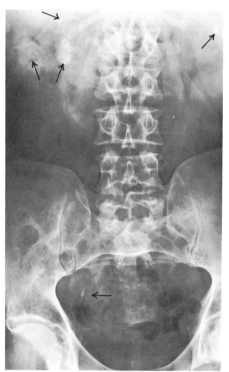

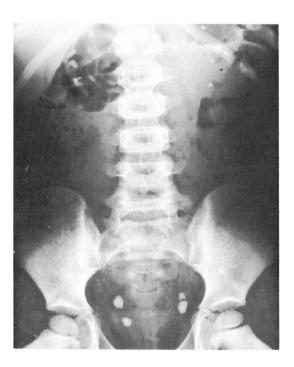

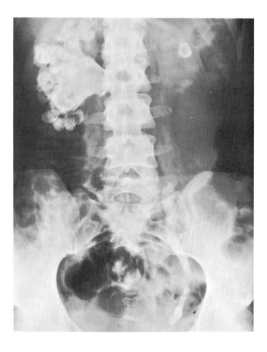

Fig 7-2. **Abnormal plain films of the abdomen. Above left:** Large soft tissue mass in left upper abdomen (simple cyst of kidney). Absence of intestinal gas (displacement of bowel) over mass (see Fig 7-17, below left and right, same patient). **Above right:** Calcification in small function-less right kidney and lower right ureter typical of advanced tuberculosis. **Below left:** Multiple renal and ureteral calcium oxalate stones in 12-year-old boy suffering from hyperoxaluria. **Below right:** Large staghorn calculus in right kidney and multiple stones in left kidney and lower half of ureter.

Duggan, H. E.: The radiological interpretation of the scout film in the acute abdomen.
S Clin North America 40:1221-40, 1960.

Elkin, M., & G. Cohen: Diagnostic value of
the psoas shadow. Clin Radiol 13:210-7,
1962.

Jafee, R.: Anterior sacral meningocele.
Obst Gynec 28:684-8, 1966.

McAfee, J. G., & M. W. Donner: Differential
diagnosis of calcifications encountered in
abnormal radiographs. Am J M Sc 243:
609-50, 1962.

Mogg, R. A.: Urinary tract displacements.
Brit J Urol 32:472-83, 1960.

Olurin, E. O., & O. Olurin: Pancreatic calcification: A report of 45 cases. Brit MJ 4:
534-9, 1969.

Salik, J. O., & B. S. Abeshouse. Calcification,
ossification and cartilage formation in the
kidney. Am J Roentgenol 88:125-43, 1962.

Stevenson, J., MacGregor, A. M., & P. Con-
nelly: Calcification of the adrenal glands
in young children. Arch Dis Childhood 36:
316-20, 1961.

EXCRETORY UROGRAMS

During the past few years, improvements
in intravenous radiographic media have been
such that they now often rival retrograde urograms in quality. This very efficiency has
impaired their usefulness as a test of renal
function. Although nausea, vomiting, and pain
in the arm are occasionally experienced after
intravenous injection of radiopaque material,
these reactions are usually less disturbing to
the patient than the sequelae of retrograde
urography (nausea and vomiting, abdominal
and renal pain). Rare allergic reactions (eg,
urticaria, asthma, shock) following intravenous
infusion of these iodized substances are apparently usually aborted by the addition of an antihistamine to the radiopaque fluid.

Excretory urograms illustrate the urinary
excretory tract in the most physiologic manner.
The renal pelves and calyces are not distorted
by the overdistention which may be produced
with retrograde filling.

The cystogram which is obtained on the
later films may reveal trabeculation, diverticula, or a space-occupying lesion. A post-
voiding film may demonstrate residual urine
in the bladder.

Note: For 1-2 hours after injection of the
radiopaque medium, the normal specific gravity of the urine is 1.040-1.060. Under these
circumstances, a specific gravity of 1.020 or
less indicates that renal function is severely
impaired.

Indications

Excretory urograms are indicated when
disease of the urinary tract is suspected. Diseases which should be investigated by this
means include cysts and tumors of the kidney
(space-occupying lesions), tuberculosis of the
kidney (ulceration of calyces), pyelonephritis,
hydronephrosis, vesicoureteral reflux, hypertension, and stone in the urinary tract.

Excretory urograms may also be of value
in patients suffering from gastrointestinal
complaints in whom no organic disease of the
gastrointestinal tract can be demonstrated.
A urologic cause for the symptoms may be
shown.

Because the radiographic fluid increases
the density of the kidneys to x-rays, the size
of the kidneys and their outlines become clearer. This is an advantage when evidence of expansion of the renal parenchyma (eg, tumor)
or change in size of the kidney is sought.

If renal injury is suspected, excretory urograms should be obtained as soon as practicable (primarily to make certain that the unin-
jured contralateral kidney is normal). This is
invaluable information if emergency removal
of the injured kidney becomes imperative as a
life-saving measure.

Excretory urograms are indispensable in
infants, particularly male infants, where cystoscopy may be unduly traumatic. During the
first month of life, delayed concentration and
prolonged excretion of urographic contrast
medium is observed. In this age group, the
usual early films should be deleted and late
films (1-2 hours) taken.

Contraindications

Excretory urograms are contraindicated if
there is evidence of hypersensitivity: history
of allergic reactions to previous intravenous
urography, iodine sensitivity, or other allergic
manifestations such as hives or asthma. Although the routine addition of an antihistamine
to the contrast medium may reduce the incidence of allergic reactions, it would be unwise
to depend upon this precaution if the patient
has manifested hypersensitivity in the past.
Excretory radiopaque material may be lethal
in patients with multiple myeloma. This risk
is markedly lessened if the patient is well hydrated beforehand. Preliminary dehydration
in patients suspected of or having primary hyperparathyroidism may precipitate irreversible
hypercalcemia. Fortunately, fairly good urograms can be obtained in association with normal fluid intake, particularly if the dose of the
opaque medium is increased.

If the PSP test is less than 30% in 1 hour
or if blood nitrogen retention is demonstrated,
it will be necessary to administer a larger
dose of radiopaque fluid (eg, double the usual
dose or use a 90% concentration of the medium)

or to perform infusion urography. Adequate films may thus be obtained when the BUN is as high as 100 mg/100 ml.

Technic

A. Preparation of the Patient: No food or fluids should be taken for at least 6 hours before the procedure is scheduled. A cathartic (eg, castor oil) taken the night before will decrease the amount of gas and fecal material in the bowel, thus ensuring clearer delineation of the urinary tract. An enema is less effective. If urgent urograms are desired and the patient is hydrated, satisfactory films are still obtainable. A 3-minute film should be added to the series, since the radiopaque material under these circumstances is excreted more promptly. A double dose of the iodide will further enhance the quality of the films.

B. Procedure:

1. Preliminary plain film - This must be taken not only to check on the quality of the radiographic technic and the position of the patient, but also to demonstrate urinary stones which might be obscured by the radiopaque medium.

2. Injection of the radiopaque fluid - The amount of fluid which should be injected varies with the type of fluid and the age of the patient. (Follow the manufacturer's directions.) One of the antihistamines should be added to the infusion material.

a. Intravenous injection - This is the method of choice if venipuncture is feasible. Since allergic reactions may occur and death may ensue (rarely), preliminary tests for hypersensitivity should be performed. If one or more tests are positive, this examination should not be done. Unfortunately, none of these tests guarantees complete safety, although the intravenous test is more reliable than the ocular or subcutaneous test.

(1) Tests for sensitivity -

(a) Ocular test - One drop of the contrast medium is instilled into the eye. If erythema is produced, the test is positive.

(b) Subcutaneous test - Inject 0.1 ml subcut. If induration and erythema develop promptly, the test is positive.

(c) Intravenous test - Inject 1 ml of the medium IV. If no signs of hypersensitivity (eg, urticaria, asthma) are observed, the test is negative.

(2) If symptoms and signs of hypersensitivity are manifested by the patient during the injection, it should be stopped immediately. Warning signs of allergic reaction include respiratory difficulty; sneezing, itching, or urticaria; nausea and vomiting; and fainting. Treatment consists of oxygen for anoxia; hypertensive drugs and intravenous dextrose solutions for shock; intravenous barbiturates for convulsions; and the intravenous injection of an antihistamine if allergic reactions are observed.

b. Extravascular infusion - This procedure is indicated if venipuncture is impossible (eg, in the infant). (See manufacturer's directions for dosage.) The ocular and intradermal tests should be performed first. If sensitivity is demonstrated by these tests, the infusion should be withheld. The ampule of radiopaque medium (to which an antihistamine has been added) is diluted to 100 ml with normal saline solution. Equal parts of the solution are given subcutaneously over the scapular areas. Excretion is maximum on the 30-60 minute films.

3. Routine urograms - Radiograms are usually taken 5, 10, and 15 minutes after the injection with the patient in the supine position. Films taken 2 and 3 minutes after the beginning of the injection (minute sequence) should be routine in all patients who are hypertensive, for these radiograms, by revealing delayed concentration of the dye in one kidney, may suggest decreased renal function and blood flow. At 25 minutes, a film is also taken with the patient erect in order to demonstrate the mobility of the kidneys, to obtain ureterograms, and to observe the efficiency with which the renal pelves and ureters drain. All films taken should include the kidney, ureter, and bladder areas. Subtle changes in the ureters which imply the presence of vesicoureteral reflux may otherwise be missed.

In infants and children the films should be taken at 3, 5, 8, and 12 minutes, for their kidneys excrete the fluid more rapidly than do those of the adult. If the renal areas are obscured by bowel content, the child should be offered 150-240 ml of a carbonated beverage. The resulting gas-filled stomach displaces the bowel and thus improves visualization of the kidneys.

Ureteral compression may be helpful if the first urogram shows poor concentration of the medium. The urine is thus held in the upper urinary tracts, affording enhanced filling. Compression, however, may cause spontaneous extravasation of urine in the region of the pelvis. This is not pathologic.

4. Supplementary urograms - As soon as the routine exposures are taken and developed, they should be viewed. Oblique or lateral films may then be indicated in order to localize calcific bodies more accurately and to gain a third dimension of the urogram; this may be helpful if calyceal distortion is suspected. Taking films in the prone position, particularly in children, may lead to improved filling of some calyces and the ureter. Troublesome gas shadows may also be displaced.

If excretion of the urographic fluid is delayed, films should be taken periodically for

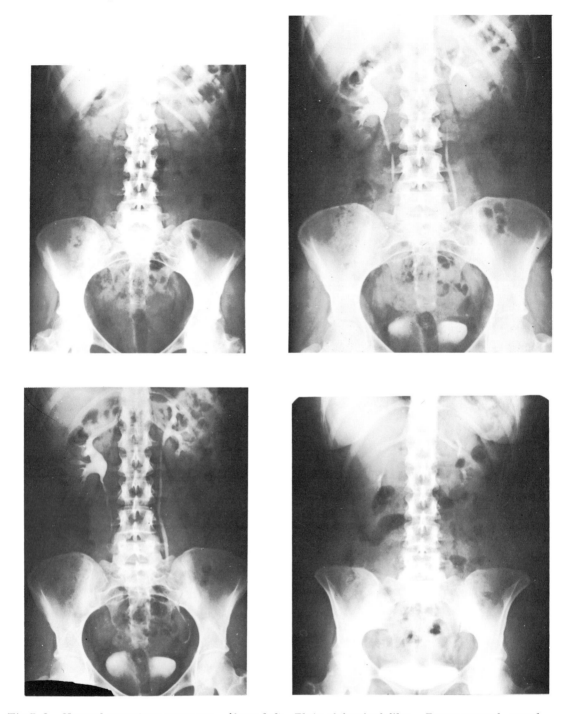

Fig 7-3. Normal excretory urogram. Above left: Plain abdominal film. Bones normal, renal shadows fairly well seen, psoas margins distinct. Black oblong shadow below coccyx is a vaginal menstrual tampon. **Above right:** Five minutes after injection of radiopaque material. Prompt excretion in good concentration. Lower calyces of left kidney indistinct, upper ureters well outlined. Note area of systole in both upper ureters. Some radiopaque material in bladder. **Below left:** Fifteen minute film. Calyces of left kidney now well filled. All calyces are well cupped. Differences in ureteral diameter are caused by systolic contractions. **Below. right:** Twenty-five minute film, upright. Excellent drainage of opaque material. Each kidney drops a distance equal to height of one-half vertebra.

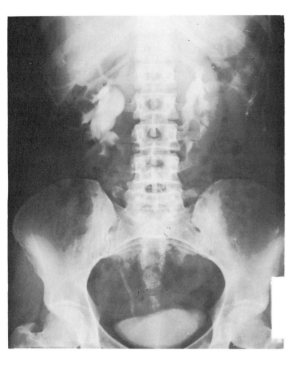
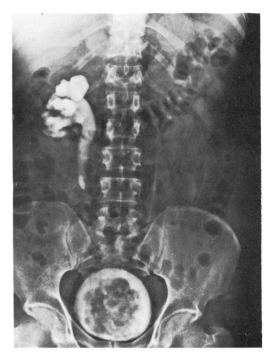
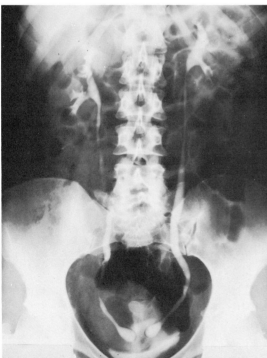
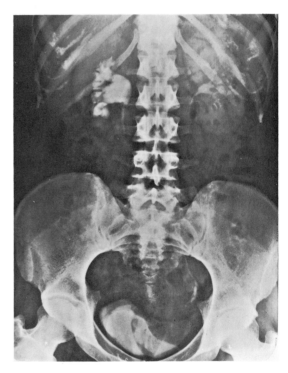

Fig 7-4. **Abnormal excretory urograms. Above left:** Horseshoe kidney. Axes of renal masses vertical, lower calyces on psoas muscles. **Above right:** Right ureteral stone causing hydronephrosis. Large irregular filling defect from unsuspected vesical neoplasm. **Below left:** Bilateral ureteroceles causing a minimum of obstruction. **Below right:** Moderate right hydronephrosis with obstruction at ureteropelvic junction due to aberrant vessel. Compression of left side of bladder from enlarged uterus.

as long as 4 hours or more after the injection. Advanced hydronephrosis and dilated ureters may become apparent only then. It is feasible to inject additional radiopaque medium if there is impaired concentration on the initial films.

5. X-ray of the bladder region after voiding - This should be routine in all urologic patients, no matter what age or sex. At the conclusion of the urographic study, the patient should be instructed to void; a film of the bladder area should be taken immediately. This will demonstrate the presence or absence of residual urine. Partial urinary retention is common but is often not suspected.

Allen, T. D.: Extensive displacement of the kidney by intraperitoneal disease. J Urol 97:823-5, 1967.

Bartley, O., Bengtsson, U., & S. Stattin: Urography in relation to renal function. Acta radiol (diag) 7:289-98, 1968.

Cerny, J. C., Kendall, A. R., & R. M. Nesbit: Subcutaneous pyelography in infants: A reappraisal. J Urol 98:405-9, 1967.

Daughtridge, T. G.: Mucosal folds in the upper urinary tract. Am J Roentgenol 107:743-5, 1969.

Feingold, M., Fine, R. N., & D. Ingall: Intravenous pyelography in infants with single umbilical artery. New England J Med 270: 1178-80, 1964.

Fletcher, E. W. L., & J. W. Lecky: The normal position of the upper ureter in lateral intravenous pyelography. Brit J Urol 41: 554-8, 1969.

Ford, W. H., Jr., & A. J. Palubinskas: Renal extravasation during excretory urography using abdominal compression. J Urol 97: 983-6, 1967.

Friedenberg, R. M., & others: Clinical significance of deviations of the lower ureter. J Urol 96:146-51, 1966.

Fulton, R. E., Witten, D. M., & R. D. Wagoner: Intravenous urography in renal insufficiency. Am J Roentgenol 106:623-34, 1969.

Geraghty, J. A.: An approach to the problem of intestinal gas in diagnostic radiology. Brit J Radiol 39:42-6, 1966.

Gilbert, E. F., & others: Hemorrhagic renal necrosis in infancy: Relationship to radiopaque compounds. J Pediat 76:49-53, 1970.

Gillenwater, J. Y.: Reactions associated with excretory urography: Current concepts. J Urol 106:122-6, 1971.

Lopez, F. A., & others: The nephrogram: A valuable indicator of renal abnormalities. Am J Roentgenol 106:614-22, 1969.

Morgan, C. J., & W. J. Hammack: Intravenous urography in multiple myeloma. New England J Med 275:77-9, 1966.

Nebesar, R. A., Pollard, J. J., & E. E. Fraley: Renal vascular impressions. Incidence and clinical significance. Am J Roentgenol 101: 719, 1967.

Nogrady, M. B., & J. S. Dunbar: Delayed concentration and prolonged excretion of urographic contrast medium in the first month of life. Am J Roentgenol 104:289-95, 1968.

Olsson, O.: Excretion of sodium metrizoate through the liver during urography. Acta radiol (diag) 11:85-90, 1971.

Pendergrass, E. P., & others: Symposium on contrast media reactions. Radiology 91: 61-95, 1968.

Pillay, V. K. G., & others: Acute renal failure following intravenous urography in patients with long-standing diabetes mellitus and azotemia. Radiology 95:633-6, 1970.

Poole, C. A., & M. Viamonte, Jr.: Unusual renal masses in the pediatric age group. Am J Roentgenol 109:368-79, 1970.

Riggs, W., Jr., Hagood, J. H., & A. E. Andrews: Anatomic changes in the normal urinary tract between supine and prone urograms. Radiology 94:107-13, 1970.

Saxton, H. M.: Urography. Brit J Radiol 42: 321-46, 1969.

Schwartz, A., & others: Spontaneous renal extravasation during intravenous urography. Am J Roentgenol 98:27-34, 1966.

Sunder, G. S., & R. D. Gardner: Drip infusion pyelography in patients with renal failure. Brit J Urol 43:540-5, 1971.

Wilson, M. C., & others: Improved excretory urograms by use of second injection of contrast medium. J Urol 87:1010-4, 1962.

INFUSION UROGRAPHY

This technic of excretory urography is indicated in patients suffering from renal insufficiency (BUN up to 100 mg/100 ml) and when maximum detail is required. Preliminary dehydration is unnecessary. One ml/lb of 50% sodium diatrizoate (Hypaque®) is added to a similar amount of normal saline. This is infused through an 18 gauge needle over a period of 5 minutes. Films are exposed at 10, 20, and 30 minutes.

The routine use of this type of urography, particularly in children, should be condemned. Preliminary hydration plus the marked osmotic diuresis stimulated by the larger dose of the radiopaque fluid causes the ureters to be completely full and somewhat dilated, thus simulating the changes compatible with vesicoureteral reflux.

If the patient is being studied for hypertension, exposure should be made at 2, 3, 4, and 5 minutes as well. This procedure also lends itself to the urea washout test, which can be done as the final step.

Duré-Smith, P.: Drip infusion and routine urography: A comparative trial. Brit J Radiol **39**:655-61, 1966.

Evans, A. T., & R. A. Knoblaugh: Routine drip infusion pyelography. Am J Surg **119**: 656-9, 1970.

Schencker, B.: Drip infusion pyelography in diagnosis. Radiology 83:12-21, 1965.

Taylor, D.A., Macken, K.L., & A.S. Fiore: Mannitol pyelography: A simplification of the drip infusion technic. Radiology **88**: 1115-20, 1967.

UREA WASHOUT TEST

Since the basic phenomenon in renal ischemia is the overreabsorption of water by the renal tubules, a hyperconcentration of the radiopaque medium in this kidney should be seen on urography. This change can be accentuated by osmotic diuresis produced by urea.

After preliminary dehydration, (1) infuse 50 ml of sodium diatrizoate (Hypaque®) rapidly through a 16 gauge needle; (2) expose films at 30 seconds and at 2, 3, 5, 8, 15, and 20 minutes; (3) give 40 gm urea and 30 ml of Hypaque® in 500 ml of normal saline in a 15 minute period; and (4) take a film every 3 minutes until one or both kidneys have "washed out" the radiopaque medium. Normally, both are washed out in 15 minutes. If one kidney retains the "dye" 6-9 minutes longer than the other kidney, the test is considered positive for renal ischemia.

Harwood-Nash, D.C.F., & E.L. Lansdown: Evaluation of the urea washout pyelogram and urography in the assessment of renovascular hypertension. Canad MAJ 96:245-56, 1967.

Schreiber, M.H., & others: The normal pyelogram urea washout test. Am J Roentgenol **98**:88-95, 1966.

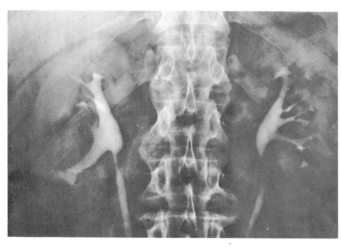

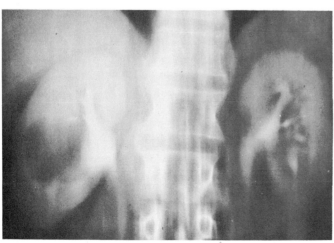

Fig 7-5. Angionephrotomogram. Above: Excretory urogram showing space-occupying lesion in the center of the right kidney; calyces distorted and displaced. **Below:** Nephrotomogram showing lack of opacification of the lesion which, therefore, is a simple cyst. Note the similarity of this urogram to that in Fig 17-3 (bottom right), which proved to be cancer.

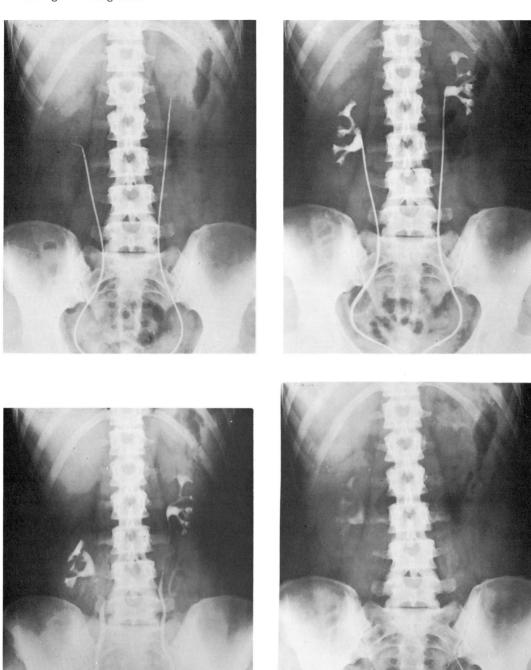

Fig 7-6. Normal retrograde urogram. Above left: Plain abdominal film showing radiopaque ureteral catheters in the renal pelves. Above right: Film taken in the supine position. Calyces are well cupped and there is no dilatation of the pelves. Below left: Urogram taken in the upright position with catheters drawn down into the lower ureters. The right kidney drops the height of $1^1/2$ vertebrae, causing some redundancy of the upper ureter. The left kidney drops the height of one vertebra. Below right: Film taken 15 minutes later, showing almost complete drainage of both kidneys.

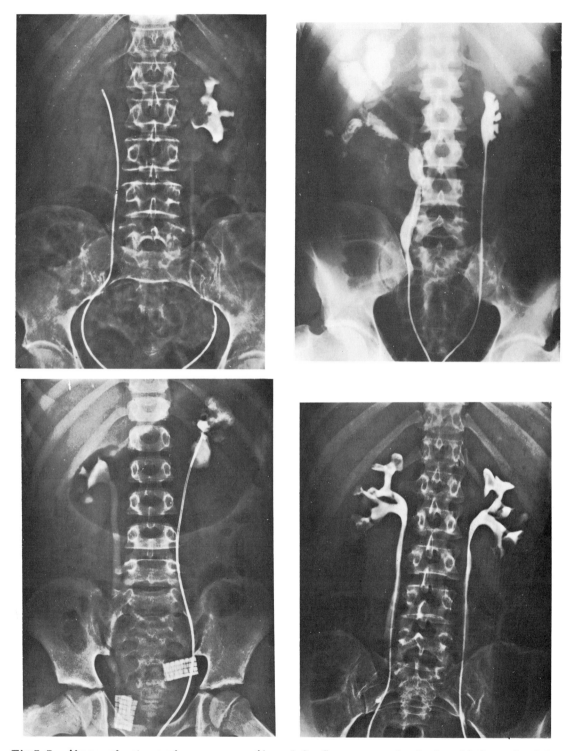

Fig 7-7. **Abnormal retrograde urograms. Above left:** Space-occupying lesion of left renal pelvis. Transitional cell carcinoma. **Above right:** Stones in right renal pelvis and upper ureter; calculus pyonephrosis. Atrophic kidney, left. **Below left:** Bilateral renal tuberculosis. Motheaten appearance of calyces of left kidney, obliteration of upper calyx, and dilated and foreshortened ureter on right. **Below right:** Bilateral papillary necrosis. All papillae have sloughed. Upper medial and lowest calyces on left show ''negative'' shadows representing retained papillae.

72

ANGIONEPHROTOMOGRAMS
(Intravenous Renal Angiograms)

Nephrotomography has its greatest usefulness in the differentiation of renal cyst and
tumor. Briefly, this technic involves the rapid
intravenous injection of a bolus of radiopaque
material which opacifies vascularized tissues
in the kidney. The space occupied by a cyst
or abscess fails to opacify (Fig 7-5); a malignant tumor shows normal or increased opacification because of its increased blood supply
(Fig 17-4). Renal angiography is more efficient in this differential diagnosis.

Technic
A. Preparation of the patient and tests
for sensitivity to the radiographic fluid are
carried out as described for excretory urograms.

B. Radiography: Take a plain film of the
renal areas, and then take test tomograms to
demonstrate the kidneys (usually 8-11 cm from
the table top). Insert a No. 12 needle into one
antecubital vein or one No. 16 needle into each
antecubital vein. Establish the circulation
time by injecting 2.5 ml of 20% sodium dehy-
drocholate (Decholin®) in 10 ml of normal
saline solution. Inject 30 ml of 50% sodium
diatrizoate (Hypaque®) to enhance the nephrogram. Rapidly inject 50 ml of 90% sodium
diatrizoate, take a plain film at the predeter-
mined circulation time, and follow immediately with 4-6 tomograms.

Becker, J.A.: The nonvisualized kidney: The
value of nephrotomography. Radiology 89:
676-81, 1967.
Kittredge, R.D., Kanick, V., & N. Finby:
The value of nephrotomography in the dif-
ferential diagnosis of abdominal masses.
Am J Roentgenol 98:935-47, 1966.
Peterson, C.C., Jr., Jackson, J.H., Jr., &
J.G. Moore: A re-evaluation of nephro-
tomography stressing limitations of the
procedure. J Urol 98:721-7, 1967.
Pfister, R.C., & T.E. Shea: Nephrotomog-
raphy: Performance and interpretation.
Radiol Clin North America 9:41-62, 1971.
Witten, D.W., Greene, L.F., & J.L. Emmett:
An evaluation of nephrotomography in uro-
logic diagnosis. Am J Roentgenol 90:115-
23, 1963.

RETROGRADE UROGRAMS

Only this type of radiography requires
special training in urologic instrumentation.

The indications, contraindications, and technic
of the preliminary cystoscopy and ureteral
catheterization are discussed in chapter 9.

After catheters have been passed to the
renal pelves, a "split" renal function test
(PSP) should be performed and urine specimens
obtained for microscopic examination and culture. Undiluted radiopaque material is then
allowed to flow up the catheters. The average
normal renal pelvis has a capacity of 3-4 ml.
Overdistention causes painful renal pelvic and
ureteral spasms (colic) and capsular (costovertebral) pain. Overfilling may also distort
the urogram; if the pelvis is extrarenal, a
normal pelvis and calyces may appear hydronephrotic (Figs 7-6 and 7-7).

Indications
A. Infection: When upper tract abnormality is suspected and pyuria is present, catheterization of the ureters affords separate urine
specimens from the kidneys for bacteriologic
study, thus establishing the site of the infection. Retrograde urograms can then be done.

B. Inadequate Excretory Urograms: If
excretory urograms (even the infusion type) do
not adequately demonstrate ureteropelvic detail, retrograde urograms may be needed.

C. Impaired Total Renal Function: If renal function is decreased to the point where
excretory urograms will prove inadequate,
retrograde filling of the renal pelves will be
necessary.

D. Assessment of Degree of Ureteral Obstruction: If excretory urograms portray ureteropelvic junction or ureteral obstruction,
its degree may be best judged by instilling
radiopaque fluid into the renal pelvis. In the
absence of significant obstruction, most of the
medium will have drained out in 15 minutes,
whereas marked stenosis may cause retention
of the iodide for hours.

E. Sensitivity to Intravenous Radiopaque
Fluid: If excretory urograms are contraindicated because of allergy, retrograde urograms
must be substituted.

F. Need for Oblique and Lateral Radiograms: Since the radiopaque medium given
intravenously is diluted by urine, the density
of the excreted fluid is less than that obtained
with retrograde filling. If oblique and lateral
films are desired, the density of the tissues
through which the x-rays must pass is increased; retrograde instillation may prove
more satisfactory.

Contraindications
Although there are contraindications to

cystoscopy and ureteral catheterization, there are none to retrograde urography itself.

Technic
A. Preparation of the Patient: Fluids can be taken as tolerated unless general anesthesia is to be employed for the procedure. The bowel should first be cleansed by catharsis (eg, castor oil).

B. Procedure:
1. Cystoscopy and ureteral catheterization are done first.
2. Preliminary plain film of abdomen (supine) - This checks on the position of the patient and the catheters and on the radiographic technic, and demonstrates calcific densities in the urinary tract which might be obscured by the radiopaque medium.
3. Instillation of the radiopaque fluid -
a. Supine urogram - If the capacity of the renal pelvis is not known, 3-4 ml of undiluted urographic medium should be instilled by gravity under low pressure (20 cm of water). A radiogram is then taken, developed, and viewed. If filling is incomplete, another x-ray film can be exposed after more fluid is introduced.
b. Oblique or lateral radiograms should then be taken as indicated.
c. Upright ureteropyelogram - The patient is then placed in the semi-erect position, and, while the urographic fluid is still being introduced, the catheters are slowly withdrawn into the lower ureters and a film taken. This affords good ureterograms and shows the degree of mobility of the kidneys.
If ureteral filling is inadequate, the patient should be placed in the Trendelenburg position and more of the contrast medium instilled; an x-ray exposure is again made.
d. "Emptying" or delayed films - If the ureteropyelograms reveal evidence of obstruction, an x-ray should be taken 15 minutes after the previous one without further introduction of radiopaque medium. If some of the medium is still retained, later films should be made in order to assess the degree of obstruction.

BULB URETEROPYELOGRAM

If optimum ureteral detail is essential, a bulb ureteropyelogram should be obtained. This is accomplished by forcing a bulbous tipped catheter tightly into the ureteral orifice. Radiopaque fluid is then instilled with a syringe.

OPACIFICATION OF RENAL CYSTS

One of the most difficult problems in diagnosis is the differentiation of renal cyst and tumor. Some urologists, fearing the complications of cancer on the wall of a cyst, tend to explore all kidneys showing evidence of a space-occupying lesion as revealed by urography. Others will not resort to surgery if the diagnosis of cyst can be established. Renal angiography (particularly of the selective type) establishes the diagnosis of vascular adenocarcinomas, but what appears to be a nonvascular mass, although almost always a cyst, could be a necrotic tumor or an abscess. In this instance, renal cystography can be performed.

Under fluoroscopic control and after administration of a radiopaque fluid intravenously (although some clinicians needle blindly, using previous urograms as a guide), a 7 inch, 18 guage needle is introduced into the presumed cyst. In most instances, clear fluid will be obtained; this should be subjected to cytologic study. Radiopaque fluid is then instilled into the cystic cavity and a film taken. If the radiopaque fluid is homogeneous, the edges of the cavity smooth, and cytology negative, the diagnosis of simple cyst is warranted, thus negating the need for surgery (Fig 21-5). The return of bloody fluid or just a little blood implies the presence of carcinoma; surgery is indicated.

This procedure should probably be reserved for the poor risk patient since seeding of the tumor in the perinephric fat has been observed.

Buttarazzi, P. J., & others: Aspiration of renal cyst. J Urol **100**:591-3, 1968.
Lalli, A. F.: Percutaneous aspiration of renal masses. Am J Roentgenol **101**:700-4, 1967.
Witherington, R., & J. R. Rinker: Percutaneous needle puncture in the diagnosis of renal cysts. J Urol **95**:733-7, 1966.

CYSTOGRAMS

Cystograms are made by instilling radiopaque fluid into the bladder through a catheter. Roentgenograms then show an outline of the bladder wall. In addition, ureteropyelograms may be obtained if the ureterovesical "valves" are incompetent (see chapter 11).

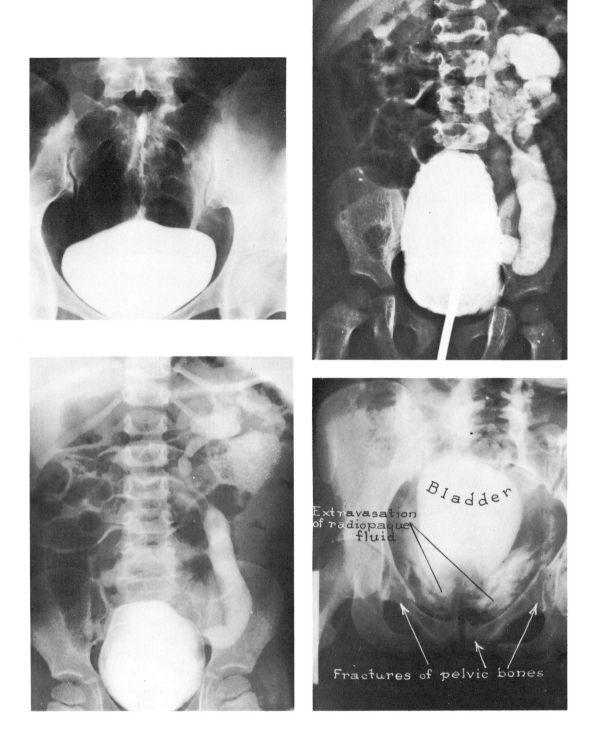

Fig 7-8. Normal and abnormal cystograms. Above left: Normal cystogram. **Above right:** Trabeculated bladder and left ureteral reflux demonstrating marked hydroureteronephrosis. **Below left:** Light iodized oil (Lipiodol®) instilled into bladder to seek evidence of residual urine. Lipiodol® refluxed up second left ureter to fill hydronephrotic lower pole (same patient as above right). **Below right:** Avulsion of prostatic urethra secondary to pelvic fracture. Extraperitoneal extravasation.

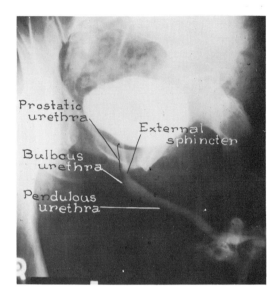

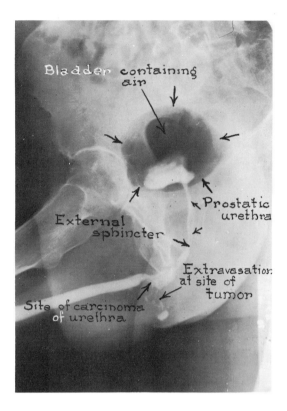

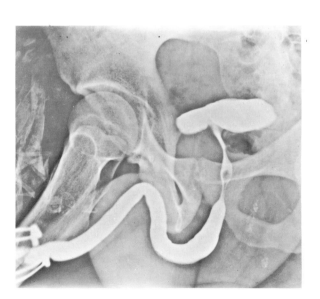

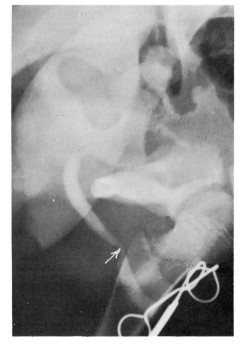

Fig 7-9. Normal and abnormal cystourethrograms and retrograde urethrograms. Above left:
Normal cystourethrogram. Above right: Cystourethrogram showing carcinoma of urethra.
Below left: Normal urethrogram. Note ''negative'' shadow over pubic bone representing the
verumontanum. Below right: Urethrogram showing congenital stricture of pendulous urethra.

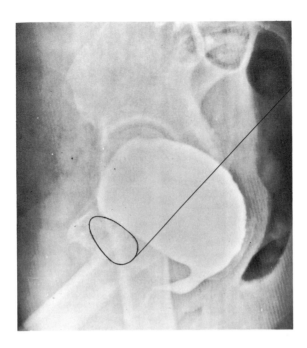

Fig 7-10. Lateral cystogram. Upright voiding film showing abnormal descent of bladder with complete loss of the posterior urethrovesical angle in patient with stress incontinence. (See Fig 23-2.) (Courtesy of J. A. Hutch, MD.)

RETROGRADE CYSTOGRAMS

Indications

A. When Cystoscopy Is Not Feasible: In male infants, the small caliber of the urethra may preclude passage of the smallest cystoscope or panendoscope. If mechanical difficulties prevent passage of an optical instrument to the bladder but a catheter can be successfully passed, a cystogram may reveal a vesical tumor, vesicoureteral reflux, or protrusion of an enlarged prostate into the vesical cavity.

If a catheter cannot be introduced through the urethra, a small plastic tube can be placed in the bladder through the barrel of a needle passed suprapubically.

B. Study of the Neurogenic Bladder: Particularly in the spastic type of neurogenic bladder, ureterovesical reflux is common. Cystograms will reveal this reflux as well as the degree of damage from hydronephrosis or pyelonephritis.

C. Rupture of the Bladder: Cystography is the best method of testing for extravasation of urine (Fig 7-8).

D. Cystography should be routine in the study of any patient suffering from recurrent infection, particularly children. Vesicoureteral reflux is one of the common causes of perpetuation of infection. This procedure may also delineate vesical fistulous communications and is of great help in the study of urinary incontinence in both males and females.

Contraindications

During acute attacks or exacerbations of chronic urinary infection, the instillation of radiopaque medium under pressure may increase the seriousness of the infection (eg, bacteremia), particularly if reflux exists.

Technic

1. Preliminary plain film of abdomen - If vesicoureteral reflux is suspected, a KUB should be made. If vesical pathology only is to be studied (eg, rupture), a film of the bladder area alone is sufficient.

2. A catheter is passed to the bladder. The urine which it contains should be drained off.

3. Introduction of radiopaque fluid - In the adult 250-350 ml is sufficient. In a child 1 year old, the normal vesical capacity is

75-100 ml. Any fluid used for excretory or retrograde urography diluted with 3 parts of water or normal saline solution can be used.

4. The catheter is then clamped off and an x-ray taken with the patient supine. This may reveal trabeculation and diverticula, intravesical protrusion of an enlarged prostate, vesical tumors, or vesicoureteral reflux.

5. Left and right oblique radiograms will visualize diverticula which lie behind the bladder or a fistulous tract into the vagina.

6. Cystograms taken in the true lateral position are helpful in delineating the cause of urinary incontinence, particularly in women (Figs 7-10 and 23-2).

7. The vesical fluid is then allowed to drain out and another x-ray film exposed. Diverticula or a fistulous tract into the vagina will still contain the radiopaque fluid and will be clearly defined. Intraperitoneal or extraperitoneal extravasation of the contrast medium behind the bladder will be shown. Fig 7-9 demonstrates the normal and some abnormal cystograms.

DELAYED CYSTOGRAMS

Simple cystography often fails to demonstrate ureterovesical reflux although incompetency of the vesicoureteral valves exists. Stewart has shown that "delayed" cystograms reveal this reflux more efficiently. If voiding cystourethrography is attempted but the patient cannot void, delayed cystograms should be resorted to.

Technic

1. Preliminary film of abdomen should be made.

2. A small catheter is passed to the bladder and the urine drained off.

3. Radiopaque fluid is then introduced into the bladder. The amount varies from 30 ml in the infant to 120 ml for a child 8 years of age and 200-300 ml for adults. The least noxious fluid is urographic medium diluted with 3 parts of water or normal saline solution.

4. The catheter is then removed.

5. Serial x-ray films are then exposed every 15-30 minutes during the next 1-3 hours. Ureteral reflux may appear on one "delayed" film only to be absent on the next. One kidney may reveal reflux, whereas on the next exposure only the opposite kidney may contain the radiopaque fluid.

VOIDING CYSTOURETHROGRAMS

This technic often shows ureteral reflux when both the simple and delayed cystograms fail to do so because of the increased intravesical pressure generated at the time of voiding. The voiding cystourethrogram may also reveal the presence of posterior urethral valves (Fig 24-2) or urethral strictures (Fig 24-4).

Immediately following the conclusion of the series of delayed cystograms or after filling the bladder with the radiopaque medium, the patient is instructed to void. During the act of urination, one or more x-rays are taken.

CYSTOURETHROGRAMS

Cystourethrograms combine simple cystography with urethrography. Vesical and urethral abnormalities are thereby visualized.

A catheter is passed to the bladder and a plain film of the bladder area is taken. About 200-300 ml of radiopaque fluid or air are then introduced into the bladder, a plain x-ray film exposed, and oblique views made. With the patient lying at a 45° angle, 20 ml of radiopaque water-soluble lubricant are injected into the urethra and a radiogram made (Fig 7-10).

Bartley, O., & C.G. Helander: Double-contrast cystography in tumors of the urinary bladder. Acta radiol **54**:161-9, 1960.

Berson, J.W., Alexander, R.L., & D.J. Mehan: Cystourethrography as a teaching aid for residents. South MJ **60**:943-7, 1967.

Currarino, G.: Narrowings of the male urethra caused by contractions or spasm of the bulbocavernosus muscle: Cystourethrographic observations. Am J Roentgenol **108**:641-7, 1970.

Hutch, J.A., & C.E. Shopfner: The lateral cystogram as an aid to urologic diagnosis. J Urol **99**:202-6, 1968.

Hyman, R.M., & G.B. Yulis: An improved technique for male urethrocystography. J Urol **93**:62-3, 1965.

Rudhe, U.: Roentgenographic diagnosis of obstructive disorders of the lower urinary tract in infancy and childhood. Postgrad Med **35**:29-39, 1964.

Shopfner, C.E.: Cystourethrography: Methodology, normal anatomy and pathology. J Urol **103**:92-103, 1970.

Stewart, C.M.: Delayed cystography and voiding cystourethrography. J Urol **74**:749-59, 1955.

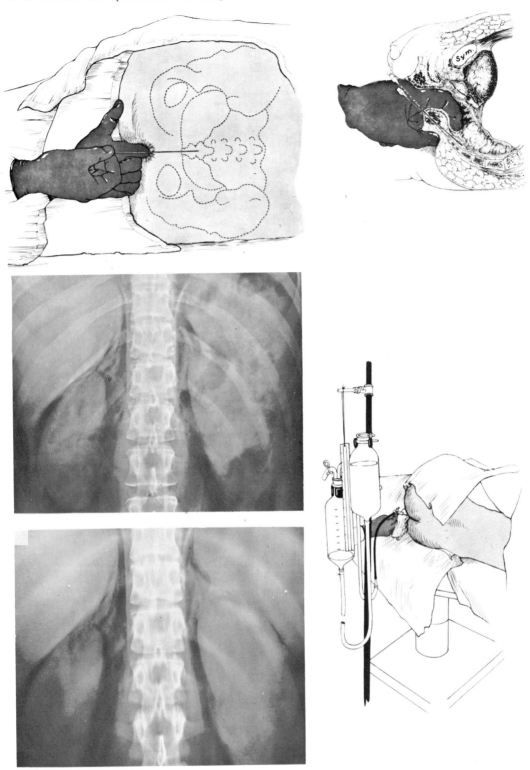

Fig 7-11. Technic of presacral retroperitoneal pneumography; normal pneumogram. **Above:** Technic of placing needle. **Below right:** Pneumothorax apparatus used for insufflation. **Center left:** Normal pneumogram showing kidneys and adrenals. **Below left:** Tomogram of same patient. Details of organs enhanced.

Tucker, A. S., & L. Persky: Cystography in childhood tumors and pseudotumors. Am J Roentgenol **109**:390-8, 1970.

Verga-Pires, J. A., & E. A. Elebute: Urethrocystography in the male. Brit J Urol **39**: 194-210, 1967.

• • •

URETHROGRAMS

Stenoses of the urethra and enlargements of the prostate and even some posterior urethral valves (Fig 24-2) can be shown on films by introducing into the urethra 20-30 ml of a water-soluble lubricant in which there is an equal amount of radiopaque fluid. Oily media (eg, Lipiodol®) are contraindicated since they may cause pulmonary emboli. The radiogram should be taken while the fluid is being injected. Oblique films of the area of the urethra and prostate will demonstrate narrowings, diverticula, fistulas, and other diseases of these organs (Fig 7-9).

McClennan, B. L., Becker, J. A., & T. Robinson: Venous extravasation at retrograde urethrography: Precautions. J Urol **106**: 412-5, 1971.

Morales, O., Nilsson, S., & R. Romands: Urethrographic studies of the posterior urethra. Acta radiol (diag) **2**:81-99, 305-15, 1964.

Shopfner, C. E., & J. A. Hutch: The normal urethrogram. Radiol Clin North America **6**:165-89, 1968.

ESTIMATION OF
RESIDUAL URINE IN CHILDREN

Instill 5 ml of ascendant Lipiodol® into the bladder. If the child does not retain urine, a film taken 24 hours later will show no retention of the opaque material. If some urinary retention does exist, the fluid may remain in the bladder for many days. If vesicoureteral reflux is present, the Lipiodol® may be visualized in the kidney (Fig 7-8).

Young, B. W., Anderson, W. G., & G. G. King: Radiographic estimation of residual urine in children. J Urol **75**:263-72, 1956.

CINERADIOGRAPHY

Cineradiography, formerly only a research tool, is now of practical value in clinical diagnosis. It reveals a higher incidence and degree of reflux than cystography and the voiding cystourethrogram and affords a dynamic picture of this abnormality.

The bladder is gradually filled with radiopaque fluid. The ureters are studied for transient or persistent reflux. Reflux may only be demonstrated during the act of voiding, when intravesical pressure is high. About half of children suffering from urinary tract infection will show vesicoureteral reflux. This phenomenon is also revealed in a significant number of adults with chronic pyelonephritis.

Mitsuya, H., & others: Cinefluorography of the upper urinary tract. Urologia Internat **13**:236-53, 1962.

Tanagho, E. A., Hutch, J. A., & E. R. Miller: Diagnostic procedures and cinefluoroscopy in vesico-ureteral reflux. Brit J Urol **38**: 435-44, 1966.

Tristan, T. A., & others: Cinefluorographic investigation of genitourinary tract function. Am J Roentgenol **90**:1-14, 1963.

PRESACRAL
RETROPERITONEAL PNEUMOGRAMS

The main value of retroperitoneal pneumograms is visualization of the adrenal glands and renal outlines. Excision of adrenal tumors or even total bilateral adrenalectomy has become a routine surgical procedure now that potent hormonal replacement preparations are available. Direct perirenal air insufflation fell into disrepute 15-20 years ago because it caused a number of deaths from gas embolus. It is safe, however, if CO_2 is used. The use of angiography has reduced the indications for this procedure.

During the past 20 years, the presacral technic has been used extensively. However, a few deaths from gas embolism have been reported where air and even oxygen have been used. Because carbon dioxide is much more soluble than oxygen in body tissues and blood, its use has recently been recommended as a safety measure. The great disadvantage of carbon dioxide is the rapidity of its absorption (20-30 minutes). Tomograms, which are essential if presacral retroperitoneal pneumograms are to attain a high degree of diagnostic accuracy, are therefore more difficult to obtain. The importance of slow low-pressure

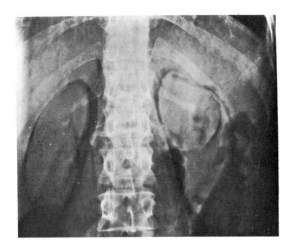

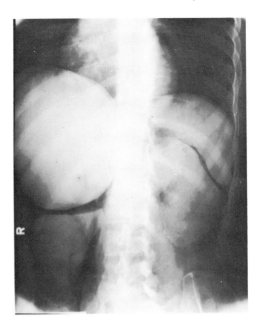

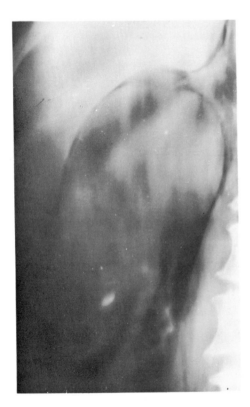

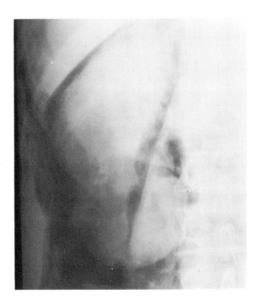

Fig 7-12. Abnormal retroperitoneal pneumograms. Above left: Presacral oxygen showing pheochromocytoma overlying upper half of left kidney. **Above right:** Massive androgenic tumor of right adrenal with downward displacement of right kidney. Spleen clearly shown above left kidney. **Below left:** Carcinoma of upper pole of right kidney. Note expansion of this pole; normal adrenal above it. **Below right:** Cyst of lower pole of right kidney overlying psoas muscle which is visible through mass.

insufflation cannot be overemphasized. The author has no personal knowledge of a death from gas embolism when oxygen has been instilled with a low-pressure apparatus as described below.

Presacral pneumograms should not be made if the proper diagnosis can be established by simpler (and possibly safer) methods (eg, plain films, tomograms, excretory urograms, angiography).

Technic

A. Preparation of the Patient: A sedative and opiate should be administered 1 hour before the procedure is to be done.

B. Procedure:

1. The patient is placed on his right side (if the physician is right-handed) with his knees drawn up on the abdomen. The skin of the sacral area is prepared with soap and water and a skin antiseptic. The area is sterilely draped.

2. A wheal of 1% procaine hydrochloride is raised on the skin just below the tip of the coccyx. The tissues deep to this point are then anesthetized.

3. A No. 18 spinal needle (stiff enough to be accurately guided) is passed to a point just below the tip of the coccyx; it is then directed upward so that its point lies just anterior to the end of the coccyx. This placement is facilitated by palpation of the area with the left index finger inserted in the rectum.

4. The needle is aspirated to be sure it has not entered a blood vessel. Ten ml of air are then introduced by syringe. It should enter with minimal resistance. If it does not, the needle should be remanipulated.

5. A pneumothorax type of machine should then be connected to the spinal needle (Fig 7-11). The upper bottle contains sterile water; the lower one is filled with oxygen. The oxygen should flow slowly when the levels of the respective bottles are about 20 cm apart. If higher pressure is required, the position of the needle should be changed. Seven ml of oxygen per kg body weight should be introduced.

If bilateral insufflation is desired, the tubing should be disconnected from the spinal needle and the patient instructed to roll slowly onto his abdomen and then onto his left side. The tubing is again connected to the needle and an equal amount of oxygen allowed to fill the right side. By changing position for each insufflation, equal distribution of the gas is obtained.

Warning: If syncope or circulatory collapse occurs, the patient should be placed immediately on his left side. If the cause is gas embolus, this position will allow the oxygen trapped in the right ventricle to pass into the lungs; death is thereby prevented.

6. The patient is then placed prone with the head of the table or cart elevated 20°; this causes the gas to rise to the perirenal area. This position should be maintained at all times except when supine x-ray films are taken.

7. Plain x-ray films of the renal area are then exposed immediately after insufflation and every 30-60 minutes thereafter until the clearest delineation of the kidney and adrenals is obtained. When visualization of the organ in question is at its maximum, tomograms should be taken. This procedure is essential since it affords optimum detail of the adrenals and kidneys (Fig 7-12).

8. Simultaneous excretory urography may further enhance the study.

C. Recovery of the Patient: Six hours after the insufflation, 75% of the oxygen has been absorbed as judged by radiography. During this period, the patient should be flat in bed. Ambulation causes the gas to rise to the mediastinum and neck, causing the patient some apprehension.

Anderson, E. E., & J. F. Glenn: Carbon dioxide contrast studies in retroperitoneal masses. J Urol **101**:530-2, 1969.

Landes, R. R., & C. L. Ransom: Presacral retroperitoneal pneumography utilizing carbon dioxide. J Urol **82**:670-3, 1959.

RENAL ANGIOGRAPHY

Although renal angiograms can be procured by direct lumbar needle puncture of the aorta, this technic has been superseded by percutaneous femoral angiography wherein a catheter is passed to the level of the renal arteries under fluoroscopic control. Percutaneous catheterization of the brachial or axillary artery is also feasible. Twelve to 24 ml of radiopaque fluid suitable for intravenous urography (eg, sodium acetrizoate [Urokon®], meglumine diatrizoate [Renographin®-76]) are rapidly introduced into the aorta, and serial films are immediately taken (midstream technic). Possibly 10 exposures are made over a period of 10 seconds, but 2 per second are exposed for the first 3 seconds. A second or even a third injection may be indicated for oblique views. Besides demonstrating the caliber of the great vessels, this procedure shows the renal arterial circulation (Fig 7-13). Fig 29-3 reveals stenosis of the renal artery as the cause of hypertension. A pheochromocytoma is shown in Fig 20-2.

Selective renal angiography is accomplished by passing a femoral catheter into one of the renal arteries under fluoroscopic control. About 8 ml of contrast medium are injected and approximately 16 exposures are made during the first few seconds (Fig 7-13). The intrarenal vascular detail demonstrated by this technic is superior to the midstream method and is therefore of particular value in the differential diagnosis of renal cyst (Fig 21-5) and tumor (Fig 17-3). The space occupied by a cyst fails to opacify. Increased density on late films is typical of tumor.

In cases where the lesion is small or obscured by overlying arteries, epinephrine can first be injected into the catheter followed by the instillation of radiopaque medium. This technic causes spasm of normal vessels but has no effect on arteries in tumors.

There is a good correlation between the renal angiogram and the technetium (camera) scan (see chapter 8).

Baum, S., & J.Y. Gillenwater: Renal artery impressions on the renal pelvis. J Urol 95:139-45, 1966.

Becker, J.A., & others: Misleading appearances in renal angiography. Radiology 88: 691-700, 1967.

Bookstein, J.J., & B.H. Stewart: The current status of renal arteriography. R Clin North America 2:461-82, 1964.

Brinsfield, D., Bland, J.W., Jr., & R.G. Sybers: Aortography in children with abdominal masses. J Pediat 73:203-11, 1968.

Bron, K.M.: Selective visceral and total abdominal arteriography via the left axillary artery in the older age group. Am J Roentgenol 97:432-7, 1966.

Caine, M., Kedar, S.S., & A. Schwartz: Renal angiography by the percutaneous non-catheter left brachial technique. Brit J Urol 39:571-6, 1967.

Crane, C.: Renal angiography. Lumbar approach. Am J Surg 107:74-7, 1964.

Foster, R.S., & others: Selective renal angiography in clinical urology. J Urol 90:631-41, 1963.

Halpern, M.: Percutaneous transfemoral arteriography. Am J Roentgenol 92:918-34, 1964.

Hotchkiss, R.S., & B.P. Sammons: Selective renal angiography. J Urol 93:309-18, 1965.

Kahn, P.C., & H.M. Wise, Jr.: The use of epinephrine in selective angiography of renal masses. J Urol 99:133, 1968.

Karras, B.G., Cannon, A.H., & J.K. Sokol: Percutaneous left brachial renal angiography. J Urol 89:101-5, 1963.

Kaufman, J.J., & M.H. Maxwell: Orthostatic renal arteriography. California Med 99: 230-3, 1963.

Killen, D.A., & J.H. Foster: Spinal cord injury as a complication of contrast angiography. Surgery 59:969-81, 1966.

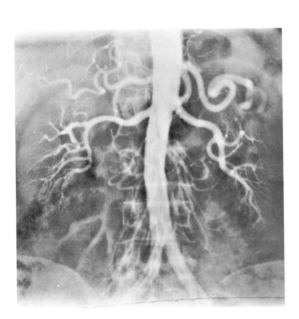
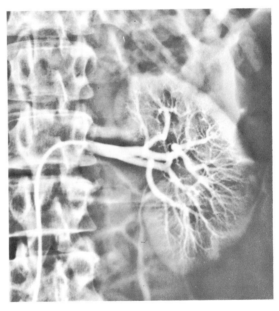

Fig 7-13. Normal percutaneous femoral renal angiograms. Left: Midstream technic. Renal arteries and their branches are of normal caliber and distribution. The celiac axis, splenic artery, and branches of the superior mesenteric arteries are well outlined. Right: Selective renal angiogram. Detail of smaller arterial branches is enhanced. They are evenly distributed throughout the kidney.

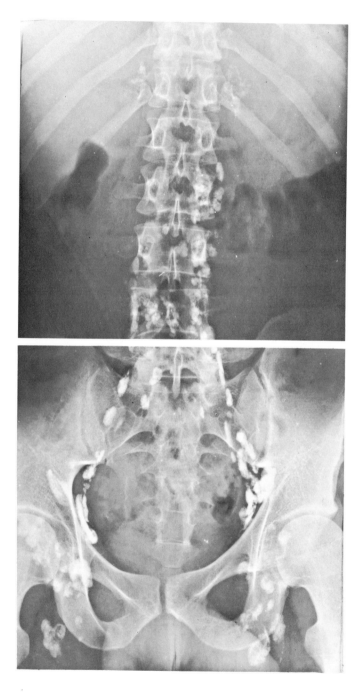

Fig 7-14. **Normal lymphangiogram.** (Composite of 2 films.) Note calcifications of both adrenal glands (cause not determined). Compare with Fig 7-15.

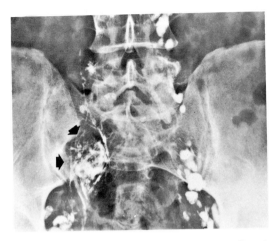

Fig 7-15. Abnormal lymphangiogram. Carcinoma of the penis with metastases to right common iliac nodes, overlying sacroiliac joint, which have blocked ascent of contrast medium.

Roy, P.: Percutaneous catheterization via the axillary artery. Am J Roentgenol 94:1-18, 1965.

VESICAL ANGIOGRAPHY

In order to judge the size and depth of penetration of vesical neoplasms, the following technic can be employed. A Seldinger catheter is passed to the bifurcation of the aorta, and the vessels are "flooded" with 30 ml of 90% contrast material. As an alternative, each hypogastric artery is selectively catheterized and into each of them are instilled 10 ml of radiopaque fluid. Films are rapidly exposed over a period of 8 seconds. The series is repeated in the oblique position, affording a tangential view of the tumor. These roentgenograms reveal the typical pattern or "stain" of an invasive tumor (Fig 17-9), thus improving accuracy of staging of the lesion. The study may be enhanced if 60 ml of CO_2 are first instilled into the bladder.

Wise, H. W., Jr., & M. H. Fainsinger: Angiography in the evaluation of carcinoma of the bladder. JAMA 192:1027-31, 1965.

LYMPHANGIOGRAPHY

Cannulation of a lymphatic vessel in an extremity and the injection of an oily contrast medium leads to x-ray opacification of the inguinal, pelvic, retroperitoneal, and supra-clavicular lymphatic systems (Fig 7-14). The main value of this procedure is the demonstration of metastatic infiltration in regional lymph nodes (Fig 7-15). It therefore lends itself to the study of patients with cancers of the testes (Fig 17-15), penis, bladder, or prostate. It can demonstrate the lymphatic connections to the kidney in patients with chyluria.

Chavez, C. M.: Lymphangiography. Am J M Sc 248:225-45, 1964.
Fraley, E. E., Clouse, M., & S. B. Litwin: The uses of lymphography, lymphadenography and color lymphadenography in urology. J Urol 93:319-25, 1965.
Oritz, F., Walzak, M. P., & V. F. Marshall: Chyluria: Lymphatic-urinary fistula demonstrated by lymphangiography. J Urol 91:608-12, 1964.
Mahaffy, R. G.: Lymphography and the urologist. Postgrad MJ 41:452-68, 1965.
Wallace, S., & others: Lymphangiographic interpretation. Radiol Clin North America 3:467-85, 1965.

VENACAVAGRAPHY

Retrograde catheterization of the femoral veins affords a route for the injection of radiopaque material into the vena cava (Fig 22-5). Evidence of masses in the right retroperitoneal area are demonstrated by encroachment on the vessel. Thus, this technic is of particular value in outlining enlarged retroperitoneal lymph nodes (eg, testicular tumor; Fig 7-16). The procedure may also reveal evidence of renal vein thrombosis (Fig 21-12).

Berdon, W. E., Baker, D. H., & T. V. Santulli: Factors producing spurious obstruction of the inferior vena cava in infants and children with abdominal tumor. Radiology 88:111-6, 1967.
Hayt, D. B.: Upright inferior vena cavagraphy. Radiology 86:865-70, 1966.
Hipona, F. A., & A. B. Crummy: The roentgen diagnosis of renal vein thrombosis. Am J Roentgenol 98:122-31, 1966.
Simon, H., Moquin, R., & W. Dameshek: The inferior venacavagram and lymphoproliferative disorders. JAMA 184:978-80, 1963.

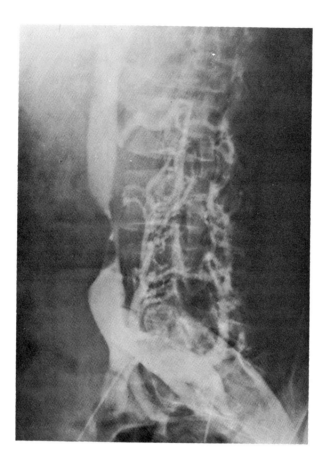

Fig 7-16. Venacavagram. Right posterior oblique exposure revealing defect caused by metastases to lumbar lymph nodes from seminoma of right testis. (See Fig 17-15 for retrograde ureterogram on same patient.)

Wendel, R. G., Evans, A. T., & J. F. Wiot: A new technique for inferior venacavagraphy. J Urol **100**:705-8, 1968.

Kahn, P. C.: Selective venography in renal parenchymal disease. Radiology **92**:345-9, 1969.

SELECTIVE RENAL VENOGRAPHY

While venacavagraphy may reveal gross extension of renal carcinoma into the vena cava, it may miss minor defects in the renal veins themselves because of the "washout" of the veins by a large volume of blood. Selective renal venography overcomes this deficiency.

The washout effect can be decreased by injection of epinephrine into the renal artery 10 seconds before the venous infusion of 35-60 ml of radiopaque material. If indicated, a blood sample from the renal vein can be subjected to analysis for renin.

OTHER X-RAY STUDIES

Roentgenograms of the gastrointestinal tract, chest, and bones may contribute to urologic diagnosis.

Gastrointestinal Series (See Fig 7-17.)

A barium enema may show displacement of the colon—a cardinal sign of retroperitoneal tumor. The stomach may also be displaced by large retroperitoneal masses (eg, kidney, spleen, pancreas).

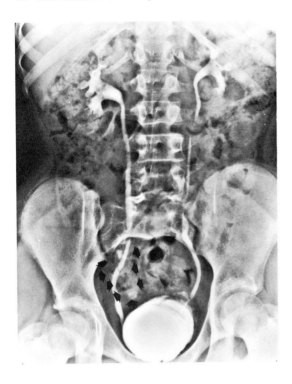
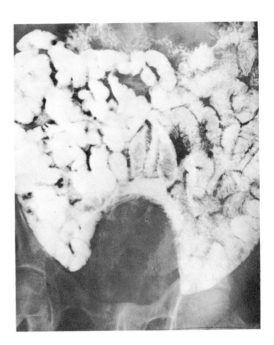
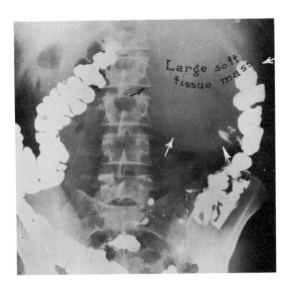
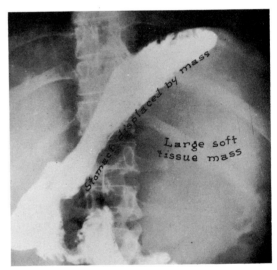

Fig 7-17. Miscellaneous x-ray studies. Above left: Study of bones reveals scimitar-shaped sacrum on the right side. Typical of anterior meningomyelocele. Patient had a neurogenic bladder. **Above right:** Patient with low midline mass and cramping abdominal pain. Gastro-intestinal series showing the cause of the symptoms—a distended bladder. **Below left:** Barium enema showing displacement of transverse colon by large cyst of left kidney. **Below right:** Gastrointestinal series (same patient) showing displacement of stomach by cyst of left kidney.

Cholecystograms

Films of the gallbladder may show evidence of gallbladder disease. Extensive renal carcinoma may invade the common duct. Cholecystitis or cholelithiasis may be the cause of pseudorenal pain.

Chest Film

An x-ray of the chest may reveal the source of a tuberculous infection of the kidney or may show metastasis from renal, testicular, or other tumors (Fig 17-4).

Osteograms

Films of bones may reveal evidence of metastases (Fig 17-4 and 17-13), spina bifida (Fig 7-17), or changes compatible with hyperparathyroidism (Fig 15-4), or osteitis fibrosa generalisata as often seen in patients with renal tubular acidosis (see p 225).

· · ·

General References

Hope, J.W., & P.F. Borns: Radiologic diagnosis of primary and metastatic cancer in infants and children. Radiol Clin North America 3:353-74, 1965.

Lowman, R.M.: Retroperitoneal tumors: A survey and assessment of Roentgen techniques. Radiol Clin North America 3:543-66, 1965.

Symposium on urinary tract (radiologic aspects). Radiol Clin North America 3:3-174, 1965.

Tucker, A.S.: The Roentgen diagnosis of abdominal masses in children. Am J Roentgenol 95:76-90, 1965.

8...

Radioisotopic Kidney Studies

Malcolm R. Powell, MD, * & Jerome M. Weiss, MD †

Radioisotopic tracer procedures provide means of studying the structure and function of internal organs without disturbing their normal physiologic processes. None of the radiopharmaceuticals used in kidney evaluation introduce the hypertonic and chemical stress of intravenous contrast media. The content of iodide in the iodinated renal radiopharmaceuticals is so low that there is not even an iodide hypersensitivity hazard. The presence of radiopharmaceuticals in the kidney is detected by an external instrument after peripheral intravenous injection, thus avoiding the instrumentation common to other methods of renal evaluation. These studies can be performed with acceptable radiation exposure in all age groups, although some methods are modified for children.

The particular advantage of radiosotopes over x-rays is the ease with which radioisotope concentration can be estimated by counting radioactive disintegrations while a simultaneous image of radioisotope distribution is produced. X-ray images are not readily susceptible to numerical quantification, but they do have higher resolution, and in this respect are greatly superior to radioisotopic images produced by current equipment. Although roentgenographic methods provide very high resolution of renovascular structures and of calyceal and pelvic anatomy, special procedures such as nephrotomography during infusion urography may be required to provide information about renal cortical structure. Images of the kidney with radionuclides, on the other hand, provide a simpler means of evaluating the renal cortex. Many of the factors that handicap roentgenographic methods for kidney evaluation, such as excessive bowel gas, marked obesity, and uremia, have little effect on the diagnostic usefulness of radioisotopic imaging studies.

Study of an internal organ by a radioactive tracer requires that the radioisotope be concentrated by the organ. The process of concentration will be referred to as "labeling." The kidney concentrates a number of radioactive labels by several mechanisms and is, therefore, readily susceptible to these study methods.

Although the exact place of radioisotopes in the diagnosis of genitourinary disorders has yet to be defined, they are versatile and provide information that cannot be obtained in other ways. The information is generally of a screening nature. The relative simplicity, the low cost, and the large amount of information provided by the radioisotopic methods has resulted in their increasing acceptance.

Current clinical evaluation of the kidney with radioisotopic tracers includes imaging radiopharmaceutical distributions within the kidney and urinary tract, function studies for determination of rates of concentration and excretion of radiopharmaceuticals by the kidneys, and blood clearance measurements.

MEANS OF RENAL EVALUATION WITH RADIOPHARMACEUTICALS

Radiopharmaceuticals

Four general types of renal radioisotopic labels are in current use. Classified according to the mechanisms of labeling, they are (1) renal cortex labels, which cause labeling of the renal tubular cells; (2) renal tubular function labels, which briefly label the renal cortex as they are accumulated by renal tubular cells but then are passed into the urine and cleared from the kidney; (3) intravascular compartment labels; and (4) substances cleared by glomerular filtration, allowing radioactive tracer determination of glomerular filtration rate. Table 8-1 lists the characteristics of the more useful radiopharmaceuticals in these categories.

Mercury-203 chlormerodrin and mercury-197 chlormerodrin are the most common-

---

*Assistant Professor of Radiology and Medicine, University of California Medical Center (San Francisco).

†Assistant Clinical Professor of Urology, University of California Medical Center (San Francisco).

Table 8-1. Radiopharmaceuticals for urologic evaluations.

Chemical Form	Radioisotopic Label	Radioisotopic Half-Life	Gamma Energy	Radiation Dose* (mrad/μc)	Use
Chlormerodrin	^{197}Hg	2.7 days	77 kev	5.4 (to kidney)	2 μc/kg for scan or 1-1.5 μc/kg for scintiphoto evaluation of renal cortical structure and perfusion.
	^{203}Hg	46.9 days	279 kev	44.-153. (to kidney)	
Hippurate	^{131}I	8.05 days	364 kev	1 (to kidney)	5 μc for renogram, 2-3 μc/kg for scintiphoto evaluation of renal function and drainage mechanisms
Pertechnetate (TcO$_4$-)	^{99m}Tc	6.05 hours	140 kev	1.5×10^{-2} (whole body)	140-200 μc/kg for scintiphoto evaluation of renal vascularization.
Iothalamate	^{125}I	60.2 days	35 kev		10 μc IV for GFR measurement.
Technetium-iron complex	^{99m}Tc	6.05 hours	140 kev		5 mc IV for renal structural evaluation by scintiphoto and for function study.

*Radiation doses are derived from data of Smith, E. M.: J Nuclear Med 6:231-251, 1965; and from Seltzer, R. A., Kereiakes, J. G., and E. L. Saenger: New England J Med 271:84-90, 1964.

ly used renal cortical labels, although a number of new renal cortical labels employing ^{99m}Tc in various compounds have been introduced. These ^{99m}Tc compounds (technetium-iron-ascorbic acid complex, technetium-gelatin, technetium-penicillamine-acetazolamide complex, and technetium caseidin) deliver a smaller absorbed radiation dose to the kidneys than do the radiomercury isotopes and improve the kidney images by providing more radioactive data for recording in the image. After intravenous injection, these tracers are accumulated in renal tubular epithelium, labeling the renal cortex, while a portion of the injected dose passes into the urine. These substances are dependent upon adequate renal blood flow for cortical labeling and, once fixed in the renal tubular cells, make it possible to record images of the renal cortex. Since the amount of uptake in the cortex is a function of blood flow, it can be used to estimate renal blood flow. The long 47-day radioactive half-life of mercury-203 chlormerodrin and the long biologic half-life of this substance in the kidney allow determination of renal position during repeat studies for several weeks after its administration. Mercury-197 chlormerodrin has a short radioactive half-life (2.7 days) which serves to reduce the radiation dose to the kidneys by this radiopharmaceutical. Its gamma ray energy is rather low, a factor that increases gamma ray absorption within the body. These internally absorbed gamma rays are then unavailable for external counting. The low ^{197}Hg gamma energy also interferes to

some extent with its efficient spatial resolution by scintillation cameras, one type of generally used radiosotope imaging equipment.

Iodide-131 hippurate is used for renal tubular function studies. It is excreted by the renal tubular epithelium into the urine and is used in radioisotope renography. A radioisotope renogram is simply a recording of the amount of radioactivity detected over each kidney from the time of injection of the labeled hippurate. After peripheral intravenous injection of hippurate, the count rate increases in a few seconds because the kidneys receive 20% of the cardiac output. The normal kidney rapidly accumulates hippurate as a function of effective renal plasma flow, and the amount of radioactivity detected over the kidney continues to rise until loss of radioactivity by urine drainage exceeds the rate of accumulation by the renal cortex. Beyond that point, if renal drainage is normal, the amount of radioactivity in the kidney continues to decrease because the radiopharmaceutical was given as a single injection and the amount available in the blood for clearance has decreased throughout the period of observation. In uremia there is slower accumulation and prolonged cortical retention of hippurate, so that late scintiphotographs usually show a useful image of the kidney. The kidney may be evaluated in severe uremia with radiohippurate when neither intravenous urograms nor radiochlormerodrin images can be obtained.

The other 2 general types of radiopharmaceuticals used in renal studies are less frequently used in general clinical practice. Technetium-99m pertechnetate is another technetium compound which, unlike the iron complex, behaves like iodide ion and is used to temporarily label the intrarenal blood pool. Pertechnetate is the agent used for brain imaging and is readily available. Any of the previously listed technetium compounds for static labeling of the renal cortex can also serve a dual role by being used for renal perfusion imaging. Since ^{99m}Tc has a 6-hour physical half-life and emits no beta radiation, very large numbers of radioactive disintegrations per second can be given without undue patient radiation exposure. The pertechnetate is rapidly injected as a bolus into a peripheral vein to produce a sudden labeling of the peripheral circulation. Organs that receive major portions of cardiac output are readily imaged in photographic exposure sequences. The appearance of pertechnetate in the kidneys during the first few seconds after injection provides a good definition of the intrarenal vascular pools. Renal blood pool imaging must be completed before the pertechnetate ion crosses capillary endothelium to label extracellular fluids. Human serum albumin labeled with ^{99m}Tc would be a longer duration label of the intrarenal blood volume, but it is sufficiently difficult to prepare that the pertechnetate ion provides a good compromise.

Similarly, xenon-133 gas in solution may be introduced into the kidney by arterial catheterization and its washout used in measuring renal blood flow.

Radioisotopic measurements of glomerular filtration rate are less frequently used in general clinical evaluations. Iothalamate is the most satisfactory substance presently available for this purpose. ^{99m}Tc DTPA, a chelated complex, can be prepared by means of a commercial radiopharmaceutical kit or by a more elaborate method, but only the latter provides 100% complexing and a true glomerular agent.

Instrumentation

All of the radiopharmaceuticals discussed above are labeled with gamma radiation emitting isotopes. Gamma radiation is necessary for external detection in in vivo studies. Gamma rays penetrate tissue as do x-rays; beta particles have charge and mass which cause rapid absorption with passage through tissue.

Table 8-2 diagrams the general types of gamma radiation detectors used in kidney tests. Several functions are common to all (Fig 8-1). Each instrument has a gamma radiation detector containing a sodium iodide crystal that converts each gamma ray to a minute flash of light. When the gamma ray is absorbed in the sodium iodide crystal, an instantaneous flash of light (scintillation) is emitted at the point of absorption. The scintillations are detected and converted to electrical pulses by photomultiplier tubes with photosensitive surfaces applied to one surface of the crystal. The magnitude of each electrical pulse is proportionate to the original gamma ray energy and can be analyzed by a spectrometer set to detect only the radiation energy characteristic of the radioisotope being studied. Since each gamma emitting radioisotope emits one or more gamma rays with characteristic radiation energies, spectrometry allows detection of one type of radioisotope in the presence of others. This is analogous to spectrophotometry in which transmission of a range of light of rather limited wavelength is measured to the exclusion of all other wavelengths of light. Once recognized as a preselected gamma ray energy, each of these gamma absorption events is recorded in one of several different ways appropriate to the instrument being used.

In addition to detectors and spectrometers, gamma radiation detecting instrumentation requires a means of limiting the radiation detected to that emitted from an area of interest. This area of interest may be the contents of a test tube, a kidney in vivo, or an even more highly restricted region of interest in vivo. Restriction of the gamma rays absorbed by the detector crystal to gamma rays coming from a selected region of interest requires that the detector crystal be protected from all other gamma rays coming from other regions. This is accomplished by lead shielding. The shielding that protects the crystal from extraneous gamma rays is referred to as ''side shielding'' or '' back shielding.'' The shielding that limits the field of view of the detector crystal is referred to as ''collimation.''

In other respects, the various gamma radiation detecting instruments used in medical diagnosis have differences which suit them to their several uses. These differences are discussed in describing the functions of the various medical types of gamma radiation detecting instrumentation.

Well counters are simple systems designed to count test tube content of radioactivity. The crystal of the detector contains a hole referred to as a ''well'' into which a test tube containing the sample is inserted for in vitro counting. In addition to the basic system, consisting of a detector with a well in the crystal and a spectrometer, the system has a ''scaler'' that registers either the number of counts detected in a preset time or the time required to reach a preset number of counts. These instruments are used for in vitro counting of the type required in glomerular filtration rate determination.

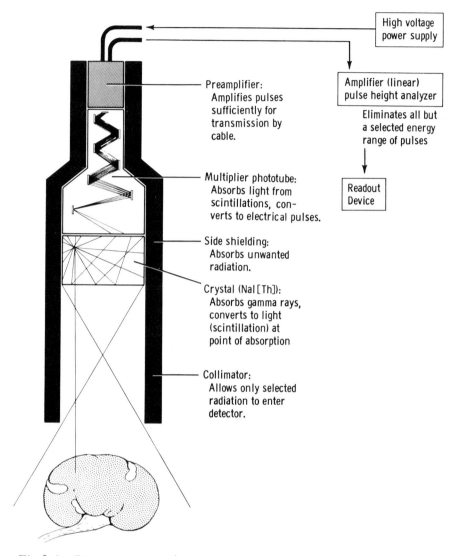

Fig 8-1. Detector. NaI(Th) = thallium-activated sodium iodide crystal.

The **probe counter** is a somewhat more complicated instrument used in radioisotope renography. It has 2 or more detectors which are used to count radioactivity in each kidney, and often a third or fourth field of view such as the bladder or the cardiac blood pool. Each detector has a scintillation crystal with a cylindrical collimator limiting the field of view to a conical geometry, as indicated in Table 8-2. After gamma spectrometry, the radioactive disintegrations detected in each field of view are continuously converted to average count rates by rate meters and then are plotted as functions of time by a recorder. When these instruments are designed principally for radioisotope renography, the collimator is designed so that the field of view will encompass an

entire kidney at the usual kidney depth. The probe counter, therefore, will provide a graphical and numerical recording of radiopharmaceutical content versus time in each kidney and perhaps the cardiac blood pool or bladder. The detectors provide information averaging the events in a whole kidney. This may prove misleading in some patients since the precise location of radioactivity within the kidney is not recorded.

Gamma-imaging instrumentation is designed to provide an image of radioisotope distribution in an organ rather than just to detect the count rate of radioactivity in the region of the organ. Two general types of radioisotope imaging equipment are now in general clinical use: radioisotope scanners and station-

Table 8-2. Differences in radiation detecting instruments.

Instrument	Well Counter	Probe Counter	Rectilinear Scanner	Gamma Camera
Function	Measures radioactivity in a test tube.	Detects radioactivity in a limited region in vivo and records quantitative changes of a radiopharmaceutical versus time.	Forms a life-sized image (planar projection) of the distribution of a radiopharmaceutical in vivo. Moving detector scans area by to and fro motion.	Forms a miniature image of radiopharmaceutical distribution in vivo; records changing distributions (stop-motion images) and numerical data.
Basic Detector Differences	**Note:** Detector orientation is inverted for well counting compared to Fig 8-1. Test tube — Well in crystal	 Cylindrical collimator	 Focused collimator	19 multiplier phototubes determine where each scintillation occurred in crystal. Parallel hole collimator Crystal 1/2 inch thick, 12 inches in diameter
Readout	Scaler: Reads either total counts in a preset time or total time to reach preset count.	Ratemeter and strip chart recorder record count rate as a function of time. (Radioisotope renogram) COUNTS PER MINUTE / TIME	Mechanical positioning of image formation; detector and image move as unit. (a) Tap scan produced by scaler and printer; one print for preset number of counts. (b) Photoscan produced by ratemeter linked x-ray film exposure.	Electronic positioning of imaged event by oscilloscope display of light flash ("dot") at position corresponding to the original gamma ray absorption in the crystal. Oscilloscope display is continuously photographed.

ary imaging devices. Of the latter, only the Anger type of scintillation camera is in general use and will be described here.

The **radioisotope scanner** is a moving detector instrument which makes an image of radiation distribution as it systematically scans the whole region of interest. It detects radiation from a rather specific focus at a distance from the surface of the detector. This is done by means of a lead collimator which has holes converging to a focal point several inches beyond the collimator. Only gamma rays originating from within the focus pass through the holes and into the detector, others being absorbed in the lead septa between the holes and in the side shielding of the detector. As a scanning detector is moved over a subject in a rectilinear raster, a systematic point to point recording of radioactivity count rate is obtained. The results are printed out by a mechanical linkage, either by a "tapper" on paper or by exposure of x-ray film proportional to the count rate detected. The resulting "scan" then shows areas of intense radioactivity as black exposure of the film, and lesser degrees of exposure are roughly proportional to lesser amounts of radioactivity. The necessity for detector motion in a scanner limits these instruments to imaging fairly static distributions of radioactivity.

The **Anger scintillation camera** or **gamma camera** is the most generally used of the newer, stationary detector gamma imaging instruments. The detector of this instrument uses a half-inch thick disk of sodium iodide 12 inches or more in diameter. The field of view is limited to a diameter approximately 2 inches less than the crystal by a lead collimator which has parallel holes perpendicular to the crystal surface. These holes allow only those gamma rays that are vertically oriented to enter the detector. The scintillations produced in the crystal are detected by an array of photomultiplier tubes that allow a computer in the instrument to "take a fix" on where the event occurred in the crystal plane. This is electronically relayed to an oscilloscope that flashes a point of light in a position approximating the originally detected event. The oscilloscope display is photographed continuously to produce photographs composed of large numbers of dots. Each dot recorded came from a gamma ray traveling vertically from its point of origin in the subject; therefore, the dots accumulate to make a pattern representative of the in vivo distribution of the radioisotope imaged. The result is referred to as a "scintiphoto" or "gammaphoto." Because the scintillation camera detector is stationary, continuous photographs can be made showing all the scintillations detected from both kidneys over an interval of time.

The scintiphotograph produced may represent an interval as brief as a few seconds or as long as many minutes. Thus, the scintillation camera allows photography either of static or of rapidly changing distributions of radioisotopic labels. Radioactivity concentration changes are imaged in rapid dynamic studies such as those showing blood flow or in slower dynamic studies such as those following concentration and excretion of a label in the urine. In addition, the information collected with a scintillation camera can be electronically processed to provide numerical information from small defined areas in the field of view. This numerical information can be subjected to computer analysis to provide quantification of regional renal function.

SCINTIPHOTOGRAPHY

Since kidney structure and function evaluation by a scintillation camera combines aspects of most of the other nuclear medicine methods, and the image sequences are efficient means of presenting clinical information, scintiphotography will be discussed first.

The scintillation camera is used to perform kidney evaluations with as many as 3 radiopharmaceuticals in sequence. The studies are performed rapidly and without patient discomfort. Gamma spectroscopy allows imaging of each radioactive label used without interference by previously injected labels. During a scintiphotography study, the patient is maintained in a constant position in relation to the scintillation camera, so that all of the scintiphotos will be exactly comparable. The patient is positioned, and initial studies are done with one of the static renal cortical labels. ("Static" denotes labeling of long duration.) The mercurial diuretics are most commonly used for this purpose.

In our laboratory, mercury-203 chlormerodrin is preferred over mercury-197 chlormerodrin because the higher gamma energy of the ^{203}Hg allows better image resolution in scintiphotography. This is considered to offset the lower radiation dose from comparable microcurie amounts of ^{197}Hg, and the latter is not used except in children. It should be pointed out that, because of the scintillation camera's sensitivity, a considerably lower radioactive dose of either isotope may be used for scintiphotography than would be used for scanning. Mercury-203 chlormerodrin is injected intravenously and the patient studied after 30 minutes or more, which is long enough to allow renal cortical labeling to occur. Later there will be increasingly apparent focal decreases of concentration of chlormerodrin in the regions of the calyceal and pelvic structures. This occurs when the content of chlormerodrin in the urine is reduced to well below the renal cortical content. The rate of accumulation of chlormerodrin in the kidney can be used as an index of renal blood flow, and the total number of counts present in the kidney after labeling has occurred can be used in the same way. The renal image obtainable with chlormerodrin affords an excellent definition of the external contours of the kidney and of the presence of any defects of cortical labeling. Decreased cortical labeling implies abnormal renal cortical metabolism, loss of cortex (scarring), or displacement of normal cortex from an area. Displacement of the cortex occurs with a mass lesion, either benign (usually a cyst) or malignant.

Iodide-131 hippurate excretion studies are also commonly performed using scintiphotography. The hippurate is injected into a peripheral vein with the patient in exactly the same position as that used for obtaining chlormerodrin scintiphotos. A series of scintiphotos is obtained using a constant exposure time and, in addition, keeping all other photographic parameters unchanged. All of the sequence of scintiphotos will then be comparable, and a simultaneous recording of count rate over the kidneys provides radioisotope renograms. If renal function is normal, hippurate scintiphotos are usually obtained at 2-minute intervals. With decreased renal function, it may be best to obtain longer exposures of 4-10 minutes to record significant numbers of counts in each photograph. After extreme reduction of renal function, there is usually insufficient chlormerodrin accumulation for renal visualization, whereas slow accumulation of hippurate often does progress without loss of counts from the kidney. Eventually, renal cortical labeling becomes sufficient that gamma imaging studies can often be conducted with hippurate despite severe reduction of renal function. Delayed views may even show sufficient detail of the renal pelvis and the ureters to rule out obstructive problems in the severely uremic patient.

Hippurate appearance in the kidneys is dependent initially upon renal blood flow. When blood levels fall as a result of renal accumulation and other extravascular loss, renal accumulation of hippurate slows. When the rate of accumulation is exceeded by hippurate loss through urine drainage from the kidney, the radioactivity count rate peaks and falls. Hippurate scintiphotos show the location of the radioactivity in the kidney during these phases of hippurate excretion. The simultaneously recorded renogram tracing is somewhat different from the conventional renogram ob-

tained with a probe detector. The gamma camera counts are obtained from a proportionally greater area surrounding each kidney than is detected by a conventional probe counter. Consequently, the content of radioisotope detected from vascular spaces is usually greater in the scintillation camera renogram than in a probe counted renogram.

Kidney scintiphotos are usually obtained with the patient prone and the abdomen compressed in order to prevent renal rotation and to position the kidneys closer to the detector. Scintiphotos can be obtained in other positions to evaluate the dynamic effects of patient position on renal function. For example, an upright position may cause ureteropelvic junction obstruction or even vascular kinking and renal ischemia in some patients. As demonstrated in Fig 8-5, accumulation of hippurate by ischemic cortex is characteristically quite different from normal accumulation and offers a means by which renal ischemia causing hypertension can be detected. During the drainage phase of a hippurate study, various obstructive problems are easily demonstrated. Even with abdominal compression in the prone position, the normal kidney is rapidly emptied of labeled urine by ureteral peristalsis. Fifteen minutes after injection, the kidney usually contains less than half the number of counts detected at the maximum count rate. Postvoiding residual urine in the bladder can be readily estimated by means of scintiphotos. Cinefluoroscopic studies can be used to detect and evaluate vesicoureteral reflux.

Technetium-99m pertechnetate or other technetium-99m compounds can be used to visualize renal blood flow directly if this additional information is considered useful. After rapid injection of a bolus of pertechnetate into a peripheral vein, a rapid sequence of scintiphotos (usually 4 seconds per photo) is used to obtain images of the sequential appearance of the isotope in the abdominal aorta, the kidneys, the spleen, and, quite late, the liver. The renal blood flow is sufficient that the kidneys are seen as well-defined images with relatively little labeling of surrounding structures. This type of study can be used to determine vascularity in any renal mass lesion. A cold area on a pertechnetate blood flow study would suggest a lack of vascularity and, if spherical, a cyst. An area well labeled by pertechnetate would suggest a vascular tumor, usually a neoplasm. Vascular tumors often fill at a time differing from the time during which the rest of the renal cortex is seen to fill. In neoplastic processes, the surrounding renal cortex and often the whole kidney show the effect of reduced blood flow, which may be due to the local pressure effect of the neoplasm or to invasion of vascular structures.

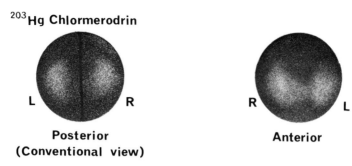

^{203}Hg Chlormerodrin

L   R

**Posterior
(Conventional view)**

R   L

Anterior

A. Horseshoe Kidney

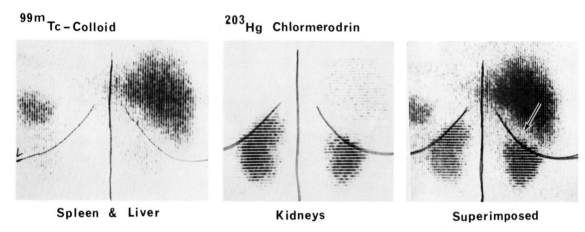

^{99m}Tc – Colloid ^{203}Hg Chlormerodrin

Spleen & Liver   **Kidneys**   **Superimposed**

B. Suprarenal Mass (Adrenal Carcinoma)

Fig 8-2. Use of mercurial diuretic labeling to demonstrate gross structure (A) and mercurial
diuretic plus 99m-technetium colloid to demonstrate abnormal position (B). A: Horseshoe
kidney. B: Suprarenal tumor (adrenal carcinoma).

On the other hand, simple cysts tend to cause
discrete spherical defects without other dis-
turbance of renal cortical blood flow. Although
direct visualization of perfusion patterns with
pertechnetate is helpful in directly determining
vascularity within defined areas of the kidney,
findings with other radiopharmaceuticals are
relied upon to provide additional information
with which to distinguish cysts from vascular
tumors.

All 3 radioisotopic studies can be performed serially in about 40 minutes. If the
patient is uremic, the chlormerodrin study is
omitted. The blood flow distribution evaluation is performed as indicated by the clinical
problem.

EXAMPLES OF
CLINICAL ABNORMALITIES STUDIED
WITH RADIOISOTOPIC TECHNICS

The value of nuclear medicine methods in
the investigation of renal structure and function can be best appreciated by a review of
common clinical findings.

Fig 8-2 illustrates 2 examples of the use
of mercurial diuretic labeling of the kidney to
demonstrate abnormal gross structure or position. In Fig 8-2A, the horseshoe kidney is
more easily identified in an anterior view because the isthmus is better visualized when
the gamma radiation passes through the low-
density tissues anteriorly rather than the
spinal column posteriorly. The spine absorbs
sufficient gamma radiation so that the narrow
band of renal cortex connecting the kidneys is

²⁰³Hg Chlormerodrin

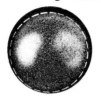

Fig 8-3. **Renal cell carcinoma.** Scintiphoto studies of renal vascular mass. m = minutes; s = seconds.

¹³¹I Hippurate

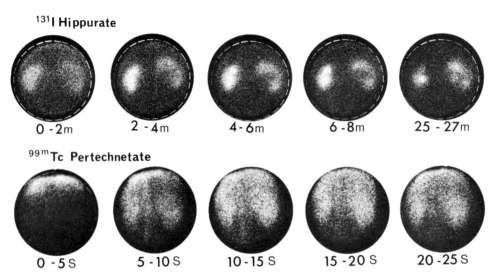

⁹⁹ᵐTc Pertechnetate

²⁰³Hg Chlormerodrin

Fig 8-4. **Renal cyst.** Scintiphoto studies showing non-vascular renal mass. m = minutes; s = seconds.

¹³¹I Hippurate

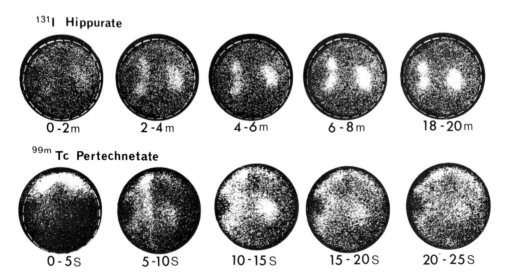

⁹⁹ᵐTc Pertechnetate

difficult to appreciate in the posterior view, although the condition may be suggested by the external contours of the images which appear separate in the posterior view and by the renal axes, which lack normal inclination.

Generally speaking, most renal imaging studies using radioisotopes are obtained with the patient prone and the kidneys viewed posteriorly. In this position, with the application of mid and lower abdominal compression, the kidneys assume a somewhat different position than that seen on the accustomed supine intravenous urograms. In the prone position, the liver shape changes with formation of a space above the right kidney, permitting this kidney to move cephalad. This is in contrast to the position of the same kidney in the supine position, when the liver shape change causes the kidney to move caudad. Fig 8-2B demonstrates kidney position evaluation with a rectilinear scan for demonstration of a suprarenal tumor in the space between the upper pole of the right kidney and the liver. In such combination scans, one radiopharmaceutical is used to label one organ and another label the second

organ, so that a space between the 2 organs may be outlined by the labeled organs.

Figs 8-3 and 8-4 demonstrate scintiphoto studies in which nonvascularized tumors are differentiated from vascular tumors involving the kidney. When the renal cortex is the site of a tumor (Fig 8-3), there are 2 ways in which a defect in a chlormerodrin image may be produced. Normal cortex may be displaced from a tumor site, or there may be interference with the mechanism of tissue labeling, or both. For normal tissue labeling to occur after intravenous introduction of a radiopharmaceutical, blood flow to the area must be normal and the tissue that accumulates the label must have the appropriate metabolic activity. Renal masses will then appear in a chlormerodrin scan or gammaphoto as "cold areas," with absent or reduced labeling surrounded by normally labeled cortex. Typically, a cyst (Fig 8-4) will be seen as a discrete spherical defect which is not associated with decreased localization of the chlormerodrin in the cortex distal to or adjacent to the cyst. Carcinomas tend to cause much more extensive change in the kidney, with large, irregular areas of de-

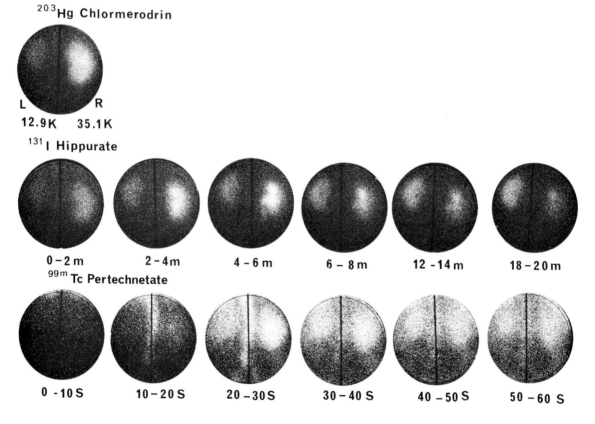

^{203}Hg Chlormerodrin

L   R

12.9K   35.1K

^{131}I Hippurate

0 - 2 m   2 - 4 m   4 - 6 m   6 - 8 m   12 - 14 m   18 - 20 m

^{99m}Tc Pertechnetate

0 - 10 S   10 - 20 S   20 - 30 S   30 - 40 S   40 - 50 S   50 - 60 S

Fig 8-5. Renovascular hypertension, secondary to arteriosclerotic vascular disease.
K = counts per 1000; m = minutes; s = seconds.

creased perfusion in the region of the neoplasm.

To evaluate vascularity of the focal defect, the patient is given a rapid peripheral intravenous injection of ^{99m}Tc-pertechnetate and a series of 5-second scintiphotographs is obtained. If the lesion is seen to be vascularized, the presumption would be that it is a neoplasm. An irregularly shaped renal cortex due to fetal lobulations would be labeled in its entirety, since it is composed of normal parenchyma. After the rapid sequence of blood flow pictures is obtained, an immediate one-minute exposure using greatly diminished dot intensity on the scintillation camera oscilloscope will produce an image of high quality (high data density), showing the renal vascular pool prior to diffusion of the label to extravascular spaces. This method can be particularly valuable in differentiating those renal tumors that have low orders of vascularity, particularly the transitional cell carcinomas.

It is essential that the relative positions of the patient and the camera detector be kept constant for each radiopharmaceutical used, so that regional findings with one radiopharmaceutical can be precisely compared with findings by others.

The camera study is limited by spatial resolution of the instrument for the number of counts detected. This is a function of radioactivity density in the area studied, intrinsic resolution of the detector system, and lack of renal motion during the study. In practice, it may not be possible to visualize renal lesions much less than 1 inch in diameter, although much smaller lesions can theoretically be identified. If a scanning instrument is used rather than a camera, comparable spatial resolution can be achieved but the study is limited to static imaging of chlormerodrin labeling. Hippurate excretion evaluation and blood flow imaging require a stationary detector, ie, a scintillation camera.

The scintiphoto renogram provides an opportunity to determine the presence of regional renal ischemia causing renal vascular hypertension. Fig 8-5 shows the sequential use of 3 radiopharmaceuticals for this purpose. Precise patient positioning is accomplished using chlormerodrin labeling of the renal cortex. The uptake of this label is related to renal blood flow. Any areas of decreased perfusion tend to have diminished chlormerodrin labeling. Next, the patient is studied with iodide-131 hippurate, and a series of gammaphotos with exactly the same photographic exposure characteristics are obtained to show accumulation and then drainage of labeled urine from the kidneys. Hippurate is seen to accumulate less rapidly in an ischemic kidney or in an area of regional renal ischemia. The hallmark of renal vascular ischemia is not the slow accumulation of radioactivity, since that occurs also in other disorders that affect renal function adversely; it is the presence of a prolonged hippurate transit time through the ischemic cortical area when other parts of the same kidney—or the other kidney—show normal transit times. The prolonged transit time results from increased water reabsorption by the ischemic area and consequent delayed washout of label from the kidney. When this occurs in the presence of normal function

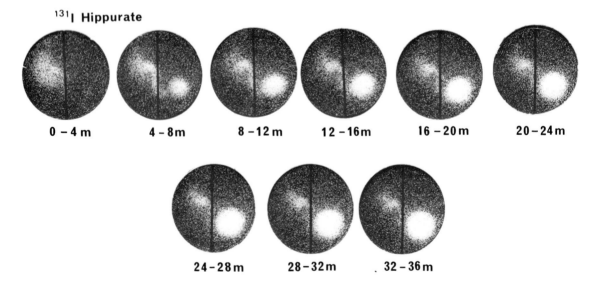

^{131}I Hippurate

| 0 – 4 m | 4 – 8m | 8 –12 m | 12 –16m | 16 – 20 m | 20 – 24 m |

| 24 – 28 m | 28 – 32 m | 32 – 36 m |

Fig 8-6. Transplanted kidney, live donor. (The left half of each scintiphoto shows the kidney, the right half the bladder.) m = minutes.

in other areas, it strongly suggests renovascular ischemia. Such late labeling must be differentiated from obstruction. Following the ^{131}I hippurate evaluation, if direct definition of renal perfusion is desirable, a pertechnetate blood flow study can be performed. Using this triple isotope technic, one can define the site of regional renal ischemia rather than just compare one entire kidney to the other. Furthermore, the hippurate study defines a characteristic physiologic abnormality, much as do the Howard, Stamey, and Rappaport tests. These other tests all require ureteral catheterization and detection of changes in solute concentration or urine volume after admixture of urine from the whole kidney, and this method of collection may mask changes present in regional renal ischemia.

The transplanted kidney study illustrated in Fig 8-6 is an example of several uses of hippurate renography by the scintillation camera. First, this study evaluates the success of the vascular and ureteral anastomoses in the period immediately following transplantation. Good labeling of the entire renal cortex attests to

normal perfusion. If urine is seen to drain normally, patency of the ureteral anastomosis is confirmed. Second, the transplant renogram often demonstrates reduction of function which may be generalized in a rejection reaction, acute tubular necrosis, or other similar process. Focal decrease of hippurate labeling may be observed if there is regional ischemia, partial infarction, or other local change. The rate at which hippurate is accumulated and subsequently drained characterizes progressive changes in renal function with change in rejection activity or other processes. Last, the hippurate scintiphoto study of a transplanted kidney is a good example of slow hippurate transit through a kidney allowing high data density scintiphotos or even scans of the renal cortex. In uremia this often allows better renal visualization than the static images obtained with chlormerodrin.

In evaluation of renal trauma, radioisotopic studies are useful in the diagnosis of extrarenal hematoma, renal lacerations, reduction of renal function secondary to contusion, or urine extravasation. Fig 8-7 demonstrates the ab-

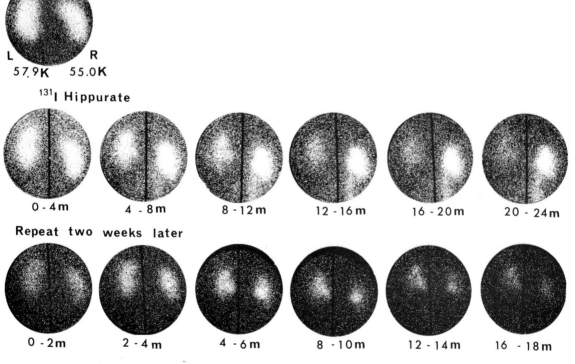

Fig 8-7. Renal trauma, dye sensitivity. K = counts per 1000; m = minutes.

normalities seen in a case of simple renal contusion and the clearing of this abnormality 2 weeks later.

The hippurate gamma-imaged urogram is also useful in studying the renal pelvis, ureters, and bladder. In renal obstructive disease, the renogram often defines structures well enough to provide a general idea of the severity of the obstruction without having to perform retrograde urography or other involved procedures. Gamma-imaged urograms may obviate the need for retrograde studies in patients hypersensitive to contrast media, since the iodide content of radioiodinated hippurate is insufficient to cause iodide sensitivity. Other uses would include screening uremics for obstructive uropathy, evaluation of male infants, and follow-up of surgically corrected obstruction for patency and functional status.

While definition of individual calyceal structure and other fine detail is not even within an order of magnitude of the resolution available on a conventional radiographic study, a gamma-photo study is sufficient for many clinical purposes. It presents enough detail so that more complicated studies may not be required. The use of hippurate in evaluation of reflux and other lower genitourinary problems has had only limited exploration, although it should be a promising method.

THE RADIOISOTOPE RENOGRAM

The radioisotope renogram is an older method for radioisotopic evaluation of the kidney. It is still useful as a screening test. The renogram consists of recording radioactive count rate over each kidney as a function of time to produce a tracing representing function in each kidney. The familiar renogram should be more readily understood after the foregoing discussion of renal scintiphotography.

In essence, the renogram consists of 3 portions which may be described as the vascular phase, the function phase, and the drainage phase. The vascular phase is simply the period during which the count rate rapidly rises in each kidney with the initial appearance of the radioiodinated hippurate in the intravascular spaces of the kidney and prior to similar labeling of other surrounding organs. The vascular phase is best understood by referring to scintiphotos of pertechnetate appearance just after injection. (See Figs 8-3, 8-4, and 8-5.) During the function phase of the renogram, the increase of count rate over the kidneys is nearly linear. The hippurate blood level is almost constant for the first few minutes after postinjection mixing, and the cortex

extracts hippurate from the blood at a constant rate for 3-8 minutes after injection of the hippurate until drainage of urine from the kidney begins to occur. As this drainage continues, it exceeds the rate of accumulation of hippurate, and the count rate tracing begins to decrease. A normally hydrated prone patient with normal urine drainage will show peaking of count rate at 3-8 minutes and then a fall of count rate to less than half of the maximum within 15 minutes. In the sitting position, the peak occurs somewhat earlier and the fall is more rapid. Because a conventional renogram detector has a limited field of view, extrarenal blood levels make a smaller contribution to the renogram count rate tracing than is the case when the scintillation camera is used to produce a renogram in conjunction with scintiphotos. Each half of the circular camera field of view is recorded separately, and a larger area surrounding the kidney is observed.

Fig 8-8 summarizes the several abnormalities which may be detected by conventional radioisotope renography using iodide-131 hippurate. It must be realized that the renogram reflects not only events from within the kidney but those of the surrounding "nontarget" structures as well. As can readily be seen from the preceding illustrations of pertechnetate renal blood flow studies, initial labeling of the area after peripheral intravenous injection of an isotope is largely renal labeling. After initial mixing, there is much greater contribution of counts from other blood vascular pools, notably the spleen and the liver. The spleen appears much earlier than the liver, due to the difference in their predominant mode of perfusion. Although the radioisotope renogram does not easily distinguish abnormality in part of a kidney from abnormality involving the whole kidney, it does provide a considerable volume of information, as may be appreciated from the outline presented with Fig 8-8. For example, the renogram in the presence of renovascular ischemia causing hypertension would be expected to show a slowed rate of count rate increase in the vascular phase plus a diminished increase of count rate compared to the other kidney; a slowed accumulation of hippurate in the function phase (greater than a 5% difference in slope when the 2 tracings are compared); a delay of the peak due to increased free water reabsorption and prolongation of hippurate transit time through the cortex and drainage structures; and a slowed drainage phase. Obstruction affecting the drainage structures might cause some renogram abnormalities that would be easily mistaken for those of renovascular ischemia, but in general the vascular phase and the function phase would be less affected than the drainage phase. The renogram is a valuable study in laboratories where it is

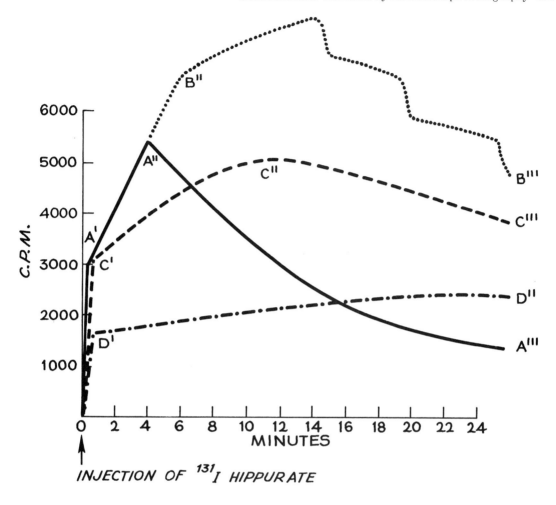

Fig 8-8. Summary of several abnormalities detected by radioisotope renography using iodide-131 hippurate. C.P.M. = counts per minute. Solid line: Normal renogram idealized as O-A′-A″-A‴. O-A′ = Vascular phase. Initial vascular labeling detected. A′-A″ = Function phase. Hippurate accumulation by renal cortical cells recorded. A″-A‴ = Drainage phase. Drainage exceeds accumulation; count rate decreases. **Dotted line:** Renogram of mild obstruction. O-A′ = No change from normal. A′-B″ = Accumulation of counts prolonged in function phase. B″-B‴ = Poorly defined broad peak and slowed drainage phase. Steps down in count rate suggest intermittent flow. **Dashed line:** Renogram of renovascular ischemia; normal renovascular volume. O-C′ = Vascular labeling delayed but similar in amount to normal. C′-C″ = Decreased function; decreased rate of accumulation. C″-C‴ = Increased water reabsorption; decreased urine volume; slowing of hippurate drainage. **Dash-dotted line:** Renogram typical of severe ischemia or nephritis and reduced function. O-D′ = Delayed and reduced vascular labeling. D′-D″ = Extreme slowing of hippurate accumulation; little drainage. The finding of normal function in one kidney and of abnormal function in the other kidney would indicate that renograms O-C‴ or O-D″ are related to unilateral disease typical of renovascular ischemia which may be functionally significant in causing hypertension. Finding of bilateral and symmetric renogram abnormality would indicate a generalized renal disease which, in terms of the renogram, could be glomerulonephritis, pyelonephritis, acute tubular necrosis, or the result of renal vascular disease.

used frequently and norms are well established. An entirely normal renogram is an excellent assurance that no major problem exists in the kidney.

CLEARANCE METHODS

Although radiopharmaceuticals and gamma detection procedures are currently used to study renal clearance more as a research tool than as a general diagnostic procedure, these methods bear considerable promise in clinical practice. In particular, the radioiodinated iothalamate test of glomerular filtration is reproducible and easy to perform, requiring only a single blood sample and a determination of count rate decrease in an intravascular space defined by a probe collimator. Hippurate clearance determinations provide information about renal blood flow, but they are less reproducible except in the presence of reduced renal function.

Radioisotopic determinations are much simpler than the chemical determinations of the standard clearance evaluation materials, inulin and para-aminohippurate. Evaluation of renal hemodynamics by these methods will no doubt become a much more frequently used clinical tool in the next few years.

BONE SCANNING

No discussion of radioisotopic methods in urology would be complete without mentioning bone scanning. ^{85}Sr, ^{18}F (Fig 8-9), and other bone-seeking radiopharmaceuticals provide means of detecting bone metastases long before radiographic bone changes are seen. Since patients with renal cell or prostatic carcinoma have a high incidence of bone metastases, bone scanning often is useful in urologic diagnosis. (See also Carcinoma of the Prostate.)

BONE SCANS WITH ^{18}F FLUORIDE

Prostatic carcinoma (roentgenograms negative)

Renal cell carcinoma

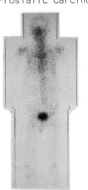 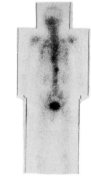 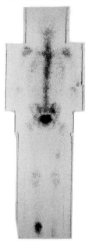

Anterior Probe   Posterior Probe   Superimposed
                                     Anterior and
                                     Posterior Scans

Superimposed
Anterior and
Posterior Scans

Fig 8-9. Bone scans with ^{18}F fluoride. Left: Three whole body scans of a patient with prostatic carcinoma metastatic to bone, predominantly the lumbar and dorsal vertebrae. Roentgenograms were negative. Note that the lesions are best shown in the posterior scan due to a laminographic effect but that the anterior and posterior scans can be superimposed to show all bone areas. **Right:** One superimposed whole body scan image of a patient with renal cell carcinoma metastatic to the distal right tibia, left mid femur, and left sacroiliac joint area. This scan illustrates the importance of long bone scanning in addition to scanning the axial skeleton.

•   •   •

General References

Andrews, G. A., Kniseley, R. M., & H. N. Wagner, Jr. (editors): Radioactive Pharmaceuticals, AEC Symposium Series No. 6. Division of Technical Information, US Atomic Energy Commission, 1966.

Hine, G. J. (editor): Instrumentation in Nuclear Medicine, Vol I. Academic Press, 1967.

Morris, J. G., & others: The diagnosis of renal tumors by radioisotope scanning. J Urol 97:40-55, 1967.

Maxwell, M. H., & others: Radioisotope renogram in renal arterial hypertension. J Urol 100:376-83, 1968.

Powell, M. R.: Clinical applications of the scintillation camera. In: Nuclear Medicine, 2nd ed. W. H. Blahd (editor). McGraw-Hill, 1971.

Powell, M. R.: Clinical uses of radionuclides: Critical comparison with other techniques. To be published in AEC Symposium Series No. 21. Evaluation of Kidney Structure and Function of Radioisotope Imaging. Division of Technical Information, US Atomic Energy Commission, 1972.

Rosenthal, L.: Ortho-iodohippurate-I^{131} kidney scanning in renal failure. Radiology 78: 298-303, 1966.

Shuler, S. E.: The scintillation camera in pediatric renal disease. Am J Dis Child 120:115-21, 1970.

9...

Instrumental Examination
of the Urinary Tract

PRELIMINARY PROCEDURES

Aseptic Technic

Instruments must be prepared and used in
an aseptic manner. Rubber catheters and
metal sounds can be boiled; silk-woven catheters, both urethral and ureteral, may be sterilized in antiseptic solutions (eg, quaternary
ammonium chlorides, mercuric oxycyanide)
or, preferably, autoclaved or gas sterilized.
Optical instruments are sterilized chemically
(never autoclaved).

The glans penis should be washed thoroughly with soap and water or an antiseptic solution.
The vulva must be cleansed and the labia held
apart as the instrument is introduced.

It should be pointed out that because of the
presence of bacteria in the distal urethra it is
impossible to pass an instrument in a completely sterile manner. Secondary cystitis rarely
occurs, however, unless there is residual
urine in the bladder.

Lubrication of Urethra

Catheters and other instruments must not
be passed into the urinary tract without proper
lubrication. In women, it is sufficient to dip
the instrument in the lubricant. In men, however, such a procedure is inadequate because
the meatus removes the lubricant and the instrument then passes over a relatively dry
mucous membrane. The male urethra can be
lubricated only by instilling at least 15 ml of a
sterile water-soluble lubricant. This is best
accomplished with a glass syringe which has
a rubber bulb on one end. It should have a
blunt tip so that it does not have to be passed
down the urethra. Oils (eg, mineral oil or
olive oil) must not be used, since fatal oil emboli have resulted from their use. The syringe
serves not only to introduce the column of lubricant into the canal but also, by virtue of the
constant, steady pressure required, to overcome the normal tone of the external sphincter
muscle. This resistance may be increased if
the patient is apprehensive. Inexperienced
instrumentalists frequently have difficulty introducing catheters against the force of this

spasm, and this has resulted in many false
diagnoses of "urethral stricture."

Anesthesia

A barbiturate administered 30-45 minutes
before instrumentation allays apprehension.
As an alternative measure, morphine, 8 mg,
or a similar narcotic can be given intravenously 5-10 minutes before the instrument is inserted.

Local anesthesia is indicated before instrumentation, although this is less effective
in men than in women. The female urethra is
best anesthetized by introducing a solution of
10% cocaine on a cotton applicator and leaving
it in the canal for 5 minutes. With this technic,
instrumentation is almost without discomfort.
In men, really effective anesthetic agents (ie,
cocaine) cannot be instilled for they are easily
absorbed through the posterior urethra and
prostate into the circulatory system and may
cause sudden collapse and even death. Less
toxic drugs must therefore be used, and these
are usually less efficient. They may be incorporated into the lubricating jelly. These
solutions or jellies are retained in the urethra
by placing a clamp on the glans for 5 minutes.
The useful anesthetic agents, in decreasing
order of efficacy, are 2% lidocaine (Xylocaine®)
or 0.5% diclonine hydrochloride (Dyclone®),
0.5% piperocaine (Metycaine®), and 5% procaine (Novocain®).

General anesthesia should be used if the
patient is apprehensive or if biopsy or other
painful manipulations are necessary. Thio-
pental (Pentothal®) is ideal for short cystoscopic procedures, but spinal anesthesia may
prove more useful if x-rays are to be taken,
since the patient can be asked to cooperate by
holding his breath at the proper time. Explo-
sive agents (eg, ether) are contraindicated if
electrocoagulation is to be employed.

Warning to Patient

Instrumentation is always uncomfortable
and may be painful. It is essential to warn all
patients that this discomfort will occur and to
warn men that the discomfort will be greater
as the instrument passes through the prostatic

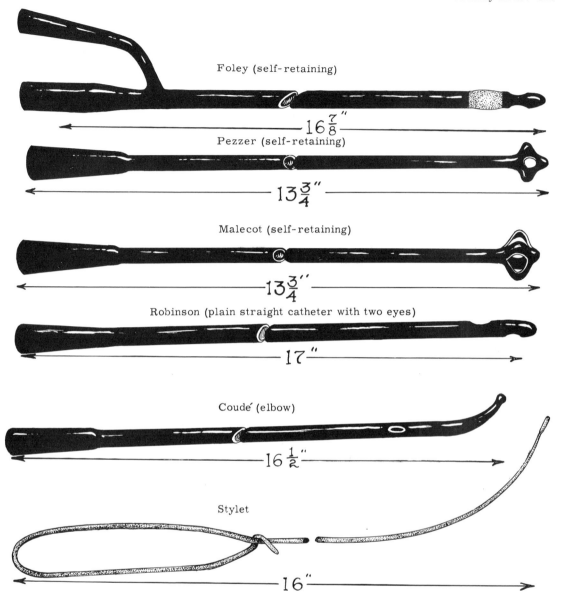

Fig 9-1. Types of catheters; catheter stylet.

urethra. No movement should be rough or abrupt; pick up the instrument slowly, introduce it gently, and advance it gradually. Failure to do these things will cause distrust and apprehension on the part of the patient. Spasm of the external sphincter may develop, in which case instrumentation is made more difficult or even impossible.

Calibration and Size of Instruments

Instruments are most commonly calibrated in the USA according to the French (F) scale. Each number on the scale equals 0.33 mm.

Therefore, a 30 F sound has a diameter of 10 mm.

Each number on the American (A) and English (E) scales equals 0.5 mm; the English scale is 2 numbers less than the American. Hence, 10 mm = 30 F = 20 A = 18 E; and 6 mm = 18 F = 12 A = 10 E.

Getzoff, P. L.: A safe and effective topical anesthetic for office cystoscopy. J Urol **99**:118-21, 1968.

Ulm, A. H., & E. C. Wagshul: Pulmonary embolization with an oily medium. New England J Med **263**:137-9, 1960.

THE CATHETER

Catheters are used for diagnostic purposes to explore the urethra for stenoses or injury, to discover residual urine in the bladder after voiding, and to introduce contrast medium into the bladder. They are used therapeutically to relieve urinary retention.

Types and Sizes of Catheters (See Fig 9-1.)

Soft rubber catheters should be used in most instances since they cause less trauma and are easier to manipulate past enlarged prostatic lobes than less flexible instruments. If for any reason a soft rubber catheter fails to pass (eg, it may impinge on the base of a lobe which occupies most of the posterior part of the bladder neck), a stiffer silk-woven coudé (elbow) catheter (which has a bent tip) should be tried. If the catheter is to be left in place (indwelling), a self-retaining (balloon) catheter should be utilized. It may be necessary or advantageous to leave a plain catheter (Robinson) in the bladder; it must then be taped in place (Fig 9-3).

In general, it is a mistake to try to pass small catheters in men (12-14 F); they lack body and are apt to coil up at the external sphincter. Catheterization is really less traumatic and more successful if instruments of adequate size (20-22 F) are used. The larger catheters are also better suited for exploring the urethra for stricture. The urethra of a girl age 6 will easily accept a 14 F catheter. The urethra of a boy of the same age will take a 12 F catheter.

Technic of Catheterization

A. In Men: After proper cleansing and anesthesia, the catheter can be manipulated with a sterile-gloved hand. It is simpler, however, to grasp the catheter near its tip with a sterile clamp and to hold the other end of the catheter between the 4th and 5th fingers of the same hand. The catheter can then be advanced with the clamp without being touched by the unsterile hand (Fig 9-2). The penis must be stretched taut with the other hand to eliminate urethral redundancy.

If an impassable stricture is encountered, it will be necessary to dilate the urethra with sounds (Fig 9-4) or with filiforms and followers (Figs 9-5 and 9-6).

If a stylet is used (Fig 9-1), the lumen of the catheter should be lubricated before the stylet is inserted; otherwise the stylet will be difficult to remove after passage of the instrument. The technic of passing a catheter with a stylet is similar to that for passing sounds. The catheter should be drawn taut over the stylet so that its tip cannot become dislodged, pass out through the "eye" of the catheter, and traumatize the urethra.

Do not partially withdraw the styleted catheter and then readvance it. The resulting drag on the catheter may allow the tip of the stylet to protrude through the distal opening of the catheter and cause urethral injury. At times it is helpful to guide stiff instruments with a finger in the rectum. When the catheter has been successfully passed, the stylet is removed.

B. In Women: A short metal catheter is more satisfactory than other types since it can be manipulated with one hand while the other holds the labia apart. Rubber catheters can also be used. Those made of glass are contraindicated; small cracks or chips may abrade the mucosa. A self-retaining (Foley) catheter can be used if constant drainage is indicated. A Pezzer or Malecot catheter introduced on a catheter stylet is also satisfactory. A plain catheter can be used for this purpose by taping it to the labial area (after shaving).

Desautels, R. E.: The causes of catheter-induced urinary infections and their prevention. J Urol **101**:757-60, 1969.

METAL SOUNDS

Metal (stainless steel or nickel-plated steel) sounds may be used instead of catheters to explore the urethra for stenoses. Their major use, however, is in the treatment of stricture.

Technic of Passing a Sound

A. In Men: With the penis stretched taut and the instrument held almost horizontally (over the groin), the tip of the sound is introduced into the urethra. When the tip reaches the bulb (at the external sphincter), the handle is brought to the vertical position, which usually enables the tip to pass through the sphincter. Moving the handle to the horizontal position (parallel to the thighs) causes the sound to advance into the bladder. (See Fig 9-4.)

The first sound passed should be a 24 F, even though the patient says he has a narrow stricture. This size has a broad tip which will not perforate a friable urethral wall and is therefore ideal for urethral exploration. If a 24 F sound cannot be passed, smaller sounds can be tried. If a 20 F will not pass, do not use the smaller sizes, for their tips are relatively sharp and may pierce the urethral wall. In this instance use filiforms and followers, which are much safer (Figs 9-5 and 9-6).

B. In Women: Because of the short and relatively straight canal of the female urethra, the passage of sounds is quite simple in women.

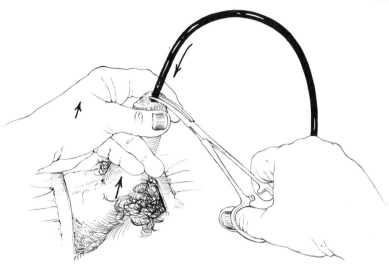

Fig 9-2. Technic of catheterization. A sterile water-soluble lubricant is first instilled into the urethra by means of a bulb syringe. The penis is drawn taut with one hand. The catheter, held near its tip with a sterile clamp, is introduced into the urethra; the other end of the catheter is held between the 4th and 5th fingers of the hand holding the clamp. The clamp is then moved up on the catheter and the catheter introduced farther into the urethra.

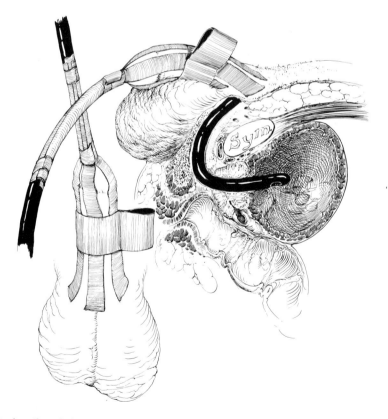

Fig 9-3. Taping the plain catheter in place in the male. Four strips of 1/2-inch adhesive tape are placed on the penis and catheter. They are bound to the catheter by 2 pieces of 1/2-inch tape just distal to the glans and at the point where they terminate on the catheter. A piece of 1-inch tape is placed about the midpenis in such manner that a loop is formed which will separate if erection occurs.

Example of a sound.

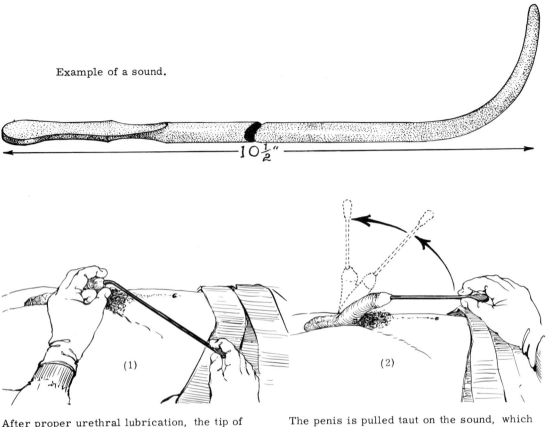

$10\frac{1}{2}"$

(1)

After proper urethral lubrication, the tip of
the sound enters the urethra. The sound
is in the horizontal position over the groin.

(2)

The penis is pulled taut on the sound, which
is advanced down the urethra and moved
simultaneously to the midline; its handle
is gradually moved to the vertical position.

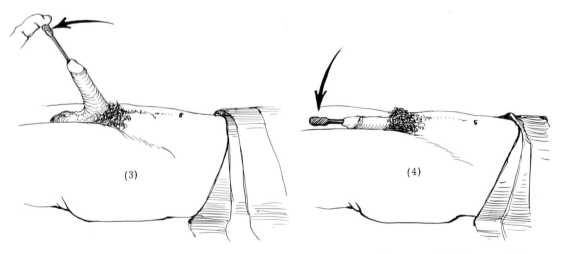

(3)

The sound will usually pass through the external urinary sphincter if pressure is
exerted on the handle at right angles to
its shaft with one finger.

(4)

When the sound has passed all the way into
the bladder it should be possible to rotate
it freely. (The curved part of the sound
is lying free in the vesical cavity.)

Fig 9-4. Passing a sound through the male urethra.

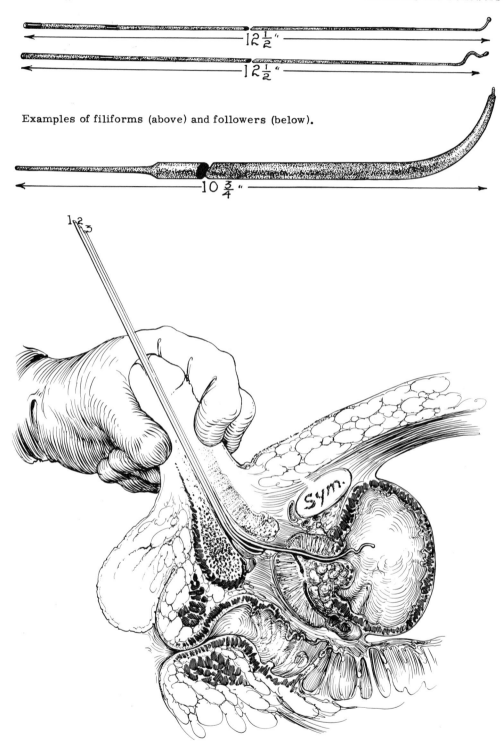

Examples of filiforms (above) and followers (below).

Fig 9-5. Technic of passage of filiforms. After proper urethral lubrication, a filiform is advanced down the urethra; the penis is held taut. If the filiform is arrested at any point, it is partially withdrawn, rotated, and advanced again. If it still fails to pass, 2 or more filiforms are inserted in the urethra. Each filiform in turn is advanced, withdrawn, rotated, and readvanced. One of them will usually pass to the bladder. (Passing of follower is shown in Fig 9-6.)

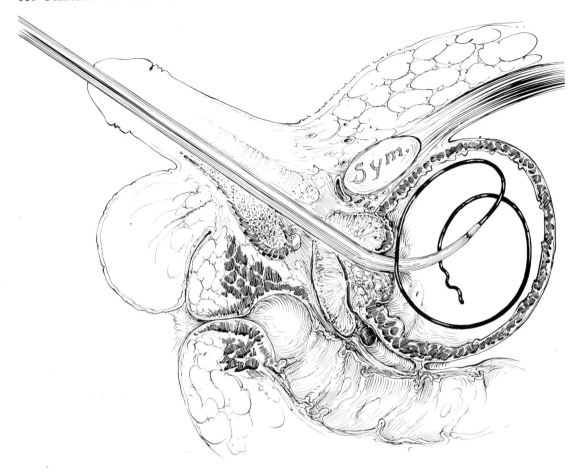

Fig 9-6. Passing the follower. When a filiform passes into the bladder, a small follower is screwed into the filiform and advanced to the bladder, using the same technic as for passage of a sound (Fig 9-5).

Significant stricture is rare, although moderate stenoses are commonly found and are often the cause of chronic or recurrent cystitis, particularly in little girls.

FILIFORMS AND FOLLOWERS

Filiforms and followers are the instruments of choice for dilating narrow strictures. Catheterizing followers may be used to catheterize men with narrow strictures.

Types and Sizes

Filiforms are made of woven silk or plastic material and must be quite pliable. Useful sizes are 3-6 F. Numerous filiform tips are available, but the coudé and corkscrew types are most useful. The free end of the filiform is equipped with a female thread.

The follower may be made of metal or of woven pliable silk. Useful sizes are 8-30 F. It may be solid or it may be hollow to allow simultaneous catheterization. Its end has a male thread which may be easily screwed into the filiform.

Technic of Passing Filiforms

After lubricant jelly has been instilled into the urethra, the filiform is introduced. If it is arrested, it must be partially withdrawn, rotated, and readvanced. If this fails, one or more filiforms should be added and all manipulated in turn. When one finally passes down to its hilt without resistance, its tip has entered the bladder. The appropriate follower is then screwed into the filiform in a clockwise direction and advanced down the urethra. (See Figs 9-5 and 9-6.)

BOUGIES À BOULE

These olive-tipped bougies (Fig 9-7) are useful in calibrating the urethra, particularly in little girls (see chapter 25). Bougies of increasing size should be used until one passes with some resistance. On withdrawal, there will be a snap as the bougie's broad shoulders pass through the stenotic area.

but the 2 most useful are the cystoscope and the panendoscope. They come in sizes varying between 12-26 F; therefore, even very young patients may be examined.

A. Cystoscope: The cystoscopic view is largely at right angles to the shaft of the instrument. It has a wide-angle lens and is therefore best for inspection of the bladder. It visualizes the prostatic urethra only fairly

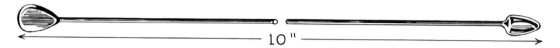

Fig 9-7. Bougie à boule.

CYSTOMETER

The cystometer is a diagnostic instrument which measures the tone of the detrusor in relation to the volume of fluid in the bladder. It evaluates both normal and pathologic physiology of bladder function and contributes much to the management of the patient suffering from vesical dysfunction secondary to disease or trauma of the nervous system. A simple cystometer is illustrated in Fig 9-8.

Technic

The apparatus is so arranged that the zero mark on the manometer is level with the symphysis pubis. Care should be taken that all air is removed from the tubing. As sterile water or normal saline solution is slowly introduced (60-120 drops/minute) into the indwelling catheter, the intravesical pressure is measured on the manometer. As each 50 ml are added, the pressure on the manometer is recorded in relation to the total volume of fluid introduced. The patient is asked to describe all sensations experienced, including the desire to void. These remarks are recorded at the appropriate points on the cystometrogram. When a strong involuntary urge to void occurs, this pressure should be noted.

Marshall, S.: A disposable cystometer. J Urol **91**:458-9, 1964.

CYSTOSCOPY AND PANENDOSCOPY

Useful Instruments

Many instruments have been devised for the visual inspection of the bladder and urethra,

well and the distal (and female) urethra not at all.

B. Panendoscope: The panendoscope has a smaller field of vision; its view is almost in line with the shaft of the instrument. Therefore, the portion of the bladder near the bladder neck cannot be seen unless a "retrograde" lens is used with it. This instrument, however, is excellent for visualization of the urethra distal to the neck of the bladder. These instruments, then, complement each other.

Uses

A. Diagnostic Uses: Complete endoscopic studies are among the most precise diagnostic tests in all medicine.

1. Direct inspection - The cystoscope and pandendoscope make possible visualization of the bladder wall for such diseases as tumor, stone, and ulcer. The configuration and position of the ureteral orifices are of paramount importance when vesicoureteral reflux is suspected. The degree of obstruction from an enlarged prostate and urethral stricture, polyp, or tumor may be seen. Biopsy of neoplasms can be made.

2. "Sterile" urine specimen, relative renal function - Through these instruments clean specimens of urine can be taken from the bladder for bacteriologic study. Catheters can be passed to the renal pelves for the collection of urine specimens and the separate measurement of renal function (ie, PSP test).

3. Through these ureteral catheters, radiopaque material can be introduced so that perfect "casts" of the calyces, pelves, and ureters can be observed on x-ray films.

4. The presence of vesicoureteral reflux can be ascertained by filling the bladder with sterile water to which indigo carmine or

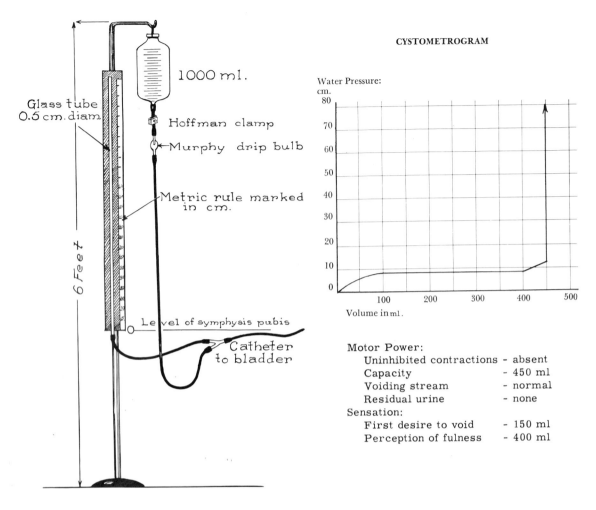

CYSTOMETROGRAM

Water Pressure:
cm.

Volume in ml.

Motor Power:
    Uninhibited contractions - absent
    Capacity   - 450 ml
    Voiding stream   - normal
    Residual urine   - none
Sensation:
    First desire to void   - 150 ml
    Perception of fulness   - 400 ml

Fig 9-8. Cystometer and normal cystogram. The pressure in the normal bladder remains at about 8-15 cm of water until capacity (350-500 ml) is reached, at which time the intravesical pressure rises sharply to or above 100 cm of water. Involuntary voiding then occurs around the catheter. No uninhibited contractions occur, and there is no residual urine.

A spastic neurogenic bladder (Fig 19-6) exhibits uninhibited contractions as demonstrated by transient increases in intravesical pressure as fluid is introduced into the bladder. In either case, involuntary voiding around the catheter occurs at relatively low volumes (50-300 ml).

The tone of the flaccid neurogenic bladder (Fig 19-8) is impaired. Thus, intravesical pressure remains low (6-10 ml), there are no uninhibited contractions, and no final involuntary voiding pressure develops even when the bladder is filled with 500 or even 1000 ml of water; vesical capacity is increased.

methylene blue has been added. After the patient voids, cystoscopy is performed. If blue fluid is seen emanating from a ureteral orifice, reflux has been demonstrated.

B. Therapeutic Uses: Many diseases of the bladder and urethra lend themselves to transurethral treatment. Tumors can be biopsied and resected. Ureteral stones can be manipulated.

The Major Indications for Cystoscopy or Panendoscopy and Ureteral Catheterization

These technics are indicated for the evaluation of hematuria, chronic or recurrent urinary infection, unexplained urologic symptoms (eg, enuresis, frequency), and evaluation of congenital anomalies, which are very commonly found in the genitourinary tract. They are useful also in any clinical situation in which excretory urograms have suggested pathologic change but have not furnished all the information necessary for definitive diagnosis and treatment.

Contraindications to Cystoscopy or Panendoscopy

Cystoscopy and panendoscopy are contraindicated in acute urinary tract infection (trauma may exacerbate the infection) and in the presence of severe symptoms of prostatic obstruction, since trauma may produce just enough edema of the bladder neck to cause complete urinary retention. Of course, if cystoscopy must be done, this risk must be taken.

Amar, A.D., & K. Chabra: Reduction of radiation exposure of children during urologic diagnosis including a non-radiographic method of demonstrating vesicoureteral reflux. Pediatrics **35**:960-6, 1965.

RESECTOSCOPE AND LITHOTRITE

Resectoscope

The resectoscope is a commonly used visual instrument with which transurethral resection of the prostate or of vesical carcinoma is performed.

Lithotrite

The lithotrite allows the urologist to crush smaller vesical calculi transurethrally.

REACTIONS TO INSTRUMENTATION

Urethra and Bladder (Sounds, Cystoscopy)

Some bleeding is to be expected in men. Burning on urination and frequency may be noted because of trauma to the mucous membrane. Acute urinary retention may develop in men suffering from moderate prostatism. This may be due to edema from the instrumentation. Exacerbation of lower tract infection may occur. Epididymitis may develop if prostatocystitis is present. "Urethral chill" (which is really due to bacteremia from an infected prostate traumatized by instrumentation or vesicoureteral reflux) may occur.

Ureters and Kidney (Ureteral Catheterization, Urography)

Nausea, vomiting, and abdominal cramps are often experienced from overdistention of the renal pelves with radiopaque material. Renal and ureteral pain and colic (from overdistention) or ureteral edema (from trauma) may ensue. Bleeding may occur if the tip of a catheter pierces the renal parenchyma. Exacerbation of kidney infection may develop, or new infection may be introduced. Temporary anuria is rare; it may be caused by excessive ureteral edema from instrumentation or sensitivity to the pyelographic medium.

• • •

10 ...
Urinary Obstruction and Stasis

Because of their damaging effect on renal function, obstruction and stasis of urinary flow are among the most important of urologic disorders. Either leads eventually to hydronephrosis, a peculiar type of atrophy of the kidney which may terminate in renal insufficiency or, if unilateral, complete destruction of the organ. Furthermore, obstruction leads to infection, which causes additional damage to the organs involved.

Etiology
Congenital anomalies, more common in the urinary tract than in any other organ system, are most commonly obstructive. In adult life many acquired obstructions occur.

A. Congenital: The common sites of congenital narrowing are just inside the external urinary meatus in little girls, posterior urethral valves, and the ureterovesical and ureteropelvic junctions. Another congenital cause of urinary stasis is damage to sacral roots 2-4 as seen in spina bifida and myelomeningocele.

B. Acquired: Acquired obstructions are numerous and may be primary in the urinary tract or secondary to extra-urologic lesions which invade or compress the urinary passages. Among the common causes are (1) urethral stricture secondary to infection or injury; (2) benign prostatic hyperplasia, or cancer of the prostate; (3) vesical tumor involving the bladder neck or one or both ureterovesical orifices; (4) local extension of cancer of the prostate or cervix into the base of the bladder, occluding the ureters; (5) compression of the ureters at the pelvic brim by metastatic nodes from malignancy of the prostate or cervix; and (6) ureteral stone.

Neurogenic dysfunction is commonly acquired and affects primarily the bladder. The upper tracts are damaged secondarily by ureterovesical obstruction or reflux and, often, complicating infection. Severe constipation in women and children can cause bilateral hydroureteronephrosis from compression of the lower ureters.

Elongation and kinking of the ureter secondary to vesicoureteral reflux commonly leads to ureteropelvic obstruction and hydronephrosis. Unless a voiding cystourethrogram is obtained in all children having this lesion, the primary cause may be missed and improper treatment applied.

Pathogenesis and Pathology
Obstruction and neurovesical dysfunction have the same effects upon the urinary tract. These changes can best be understood by considering (1) the effects upon the lower tract (distal to the bladder neck) of severe external urinary meatal stricture, and (2) the effects upon the mid tract (bladder) and upper tract (ureter and kidney) of benign prostatic hyperplasia.

A. Lower Tract: Hydrostatic pressure proximal to the obstruction causes dilatation of the urethra. The wall of the urethra may become thin, and a diverticulum may form. If the urine becomes infected, spontaneous urethral rupture with urinary extravasation may occur. The prostatic ducts may become widely dilated.

B. Mid Tract: In the earlier stages (compensatory phase), the muscle wall of the bladder becomes thickened. With decompensation, it may be thinned and, therefore, weakened.

1. Stage of compensation - In order to balance the increasing urethral resistance, the bladder musculature hypertrophies. Its thickness may double. Complete emptying of the bladder is thus made possible.

Little more than hypertrophied muscle may be seen microscopically, although the effects of infection are often superimposed. In case of secondary infection, there may be edema of the submucosa, which may be infiltrated with plasma cells, lymphocytes, and polymorphonuclear cells.

At cystoscopy, surgery, or autopsy, visual evidence of this compensation is demonstrated in the following ways (Fig 10-1):

a. Trabeculation of the bladder wall - The wall of the distended bladder is normally quite smooth. With hypertrophy, individual muscle bundles stand out taut and give a coarsely interwoven appearance to the mucosal surface. The

114

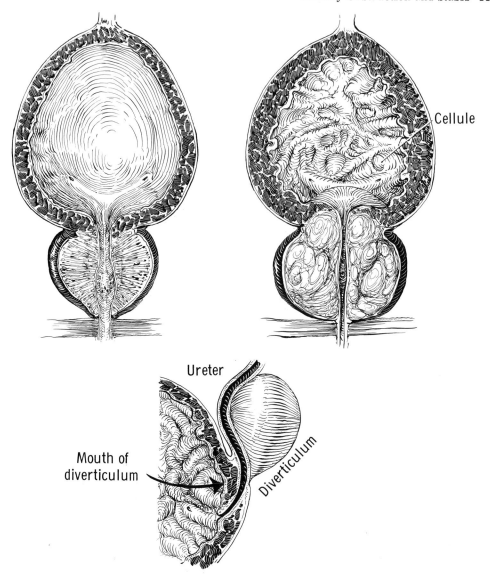

Fig 10-1. Changes in the bladder developing from obstruction. Above left: Normal bladder and prostate. **Above right:** Obstructing prostate causing trabeculation, cellule formation, and hypertrophy of the interureteric ridge. **Below:** Marked trabeculation (hypertrophy) of the vesical musculature; diverticulum displacing left ureter.

trigonal muscle and the interureteric ridge, which normally are only slightly raised above the surrounding tissues, respond to obstruction by hypertrophy of their smooth musculature. The ridge then becomes a prominent structure. This trigonal hypertrophy causes increased resistance in the intravesical ureteral segments due to accentuated downward pull upon them. It is this mechanism that causes relative stenosis of the ureterovesical junctions leading to hydroureteronephrosis. In the presence of significant residual urine,

which further stretches the ureterotrigonal complex, further obstruction ensues. (A urethral catheter will relieve this somewhat; definitive prostatectomy leads to reduction of trigonal hypertrophy with relief of the uretero-vesical obstruction.)

b. Cellules - Normal intravesical pressure is about 30 cm of water at the beginning of micturition. Pressures 2-4 times as great may be reached by the trabeculated (hypertrophied) bladder in its attempt to force urine past the obstruction. This pressure tends to push mucosa between the superficial muscle bundles, causing the formation of small pockets, or cellules (see Fig 10-1).

c. Diverticula - If cellules force their way entirely through the musculature of the bladder wall, they become diverticula, which may be embedded in perivesical fat or covered by peritoneum, depending upon their location. They have no muscle wall and are therefore unable to expel their contents into the bladder efficiently even after the primary obstruction has been removed. When this occurs, secondary infection is difficult to eradicate, and surgical removal of the diverticula may be required. Should the diverticulum push through the bladder wall on the anterior surface of the ureter, the ureterovesical junction will become incompetent.

d. Mucosa - In the presence of acute infection, the mucosa may be reddened and edematous. This may lead to temporary ureterovesical reflux in the presence of a "borderline" junction. The chronically inflamed membrane may be thinned and pale.

2. Stage of decompensation - The compensatory power of the bladder musculature varies greatly. This is commonly seen with prostatic enlargement; one patient may have only mild symptoms of prostatism yet have a large obstructing gland both rectally and cystoscopically; another may suffer acute retention and yet have a gland of normal size on rectal palpation and what appears to be only a mild obstruction cystoscopically.

In the face of progressive urethral obstruction, possibly aggravated by prostatic infection with edema, or congestion from lack of intercourse, decompensation of the detrusor may occur, resulting in the presence of residual urine after voiding. The amount may range up to 500 ml or more.

C. Upper Tract:

1. Ureter - In the early phases of obstruction, intravesical pressure, even when it is increased, is not transmitted to the ureters and renal pelves because of the competence of the ureterovesical "valves." (A true valve is not present; the ureterotrigonal unit, by virtue of its intrinsic structure, resists the retrograde flow of urine.) Eventually, with decompensation of the ureterotrigonal complex, the valve-like action may be lost, vesicoureteral reflux occurs, and the increased intravesical pressure is then transmitted to the renal pelves.

Secondary to the back pressure from reflux or obstruction from the hypertrophied and stretched trigone or a ureteral stone, the ureteral musculature thickens in its attempt to push the urine downward by increased peristaltic activity (stage of compensation). This causes elongation and some tortuosity of the

ureter (Fig 10-2). At times this change becomes marked; bands of fibrous tissue develop which on contraction further angulate the ureter so that secondary ureteral stenosis develops. Under these circumstances, removal of the obstruction below may not prevent the kidney from undergoing complete destruction from the acquired ureteral obstruction.

Finally, because of increasing pressure, the ureteral wall becomes attenuated and therefore loses all of its contractile power (stage of decompensation). Dilatation may be so extreme that the ureter resembles a loop of bowel (Figs 10-3 and 11-7, top right).

2. Kidney - The pressure within the renal pelvis is normally close to zero. When this pressure increases because of obstruction or reflux, the pelvis and calyces dilate. The degree of hydronephrosis which develops depends upon the duration, degree, and site of the obstruction. The higher the obstruction, the greater the effect upon the kidney. If the renal pelvis is entirely intrarenal and the obstruction is at the ureteropelvic junction, all the pressure will be exerted upon the parenchyma. If the renal pelvis is extrarenal, a ureteropelvic stenosis will exert only part of the resulting pressure on the parenchyma. The pelvis, being embedded in fat, dilates more readily, thus "decompressing" the calyces (Fig 10-2).

In the earlier stages, the pelvic musculature undergoes compensatory hypertrophy in its effort to force urine past the obstruction. Later, however, the muscle becomes attenuated (and decompensated).

The progression of hydronephrotic atrophy is as follows:

(1) The earliest changes in the development of hydronephrosis are seen in the calyces. The end of a normal calyx (as seen on a urogram, Fig 7-6) is concave because of the papilla which projects into it; with a chronic increase in intrapelvic pressure, it becomes flattened then convex (clubbed) from ischemia, necrosis, and absorption of the papilla. The parenchyma between the calyces is affected to a lesser extent.

This spotty atrophy is caused by the nature of the blood supply of the kidney. The arterioles are "end arteries"; therefore, ischemia is most marked in the areas farthest from the interlobular arteries. As the back pressure increases, hydronephrosis progresses, with the cells nearest the main arteries exhibiting the greatest resistance.

This increased pressure is transmitted up the tubules. The tubules become dilated, and their cells atrophy from ischemia.

(2) Only in unilateral hydronephrosis are the advanced stages of hydronephrotic atrophy seen. Eventually the kidney is completely destroyed and appears as a thin-walled sac filled

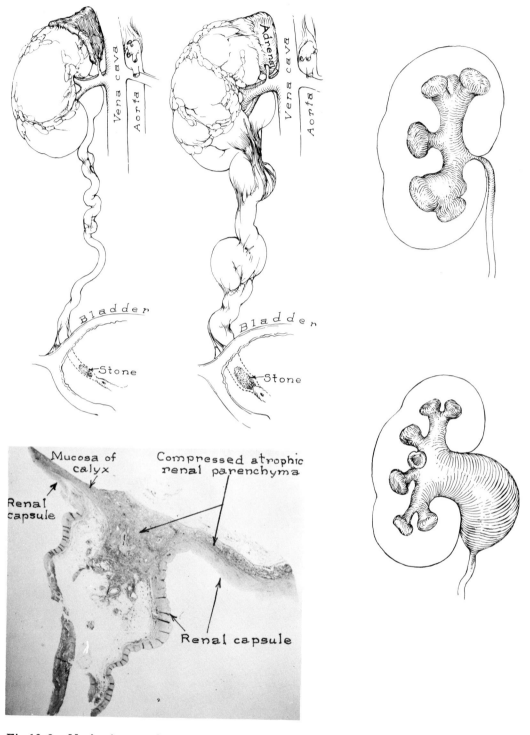

Fig 10-2. **Mechanisms and results of obstruction. Above left:** Early stage. Elongation and dilatation of ureter due to mild obstruction. **Above center:** Later stage. Further dilatation and elongation with kinking of the ureter; fibrous bands cause further kinking. **Below left:** Photomicrograph of advanced hydronephrosis. Thin layer of renal parenchyma covered by fibrous capsule. **Above right:** Intrarenal pelvis. Obstruction transmits all back pressure to parenchyma. **Below right:** Extrarenal pelvis, when obstructed, allows some of the increased pressure to be dissipated by the pelvis.

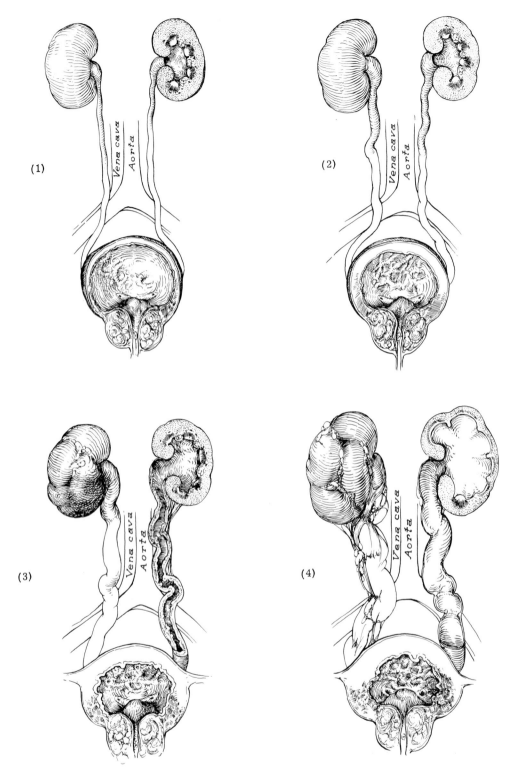

Fig 10-3. Pathogenesis of bilateral hydronephrosis. Progressive changes in bladder, ureters, and kidneys from obstruction of an enlarged prostate: thickening of bladder wall, dilatation and elongation of ureters, and hydronephrosis.

with clear fluid (water and electrolytes) or pus (Fig 10-4).

If obstruction is unilateral, the increased intrarenal pressure will cause some suppression of renal function on that side. The closer the intrapelvic pressure approaches the glomerular filtration pressure (30-40 mm Hg), the less urine can be secreted. Glomerular filtration rate and renal plasma flow are reduced. Concentrating power is gradually lost. The urine urea-creatinine concentration ratio is low when compared to the normal kidney (see p 54).

Hydronephrotic atrophy is an unusual type of pathologic change. Other secretory organs (eg, the submaxillary gland) cease secreting when their ducts are obstructed. This causes primary (disuse) atrophy. The completely obstructed kidney, however, continues to secrete urine. (If this were not so hydronephrosis could not occur, since it depends upon increased intrarenal pressure.) As urine is excreted into the renal pelvis, fluid and, particularly, soluble substances are reabsorbed, either through the tubules or the lymphatics. This has been demonstrated by injecting phenolsulfonphthalein into the obstructed renal pelvis. It disappears (is reabsorbed) in a few hours and is excreted by the other kidney. Other evidence is the fact that the markedly hydronephrotic kidney does not contain urine in the true sense; only water and a few salts are present.

Functional impairment in unilateral hydronephrosis, as measured by PSP or excretory urograms, will be greater and will increase faster than that seen in bilateral hydronephrotic kidneys showing comparable damage on pyelography. As unilateral hydronephrosis progresses, the normal kidney undergoes compensatory hypertrophy of its nephrons (renal counterbalance), thereby assuming the function of the diseased kidney in order to maintain normal total renal function. For this reason, successful anatomic repair of the ureteral obstruction of such a kidney may not only fail to improve its powers of waste elimination, but it may even continue to lose function.

If both kidneys are equally hydronephrotic, a strong stimulus is continually being exerted on both to maintain maximum function. This is also true of a solitary hydronephrotic kidney. Because of this, the return of function in these kidneys, after repair of their obstructions, is at times remarkable.

Physiologic Explanation of Symptoms of Bladder Neck Obstruction

The following hypothesis has been brought forward to explain the syndrome known as "prostatism" which occurs with progressive vesical obstruction:

The bladder, like the heart, is a hollow muscular organ which receives fluid and forcefully expels it. And, like the heart, it reacts to an increasing work load by going through the successive phases of compensation and finally decompensation.

Normally, contracture of the detrusor muscle and the trigone pulls the bladder neck open and forms a funnel through which the urine is expelled. The intravesical pressure generated in this instance varies between 20-40 cm of water; this force further widens the bladder neck.

With bladder neck obstruction, hypertrophy of the vesical musculature develops, allowing intravesical pressure to rise to 50-100 cm or more of water in order to overcome the increased urethral resistance. Despite this, the encroaching prostate appears to interfere with the mechanisms which ordinarily open the internal orifice. In addition, the contraction phase may not last long enough for all of the urine to be expelled; "exhaustion" of the muscle occurs prematurely. The refractory phase then sets in, and the detrusor is temporarily unable to respond to further stimuli. A few minutes later, voiding may again be initiated and completed.

A. Compensation Phase:

1. Stage of irritability - In the earliest stages of obstruction of the bladder neck, the vesical musculature begins to hypertrophy. The force and size of the urinary stream remain normal because the balance is maintained between the expelling power of the bladder and urethral resistance. During this phase, however, the bladder appears to be hypersensitive. As the bladder is distended, the need to void is felt. In the individual with a normal bladder these early urges can be inhibited, and the bladder relaxes and distends to receive more urine. However, in the patient with hypertrophied detrusor, the contraction of the detrusor is so strong that it virtually goes into spasm, producing the symptoms of an irritable bladder. The earliest symptoms of bladder neck obstruction, therefore, are urgency (even to the point of incontinence) and frequency, both day and night.

2. Stage of compensation - As the obstruction increases, further hypertrophy of the muscle fibers of the bladder occurs and the power to empty the bladder completely is thereby maintained. During this period, in addition to urgency and frequency, the patient notices hesitancy in initiating urination while the bladder develops contractions strong enough to overcome resistance at the bladder neck. The obstruction causes some loss in the force and size of the urinary stream, and the stream becomes slower as vesical emptying nears com-

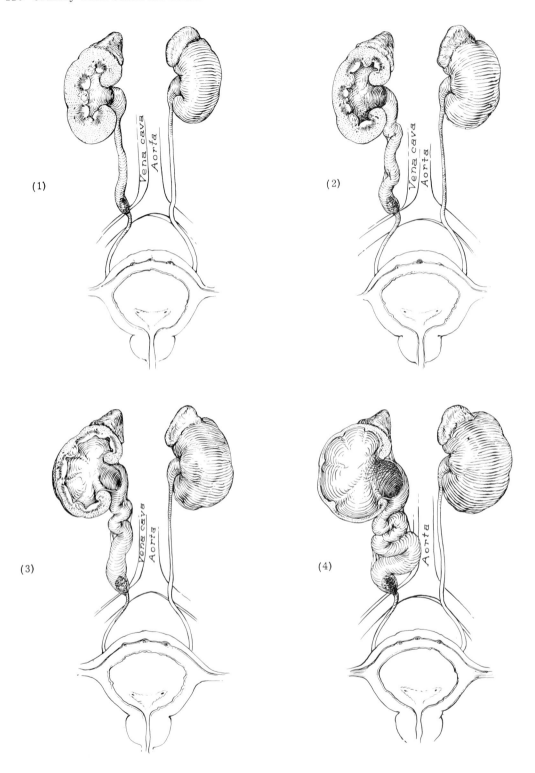

Fig 10-4. Pathogenesis of unilateral hydronephrosis. Progressive changes in ureter and kidney secondary to obstructing calculus. As the right kidney undergoes gradual destruction, the left kidney gradually enlarges (compensatory hypertrophy).

pletion (exhaustion of the detrusor as it nears the end of the contraction phase).

B. Decompensation Phase: If vesical tone becomes impaired or if urethral resistance exceeds detrusor power, some degree of decompensation (imbalance) occurs. The contraction phase of the vesical muscle becomes too short to completely expel the contents of the bladder, and residual urine is the result.

1. Acute decompensation - The tone of the compensated vesical muscle can be temporarily embarrassed by rapid filling of the bladder (high fluid intake) or by overstretching of the detrusor (postponement of urination though the urge is felt). This may cause increased difficulty of urination, with marked hesitancy and the need for straining to initiate urination a very weak and small stream, and termination of the stream before the bladder completely empties (residual urine). Acute and sudden complete urinary retention may also occur.

2. Chronic decompensation - As the degree of obstruction increases, a progressive imbalance between the power of the bladder musculature and urethral resistance develops. Therefore it becomes increasingly more difficult to expel all the urine during the contraction phase of the detrusor. The symptoms of obstruction become more marked. This residuum gradually increases, thus diminishing the functional capacity of the bladder. Progressive frequency of urination is noted. On occasion, as the bladder decompensates, it becomes overstretched and attenuated. It may contain 1000-3000 ml of urine. It loses its power of contraction, and overflow (paradoxical) incontinence results.

Clinical Findings

A. Symptoms:

1. Lower and mid tract (urethra and bladder) - Symptoms of obstruction of the lower and mid tract are typified by the symptoms of urethral stricture, benign prostatic hyperplasia, neurogenic bladder, and tumor of the bladder involving the vesical neck. The principal symptoms are hesitancy in starting urination, lessened force and size of the stream, terminal dribbling; hematuria, which may be initial with stricture, total with prostatic obstruction or vesical tumor; burning on urination, cloudy urine (complicating infection), and acute urinary retention.

2. Upper tract (ureter and kidney) - Symptoms of obstruction of the upper tract are typified by the symptoms of congenital ureteral stenosis or ureteral or renal stone. The principal complaints are pain in the flank radiating along the course of the ureter, gross total hematuria (from stone), gastrointestinal symptoms, chills, fever, burning on urination, and cloudy urine with onset of infection, which is

the common sequel to obstruction or vesicoureteral reflux. Nausea, vomiting, loss of weight and strength, and pallor are due to uremia secondary to bilateral hydronephrosis.

Obstruction of the upper tract may be silent even when uremia supervenes.

B. Signs:

1. Lower and mid tract - Palpation of the urethra may reveal induration about a stricture. Rectal examination may show atony of the anal sphincter (damage to the sacral nerve roots) or benign or malignant enlargement of the prostate. Vesical distention may be found.

Although observation of the force and caliber of the urinary stream affords a rough estimate of maximum flow rate, the rate can be measured accurately with a urine flow-meter or, even more simply, by the following technic: Have the patient begin to void. When observed maximum flow has been reached, interpose a container to collect the urine, and simultaneously start a stop watch. When urine flow begins to fade, remove the container and stop the watch. The flow in milliliters per second can then be calculated. The normal maximum urine flow rate is 15 ml or more/sec. Flow rates associated with an atonic neurogenic bladder (diminished detrusor power), urethral stricture, or prostatic obstruction (increased urethral resistance) may be as low as 3-5 ml/sec. A cystometrogram will differentiate between these 2 causes of impaired flow rate. After definitive treatment of the cause, flow rate should return to normal.

In the presence of a vesical diverticulum or vesicoureteral reflux, although detrusor power is normal, the urinary stream may be impaired because of the diffusion of intravesical pressure into the diverticulum and vesicoureteral junctions as well as the urethra. Excision of the diverticulum or repair of the vesicoureteral junctions leads to efficient explusion of urine via the urethra.

2. Upper tract - An enlarged kidney may be discovered by palpation or percussion. Renal tenderness may be elicited if infection has supervened. Cancer of the cervix may be noted; it may invade the base of the bladder and occlude one or both ureteral orifices, or its metastases to the iliac lymph nodes may compress the ureters. A large pelvic mass (tumor, pregnancy) can displace and compress the ureters. Children with advanced urinary tract obstruction (usually due to posterior urethral valves) may develop ascites. Rupture of the renal fornices allows leakage of urine which passes into the peritoneal cavity through a tear in the peritoneum.

C. Laboratory Findings: Anemia may be found secondary to chronic infection or in ad-

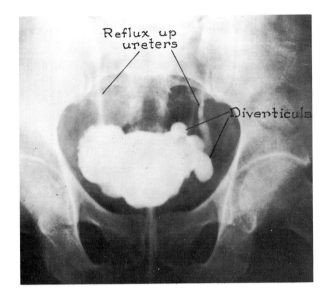

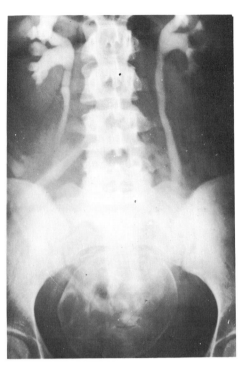

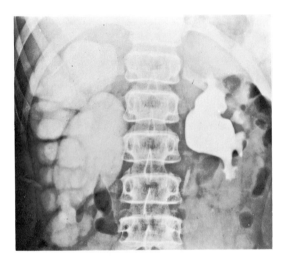

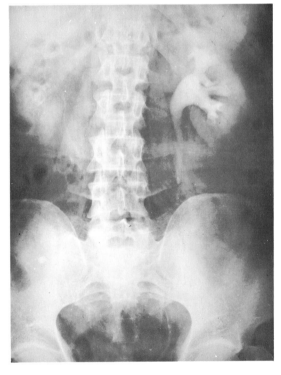

Fig 10-5. **Changes in bladder, ureters, and kidneys caused by obstruction.** **Above left:** Cystogram. Benign prostatic hyperplasia. Trabeculation of bladder wall, diverticula, ureteral reflux. **Above right:** Pregnancy. Mild dilatation of ureters, renal pelves, and calyces. **Below left:** Excretory urogram, 70 minutes after injection. Advanced right hydronephrosis secondary to ureteropelvic obstruction. Mild ureteropelvic obstruction on left. **Below right:** Mild left hydroureteronephrosis caused by stone opposite L4.

vanced bilateral hydronephrosis (stage of ure-mia). Leukocytosis is to be expected in the acute stage of infection. Little if any eleva-tion of the white blood count accompanies the chronic stage.

Large amounts of protein are usually not found in the obstructive uropathies. Casts are not common from hydronephrotic kidneys. Microscopic hematuria may indicate renal or vesical infection, tumor, or stone. Pus cells and bacteria may or may not be present.

In the presence of unilateral hydronephro-sis the PSP test will be normal because of the contralateral renal hypertrophy. Suppression of the PSP indicates bilateral renal damage, residual urine (vesical or bilateral uretero-renal), or vesicoureteral reflux.

In the presence of significant bilateral hydronephrosis, urine flow through the renal tubules is slowed. Thus, urea is significantly absorbed, but creatinine is not. Blood chem-istry therefore reveals a urea-creatinine ratio well above the normal 10:1 relationship.

D. X-ray Findings: (Fig 10-5.) A plain film of the abdomen may show enlargement of renal shadows, calcific bodies suggesting ure-teral or renal stone, or metastases to the bones of the spine or pelvis. If metastases are present in the spine, they may be the cause of spinal cord damage (neurogenic bladder). If osteoblastic, cancer of the prostate is almost certainly the cause.

Excretory urograms will reveal almost the entire story unless renal function is se-verely impaired. They are more informative when obstruction is present, because the opaque material is retained. These urograms will demonstrate the degree of dilatation of the pelves, calyces, and ureters. The point of ureteral stenosis will be revealed. Segmental dilatation of the lower end of a ureter implies the possibility of vesicoureteral reflux (Fig 11-6), which can be revealed by cystography. The accompanying cystogram may show tra-beculation as an irregularity of the vesical out-line and may show diverticula. Vesical tu-mors, nonopaque stones, and large intravesical prostatic lobes may cause radiolucent shadows. A film taken immediately after voiding will show residual urine. Few tests that are as simple and inexpensive give the physician so much information.

Retrograde cystography shows changes of the bladder wall caused by distal obstruction (trabeculation, diverticula) or demonstrates the obstructive lesion itself (enlarged prostate, posterior urethral valves, vesical neoplasm). If the ureterovesical valves are incompetent, ureteropyelograms will be obtained by reflux (Fig 7-9).

Retrograde urograms may show better detail than the excretory type, but care must be taken not to overdistend the passages with too much opaque fluid; small hydronephroses can be made to look quite large. The degree of ureteral or ureterovesical obstruction can be judged by the degree of delay of drainage of the radiopaque fluid instilled.

E. Isotope Scanning: In the presence of obstruction, the radioisotope renogram may show depression of both the vascular and sec-retory phases, and a rising rather than a falling excretory phase due to retention of the radiopaque urine in the renal pelvis.

The ^{131}I activity recorded on the gamma camera will reveal poor uptake of the isotope, slow transport of the isotope through the par-enchyma, and accumulation of scintillations in the renal pelvis. (See chapter 8.)

F. Instrumental Examination: Explora-tion of the urethra with a catheter or other instrument is a valuable diagnostic measure. Passage may be blocked by a stricture or tu-mor. External sphincter spasm may make passage difficult. Passage of the catheter im-mediately after voiding allows estimation of the amount of residual urine in the bladder. Residual urine is common in bladder neck ob-struction (enlarged prostate, cystocele, and neurogenic bladder. Even though the urinary stream may be markedly impaired with ure-thral stricture, residual urine is absent.

Measurement of vesical tone by means of cystometry is helpful in diagnosing the neuro-genic bladder and in differentiating between bladder neck obstruction and vesical atony.

Inspection of the urethra and bladder by means of cystoscopy and panendoscopy may reveal the primary obstructive agent. Cathe-ters may be passed to the renal pelves and urine specimens obtained. Measurement of the function of each kidney may be done (PSP test), and retrograde ureteropyelograms can be made.

Differential Diagnosis

A thorough examination usually leaves no doubt about the diagnosis. The differential diagnosis under these circumstances is rarely difficult. If seemingly simple infection does not respond to medical therapy, or if infection recurs, obstruction or vesicoureteral reflux is the probable cause and complete study of the urinary tract is indicated.

Complications

Stagnation of urine leads to infection, which then may spread throughout the entire urinary system. Once established, infection is difficult and at times impossible to eradicate even after the obstruction has been relieved.

Often the invading organisms are urea-splitting (proteus, staphylococci). This causes the urine to become alkaline, in which case calcium salts precipitate and form bladder or kidney stones more easily.

If both kidneys are affected, the result may be renal insufficiency. Secondary infection increases renal damage.

Pyonephrosis is the end stage of a severely infected and obstructed kidney. The kidney is functionless and is filled with thick pus.

Treatment

A. Relief of Obstruction: The treatment of the main causes of obstruction and stasis are described in detail elsewhere: benign prostatic hyperplasia, cancer of the prostate, neurogenic bladder, ureteral stone, posterior urethral valves, and ureteral stenosis.

1. Lower tract obstruction (distal to the bladder) - With patients in whom secondary renal or ureterovesical damage (reflux in the latter) is minimal or nonexistent, correction of the obstruction is sufficient. If significant reflux is demonstrated, "triple voiding" should be instituted once a day. This consists of voiding with strain; walking around, voiding with strain; walking around and then voiding again. This technic will usually empty the entire urinary tract completely, thus increasing the chances of sterilizing the urine and keeping it sterile. However, if there is considerable hydronephrosis in addition to reflux, drainage of the bladder by indwelling catheter or cystostomy is indicated in order to preserve or improve renal function. If, after many months of drainage, reflux persists, surgical repair of the incompetent intravesical portion of the ureter should be done.

2. Upper tract obstruction (above the bladder) - If tortuous, kinked, dilated, or atonic ureters have developed secondary to lower tract obstruction (so that they are themselves obstructive), vesical drainage will not protect the kidneys from further damage; the urine proximal to the obstruction must be diverted by nephrostomy or ureterostomy. The kidneys then may regain some function. Over a period of many months, the ureter may become less tortuous and less dilated; its obstructive areas may open up. If radiopaque material instilled into the nephrostomy tube passes readily to the bladder, it may be possible to remove the nephrostomy tube. If obstruction persists, surgical repair is indicated.

If one kidney has been badly damaged, as measured by tests of function and urography, nephrectomy may be necessary.

B. Eradication of Infection: Once the obstruction is removed, every effort should be made to eradicate infection. If it has been severe and prolonged, antibiotics may fail to sterilize the urinary tract.

Prognosis

No simple statement can be made about the prognosis in this group of patients. The outcome depends upon the etiology, site, degree, and duration of the obstruction. The prognosis is also definitely influenced by complicating infection, particularly if it has been present for a long time.

If renal function is fair to good, if the obstruction or other causes for stasis can be corrected, and if complicating infection can then be eradicated, the prognosis is generally excellent.

Bellina, J.H., Dougherty, C.M., & A. Mickal: Pyeloureteral dilation and pregnancy. Am J Obst Gynec 108:356-63, 1970.

Berdon, W.E., & others: Hydronephrosis in infants and children. Value of high dosage excretory urography in predicting renal salvageability. Am J Roentgenol 109:380-9, 1970.

Bourne, R.B.: Intermittent hydronephrosis as a cause of abdominal pain. JAMA 198: 1218-9, 1966.

Chovnick, S.D.: Anterior sacral meningocele as a cause of urinary retention. J Urol 106: 371-4, 1971.

Cook, G.T.: Appendiceal abscess causing urinary obstruction. J Urol 101:212-5, 1969.

Culp, D.A.: Acute urinary retention. Postgrad Med 31:252-62, 1962.

Culp, O.S., & others: Hydronephrosis and hydroureter in infancy and childhood: A panel discussion. J Urol 88:443-50, 1962.

Dure-Smith, P.: Pregnancy dilatation of the urinary tract. The iliac sign and its significance. Radiology 96:545-50, 1970.

Earlam, R.J.: Recovery of renal function after prolonged ureteric obstruction. Brit J Urol 39:58-62, 1967.

Eckstein, H.B., & L. Kapila: Cutaneous ureterostomy. Brit J Urol 42:306-15, 1970.

Edelmann, C.M., Jr., & A. Spitzer: The maturing kidney: A modern view of well-balanced infants with imbalanced nephrons. J Pediat 75:509-17, 1969.

Feminella, J.G., & J.K. Lattimer: A retrospective analysis of 70 cases of cutaneous ureterostomy. J Urol 106:538-40, 1971.

Flinn, R.A., & others: Cutaneous ureterostomy: An alternative urinary diversion. J Urol 105:358-64, 1971.

Garrett, R.A., & E.A. Franken, Jr.: Neonatal ascites: Perirenal urinary extravasation with bladder outlet obstruction. J Urol 102:627-32, 1969.

Glen, E. S.: Spontaneous intraperitoneal rupture of hydronephrosis. Brit J Urol **41**: 414-6, 1969.

Green, N., Fingerhut, A. G., & S. French: Mechanism of renovascular backflow. A pathophysiologic study. Radiology **92**:531-6, 1969.

Guyer, P. B., & D. Delany: Urinary tract dilatation and oral contraceptives. Brit MJ **4**:588-90, 1970.

Harrow, B. R., Sloane, J. A., & L. Shalhanick: Etiology of the hydronephrosis of pregnancy. Surg Gynec Obst **119**:1042-8, 1964.

Hinman, F., Jr.: Flowmeter for automatically timed void. J Urol **94**:89-91, 1965.

Hutch, J. A., & E. A. Tanagho: Etiology of non-occlusive ureteral dilatation. J Urol **93**:177-84, 1965.

Joekes, A. M., & D. R. Rellan: Radioactive renography in diagnosis and treatment of acute obstructive renal failure. Lancet **2**: 96-6, 1965.

Johnston, J. H.: The pathogenesis of hydronephrosis in children. Brit J Urol **41**:724-34, 1969.

Kelalis, P. P., & others: Ureteropelvic obstruction in children: Experiences with 109 cases. J Urol **106**:418-22, 1971.

Kelalis, P. P., & P. McLean: The treatment of diverticulum of the bladder. J Urol **98**: 347-52, 1967.

Kendall, A. R., & L. Karafin: Intermittent hydronephrosis: Hydration pyelography. J Urol **98**:653-6, 1967.

King, L. R., Mellens, H. Z., & H. White: Measurement of the intravesical pressure during voiding: An analysis of pressure recordings made by 3 different techniques with comment on diagnostic significance of such studies in the evaluation of bladder outflow. Invest Urol **2**:303-22, 1965.

Krohn, A. G., & others: Compensatory renal hypertrophy: The role of immediate vascular changes in its production. J Urol **103**: 564-8, 1970.

Maloney, J. D., & J. P. Smith: Temporary cutaneous loop ureterostomy. J Urol **103**: 790-4, 1970.

Marshall, S.: Urea-creatinine ratio in obstructive uropathy and renal hypertension. JAMA **190**:719-20, 1964.

Moncada, R., & others: Neonatal ascites associated with urinary outlet obstruction (urine ascites). Radiology **90**:1165-70, 1968.

Morillo, M. M.: Intravesical pressure before and after surgery for bladder neck obstruction. J Urol **91**:361-3, 1964.

Roberts, J. B. M., & N. Slade: The natural history of primary pelvic hydronephrosis. Brit J Surg **51**:759-62, 1964.

Shopfner, C. E.: Nonobstructive hydronephrosis and hydroureter. Am J Roentgenol **98**: 172-80, 1966.

Shopfner, C. E.: Ureteropelvic junction obstruction. Am J Roentgenol **98**:148-59, 1966.

Shopfner, C. E.: Urinary tract pathology associated with constipation. Radiology **90**:865-77, 1968.

Smart, W. R.: Chapter 55 in: Urology, 3rd ed. Campbell, M. F., & J. H. Harrison (editors). Saunders, 1970.

Stephens, F. D.: Treatment of megaloureters by multiple micturition. Australian & New Zealand J Surg **27**:130-4, 1957.

Straffon, R. A., Kyle, K., & J. Corvalan: Techniques of cutaneous ureterostomy and results in 51 patients. J Urol **103**:138-46, 1970.

Susset, J. G., Rabinovitch, H., & K. J. MacKinnon: Parameters of micturition: clinical study. J Urol **94**:113-21, 1965.

Tanagho, E. A., & F. H. Meyers: Trigonal hypertrophy: a cause of ureteral obstruction. J Urol **93**:678-83, 1965.

Tanagho, E. A., Smith, D. R., & T. H. Guthrie: Pathophysiology of functional ureteral obstruction. J Urol **104**:73-88, 1970.

Wedge, J. J., Grosfeld, J. L., & J. P. Smith: Abdominal masses in the newborn: 63 cases. J Urol **106**:770-5, 1971.

Williams, D. I., & C. M. Karlaftis: Hydronephrosis due to pelvic-ureteric obstruction in the newborn. Brit J Urol **38**:138-44, 1966.

Williams, D. I., & I. Hulme-Moir: Primary obstructive megaureter. Brit J Urol **42**: 140-9, 1970.

UREMIA

Uremia is due to renal insufficiency from any cause, and is characterized by disturbances of electrolyte balance and retention of nitrogenous and other metabolic end products. It is reversible when caused by decreased renal blood flow (eg, as a result of dehydration), acute tubular necrosis, or lower urinary tract obstruction; but is irreversible and ultimately fatal when due to destruction of the renal parenchyma (eg, as in the terminal stages of chronic glomerulonephritis, pyelonephritis, and hypertensive renal disease). The impediment to urine flow in obstruction or the decrease in glomerular filtration rate which occurs in renal parenchymal disease leads to elevation of the serum phosphate, sulfate, and other acid radicals, and the serum creatinine, which in turn produces a metabolic acidosis. As the serum phosphate rises the serum calcium falls. The electrolyte abnormalities which occur as a result of the accumulation of organic acids are hypokalemia, hyponatremia, hypocalcemia, and hyperchloremia.

The clinical manifestations of uremia are variable; the diagnosis is made on the basis of elevated blood NPN and serum creatinine levels and the electrolyte abnormalities. In the early stages, weakness, drowsiness, and lethargy are the most significant findings; headache and generalized pruritus may be present. In the later stages of irreversible uremia, the signs of dehydration appear as a result of increased urine output; tetany occurs as the serum calcium falls; and the rate and depth of respirations increase. Coma ultimately supervenes, and at times a characteristic "uremic frost" may be seen on the patient's face.

In reversible cases treatment is directed at the underlying cause: relief of obstruction, rehydration, or fluid restriction in the patient with acute tubular necrosis. In the patient with irreversible uremia treatment must be limited to restoring electrolyte balance. Treatment in the terminal stage is symptomatic and supportive: calcium to control tetany, and antinauseant and sedative drugs. Intermittent hemodialysis or renal homotransplantation may also be considered.

Eschbach, J.W., Jr., & others: Hemodialysis in the home. A new approach to the treatment of chronic uremia. Ann Int Med **67**: 1149-62, 1967.

Hume, D.M.: Renal homotransplantation in man. Ann Rev Med **18**:229-68, 1967.

Martin, D.C., & others: Kidney transplants: 92 cases. Results, lessons learned, future prospects. J Urol **100**:227-32, 1968.

Schwartz, W.B., & J.P. Kassirer: Medical management of chronic renal failure. Am J Med **44**:786-802, 1968.

Straffon, R.A., & others: Four years' experience with 138 kidney transplants. J Urol **99**:479-85, 1968.

Symposium on renal transplantation. Arch Int Med **123**:483-567, 1969.

Thomson, G.E., & others: Hemodialysis for chronic renal failure. Arch Int Med **120**: 153-67, 1967.

•   •   •

11 . . .

Vesicoureteral Reflux

Under normal circumstances, the uretero-vesical junction allows urine to enter the bladder but prevents urine from regurgitating into the ureter, particularly at the time of voiding. In this way, the kidney is protected from high pressure in the bladder and from contamination by infected vesical urine. When this valve is incompetent, although some degree of hydro-ureteronephrosis may ensue, the chance for the development of urinary infection is significantly enhanced and pyelonephritis is then inevitable. With few exceptions, pyelonephritis-acute, chronic, or healed—is secondary to ves-icoureteral reflux.

ANATOMY OF THE
URETEROVESICAL JUNCTION

An understanding of the etiology of vesi-coureteral reflux requires a knowledge of the anatomy of the ureterovesical valve. Anatomic studies performed by Hutch & others and by Tanagho and Pugh are incorporated into the following discussion (Fig 11-1).

Mesodermal Component
This structure, which arises from the Wolffian duct, is made of 2 parts which are innervated by the sympathetic nervous system:

A. The Ureter and the Superficial Trigone: The smooth musculature of the renal calyces, pelvis, and extravesical ureter is composed of longitudinal and spirally oriented fibers. So constituted, they can undergo peristaltic activity. As these fibers approach the vesical wall, they are reoriented into the longitudinal plane. The ureter passes obliquely through the vesical wall; the intravesical ureteral segment is thus composed of longitudinal muscle fibers only and thus cannot undergo peristalsis. As these smooth muscle fibers approach the ureteral orifice, those that form the roof swing dorsally and join those fibers forming the floor of the ureter. They then spread out and join those muscle bundles from the other ureter and also

continue caudally, thus forming the superficial trigone, which then passes over the neck of the bladder, ending at the verumontanum in the male and just inside the external urethral orifice in the female. Thus, the ureterotrigonal complex is one structure. Above the ureteral orifice, it is tubular; below that point, it is flat.

B. Waldeyer's Sheath and the Deep Trigone: Beginning at a point about 2-3 cm above the bladder, an external layer of longitudinal smooth muscle surrounds the ureter. These fibers pass through the vesical wall, to which they are connected by a few detrusor fibers. As this muscular sheath enters the vesical lumen, its roof fibers also diverge to join their floor fibers, which then spread out, joining muscle bundles from the contralateral ureter and thus forming the deep trigone which ends at the bladder neck.

Endodermal Component
The vesical detrusor muscle bundles are intertwined and run in various directions. However, as they converge upon the internal orifice of the bladder, they tend to become oriented into 3 layers:

A. Internal Longitudinal Layer: This layer continues into the urethra submucosally and ends just inside the external meatus in the female and at the caudal end of the prostate in the male.

B. Middle Circular Layer: This layer is thickest anteriorly and stops at the vesical neck.

C. Outer Longitudinal Layer: These muscle bundles take a circular and spiral course about the external surface of the urethra, thus constituting the true vesicourethral sphincter. These latter fibers are incorporated within the glandular prostatic tissue in the male.

The vesical detrusor muscle is innervated by the parasympathetic nerves (S2-4).

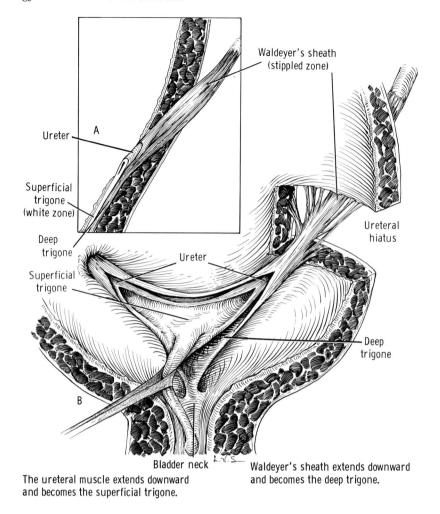

Ureter

A

Waldeyer's sheath
(stippled zone)

Ureter

Superficial
trigone
(white zone)

Ureteral
hiatus

Deep
trigone

Superficial
trigone

Ureter

Deep
trigone

B

Bladder neck

The ureteral muscle extends downward
and becomes the superficial trigone.

Waldeyer's sheath extends downward
and becomes the deep trigone.

Fig 11-1. Normal ureterotrigonal complex. A: Side view of ureterovesical junction. Waldeyer's muscular sheath invests the juxtavesical ureter and continues downward as the deep trigone, which extends to the bladder neck. The ureteral musculature becomes the superficial trigone, which extends to the verumontanum in the male and stops just short of the external meatus in the female. **B: Waldeyer's sheath is connected by a few fibers to the detrusor muscle in the ureteral hiatus.** This muscular sheath, inferior to the ureteral orifices, becomes the deep trigone. The musculature of the ureters continues downward as the superficial trigone. (Redrawn and modified, with permission, from Fig 1 in Tanagho, E.A., & R.C.B. Pugh: The Anatomy and Function of the Ureterovesical Junction. Brit J Urol **35**:151-65, 1963.)

PHYSIOLOGY OF THE
URETEROVESICAL JUNCTION

While many investigators had suspected that normal trigonal tone tended to occlude the intravesical ureter, it remained for Tanagho, Hutch, Myers, and Rambo to prove this tenet. Using nonrefluxing dogs, they demonstrated the following:

(1) Interruption of the continuity of the trigone resulted in reflux. An incision was made in the trigone 3 mm below the ureteral orifice, resulting in an upward and lateral migration of the ureteral orifice with shortening of the intravesical ureter. Reflux was demonstrable. After the incision healed, reflux ceased.

(2) Unilateral lumbar sympathectomy resulted in paralysis of the ipsilateral trigone. This led to lateral and superior migration of the ureteral orifice and reflux.

(3) Electrical stimulation of the trigone caused the ureteral orifice to move caudally, thus lengthening the intravesical ureter. This maneuver caused a marked rise in resistance

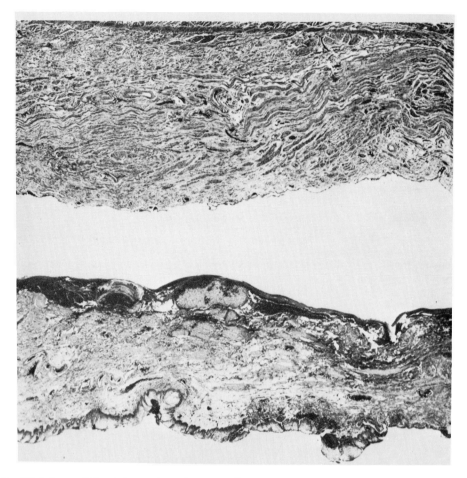

Fig 11-2. Histology of the trigone in primary reflux. Above: Normal trigone demonstrating wealth of closely packed smooth muscle fibers. **Below:** The congenitally attenuated trigonal muscle that accompanies vesicoureteral reflux. Note absence of inflammatory cells. (Reproduced, with permission, from Fig 15 in Tanagho, E.A., & others: Primary vesicoureteral reflux: Experimental studies of its etiology. J Urol **93**:165-76, 1965.)

to flow through the ureterovesical junction. Ureteral efflux of urine ceased. The intravenous injection of epinephrine caused the same reaction. On the other hand, isoproterenol caused the degree of occlusion to drop below normal. If, however, the trigone was incised, electrical stimulation of the trigone or the administration of epinephrine failed to increase ureteral occlusive pressure.

(4) During gradual filling of the bladder, intravesical pressure increased but little, whereas the pressure within the intravesical ureter rose progressively—due, apparently, to increasing trigonal stretch. A few seconds before the expected sharp rise in intravesical pressure generated for voiding, the closure pressure in the intravesical ureter rose sharply and was maintained for 20 seconds after detrusor contracture had ceased. This experiment demonstrated that ureterovesical competence is independent of detrusor action and is governed by the tone of the trigone, which, just before voiding, contracts vigorously and thus helps to open and funnel the vesical neck. At the same time, significant pull is placed upon the intravesical ureter, thus occluding it during the period when intravesical pressure is high. During the voiding phase, there is naturally no efflux of ureteral urine.

One may liken this function to the phenomenon of the Chinese thimble: the harder the finger (trigone) pulls, the tighter the thimble (intravesical ureter). Contrariwise, a deficient pull may lead to incomplete closure of the ureterovesical junction.

It was concluded from these experiments that normal ureterotrigonal tone prevents vesicoureteral reflux. Electrical or pharma-

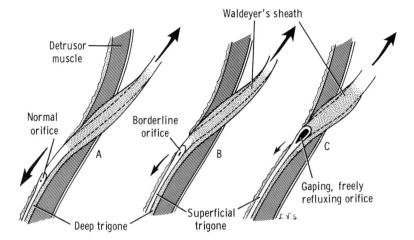

Fig 11-3. The effect of trigonal tone on the competency of the ureterovesical junction. A: Normal ureterotrigonal complex. Normal upper ureteral and ureterotrigonal muscles exert equal pull as shown by arrows. Trigonal tone occludes ureteral orifice and protects length of intravesical ureteral segment. **B: Trigonal musculature moderately attenuated.** The occlusive force on the orifice is subnormal and the tone and peristaltic action of the normal upper ureter may cause some cephalad migration of the ureter, thus decreasing the length of the intravesical ureter. This is a "borderline" valve that may reflux if the bladder becomes infected. **C: Severe attenuation of intravesical-trigonal musculature.** Little occlusive force exerted on ureteral orifice. Lumbar ureteral muscle has pulled ureteral orifice up to the ureteral hiatus. Valve action destroyed; low pressure reflux occurs.

cologic stimulation or voiding caused increased occlusive pressure in the intravesical ureter and increased resistance to flow down the ureter. Contrariwise, incision or paralysis of the trigone led to reflux. The theory that ureterovesical competence was maintained by intravesical pressure crushing the intravesical ureter against its backing of detrusor muscle was thereby disproved.

Biopsy of the trigone (and the intravesical ureter) in patients with primary reflux revealed marked deficiency in the development of its smooth muscle (Fig 11-2). Electrical stimulation of such a trigone caused only a minor contraction of the ureterotrigonal complex. This work led to the conclusion that the common cause of reflux, particularly in children, is congenital attenuation of the ureterotrigonal musculature.

THE ETIOLOGY OF REFLUX

The major cause of vesicoureteral reflux is attenuation of the trigone and its contiguous intravesical ureteral musculature. Any condition that shortens the intravesical ureter may also lead to reflux, but this is less common.

Congenital Causes

A. Trigonal Weakness ("Primary Reflux"): This is by far the most common cause of ureteral regurgitation. It is most often seen in little girls, though it is observed occasionally in boys. Reflux in adults—usually women—probably represents the same congenital defect. Weakness of one side of the trigone leads to decrease in the occlusive pressure in the ipsilateral intravesical ureter. Diffuse ureterotrigonal weakness causes bilateral reflux.

In the normal state, the intravesical ureterotrigonal muscle tone exerts a downward pull whereas the extravesical ureter tends to pull cephalad (Fig 11-3). If trigonal development is deficient, not only is its occlusive power diminished but the ureteral orifice tends to gravitate upward toward the ureteral hiatus. The degree of this retraction relates to the degree of incompetence of the junction. If the ureteral orifice lies over the ureteral hiatus in the bladder wall (so-called golf-hole orifice), it is completely incompetent. The degree of incompetency is judged by the findings on excretory urography and on cystography, and the cystoscopic appearance of the ureteral orifices.

B. Ureteral Abnormalities:
1. Complete ureteral duplication (Fig 11-4) - The intravesical portion of the ureter to

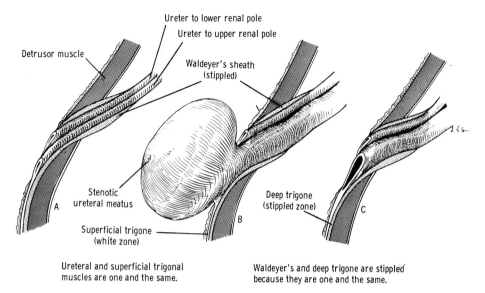

Ureter to lower renal pole

Ureter to upper renal pole

Detrusor muscle

Waldeyer's sheath
(stippled)

Stenotic
ureteral meatus

Deep trigone
(stippled zone)

Superficial trigone
(white zone)

Ureteral and superficial trigonal
muscles are one and the same.

Waldeyer's and deep trigone are stippled
because they are one and the same.

Fig 11-4. Ureteral duplication and ureterocele as causes of vesicoureteral reflux. A: Ureteral
duplication showing juxtavesical and intravesical ureters encased in common sheath
(Waldeyer's). The superior ureter, which always drains the lower renal pole, has a shorter
intravesical segment; in addition, it is somewhat devoid of muscle. It therefore tends to allow
reflux. **B:** Duplication with ureterocele that always involves caudal ureter which drains upper
renal pole. Pinpoint orifice is obstructive, causing hydroureteronephrosis. Resulting wide
dilatation of ureter and ureteral hiatus shortens the intravesical segment of the other ureter,
often causing it to reflux. **C:** Resection of ureterocele allows reflux into that ureter.

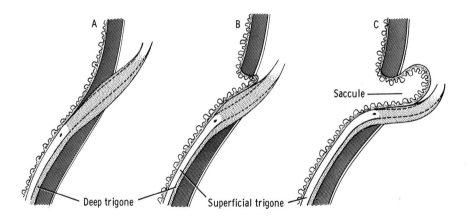

Saccule

Deep trigone

Superficial trigone

Fig 11-5. The effect of trabeculation of the bladder on the ureterovesical junction. A: Trabeculated bladder caused by upper motor neuron lesion or vesical neck obstruction. Normal and
competent ureterovesical junction protected from reflux by hypertrophied trigonal muscle.
B: High intravesical voiding pressure forces a nipple of vesical mucosa into the ureteral hiatus.
This has the effect of shortening the intravesical ureter; reflux may occur. **C:** A large saccule
or diverticulum may form with complete destruction of valvular action. (Modified from Hutch,
J.A., & A.D. Amar: Vesicoureteral Reflux. Volume 7, Encyclopedia of Urology. Berlin-
Heidelberg-New York: Springer, 1968.)

the upper renal segment is usually of normal length, whereas that of the ureter to the lower pole is abnormally short; this orifice is commonly incompetent. However, Stephens has demonstrated that the musculature of the superiorly placed orifice is attenuated and this further contributes to its weakness.

2. Ectopic ureteral orifice - A single ureter or one of a pair may open well down on the trigone, at the vesical neck or in the urethra. In this instance, vesicoureteral reflux is the rule. This observation makes it clear that the length of the intravesical ureter is not the sole factor in reflux. Stephens has observed that such intravesical ureteral segments are usually devoid of smooth muscle. Thus, it has no occlusive force.

3. Ureterocele - A ureterocele involving a single ureter rarely allows reflux, but this lesion usually involves the ureter that drains the upper pole of a duplicated kidney. Since the ureteral orifice is obstructed, the intramural ureter becomes dilated. This increases the diameter of the ureteral hiatus, thus further shortening the intravesical segment of the other ureter, which therefore may become incompetent. Resection of the ureterocele usually causes its ureter to reflux freely as well.

Vesical Trabeculation

Occasionally, a heavily trabeculated bladder may be associated with reflux. The causes include the spastic neurogenic bladder and severe obstruction distal to the bladder. These lesions, however, are associated with trigonal hypertrophy as well; the resultant extra pull on the ureterotrigonal muscle tends to protect the junction from incompetency. In a few such cases, however, the vesical mucosa may protrude through the ureteral hiatus just above the ureter, thus forming a diverticulum or saccule (Fig 11-5). The resulting dilatation of the hiatus shortens the intravesical segment; reflux may then occur.

Edema of the Vesical Wall Secondary to Cystitis

As noted above, valves vary in their degrees of incompetency. A "border-line" junction may not allow reflux when the urine is sterile, but the edema involving the trigone and intravesical ureter associated with cystitis may impair valvular function, in which case secondary pyelonephritis may ensue. After cure of the infection, cystography again reveals no reflux. It is believed that a completely normal junction will not decompensate even under these circumstances.

It has been shown that pyelonephritis of pregnancy is associated with vesicoureteral reflux. Many of these women give a history of urinary tract infections during childhood. The implication is that they "outgrew" their reflux at puberty but that if bacteriuria becomes established during pregnancy, their "border-line" valves may become incompetent. This may be enhanced by the circulating hormones of pregnancy that may contribute to a further loss of tone of the ureterotrigonal complex. After delivery the reflux is usually no longer demonstrable.

Iatrogenic Causes

Certain operative procedures may lead to either temporary or permanent ureteral regurgitation.

A. Prostatectomy: With any type of prostatectomy, the continuity of the superficial trigone is interrupted at the vesical neck. If the proximal trigone moves upward, temporary reflux may occur. This mechanism may account for the high fever (even bacteremia) that is sometimes observed when the catheter is finally removed. Fortunately, in 2-3 weeks the trigone again becomes anchored and reflux ceases.

B. Wedge Resection of the Posterior Vesical Neck: This procedure, often performed in conjunction with plastic revision of the vesical neck for supposed vesical neck stenosis or dysfunction, may also upset trigonal continuity and allow reflux.

C. Ureteral Meatotomy: Ureteral meatotomy occasionally is followed by reflux if it is extensive. Fortunately, however, limited incision of the roof of the intravesical ureter divides few muscle fibers since they have left the roof to join those fibers on the floor. Wide resection in the treatment of vesical neoplasm is often followed by ureteral regurgitation.

D. Resection of Ureterocele: If the ureteral hiatus is widely dilated, this procedure is often followed by reflux.

Miscellaneous Causes

A bladder that is contracted secondary to interstitial cystitis, tuberculosis, carcinoma, or schistosomiasis may be associated with ureteral reflux.

The child with congenital attenuation of the abdominal musculature (prune-belly syndrome) has bilateral hydroureteronephrosis secondary to ureteral reflux. Significant maldevelopment of the uretero-ureterotrigonal muscle has been documented.

COMPLICATIONS OF
VESICOURETERAL REFLUX

Vesicoureteral reflux damages the kidney through one or both of 2 mechanisms: (1) pyelonephritis and (2) hydroureteronephrosis.

Pyelonephritis

Vesicoureteral reflux is one of the common contributing factors leading to the development of cystitis, particularly in females. In the presence of vesicoureteral reflux, the bacteria reach the kidney. In the face of reflux, the urinary tract cannot empty itself completely and the infection is perpetuated. (See chapter 12 for a discussion of this phenomenon.)

Hydroureteronephrosis

Some degree of dilatation of the ureter, renal pelvis, and calyces is usually observed in association with reflux. Its degree may be extreme (Fig 11-7). Such changes are often seen in the absence of infection in the male because of the relatively long segment of sterile urethra in that sex. Sterile reflux is less damaging than infected reflux.

Intravesical pressure is transmitted through the incompetent ureteral orifice. This back pressure is quite high at the time of voiding. Furthermore, the ureteropelvic and ureterovesical junctions are less distensible than the rest of the ureter. Either junction may have trouble passing the volume of normal urinary secretion plus the refluxed urine; functional obstruction may result. The common cause of ureteropelvic and ureterovesical "obstruction" is vesicoureteral reflux. Such changes indicate the need for cystography.

THE INCIDENCE OF REFLUX

Incompetency of the ureterovesical junction is an abnormal condition. Peters and others found no reflux in 66 premature infants; Lich and co-workers found none in 26 infants studied during the first 2 days of life. Leadbetter and others noted normal cystograms in 50 adult males.

The incidence of vesicoureteral reflux is 50% in children with urinary tract infection but only 8% in adults with bacteriuria. This discrepancy is explained by the fact that the female child usually has pyelonephritis whereas the adult female usually has cystitis only. The concept that bacteriuria implies the presence of pyelonephritis must be condemned.

The fairly competent ("borderline") valve only refluxes during an acute attack of cystitis. Since cystography is only performed

in this group after the infection has been eradicated, the incidence of reflux is abnormally low. On the other hand, in patients whose excretory urograms reveal significant changes typical of healed pyelonephritis, reflux is demonstrable in 85%.

CLINICAL FINDINGS

A story compatible with acute pyelonephritis implies the presence of vesicoureteral reflux. This is most commonly seen in females, particularly little girls. Persistence of recurrent "cystitis" should suggest the possibility of reflux. Often, in these instances, the patient has an asymptomatic low grade pyelonephritis.

Symptoms Related to Reflux

A. Symptomatic Pyelonephritis: The usual symptoms in the adult are chills and high fever, renal pain, nausea and vomiting, and symptoms of cystitis. In children, only fever and vague abdominal pains and sometimes diarrhea are apt to be experienced.

B. Asymptomatic Pyelonephritis: The patient may have no symptoms whatsoever. The incidental finding of pyuria and bacteriuria may be the only clue.

C. Symptoms of Cystitis Only: In these patients, the bacteriuria is resistant to antimicrobials, or, if bacteriuria clears, relapse quickly occurs. These patients may have reflux with asymptomatic chronic pyelonephritis.

D. Renal Pain on Voiding: Surprisingly, this is a rare complaint in the refluxing patient.

E. Uremia: The last stage of bilateral reflux is uremia due to destruction of the renal parenchyma by hydronephrosis or pyelonephritis (or both). The patient may often adjust to renal insufficiency and may appear quite healthy. Many renal transplants are performed in patients whose kidneys have deteriorated secondarily to reflux and accompanying infection.

F. Hypertension: In the later stages of atrophic pyelonephritis, a significant incidence of hypertension is observed.

Symptoms Related to the Underlying Disease

The clinical picture is often dominated by the signs and symptoms of the primary disease.

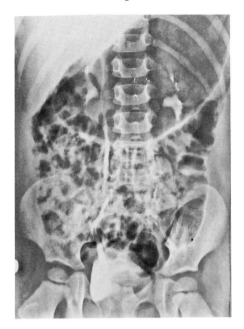 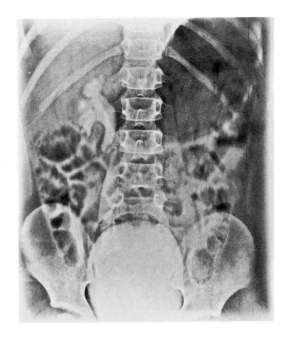

Fig 11-6. Excretory urogram with changes that imply right vesicoureteral reflux. Left: Excretory urogram showing normal right urogram and a ureter which is mildly dilated and remains full through its entire length. The ureteral change implies reflux. **Right:** Cystogram demonstrates the reflux. Note, now, the degree of dilatation of the ureter, pelvis and calyces.

A. Urinary Tract Obstruction: The little girl may be noted to have hesitancy in initiating the urinary stream and an impaired or intermittent stream secondary to spasm of the periurethral striated muscle (see p 385). In males, the urinary stream may be slow as a result of posterior urethral valves (infants) or prostatic enlargement (men over 50).

B. Spinal Cord Disease: The patient may be grossly deformed by a serious neurogenic disease such as paraplegia, quadriplegia, multiple sclerosis, or meningomyelocele. Symptoms may be limited to those of neurogenic bladder: incontinence of urine, urinary retention, and vesical urgency.

Physical Findings

During an attack of acute pyelonephritis, renal tenderness may be elicited. Absence of such a finding does not rule out chronic renal infection.

Palpation and percussion of the suprapubic area may reveal a distended bladder secondary to obstruction or neurogenic disease.

The finding of a hard midline mass deep in the pelvis in a male infant is apt to represent a markedly thickened bladder caused by posterior urethral valves.

Examination may reveal a neurologic deficit compatible with a paretic bladder.

Laboratory Findings

The most common complication, particularly in the female, is infection. Bacteriuria without pyuria is not uncommon. In the male, because of his long, sterile urethra, the urine may be normal.

PSP excretion will be diminished in the face of uremia. The curve, even when renal function is normal, may be "flat" because some of the first half-hour excretion may be refluxed back up to the kidneys; with gross bilateral reflux, the total PSP may be alarmingly low. The serum creatinine may be elevated in the advanced stage of renal damage, but it may be normal even when the degree of reflux and hydronephrosis is marked (Fig 11-7, above right). The PSP test is the superior screening test in this instance.

X-ray Findings

The plain film may reveal evidence of spina bifida, meningomyelocele, or absence of the sacrum, thus pointing to a neurologic deficit. Even in the face of vesicoureteral reflux, excretory urograms may be normal, but usually one or more of the following clues to the presence of reflux may be noted (Fig 11-6): (1) A persistently dilated lower ureter. (2) Areas of dilatation in the ureter. (3) Ureter visualized throughout its entire length. (4) Presence of hydroureteronephrosis with a narrow juxta-

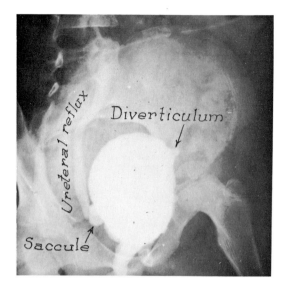

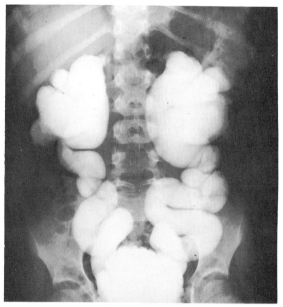

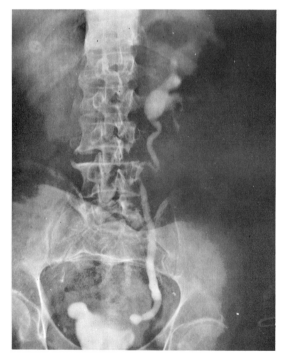

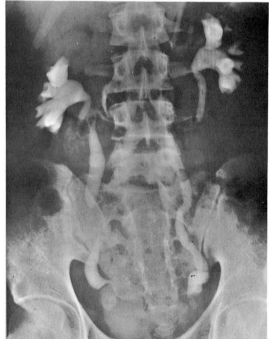

Fig 11-7. **Cystograms revealing vesicoureteral reflux.** **Above left:** Saccule at right uretero-vesical junction. **Above right:** Reflux with severe bilateral ureterohydronephrosis; serum creatinine, 0.6 mg/100 ml; PSP excretion, 5% in 1 hour. **Below left:** Postprostatectomy patient with reflux on left and bilateral saccules. **Below right:** Ten-year-old boy with meningomyelocele. Bladder has been emptied. Impairment of drainage at ureterovesical junctions is demonstrated. (Courtesy of John A. Hutch, MD.)

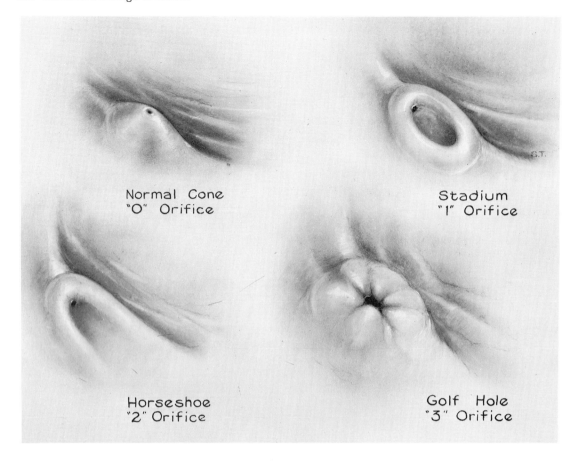

Normal Cone
"O" Orifice

Stadium
"1" Orifice

Horseshoe
"2" Orifice

Golf Hole
"3" Orifice

Fig 11-8. Cystoscopic appearance of the normal ureteral orifice and three degrees of incompetency of the ureterovesical junction. (Reproduced with permission, from Lyon, R.G., Marshall, S., & E.A. Tanagho: J Urol **102**:504-9, 1969.)

vesical ureteral segment. (5) Changes of healed pyelonephritis: calyceal clubbing with narrowed infundibula or cortical thinning.

The presence of ureteral duplication suggests the possibility of reflux into the lower pole of the kidney. In this instance, hydronephrosis or changes compatible with pyelonephritic scarring may be noted. Abnormality of the upper segment of a duplicated system can be caused by the presence of an ectopic ureteral orifice with reflux or by obstruction secondary to a ureterocele.

Reflux is diagnosed by demonstrating its existence with one of the following technics (Fig 11-6): simple or delayed cystography, voiding cystourethrography, or voiding cinefluoroscopy. In general, reflux that is demonstrated only with voiding implies a more competent valve than that which allows low pressure regurgitation. As has been pointed out, failure to demonstrate reflux on one study does not rule out intermittent reflux.

The voiding phase of the cystogram may reveal changes compatible with distal urethral stenosis with secondary spasm of the voluntary periurethral muscles in the female child or changes in the small boy that are diagnostic of posterior urethral valves.

Instrumental Examination

A. Urethral Calibration: In females, urethral calibration, using bougies. á boule, should be done. Distal urethral stenosis is almost routinely found in little girls suffering from urinary infection. Destruction of the ring is an important step in improving the hydrodynamics of voiding: lowered intravesical voiding pressure and the abolition of vesical residual urine (see p 385). Less commonly, urethral stenosis is discovered in the adult female. It, too, should be treated.

B. Cystoscopy: Most little girls with reflux have smooth-walled or only slightly trabeculated bladders. Evidence of chronic cystitis may be noted. Ureteral duplication may be seen. A ureterocele may be evident. An orifice may be found to be ectopic at the bladder neck or even in the urethra. These findings imply the possibility of reflux. The major contribution of cystoscopy is to allow study of the morphology of the ureteral orifice and its position in relation to the vesical neck (Fig 11-8).

1. Morphology - The normal ureter has the appearance of a volcanic cone. The orifice of a slightly weaker valve looks like a football stadium; an even weaker one has the appearance of a horseshoe with its open end pointing toward the vesical neck. The completely incompetent junction has a "golf hole" orifice which lies over the ureteral hiatus.

2. Position - By and large, the more defective the appearance of the ureteral orifice, the farther from the vesical neck it lies. The degree of retraction of the orifice reflects the degree of ureterotrigonal deficiency.

DIFFERENTIAL DIAGNOSIS

Functional (nonocclusive) vesicoureteral obstruction may cause changes similar to those suggesting the presence of reflux on excretory urography. Multiple cystograms fail to show reflux. Creevy has termed this condition "ureteral achalasia." Tanagho & others have shown that this congenital obstruction is due to a heavy layer of circularly oriented smooth muscle fibers surrounding the ureter at this point. Its action is sphincteric.

Significant obstruction distal to the vesical neck leads to hypertrophy of both the detrusor and trigonal muscles. The latter exert an exaggerated pull upon the intravesical ureter, thus causing functional obstruction (Tanagho & others). Ureterohydronephrosis is therefore to be expected; vesicoureteral reflux is uncommon.

Other lesions that may cause ureterohydronephrosis without reflux include low ureteral stone, ureteral occlusion by cervical or prostatic cancer, urinary tract tuberculosis, and schistosomiasis.

TREATMENT

It is impossible to give a concise and definitive discourse on the treatment of vesicoureteral reflux because of the many factors involved and because there is no unanimity of opinion among urologists on this subject. In general, probably more than half of children with primary reflux can be controlled by nonsurgical means and the rest will require some form of operative procedure. Adults exhibiting reflux will usually require vesicoureteroplasty.

Medical Treatment

A. Indications: The child with primary reflux (attenuated trigone) who has fairly normal upper tracts on urographic study and whose ureterovesical valves on cystoscopy appear fair to good has an excellent chance of "outgrowing" the defect, particularly if cystograms show only transient or "high pressure" reflux.

The male child with posterior urethral valves may cease to reflux once these valves are destroyed.

The adult female who occasionally develops acute pyelonephritis following intercourse but whose urine quickly clears on antimicrobial therapy will probably be controlled if she takes steps to prevent vesical infections (see p 163). This is particularly true if, when her urine is sterile, reflux cannot be demonstrated on cystography. The maintenance of sterile urine will allow her "borderline" valve to remain competent.

B. Methods of Treatment: Destruction of the ring of distal urethral stenosis in little girls, or posterior urethral valves in boys, has an excellent chance of reducing voiding intravesical pressure, abolishing vesical residual urine and reflux.

Definitive treatment of the urinary infection with bactericidal drugs should be given, followed by chronic suppressive therapy for 6 months or more.

Triple voiding. Since vesicoureteral reflux prevents the urinary tract from emptying itself completely, thus destroying the vesical defense mechanism, triple voiding once a day is helpful if the child is old enough to be trained. When reflux is present, the bladder empties itself on voiding, but some urine ascends to the kidneys and then returns to the bladder. Voiding again a few minutes later will push less urine into the ureters. A third voiding will usually completely empty the urinary tract. Thus the patient's own natural resistance can operate to a maximum degree.

Children with reflux often have thin-walled bladders and do not perceive the normal urge to void when the bladder is full. Further detrusor tone is lost with overfilling, thus contributing to residual urine. Such children should "void by the clock" every 3-4 hours whether they have the urge or not. Vesical residual urine may then be minimized.

The infant female with markedly dilated upper urinary tracts may be tided over by means of an indwelling urethral catheter. Over a period of months, the ureteral dilatation and elongation may regress; renal function is protected. At a convenient and strategic time, more definitive therapy can then be accomplished.

C. Evaluation of Success of Medical Treatment: Urinalysis should be done at least once a month for a year or more. Maintenance of sterile urine is an encouraging sign.

Cystograms should be repeated every 4-6 months, hoping for disappearance of the reflux.

Excretory urography should be ordered at 6 and 12 months to be sure that renal deterioration does not occur.

Surgical Treatment

A. Indications: Reflux caused by the following abnormalities will not disappear spontaneously: (1) Ectopic ureteral orifice, (2) ureteral duplication, (3) ureterocele associated with ureteral duplication and reflux into the uninvolved ureter, (4) "golf hole" ureteral orifice, and (5) low pressure reflux with significant hydroureteronephrosis.

Surgery is indicated (1) if it is not possible to keep the urine sterile and reflux persists; (2) if acute pyelonephritis recurs despite a strict medical regimen and chronic suppressive antimicrobial therapy; (3) if there is increased renal damage as portrayed by serial excretory urograms; or (4) if reflux persists for 1 year after institution of therapy.

B. **Types of Surgical Therapy:** Surgical treatment may require preliminary urinary diversion to improve renal function and to allow dilated ureters to regain tone. Later, definitive relief of obstruction (eg, posterior urethral valves) and ureterovesicoplasty can be performed at the optimum time. Some patients with irreversible lesions causing reflux (eg, meningomyelocele) or badly damaged and atonic ureters may require permanent diversion of the urine (ie, uretero-iliocutaneous anastomosis).

1. Temporary urinary diversion - If drainage of refluxed urine into the bladder is free, cystostomy (or an indwelling urethral catheter in girls) may prove helpful. If the ureters are dilated and kinked, a redundant loop can be brought to the skin. The ureter is opened at this point and urine collected into an iliostomy bag. Later, the loop can be resected and its ends anastomosed. Nephrostomy may be necessary if ureteral redundancy is absent.

2. Permanent urinary diversion - If it is felt that successful ureterovesicoplasty cannot be accomplished, a Bricker type of diversion

is indicated. If renal function is poor and the ureters are widely dilated and atonic, ureterocutaneous diversion may be the procedure of choice.

3. Other surgical procedures -

a. If reflux is unilateral and the kidney badly damaged and the other kidney is normal, nephrectomy is indicated.

b. If one renal pole of a duplicated system is essentially functionless, heminephrectomy with removal of its entire ureter should be done. If there is moderate hydronephrosis of one renal pole with duplication, an alternative is anastomosis of the dilated ureter or pelvis to the normal ureter or pelvis. The remainder of the dilated refluxing ureter should be removed.

c. In the face of unilateral reflux, anastomosis of the lower end of the refluxing ureter into the side of its normal mate (transureteroureterostomy) has a few proponents.

4. Definitive repair.

Definitive Repair of Ureterovesical Junction (Ureterovesicoplasty)

A. Principles of Repair:

1. Resect the lower 2-3 cm of the ureter whose muscle is underdeveloped.

2. Free up enough extravesical ureter so that an intravesical segment 2.5 cm long can be formed.

3. Place the intravesical ureter in a submucosal position.

4. Suture the wall of the new ureteral orifice to the cut edge of the trigonal muscle.

B. **Types of Operation:** The following procedures satisfy the above principles and have afforded success in a high percentage of cases: The advancement operation (Williams; Hutch; Glenn and Anderson), and the Politano-Leadbetter and the Paquin operations.

C. Results of Ureterovesicoplasty: About 93% of the patients no longer show reflux after ureterovesicoplasty. About 3% develop ureterovesical stenosis which requires reoperation. At least 75% will have and maintain sterile urine without antimicrobials 3-6 months after surgery. Many patients in whom bacteriuria persists have cystitis only. These are impressive results considering that only the most severe and advanced cases are submitted to surgical repair, and they exceed by far the cure rates reported when only antimicrobials are used (10-15%). This operation is rightly considered one of the most significant accomplishments of modern urology.

PROGNOSIS

In patients with reflux who are judged to have fairly competent valves, conservative therapy as outlined above is highly successful in the cure of reflux and therefore infection.

The patients with very incompetent ureterovesical valves subjected to surgical repair also have an excellent prognosis. A few children, however, have such badly damaged urinary tracts when finally submitted to diagnostic procedures that little help other than permanent urinary diversion can be offered.

•   •   •

General References

Ambrose, S. S.: Reflux pyelonephritis in adults secondary to congenital lesions of the ureteral orifice. J Urol 102:302-4, 1969.

Blight, E. M., Jr., & E. J. O'Shaughnessy: Vesicoureteral reflux in children: A prospective study. J Urol 102:44-6, 1969.

Burkholder, G. V., Harper, R. C., & P. D. Beach: Congenital absence of the abdominal muscles. Am J Clin Path 53:602-8, 1970.

Burko, H., & R. K. Rhamy: Lower urinary tract problems related to infection: Diagnosis and treatment. P Clin North America 17:233-53, 1970.

Burns, A., & M. Palken: Ureteroureterostomy for reflux in duplex systems. J Urol 106: 290-4, 1971.

Cremin, B. J.: The urinary tract anomalies associated with agenesis of the abdominal walls. Brit J Radiol 44:767-72, 1971.

Cussen, L. J.: The structure of the normal human ureter in infancy and childhood. Invest Urol 5:179-94, 1967.

Daines, S. L., & N. B. Hodgson: Management of reflux in total duplication anomalies. J Urol 105:720-4, 1971.

Elo, J.: Vesicoureteral reflux in children. J Urol 106:603-5, 1971.

Estes, R. C., & R. J. Brooks: Vesicoureteral reflux in adults. J Urol 103:601-5, 1970.

Fein, R. L., Young, J. G., & K. E. van Buskirk: The case for loop ureterostomy in the infant with advanced lower urinary tract obstruction. J Urol 101:513-9, 1969.

Garrett, R. A.: Conservative management of reflux: Indications, objectives, technique, follow-up, and results. Proceedings of a workshop on ureteral reflux in children. National Academy of Sciences—National Research Council, Washington, D. C., 1967.

Glenn, J. F., & E. E. Anderson: Distal tunnel ureteral reimplantation. J Urol 97:623-6, 1967.

Haran, P. J., Darling, D. B., & J. H. Fisher: The excretory urogram in children with ureterorenal reflux. Am J Roentgenol 99: 585-92, 1967.

Heidrick, W. P., Mattingly, R. F., & J. R. Amberg: Vesicoureteral reflux in pregnancy. Obst Gynec 29:571-8, 1967.

Hendren, W. H.: Functional restoration of decompensated ureters in children. Am J Surg 119:477-82, 1970.

Hodson, C. J.: The radiological contribution toward the diagnosis of chronic pyelonephritis. Radiology 88:857-71, 1967.

Hutch, J. A., & A. D. Amar: Vesicoureteral reflux. In: Encyclopedia of Urology. Vol 7-1: Malformations. C. E. Aiken & others (editors). Springer-Verlag, 1968.

Hutch, J. A., Ayers, R. D., & G. S. Loquvam: The bladder musculature, with special reference to the ureterovesical junction. J Urol 85:531-9, 1961.

Hutch, J. A., Smith, D. R., & R. Osborne: Review of a series of ureterovesicoplastics. J Urol 100:285-9, 1968.

Hutch, J. A.: Ureteric advancement operation: Anatomy, technique, and early results. J Urol 89:180-4, 1963.

Johnston, J. H.: Reconstructive surgery of mega-ureter in childhood. Brit J Urol 39: 17-21, 1967.

Kern, H. B., & M. Malament: Vesicoureteral reflux and the adult male. Brit J Urol 41: 295-306, 1969.

Leadbetter, W. F.: Surgical management of simple reflux: Indications, objectives, techniques, follow-up and results. Proceedings of a workshop on ureteral reflux in children. National Academy of Sciences—National Research Council, Washington, D. C., 1967, pp. 157-63.

Lipsky, H., & G. D. Chisholm: Primary vesico-ureteric reflux in adults. Brit J Urol 43:277-83, 1971.

Lyon, R. P., Marshall, S., & E. A. Tanagho: The ureteral orifice: Its configuration and competency. J Urol 102:504-9, 1969.

Lytton, B., Weiss, R. M., & R. R. Berneike: Ipsilateral ureteroureterostomy in the management of vesicoureteral reflux in duplication of the upper urinary tract. J Urol 105: 507-10, 1971.

MacGregor, M.: Pyelonephritis lenta. Consideration of childhood urinary infection as the forerunner of renal insufficiency in later life. Arch Dis Childhood 45:159-72, 1970.

McGovern, J.H., & V.F. Marshall: Reimplantation of ureters into the bladders of children. Trans Am Ass Genitourin Surg 59:116-8, 1967.

O'Donnell, B., Moloney, M.A., & V. Lynch: Vesico-ureteric reflux in infants and children. Brit J Urol 41:6-13, 1969.

Palken, M.: Surgical correction of vesicoureteral reflux in children: Results with the use of a single standard technique. J Urol 104:765-8, 1970.

Paquin, A.J., Jr.: Ureterovesical anastomosis: The description and evaluation of a technique. J Urol 82:573-83, 1959.

Politano, V.A., & W.F. Leadbetter: An operative technique for correction of vesicoureteral reflux. J Urol 79:932-41, 1958.

Price, S.E., Jr., Johnson, S.H. III, & M. Marshall, Jr.: Experience with ureteral reimplantation in the treatment of recurring urinary infections in childhood. J Urol 103:485-90, 1970.

Rees, R.W.M.: The effect of transurethral resection of the intravesical ureter during the removal of bladder tumours. Brit J Urol 41:2-5, 1969.

Servadio, C., & A. Shachner: Observations on vesicoureteral reflux and chronic pyelonephritis in adults. J Urol 103:722-6, 1970.

Smith, D.R.: Vesicoureteral reflux and other abnormalities of the ureterovesical junction. Chap 10 in: Urology, 3rd ed. Campbell, M.F., & J.H. Harrison (editors). Saunders, 1970.

Stephens, F.D.: Intramural ureter and ureterocele. Postgrad MJ 40:179-83, 1964.

Stephens, F.D.: Treatment of megaloureters by multiple micturition. Australian New Zealand J Surg 27:130-4, 1957.

Stickler, G.B., & others: Primary interstitial nephritis with reflux: A cause of hypertension. Am J Dis Child 122:144-8, 1971.

Tanagho, E.A., & F.H. Meyers: Trigonal hypertrophy: A cause of ureteral obstruction. J Urol 93:678-83, 1965.

Tanagho, E.A., Guthrie, T.H., & R.P. Lyon: The intravesical ureter in primary reflux. J Urol 101:824-32, 1969.

Tanagho, E.A., Hutch, J.A., & E.R. Miller: Diagnostic procedures and cinefluoroscopy in vesicoureteral reflux. Brit J Urol 38:435-44, 1966.

Tanagho, E.A., & J.A. Hutch: Primary reflux. J Urol 93:158-64, 1965.

Tanagho, E.A., & others: Primary vesicoureteral reflux: Experimental studies of its etiology. J Urol 93:165-76, 1965.

Tanagho, E.A., & R.C.B. Pugh: The anatomy and function of the ureterovesical junction. Brit J Urol 35:151-65, 1963.

Tanagho, E.A., Smith, D.R., & T.H. Guthrie: Pathophysiology of functional ureteral obstruction. J Urol 104:73-88, 1970.

Tanagho, E.A.: Surgical revision of the incompetent ureterovesical junction: A critical analysis of techniques and requirements. Brit J Urol 42:410-24, 1970.

Tanagho, E.A.: Ureteral tailoring. J Urol 106:194-7, 1971.

Timothy, R.P., Decter, A., & A.D. Perlmutter: Ureteral duplication: Clinical findings and therapy in 46 children. J Urol 105:445-51, 1971.

Waldbaum, R.S., & V.F. Marshall: The prune belly syndrome: A diagnostic therapeutic plan. J Urol 103:668-74, 1970.

Weber, A.L., & W.T. Weylman: Evaluation of vesicoureteral reflux by intravenous pyelography and cinecystography. Radiology 87:489-94, 1966.

Williams, D.I., & H.H. Rabinovitch: Cutaneous ureterostomy for the grossly dilated ureter of childhood. Brit J Urol 39:696-9, 1967.

Williams, G.L., & others: Vesicoureteric reflux in patients with bacteriuria in pregnancy. Lancet 2:1202-5, 1968.

12...

Nonspecific Infections of the Urinary Tract

The "nonspecific" infections of the genito-urinary tract are a group of diseases having similar manifestations and caused by the gram-negative rods (eg, E coli and P vulgaris) and gram-positive cocci (staphylococci and streptococci). They are to be distinguished from infections caused by "specific" organisms, each of which causes a clinically unique disease (eg, tuberculosis, gonorrhea, actinomycosis). In acute infections, a single organism is usually found; mixed infections are often seen in chronic stages.

By far the most common invaders are the gram-negative bacteria, particularly E coli. Others in this group are A aerogenes, P vulgaris and mirabilis, and Ps aeruginosa. Str faecalis (enterococcus) and S aureus are found on occasion. A pure coccal infection may suggest renal stone.

These infections can involve any of the urinary organs (or genital organs in the male), and can spread from a given locus to any or all of the others. Renal infections are of the greatest importance because of the parenchymal destruction caused by them.

Identification of the type of bacteria (ie, rods or cocci) may be important in the empirical selection of medication.

PATHOGENESIS

Four Main Pathways of Entry Into the Urinary Tract

It is not always possible to trace the mode of entry of bacteria into the genitourinary tract. There are 4 major possibilities.

A. Ascending Infection: There is increasing evidence that ascending infection is the most common cause of urinary tract infection. The incidence of urinary infection—judged by age group and sex—permits certain inferences. Urosepsis is common from birth to age 10. At least 80% of these affect the female, and the incidence of pyelonephritis is relatively high. New infections are seldom seen from this age until age 20, at which time urinary infection again becomes common. Again, the great majority affect women, and the incidence parallels the years of sexual activity. This high incidence appears to be related to the short urethra of the female, which often harbors urinary pathogens. Most of these infections involve the bladder only. At age 60 and beyond, the incidence of infection again increases; and because bladder neck obstruction and the inevitable vesical residual urine commonly affect males of this age, most of these patients are men. Secondary pyelonephritis in this group is not uncommon.

These data strongly support the inference that the most common route of infection is up the urethra, particularly in the female. The high incidence of pyelonephritis in the very young patient is usually associated with demonstrable vesicoureteral reflux. Infection in older men is usually secondary to prostatitis or obstruction with or without reflux.

B. Hematogenous Spread: This is an uncommon pathway of bacterial invasion of the kidneys, prostate, and testes. During the course of many infections elsewhere in the body, bacteria are apt to enter the blood stream; in fact, this may occur in the healthy person. Ordinarily these invaders are destroyed by normal body processes; but if the number of bacteria is great, if they are virulent, and particularly if the field is receptive (ie, renal stone), infection of the genitourinary tract may occur. In experimental animals, intravenous injection of urinary pathogens only leads to pyelonephritis if the ureter is temporarily obstructed or the kidney traumatized. It seems conceivable that ureteral or ureteropelvic obstruction or vesicoureteral reflux could prepare the ground for hematogenous pyelonephritis by this mechanism.

The most obvious examples of renal infection via hematogenous invasion are tuberculosis (metastatic from the lungs) and renal carbuncle (metastatic from skin infection). Conversely, in the course of acute infections of the kidney or prostate, bacteria often enter the blood stream.

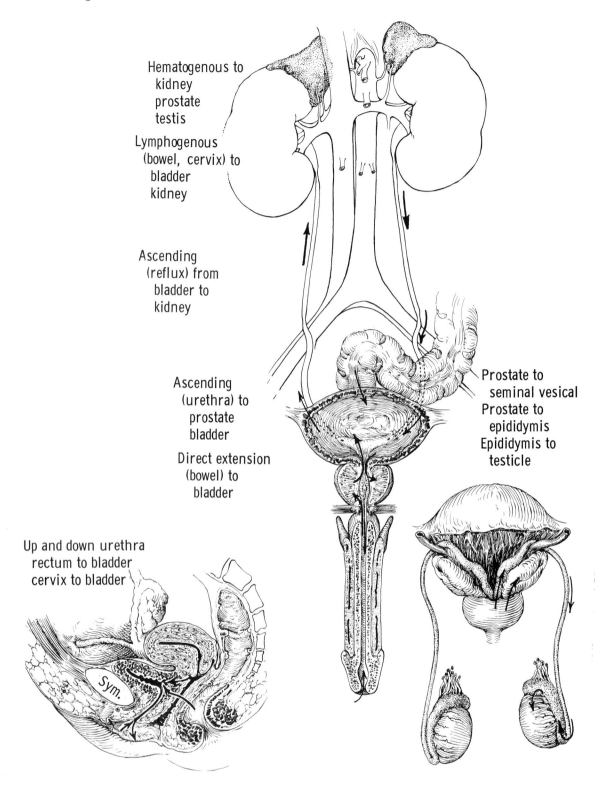

Hematogenous to
kidney
prostate
testis

Lymphogenous
(bowel, cervix) to
bladder
kidney

Ascending
(reflux) from
bladder to
kidney

Ascending
(urethra) to
prostate
bladder

Direct extension
(bowel) to
bladder

Up and down urethra
rectum to bladder
cervix to bladder

Prostate to
seminal vesical
Prostate to
epididymis
Epididymis to
testicle

Sym.

Fig 12-1. Routes of infection in the genitourinary tract.

C. Lymphogenous Spread: Undoubted evidence has been brought forward to show that infection can spread to the urinary tract through the lymphatic channels, but this probably occurs only rarely. A few investigators believe that infections spread from the large bowel to the urinary tract through the lymphatics. Others think that cervicitis may cause vesical or renal infection by the spread of bacteria via the periureteral lymph vessels. Blood stream infections of lymphatic origin are also a theoretical possibility.

D. Direct Extension From Another Organ: Intraperitoneal abscesses (appendiceal abscess, diverticulitis of the sigmoid) may involve and infect the urinary organs (bladder).

Factors Contributing to Infection

Other factors which contribute to the establishment of bacteria in the genitourinary organs include the following:

A. Stasis and Obstruction: Bacteria are better able to gain a foothold if there is stasis or obstruction as seen with distal urethral stenosis in little girls, enlarged prostate, and vesicoureteral reflux. Under these circumstances, pathogenic urethral bacteria ascending to the bladder become established in the bladder because the vesical defense mechanism is made inoperative by the presence of vesical residual urine.

B. Presence of a Foreign Body: A kidney containing a stone is apt to become infected even in the absence of obstruction. A foreign body introduced into the bladder (eg, indwelling catheter) will lead to infection. Such objects seem to lower the normal resistance to successful invasion by bacteria.

C. General Body Resistance: Resistance may be lowered in the course of debilitating illnesses and during periods of chronic or excessive fatigue, in which case infection gains a foothold more easily. Diabetes predisposes to urinary infection.

Organs and Pathways of Infection Within the Urinary Tract (See Fig 12-1.)

A. Kidney: It is becoming increasingly clear that the most common cause of renal infection is ureterovesical reflux. Reflux is found in association with most instances of atrophic pyelonephritis. Hematogenous invasion is a rare route of infection.

B. Bladder: The bladder may become involved by bacteria descending from the kidney or, more commonly, ascending from the urethra. Direct blood stream invasion of the bladder is undoubtedly rare. Lymphogenous spread from cervical or uterine infection seems possible. Infections of the bowel may spread to the bladder by contiguity (diverticulitis of the sigmoid colon).

C. Prostate: The prostate is most commonly infected by ascent of the urethral flora, whose numbers are increased in urethritis. Hematogenous invasion is a possibility.

D. Urethra: The urethra in both sexes usually becomes infected by ascending bacteria. These infections are usually nonvenereal. Deep ascent of these bacteria may cause cystitis and, if there is ureteral reflux, pyelonephritis. Infection may also descend to the urethra from prostate or bladder.

E. Epididymis: Infection usually reaches the epididymis by descent (reflux of urine) along the vas or the perivasal lymphatics from an infected prostate.

F. Testis: The testis is commonly invaded hematogenously by bacteria (pneumococci, brucellae, etc) or viruses (mumps, etc). Occasionally it becomes infected by direct extension from epididymal inflammation (both tuberculous and nonspecific).

Relation of Symptoms to Onset of Infection

If lower tract symptoms precede the onset of chills, fever, and renal pain, a primary (ascending) urologic infection is probably present. In this instance, vesicoureteral reflux should be suspected. If, however, the systemic symptoms precede the complaints referable to the lower urinary tract, metastatic infection or spread from some other area of infection may have occurred. In the latter instance, the extra-urologic focus must be identified if possible.

Correlation of Factors That Cause and Perpetuate Urinary Tract Infections

The cause of urinary tract infections and their perpetuation can now be explained on a scientific basis. With few exceptions, the offending organism ascends the urethra and gains a foothold in the presence of vesical residual urine. The complication of pyelonephritis implies incompetency of the ureterovesical junction.

A. Source of Bacteria: Years ago, Helmholz showed that, with few exceptions, bacteria are found in significant numbers only in the distal 3-4 cm of the male urethra. Furthermore, it is unusual to find urinary pathogens in the male urethra. It is for these reasons that bladder or kidney infection develops late or not at all in males even in the presence of significant vesical residual urine (posterior urethral valves, enlarged prostate). It may be that anything that slows voiding flow rate might allow further ascent of bacteria in males so that the organisms finally reach the bladder.

In the female, however, the short urethra presents an entirely different problem. Cox studied the urethral flora in women. In those without a history of urinary tract infections, 50% had bacteria in the proximal 4th of the urethra; of these bacteria, 27% were urinary pathogens. These organisms have their source from the perineum. In a group of women suffering from recurrent infections, 77% had bacteria in the proximal 1 cm of the urethra and 55% of the organisms were pathogenic to the urinary tract. Unfortunately, successful eradication of the urinary infection is not accompanied by sterilization of the urethra. The same organism may remain, in which case the next infection is caused by that bacterium; or a new pathogen may become established and cause a new infection.

These findings readily explain the common mistaken observation that urinary infections are "difficult to cure." Infection usually is eradicated, but new infections develop in a high percentage of cases. Certainly, a new organism represents a new infection but the reappearance of the same bacterium does not necessarily imply relapse. The urethral flora govern the bacteriologic findings in the urine. Methods taken to correct vesical outlet obstruction (posterior urethral valves, distal urethral stenosis in little girls) usually stop recurrent urinary infection, but the pathogenic urethral bacteria are still present.

We may say, then, that with few exceptions the bacteria infecting the bladder ascend from the urethra.

B. The Vesical Defense Mechanism: Clinical experience dictates that the bladder has an intrinsic defense against bacteria. It is impossible to pass a catheter to the bladder without carrying bacteria into the bladder, but cystitis secondary to this procedure is rare unless there is vesical residual urine. Cox and Hinman showed that, though significant numbers of bacteria were introduced into the bladders of normal young men by catheter, all had sterile urine within 72 hours. A similar observation was made in a group of women who required indwelling catheters for some days following certain gynecologic operations. Without the use of antimicrobials, their urine became sterile spontaneously. They were able to show experimentally that a bladder that completely empties itself seldom becomes infected. Complete voiding washes out most of the bacteria.

Those few left in a film of urine on the vesical mucosa are killed. The implication is that the mucosa represents the intrinsic vesical defense mechanism against bacteria.

C. Factors Causing Perpetuation of Urinary Infection: The urinary tract that completely empties itself at the time of voiding tends to remain sterile even though bacteria ascend to the bladder. If, however, there is some urologic abnormality which defeats this normal mechanism, the bacteria not only gain a foothold but the infection is perpetuated.

1. Vesical residual urine - Any defect that causes residual urine contributes to persistence of infection. Such diseases include neurogenic bladder, urethral obstruction, enlarged prostate, and cystocele. Although drugs may fail to keep the urine sterile, correcting the urologic disease process will often cause the urine to clear spontaneously. If it does not, antimicrobials will usually bring about cure.

2. Foreign bodies in the bladder - Even though meticulous hygiene and antibiotic coverage are practiced when an indwelling catheter is in place, after 3-10 days bacteriuria is almost always found. It cannot be eradicated until the catheter is removed. The presence of a stone in the bladder will cause infection to persist.

3. Vesicoureteral reflux - At the time of voiding, in the presence of vesicoureteral reflux, the bladder usually empties itself completely but some urine is forced into the ureter and kidney. Within a few minutes after voiding, this urine drains back to the bladder; in essence, the patient has not emptied the bladder. This defeats the vesical defense mechanism.

4. Residual urine in the upper urinary tract - Any disease causing retention of urine in the renal pelvis (ureteral stone, ureteropelvic junction obstruction) will perpetuate infection once it gains a foothold.

5. Foreign bodies in the kidney - Once renal infection ensues, the presence of a stone will tend to defeat efforts to sterilize the urine.

Allen, T. D.: Pathogenesis of urinary-tract infections in children. New England J Med **273**:1421-4, 1472-7, 1965.

Cox, C. E.: The urethra and its relationship to urinary tract infection: The flora of the normal female urethra. South MJ **59**:621-6, 1966.

Cox, C. E., Lacy, S. S., & F. Hinman, Jr.: The urethra and its relationship to urinary tract infection. II. The urethral flora of the female with recurrent urinary infection. J Urol **99**:632-8, 1968.

Domingue, G. J., & J. U. Schlegel: The possible role of microbial L-forms in pyelonephritis. J Urol **104**:790-8, 1970.

Fair, W. R.: Bacteriologic and hormonal observations of the urethra and vaginal vestibule in normal, premenopausal women. J Urol **104**:426-31, 1970.

Glynn, A. A., Brumfitt, W., & C. J. Howard: K antigens of Escherichia coli and renal involvement in urinary tract infections. Lancet **2**:514-6, 1971.

Heidrick, W. P., Mattingly, R. F., & J. R. Amberg: Vesicoureteral reflux in pregnancy. Obst Gynec **29**:571-8, 1967.

Hinman, F., Jr.: Bacterial elimination. J Urol **99**:811-25, 1968.

Hodson, C. J., & S. Wilson: Natural history of chronic pyelonephritic scarring. Brit MJ **2**:191-4, 1965.

Hutch, J. A., Ayers, R. D., & L. E. Noll: Vesicoureteral reflux as cause of pyelonephritis of pregnancy. Am J Obst Gynec **87**:478-85, 1963.

Hutch, J. A., Miller, E. R., & F. Hinman, Jr.: Perpetuation of infection in unobstructed urinary tracts. J Urol **90**:88-91, 1963.

Kunin, C. M., & R. C. McCormack: Prevention of catheter-induced urinary-tract infections by sterile closed drainage. New England J Med **274**:1155-61, 1966.

Kunin, C. M.: The natural history of recurrent bacteriuria in school girls. New England J Med **282**:1443-8, 1970.

MacGregor, M.: Pyelonephritis in children. Postgrad MJ **41**:485-96, 1965.

Marshall, V. F.: Editorial. Treatment of girls with urinary infection and nothing else. J Urol **106**:441-2, 1971.

Stamey, T. A., & others: Recurrent urinary infections in adult women. The role of introital enterobacteria. California Med **115**:1-19, July 1971.

Stamey, T. A., & A. Pfau: Urinary infections: A selective review and some observations. California Med **113**:16-35, Dec. 1970.

Thornton, G. F., Lytton, B., & V. T. Andriole: Bacteriuria during indwelling catheter drainage. JAMA **195**:179-83, 1966.

Turck, M., Ronald, A. R., & R. G. Petersdorf: Relapse and reinfection in chronic bacteriuria. The correlation between site of infection and pattern of recurrence in chronic bacteriuria. New England J Med **278**:422-7, 1968.

NONSPECIFIC INFECTIONS OF THE KIDNEYS

ACUTE PYELONEPHRITIS

The term "pyelonephritis" is used because infections of the renal pelvis alone ("pyelitis") do not occur; however, it is the "nephritis" that is important.

Bacteria can reach the kidney through the blood stream, or they may travel up a ureter which has an incompetent ureterovesical valve. The latter mechanism is by far the most common. It has been shown that vesicoureteral reflux may occur during acute cystitis but ceases when the infection has been cured. This explains the onset of secondary pyelonephritis. If obstruction, reflux, or stasis is present, the chances for the bacteria to gain a foothold are increased. These factors also tend to perpetuate the infection.

One-third of pregnant women with pyelonephritis will exhibit reflux. After termination of the pregnancy, reflux disappears. It is for this reason that the not uncommon bacteriuria seen in pregnancy (6% incidence) is potentially dangerous.

Pathology

A. Gross: The kidney may be greatly enlarged as a result of edema. The surface may be dull. On cut section, the sharp demarcation between cortex and medulla is lost; multiple small abscesses may be visible. The pelvic mucosa is often injected and roughened.

B. Microscopic: There is diffuse or spotty inflammation characterized by leukocytic infiltration, edema, and small hemorrhagic areas. The tubular epithelium may desquamate if the infection is severe. The glomeruli are much less involved; in fact, they are peculiarly immune to inflammatory change except in the most severe cases.

Pathogenesis (See Fig 12-2.)

With few exceptions, acute pyelonephritis develops from infection in the bladder through the mechanism of vesicoureteral reflux. If the ureterovesical junction, anatomically and physiologically, is of "borderline" quality, cure of the infection will cause the "valve" to revert to competency; a cystogram taken at this time will fail to reveal reflux. When the junction is grossly abnormal, response to antimicrobial therapy may be slow; sterilization of the urine may not be possible. Even in the presence of sterile urine, reflux persists. This inability to completely empty the urinary

Route of Infection

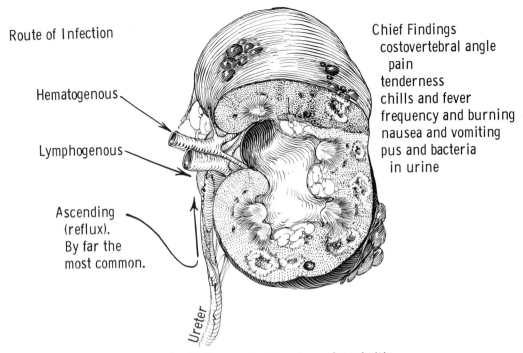

Chief Findings
costovertebral angle
     pain
tenderness
chills and fever
frequency and burning
nausea and vomiting
pus and bacteria
     in urine

Hematogenous

Lymphogenous

Ascending
(reflux).
By far the
most common.

Ureter

Fig 12-2. Pathogenesis of acute pyelonephritis.

tract makes the vesical defense mechanism inoperative; recurring infections are, therefore, to be expected.

If the urine becomes sterile, the renal lesion has been healed, although new infections may occur. Some of these patients may become afebrile although bacteriuria persists. This represents the asymptomatic stage of chronic pyelonephritis.

Each acute infection leads to healing by scar. The kidney becomes smaller and its edge irregular. In the past, these radiographic findings have been called "chronic pyelonephritis." This is not correct since these scars represent evidence of previous infections and such a patient may have had sterile urine for many years. The radiogram, then, is of no help in judging whether active infection exists, although the findings of bacteriuria and reflux imply the presence of chronic pyelonephritis.

Clinical Findings

A. Symptoms: At the onset, there is a severe constant ache over one or both kidneys (flank and back) due to the distention of the renal capsule caused by edema. The pain may radiate to the lower abdominal quadrant. Young children seldom complain of localized renal pain, which is apt to be reflected as ill-localized abdominal discomfort. Symptoms of cystitis develop: frequency, nocturia, urgency, and burning on urination. The temperature

reaches 39-40° C (102-104° F) and is often accompanied by chills. The patient is quite prostrated and usually suffers from nausea and vomiting.

B. Signs: The patient appears to be quite sick. Intermittent high fever is to be expected. The pulse rate is, however, the best index of judging the severity of the infection. If the infection is due to E coli, the pulse may be only 90/minute; with staphylococci, it may reach 140. Tenderness is present over the affected kidney, which is usually not palpable because of muscle spasm. Fist percussion over the costovertebral angle will be quite painful. Abdominal distention may be marked and rebound tenderness may be present, suggesting an intraperitoneal lesion. Auscultation usually reveals a quiet intestine.

C. Laboratory Findings: The white blood count may reach 40,000/μl, and the neutrophil count is elevated. Sedimentation rate is increased. The urine is usually cloudy and shows a little protein, and contains large amounts of pus and bacteria. A few red cells may also be noted. Quantitative cultures will be positive and may be helpful in treatment in refractory infections, in which case sensitivity studies should be done. Renal function as measured by specific gravity of urine or PSP will be only slightly affected unless there is overwhelming sepsis with bilateral multiple cortical abscesses or necrotizing papillitis. Serial blood cultures should be done on any patient with urinary tract infection who has chills and fever. Bacteremia is not uncommon.

D. X-ray Findings: A plain film of the abdomen may show some obliteration of the renal shadow due to edema of the kidney and perinephric fat. Suspicious calcifications (stones) should be sought. Excretory urograms during the acute stage usually show little diminution in function, although the pelvis and calyces on the affected side may be small because of secretion of a small volume of urine as compared to the uninvolved kidney. These films are most valuable in surveying the tract for the presence of obstruction or possible vesicoureteral reflux.

While cystography might reveal vesicoureteral reflux during the acute stage of infection, such an examination is contraindicated at this time. Later, excretory urography and cystography should be done after the infection is controlled.

Differential Diagnosis

Pancreatitis causes pain which may be posterior, and its position and degree may be confused with that of pyelonephritis. Blood amylase, however, will be elevated and pyuria will not be found.

Basal pneumonia may cause pain in the subcostal area, but it is usually pleuritic in type. Examination of the chest should make that diagnosis.

Acute appendicitis or acute disease of the gallbladder may be suggested if the patient's pain is largely anterior and if there is muscle spasm and rebound tenderness in the right upper or lower quadrants. Careful palpation over the kidney should reveal some tenderness, and proper urinalysis should be definitive.

Acute diverticulitis of the descending colon may cause pain in the left flank. Usually, however, a history of change in bowel habits may be elicited. The urine is normal. A barium enema will reveal evidence of changes in the bowel.

Herpes zoster affecting the somatic segments of the renal area (T12, L1) can simulate pain arising from the kidney. However, the pain is superficial and skin hypersensitivity can be demonstrated. The onset of the typical skin changes of shingles will settle the problem.

Complications

If diagnosis is delayed and treatment inadequate, the infection may become chronic. This is particularly true if vesicoureteral reflux is present. The chronic form is seldom recognized because it is usually silent and because few or no pus cells are found in the urine. The bacteria can be found, however, if they are diligently sought for. The chronic infection may lead to (1) renal insufficiency; (2) secondary arteriolar sclerosis, which may cause renal ischemia and, in turn, hypertension; or (3) stone formation and further renal damage.

Bacteremia or septicemia of renal origin may develop in the acute stage of fulminating pyelonephritis and may cause infection or even multiple cortical abscesses of the other kidney. Metastatic abscesses may develop in other organs. Bacteremic shock is occasionally seen, especially when gram-negative rods invade the blood stream.

Treatment

A. Specific Measures: Urine should first be obtained for microscopy, cultures, and sensitivity tests. Based upon the findings gained from the stained smear of the sediment, a relatively nontoxic drug, chosen empirically, should be started. Preferably it should afford both a high urine and tissue concentration (eg, one of the tetracyclines, ampicillin). Ureteral obstruction may have to be relieved by cystoscopic means. This may mean extraction of a ureteral stone or temporary drainage with an indwelling ureteral catheter, as in acute ureteral obstruction due to pregnancy or to extrinsic pressure on the ureter from cancer.

If other methods fail, surgical treatment of obstruction may be necessary (eg, removal of a ureteral stone).

B. General Measures: Pain must be relieved by appropriate drugs. Vesical irritability can be minimized by alkalinizing the urine (which may require 12-20 gm/day of sodium bicarbonate) or giving an antispasmodic such as belladonna or atropine with phenobarbital. Bed rest is definitely indicated during the acute phase of the infection. Adequate urinary output (1000 ml/day) should be maintained, but indiscriminate forcing of fluids only leads to urinary dilution of the antimicrobial drug being administered. Nausea and vomiting may necessitate the administration of parenteral fluids.

C. Failure of Response: If no clinical improvement occurs in 48-72 hours, either the wrong drug is being used or obstruction or stasis is present. Obtain excretory urograms, and look for changes suggesting vesicoureteral reflux or obstruction. Obtain a report on the culture and sensitivity test and switch to an appropriate bactericidal drug, observing the usual precautions against toxicity.

D. Follow-up Care: Even after clinical response, the urinary sediment must be ex-

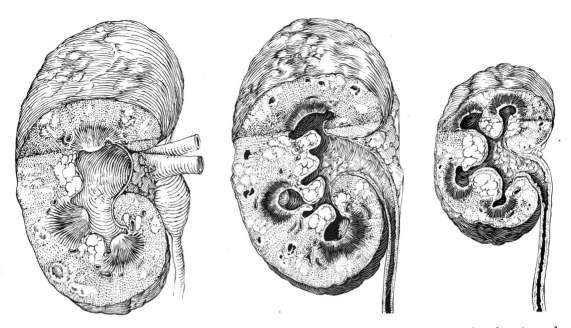

Fig 12-3. **Progressive pathologic changes in kidney suffering from repeated attacks of acute pyelo-nephritis with progressive scarring.** **Left:** Early stage of focal parenchymal scarring. **Center:** Progressive scarring with narrowing of the necks of the calyces, which therefore become dilated (Fig 12-4). **Right:** End stage of recurrent pyelonephritis (stage of atrophy).

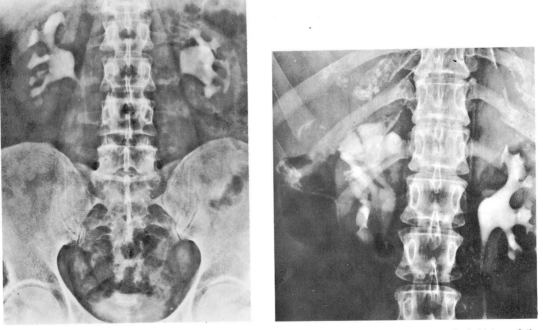

Fig 12-4. **Healed pyelonephritis.** **Left:** Excretory urogram showing flattening and clubbing of the calyces, edge of renal shadow close to ends of the calyces. These changes reflect numerous past episodes of acute pyelonephritis. **Right:** Excretory urogram showing marked atrophy of parenchyma of right kidney with calyces of upper pole extending to renal capsule. Left kidney normal.

amined for pathogens periodically for 2 months. Absence of symptoms is not proof of cure, nor is lack of pus cells in the urine.

Prognosis

The prognosis is good if response to antibiotics is complete, ie, if all infectious organisms are eliminated. If obstruction or reflux is present but is not discovered, recurrences are to be expected. Persistence of bacteriuria requires explanation. Estimation of vesical residual urine, excretory urograms, and cystograms must then be done.

CHRONIC PYELONEPHRITIS

Etiology and Pathogenesis

The term "chronic pyelonephritis" implies the persistent presence of bacteria in the kidney. An outdated medical tenet states that once a kidney becomes infected it is difficult to cure by medical means. The implication is that renal infection is not often curable by the administration of appropriate drugs as are infections of the lungs, meninges, and other organs and structures. It has become increasingly clear that if the urine of such a patient can be rendered sterile, another attack represents a new infection. The failure of medical treatment is readily explained by the omission of a proper urologic work-up seeking evidence of stasis of urine and, particularly, vesicoureteral reflux. The cure rate of recurrent or chronic pyelonephritis is at least 80% if refluxing ureterovesical valves are corrected surgically, whereas medical treatment alone permanently cures only 10-15% of a similar group of patients. The cure of a disease requires understanding of its cause.

The source of the bacteria is, with few exceptions, in the urethra; they ascend to the bladder with ease, particularly in females following sexual intercourse. If the ureterovesical valves are entirely normal, the infection is confined to the bladder. In the presence of a "borderline" valve, acute cystitis may cause such a valve to become temporarily incompetent, thus causing pyelonephritis. Cure by antibiotics again leads to competency of the ureterovesical junction. If the vesical urine can be kept sterile, pyelonephritis is prevented. If, however, the ureterovesical junction is grossly abnormal, bacteria in the bladder reach the kidney, and, since the infection is then perpetuated, true chronic pyelonephritis persists. Recent observations have made it clear that healed or atrophic pyelonephritis, portrayed on x-rays, is usually associated with vesicoureteral reflux.

In the absence of reflux, hematogenous pyelonephritis may occur secondary to ureteral obstruction or the presence of a renal stone. Again, treatment of the cause must be considered if infection is to be permanently relieved.

It should be pointed out that chronic pyelonephritis cannot be diagnosed on urograms. Evidence of scarring may be noted, but this represents healing from previous infections and tells us nothing about the presence or absence of renal bacteriuria. These changes should be read as "healed pyelonephritis."

Pathology

Grossly, the kidney is of normal size or small, depending upon the stage and duration of the disease. The capsule is pale and strips poorly. The surface of the kidney is often pitted and depressed; scarred areas are usual. The cut surface may show fairly well defined cortical and medullary zones, but in a more advanced stage the tissues may be pale and scarred. The pelvic mucosa is pale and fibrotic (Fig 12-3).

Microscopically, the parenchyma is diffusely infiltrated with plasma cells and lymphocytes. The tubules show varying stages of degeneration; some may show considerable dilatation and may contain proteinaceous casts. The glomeruli may be fibrosed, even hyalinized. Considerable thickening of arteries and arterioles is obvious. Not infrequently, the kidney will show areas of acute as well as varying degrees of healed disease.

It is often stated that evidence of pyelonephritis is found in 10-15% of autopsies. As diagnostic criteria for this entity are tightened, the incidence is now considered to be in the range of 1-2% (Freedman).

Many instances of xanthogranulomatous pyelonephritis have been reported. The kidney is usually functionless. It is enlarged, often nodular, and may suggest carcinoma. Sheets of lipid-filled histiocytes, plasma cells, and lymphocytes in a fibrous stroma are microscopically visible; these signs may be confused with those of renal cancer.

Clinical Findings

A. Symptoms: Except at the time of acute exacerbation, there are apt to be few symptoms. There may be mild discomfort over the kidney and some degree of vesical irritability. These, however, may be entirely absent. Vague gastrointestinal complaints may be noted, particularly in children. Unexplained low-grade fever or anemia may be the only clue to the presence of disease. Hypertension is common, particularly in children.

When acute exacerbations occur, localized renal pain may be present and the patient may complain of vesical symptoms. This clinical picture may be misinterpreted as a recurrent acute infection rather than an acute stage of chronic infection.

If the disease is advanced and bilateral (atrophic pyelonephritis), the presenting symptoms may be those of uremia.

B. Signs: There are usually no physical findings unless exacerbation is present, in which case some degree of localized renal tenderness may be elicited. Hypertension may be discovered.

C. Laboratory Findings: Anemia may be found, especially if the patient is uremic. The white blood count may be elevated during an acute stage but otherwise is usually normal.

The urinary sediment may or may not contain white cells, but some bacteria can almost always be demonstrated in the stained smear or culture. The degree of seriousness of an infection cannot be gauged by numbers of pus cells or organisms.

Quantitative cultures should be obtained and sensitivity tests performed.

Some type of renal function test should be done. If the PSP is low, bilateral renal damage, residual urine, or reflux should be suspected.

D. X-ray Findings: A plain film of the abdomen may show that one or both kidneys are small (atrophic). Evidence of stone may be noted. Excretory urograms may be normal, but changes are usually seen that suggest scarring from repeated attacks of renal infection (small kidney, narrowing of the infundibula where they join the pelvis, dilatation and roughening of the calyces, delayed excretion and poor concentration of the medium; Figs 12-3 and 12-4). Dilatation or fullness of the ureter may imply the presence of vesicoureteral reflux (Fig 11-6).

Retrograde urograms will show similar changes. Voiding cystourethrography demonstrates vesicoureteral reflux in at least half of patients with scarred kidneys.

E. Instrumental Examination: On cystoscopy the bladder wall may show evidence of chronic infection. Abnormal configuration and position of a ureteral orifice may be compatible with a refluxing ureterovesical junction. Stained smears and cultures of vesical and renal urine specimens will place the site of infection accurately. Only in this way can the presence of active renal infection be established. Renal function tests (PSP) will measure function of each kidney separately. Diminution may be noted in advanced disease.

Differential Diagnosis

Recurrent acute cystitis may cause symptoms identical to those of a mild attack of pyelonephritis. A history of recurrent attacks of vesical irritability associated with bacteriuria indicates the need for excretory urograms and possibly cystograms. These should allow differentiation.

Chronic cystitis can only be differentiated from chronic pyelonephritis by the absence of renal infection as demonstrated by ureteral catheterization. Urograms are normal in cystitis but show evidence of scarring in pyelonephritis.

Tuberculosis may mimic chronic pyelonephritis perfectly. The absence of bacteria on the methylene blue stain of sediment containing pus cells should suggest tuberculosis. Further bacteriologic studies will confirm this. Pyelography may reveal parenchymal calcifications and moth-eaten (ulcerated) calyceal changes which are typical of tuberculosis.

Xanthogranulomatous pyelonephritis and cancer of the kidney may be confused on urography. The former is usually functionless, whereas the latter can almost always be visualized by means of excretory urography. Angiography or a triple scan (see chapter 8) should differentiate the two.

Complications

A. Unilateral Infection: In the atrophic stage, hypertension may develop due to renal ischemia from severe arteriolar sclerosis. During the stage of exacerbation, bacteremia may occur with involvement of the other kidney.

B. Bilateral Infection: In the late stage of bilateral renal infection, the incidence of hypertension is high. The end stage is often uremia.

C. General: Stone formation is enhanced in the presence of urea-splitting organisms, which produce an alkaline urine, since calcium salts are less soluble in an alkaline medium.

Treatment

The finding of pus and bacteria in the urine does not establish the diagnosis of pyelonephritis. The most common cause of these abnormal elements is acute or chronic cystitis, particularly in adults.

A. Specific Measures:

1. Medical - Intensive chemotherapeutic and antibiotic therapy is needed. Choice of the drug depends upon antimicrobial sensitivity tests prepared from cultures of the urine. The drug should be given for 2-3 weeks. This should be followed by suppressive therapy for

months or years. Suitable drugs include the sulfonamides, methenamine plus a urinary acidifier, or nitrofurantoin.

2. Local - The eradication of chronic prostatic infection or the treatment of a urethral stricture may contribute to the ultimate control of the renal infection.

3. Surgical - Correction of obstructive lesions may be indicated. If vesicoureteral reflux has been demonstrated and sterilization of the urine cannot be gained or maintained, repair of the ureterovesical junction must be considered. If one kidney is badly damaged, nephrectomy may be the procedure of choice.

B. Treatment of Complications: If the disease is bilateral and function is impaired (loss of concentrating power), a urine output of 1000-1500 ml is necessary to facilitate the removal of metabolic waste products. If hypertension is present in association with a unilateral atrophic kidney (and provided the other kidney functions perfectly), nephrectomy should be considered.

Prognosis

If diagnosis is delayed until both kidneys are badly scarred, only medical therapy is indicated in the hope of conserving what functioning tissue is left. Fortunately, repair of the incompetent ureterovesical junction leads to permanent sterilization of the urine in a high percentage of patients with chronic pyelonephritis.

Angell, M. E., Relman, A. S., & S. L. Robbins: "Active chronic pyelonephritis" without evidence of bacterial infection. New England J Med 278:1303-8, 1968.

Anhalt, M. A., Cawood, C. D., & R. Scott, Jr.: Xanthogranulomatous pyelonephritis: A comprehensive review with a report of 4 additional cases. J Urol 105:10-7, 1971.

Aoki, S., & others: "Abacterial" and bacterial pyelonephritis. New England J Med 281:1375-82, 1969.

Carter, M. J., & others: Serologic responses to heterologous Escherichia serogroups in women with pyelonephritis. New England J Med 279:1407-12, 1968.

Freedman, L. R.: Chronic pyelonephritis at autopsy. Ann Int Med 66:697-710, 1967.

Heptinstall, R. H.: Pathology of end-stage kidney disease. Am J Med 44:656-63, 1968.

Hinman, F., Jr., & J. A. Hutch: Atrophic pyelonephritis from ureteral reflux without obstructive signs. J Urol 87:230-42, 1962.

Hodson, C. J.: The radiological contribution toward the diagnosis of chronic pyelonephritis. Radiology 88:857-71, 1967.

Jackson, G. G., & others: Profiles of pyelonephritis. Arch Int Med 110:663-75, 1962.

Jensen, M. M.: Viruses and kidney disease. Am J Med 43:897-911, 1967.

Kimmelstiel, P.: The nature of chronic pyelonephritis. Geriatrics 19:145-54, 1964.

Little, P. J.: The incidence of urinary infection in 5000 pregnant women. Lancet 2: 925-8, 1966.

McCabe, W. R., & G. G. Jackson: Treatment of pyelonephritis. New England J Med 272: 1037-44, 1965.

Noyes, W. E., & A. J. Palubinskas: Xanthogranulomatous pyelonephritis. J Urol 101: 132-6, 1969.

Smith, J. F.: The diagnosis of the scars of chronic pyelonephritis. J Clin Path 15:522-6, 1962.

Spence, H. M., & others: Urinary tract infections in infants and children. J Urol 91: 623-38, 1964.

Still, J. L., & D. Cottom: Severe hypertension in childhood. Arch Dis Childhood 42:34-9, 1967.

Symposium on pyelonephritis. J Infect Dis 120:1-140, 1969.

Vinik, M., & others: Xanthogranulomatous pyelonephritis: angiographic considerations. Radiology 92:537-40, 1969.

Williams, D. I.: Urinary infection. Brit MJ 1:1043-6, 1965.

Zinner, S. H., & E. H. Kass: Long-term (10 to 14 years) follow-up of bacteriuria of pregnancy. New England J Med 285:820-4, 1971.

BACTEREMIC SHOCK

Etiology

Shock is caused by (1) cardiac decompensation, (2) inadequate blood volume, or (3) an enlargement of the vascular space. It reflects a failure of blood flow; the hypotension is merely secondary.

Pathogenesis and Pathology

Shock due to any cause is associated with diminished cardiac output. The latter may be primary (cardiac failure) or secondary (diminished circulating blood volume). About 25% of patients with gram-negative bacteremia will have the complication of shock. The bacteria liberate an endotoxin which causes a marked increase in circulating catecholamines, serotonin, histamine, bradykinin, and acetylcholine. This leads to disseminated intravascular coagulation, severe peripheral vasoconstriction, and pooling of plasma, particularly in the wall of the bowel, which may undergo necrosis. In essence, circulating blood volume decreases and cardiac output drops; hypotension thus occurs. Hypoxia and acidosis develop. Evidence of impaired perfusion of vital organs is noted (eg, oliguria, impaired cerebration). The problem, then, is to attack the cause of the shock (ie, bacteremia) and the shock itself.

Clinical Findings

A. Symptoms: The patient develops fever ranging from 38.5-40° C (101-104° F) and may have associated chills. There is evidence of bacterial infection (eg, peritonitis, urinary infection). At times the febrile response follows shortly after urethral instrumentation. In this instance the source of bacteremia may be the prostate or the kidney secondary to vesico-ureteral reflux. Vomiting and diarrhea are common. Stools may be bloody.

B. Signs: Cloudy mentation is usual. Peripheral cyanosis may be noted. The extremities may be cool but are often warm. The blood pressure is apt to be in the range of 70/30 mm Hg. The pulse rate may be slow or rapid; pulse pressure is diminished. Respiration is rapid and shallow. Findings consistent with ileus are usual. Oliguria is the rule.

C. Laboratory Findings: The white blood count is usually elevated. The PCV is increased due to loss of plasma from the vascular tree. Blood volume determinations are of no value and, indeed, may be misleading.

Since the source of the bacteremia is often the urinary tract, pyuria and bacteriuria may be found. It is essential to obtain cultures and sensitivity tests immediately as a guide to antimicrobial therapy. E coli is the most common offending organism; proteus is the most dangerous. Serial blood cultures are essential for diagnosis and for sensitivity tests. Because of diminished renal blood flow, the specific gravity of the urine is elevated; PSP excretion is depressed. Oliguria leads to retention of nitrogenous waste products in the blood. Because of urinary stasis in the renal tubules, the ratio of BUN to creatinine will exceed the usual 10:1 ratio. In most instances, an ECG will suggest the diagnosis of myocardial ischemia. The ECG changes merely reflect diminished coronary artery blood flow.

Differential Diagnosis

Simple bacteremia is accompanied by chills and fever, but hypotension and oliguria do not occur. This is particularly true in coccal infections. Secondary heart failure may lead to hypotension, thus obscuring the diagnosis. Estimation of central venous pressure will facilitate differentiation (see below).

Acute cardiac failure, especially when secondary to myocardial infarction, may cause sudden hypotension. Evidence of overwhelming infection is absent.

Hypovolemic shock may be caused by marked dehydration or hemorrhage. Symptoms and signs of infection are absent. Basically, the treatment of these conditions is the same as for bacteremic shock, ie, restoration of circulating blood volume.

Complications

The primary infection may not respond to antibiotic therapy; shock may become irreversible. Prolonged hypoxia and hypotension may lead to acute renal tubular necrosis or myocardial infarction. Bowel ulceration may develop. Heart failure may ensue. Increasing levels of blood lactic acid may make reversal difficult.

Treatment

The aim of treatment is to combat the infection, restore blood volume, and improve cardiac output and perfusion of other vital organs (eg, kidneys, brain).

A. Specific Measures:
1. Initial steps -
a. Insert a urethral catheter to monitor the urine flow. Urine flow is the index of renal perfusion.
b. Introduce a small plastic catheter into the superior vena cava so that central venous pressure can be estimated. Pressures of 0-4 cm of water imply diminished circulating blood volume; levels of 6-10 cm of water are compatible with normal blood volume but can occur if both cardiac failure and diminished blood volume are present. A pressure above 15 cm of water is diagnostic of heart failure.
2. Antibiotics - If the organism from the primary site of infection has been identified, sensitivity tests will dictate the choice of drugs. If the offending organism is not known, the assumption should be made that a gram-negative rod is involved. Either kanamycin, one of the cephalosporins, or gentamicin would be good empirical choices initially. The addition of penicillin, 20-40 million units/day, might also be considered. Subsequent bacteriologic reports may suggest the use of other antimicrobials.
3. Steps to improve circulating blood volume, cardiac output, and perfusion of vital organs -
a. Cortisone appears to reduce peripheral resistance, improve cardiac output, and suppress the increased level of catecholamines. It may also protect the cell from the effects of

ischemia. Give 500 mg of hydrocortisone (or comparable corticosteroid) IV over a period of 3 minutes. This should be repeated every 6 hours. Abrupt cessation of the drug 2 or 3 days later can be ordered without fear.

b. Parenteral fluids - If the central venous pressure is very low, rapid infusion of low-viscosity dextran, plasma, or albumin is essential in order to restore circulating plasma volume. It should be continued until the central venous pressure reaches 6-12 cm of water, which implies improved cardiac output. Increase in secretion of urine is a favorable sign even though the peripheral blood pressure rises only moderately. Evidence of efficient organ perfusion is more important than an increase in peripheral blood pressure.

If the initial central venous pressure is 15 cm of water or more, the diagnosis is cardiac failure. Appropriate treatment is indicated.

c. Vasoconstricting (pressor) agents - These drugs are contraindicated in the treatment of shock. They merely treat the blood pressure cuff by further constricting already severely constricted arterioles and veins.

d. Vasodilating agents - If restoration of circulating blood volume fails to relieve the signs of shock (eg, increase in urinary output), vasodilating drugs should be used. In addition to overcoming intense peripheral and visceral vasoconstriction, some of these drugs increase cardiac output and block serotonin and catecholamines. These include both alpha- and beta-adrenergic drugs. The latter have proved the most effective. Isoproterenol (Isuprel®) decreases venous pooling and arterial tone and increases venous return. 2.5 mg of the drug are added to 500 ml of 5% dextrose in water and the infusion is run at about 1 ml/minute. If there is no change in central venous pressure, pulse pressure, or urine output, the rate of drip should be increased. The dosage is not critical.

The alpha-adrenergic blocking agent phenoxybenzamine (Dibenzyline®) blocks the vasoconstricting action of the catecholamines, which are circulating in large amounts during shock, yet allows vasodilatation and cardiac stimulation to persist. The usual dose is 1 mg/kg/hour in 200 ml of saline given over a period of 2 hours. Since it is a long-acting drug, titration cannot be done.

The vasodilating effects of these drugs may increase the volume of the vascular space as much as 25%, thus lowering central venous pressure. This must be covered by more plasma or plasma expanders to maintain the central venous pressure at 6-10 cm of water.

e. Treatment of hypoxia - Administration of oxygen is helpful. Hyperbaric oxygen has been suggested. Hypothermia has its advocates.

f. Acidosis requires the utilization of alkalis (eg, bicarbonate or lactate solutions).

Prognosis

Recovery is to be expected if the infection can be controlled and organ perfusion reestablished. Within 48 hours after therapy is begun, the degree of therapeutic success is usually obvious. Encouraging signs include clearing cerebration, establishment of good urine flow, and control of fever. When the patient's condition has become stabilized, all therapy except maintenance fluids and electrolytes and antibiotics can be stopped.

Despite these measures, the mortality rate of bacteremic shock is about 50%—though Christy has recently reported a cure rate of 90% in 21 patients (see reference below). Earlier and more intensive therapy may improve the outlook.

Anderson, R.W., & others: Phenoxybenzamine in septic shock. Ann Surg **165**:341-50, 1967.

Baker, R.J., & W.C. Shoemaker: Changing concepts in treatment of hypovolemic shock. M Clin North America **51**:83-96, 1967.

Blair, E., Wise, A., and Al. E. Mackay: Gram-negative bacteremic shock. JAMA **207**:333-6, 1969.

Borow, M., & others: Central venous pressure as an accurate guide for body fluid replacement. Surg Gynec Obst **120**:545-52, 1965.

Carey, J.S., & others: Circulatory response to low viscosity dextran in clinical shock. Surg Gynec Obst **121**:563-70, 1965.

Christy, J.H.: Treatment of gram-negative shock. Am J Med **50**:77-88, 1971.

Crowder, J.G., Gilkey, G.H., & A.C. White: Serratia marcescens bacteremia. Clinical observations and studies of precipitin reactions. Arch Int Med **128**:247-53, 1971.

Hardaway, R.M., & others: Intensive study and treatment of shock in man. JAMA **199**:779-91, 1967.

Johnson, D.G., & W.M. Parkins: Effects of isoproterenol and levarterenol in blood flow and oxygen use in hemorrhagic shock. Arch Surg **92**:277-85, 1966.

Kardos, G.G.: Isoproterenol in the treatment of shock due to bacteremia with gram-negative pathogens. New England J Med **274**:868-73, 1966.

Kwaan, H.M., & M.H. Weil: Differences in the mechanism of shock caused by bacterial infections. Surg Gynec Obst **128**:37-45, 1968.

Longerbeam, J.K., & others: Central venous pressure monitoring. Am J Surg **110**:220-9, 1965.

MacLean, L.D., & others: Patterns of septic shock in man - a detailed study of 56 patients. Ann Surg **166**:543-58, 1967.

Petersdorf, R.G., & H.N. Beaty: The role of antibiotics, vasoactive drugs and steroids in gram-negative bacteremia. Ann New York Acad Sc **145**:319-27, 1967.

Roberts, J.M., & R.K. Laros, Jr.: Hemorrhagic and endotoxic shock: A pathophysiologic approach to diagnosis and management. Am J Obst Gynec **110**:1041-9, 1971.

Schumer, W., & R. Sperling: Shock and its effect on the cell. JAMA **205**:215-9, 1968.

Siegel, J.H., Greenspan, M., & L.R. Del Guercio: Abnormal vascular tone, defective oxygen transport and myocardial failure in human septic shock. Ann Surg **165**:504-17, 1967.

Siegel, J.H., & M. Fabian: Therapeutic advantages of inotropic vasodilator in endotoxic shock. JAMA **200**:696-704, 1967.

Weil, M.H., and H. Shubin: The "VIP" approach to the bedside management of shock. JAMA **207**:337-40, 1969.

NECROTIZING PAPILLITIS
(Papillary Necrosis)

Etiology

This is an uncommon type of renal inflammation, though Harrow believes that the necrosis is primary and the infection secondary. Formerly, it was usually a complication of pyelonephritis in diabetics or in patients suffering from urinary obstruction. Today, most patients with papillitis give a history of excessive and prolonged ingestion of analgesics containing acetophenetidin (phenacetin) and aspirin. Patients with sickle cell trait may develop papillary necrosis. The combination of infection and vesicoureteral reflux may also cause this lesion. The association of papillary necrosis and cirrhosis has been cited. Papillary necrosis appears to be caused by ischemic necrosis of the papilla or the entire pyramid, leading to the diagnostic urographic changes.

Pathogenesis and Pathology (See Figs 12-5 and 12-6.)

The disease is usually bilateral; a few or all of the calyces may become progressively involved. While most patients have pyelonephritis as well, a few are found to have sterile urine. This latter group has associated chronic interstitial nephritis which is seen in association with analgesic abuse.

Some degree of renal atrophy secondary to infection may be noted. One or more papillae are absent. The line of demarcation is shaggy. Retained or calcified papillae may be found free in the pelvis. Infiltration of neutrophils, small round cells, and plasma cells is microscopically visible at the site of papillary slough. Changes typical of chronic pyelonephritis are usually evident. In the case of analgesic abuse, the interstitial tissues are infiltrated by fibrous tissue and round cells (chronic interstitial nephritis). Severe ischemia of the pyramids may be noted.

Clinical Findings

A. Symptoms: In the rare fulminating type of papillitis, severe sepsis may come on abruptly. Renal pain may be noted. Oliguria with uremic coma may develop rapidly, culminating in death. More commonly the patient complains of symptoms of chronic cystitis, often with exacerbations of pyelonephritis. Attempts at sterilization of the urine usually fail. Recurrent renal colic may be experienced as sloughed papillae are passed. Known sickle cell trait, vesicoureteral reflux, diabetes, cirrhosis, or a history of prolonged use of analgesics (6-60 pills a day for years) may be significant.

B. Signs: In acute papillitis, fever is high and prostration marked. Renal tenderness may be noted. In the chronic form, no abnormal signs are usually elicited. At the time of flare-up, renal tenderness may be found.

C. Laboratory Findings: In the fulminating form, the white blood count is significantly elevated. Urinalysis reveals pyuria and bacteriuria. Glycosuria and acidosis will be noted in the uncontrolled diabetic. Progressive azotemia is to be expected. Blood cultures may be positive.

Most of the patients in the chronic phase have infected urine. Anemia may be found in association with renal insufficiency. The PSP excretion is usually depressed, often below 30% in one-half hour. At this level, tests of nitrogen retention will be elevated.

D. X-ray Findings: Satisfactory excretory urograms in the uremic patient may only be obtained by infusing increased amounts of radiopaque material. In the earliest stages, before papillary slough, the urograms may show no anatomic abnormality. Later, ulceration of the central portion of a papilla (medullary necrosis; see Fig 12-5) or delineation of cavities, caused by sloughed papillae, may be seen (Fig 12-6). "Negative" shadows representing retained papillae may be noted. During the later phase, irregular calcified bodies containing radiolucent centers (the papillae) are diagnostic.

If the degree of uremia precludes excretory urography, retrograde urography is indicated. Retrograde urography will either establish the diagnosis or, it is hoped, will reveal a reversible urologic lesion amenable to therapy.

Route of Infection

Ascending or
  hematogenous

Chief Findings
  sepsis
  costovertebral angle
    pain or colic
  tenderness
  frequency and burning
  pus and bacteria
    in urine in a
    diabetic or a
    phenacetin addict

Abscesses

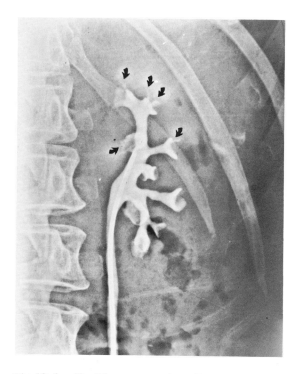

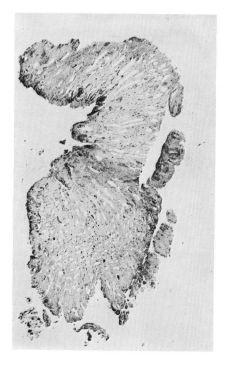

Fig 12-5. Papillary necrosis. **Above:** Pathogenesis. **Left:** Arrows point to "cracks" into paren-chyma in a patient in the earliest stage of papillitis (medullary type). **Right:** Papilla passed spontaneously in urine, recovered by patient. (Reduced 30% from × 10.)

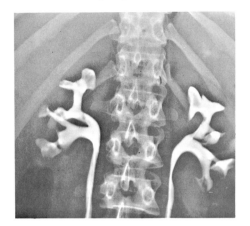 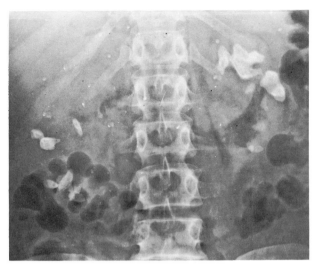

Fig 12-6. Papillary necrosis. Left: Retrograde urogram showing bilateral papillary necrosis. Calyces seem enlarged because of sloughed papillae. "Negative" shadows in upper medial calyces and in lowest calyces on left represent sloughed papillae. **Right:** Multiple renal stones caused by calcification of retained sloughed papillae. (Same patient 5 years later.) The papillae are represented by the relatively translucent centers in peculiarly shaped stones.

Differential Diagnosis

Uncomplicated diabetic coma can be diagnosed on the basis of blood sugar and serum electrolytes. Treatment of the coma should cause prompt response. If bilateral necrotizing papillitis is present as a complication, the diabetic patient will not improve under insulin therapy; progressive renal impairment will be observed, and death from renal failure and sepsis may ensue. Patients with acute pyelonephritis are not so prostrated, nor does acute renal failure develop.

Bilateral renal cortical abscesses secondary to bacteremia may simulate acute papillitis clinically. Both may show progressive loss of renal function. Urograms made early in the course of either disease may be normal or may show evidence of chronic infection. After 2 or 3 weeks, when the necrotic papillae have sloughed, the urographic demonstration of necrotizing papillitis is diagnostic.

Complications

If the patient with bilateral papillary necrosis recovers, persistent chronic pyelonephritis is usually seen; bacteriuria resists antimicrobial therapy.

If the sloughed papillae are not passed down the ureter, they may undergo peripheral calcification. The clinical picture is then compatible with nephrolithiasis or ureterolithiasis.

Treatment

A. Specific Therapy: Intensive treatment with an appropriate antibiotic is indicated, although the results have been disappointing. The choice of drug depends upon the type of bacteria found in the urine and the results of antibiotic sensitivity studies.

B. General Measures: Diabetes must be carefully controlled. The aspirin-phenacetin addict must stop taking the drug.

C. Surgical Therapy: If the disease is unilateral and fulminating (as demonstrated by physical examination, urography, and renal function tests) and if drug therapy does not result in prompt improvement, nephrectomy must be considered. This procedure must be approached with caution, however, since the other kidney may later become involved.

Prevention

Because of the relatively high incidence of papillitis in diabetics and cirrhotics, careful urinalyses and periodic urine cultures should be obtained whether symptoms of urologic infection are present or not. Infection, once discovered, should be treated vigorously. Pharmaceutical compounds containing aspirin and phenacetin should be considered nephrotoxic; their long-term and persistent use must be condemned.

Prognosis

The rare fulminating form is rapidly fatal. Patients with the chronic type usually do fairly well. Although renal function may be depressed, progressive uremia is unusual if chronic suppression antimicrobial therapy is instituted.

Chrispin, A. R., & others: Renal tubular necrosis and papillary necrosis after gastroenteritis in infants. Brit MJ 1:410-2, 1970.

Edmondson, H. A., Reynolds, T. B., & H. G. Jacobson: Renal papillary necrosis with special reference to chronic alcoholism. Arch Int Med **118**:255-64, 1966.

Fellner, S. K., & E. P. Tuttle: The clinical syndrome of analgesic abuse. Arch Int Med **124**:379-82, 1969.

Harrow, B. R.: Renal papillary necrosis: A critique of pathogenesis. J Urol **97**:203-8, 1967.

Kay, C. J., & others: Renal papillary necrosis in hemoglobin SC disease. Radiology **90**:897-9, 1968.

Liebman, N. C.: Renal papillary necrosis and sickle cell disease. J Urol **102**:294-7, 1969.

Lindvall, N.: Renal papillary necrosis. A roentgenographic study of 155 cases. Acta radiol Suppl **192**, 1960.

Longacre, A. M., & G. L. Popky: Papillary necrosis in patients with cirrhosis: A study of 102 patients. J Urol **99**:391-5, 1968.

Murray, R. M., Lawson, D. H., & A. L. Linton: Analgesic nephropathy: Clinical syndrome and prognosis. Brit MJ 1:479-82, 1971.

Nanra, R. S., & P. Kincaid-Smith: Papillary necrosis in rats caused by aspirin and aspirin-containing mixtures. Brit MJ **3**: 559-61, 1970.

Prescott, L. F.: Effects of acetylsalicylic acid, phenacetin, paracetamol, and caffeine on renal tubular epithelium. Lancet **2**: 91-5, 1965.

RENAL CARBUNCLE

Etiology

Renal carbuncle is due to a unilateral hematogenous infection complicating a pyogenic skin lesion. The infecting organism is usually hemolytic Staphylococcus aureus.

Pathogenesis and Pathology (See Fig 12-7.)

Although a diffuse acute pyelonephritis may be simultaneously present, the infection is usually localized in a single zone of the parenchyma. Development of a multilocular abscess takes place as necrosis advances. The abscess may rupture, giving rise to a perinephric abscess.

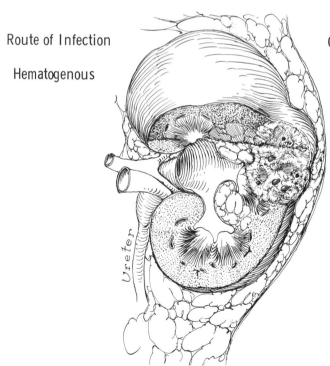

Route of Infection

Hematogenous

Chief Findings
fever (high or
low grade)
costovertebral
angle pain
tenderness or no
localizing signs
or bladder symptoms
normal urine

Ureter

Fig 12-7. Pathogenesis of renal carbuncle.

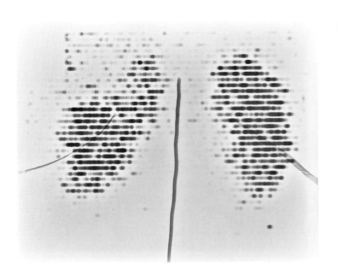

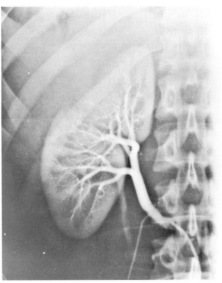

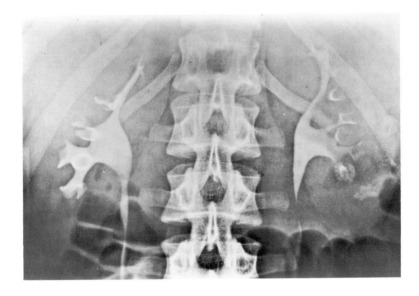

Fig 12-8. Renal carbuncle. Above left: Renal scan revealing absence of functional renal tissue in superolateral portion, right kidney. Above right: Selective renal angiogram, same patient, showing avascular mass in superolateral portion, right kidney. Surgical diagnosis: renal carbuncle. Below: Excretory urogram. Elongation of upper calyx, right kidney. Carbuncle was a complication of measles.

Clinical Findings

A. Symptoms: Renal carbuncle may have an abrupt onset with well-localized symptoms associated with marked sepsis, or its course may be mild with no symptoms other than low-grade fever.

B. Signs: In the acute case, the localized signs are flank tenderness and possibly a palpable mass, as well as, at times, edema of the skin of the costovertebral area. In the mild cases few signs may be discovered over the affected kidney.

C. Laboratory Findings: If staphylococci are the cause, the urine is free of formed sediment (cells, bacteria, etc) and the cultures negative until the abscess breaks into the pelvis. The white blood count is high, with an absolute increase in polymorphonuclear neutrophils. If there are chills and fever, blood cultures should be obtained.

D. X-ray Findings: The plain film may show an enlarged kidney or absence of renal shadow. The psoas shadow may be obliterated. The abscess may be seen as a bulge of the external contour of the kidney. Excretory or retrograde urograms often demonstrate a space-occupying lesion. Angiography will reveal an avascular mass (Fig 12-8).

E. Isotope Scanning: The rectilinear scan will depict a space-occupying lesion (Fig 12-8). The triple scan using the camera will show (1) a "cold" area with ^{203}Hg, (2) a "cold" zone with ^{131}I, and (3) an avascular space-occupying lesion with ^{99m}Tc. These findings are also compatible with simple cyst. (See chapter 8.)

Differential Diagnosis

In acute pyelonephritis the urinary sediment shows pus and bacteria (usually rods). No space-occupying lesion is seen on urography.

Acute cholecystitis may resemble renal carbuncle. The presence of a tender and palpable gallbladder may make the diagnosis. Radiographic visualization of the gallbladder and kidneys should be definitive.

Acute appendicitis may be confused with renal carbuncle since renal pain often radiates to the lower abdominal quadrant. However, signs and symptoms in the flank should suggest renal disease. Excretory urograms make the diagnosis.

Since x-ray findings of a space-occupying lesion of the kidney can be due to one of 3 diseases (tumor, cyst, or carbuncle), the differentiation may be impossible until the kidney is explored surgically.

Complications

Bacteremia with general sepsis; rupture of carbuncle leading to perinephric abscess.

Treatment

A. Specific Measures: In staphylococcal infections, large doses of the most potent drug or combination of drugs (as determined by culture and sensitivity tests) should be given. If a frank abscess develops in the kidney, surgical drainage of the carbuncle is the treatment of choice but heminephrectomy or even removal of the kidney may be necessary.

B. General Measures: Pain should be relieved by appropriate drugs and heat to the flank. An adequate urinary output must be maintained.

C. Treatment of Complications: Perinephric abscess requires surgical drainage.

Prognosis

Administration of the appropriate drug early in the course of the disease usually aborts the infection. If diagnosis is late or treatment inadequate, surgical intervention may be necessary.

Caplan, L. H., Siegelman, S. S., & M. A. Bosniak: Angiography in inflammatory space-occupying lesions of the kidney. Radiology **88**:14-23, 1967.

Cobb, O. E.: Carbuncle of the kidney. Brit J Urol **38**:262-7, 1966.

Fair, W. R., & M. H. Higgins: Renal abscess. J Urol **104**:179-83, 1970.

Moore, C. A., & M. P. Gangai: Renal cortical abscess. J Urol **98**:303-6, 1967.

Salmon, R. B., & P. R. Koehler: Angiography in renal and perirenal inflammatory masses. Radiology **88**:9-13, 1967.

PERINEPHRIC ABSCESS

Etiology

Perinephric abscess can be secondary to a staphylococcal infection of the kidney but is usually a complication of an advanced chronic renal infection.

Pathogenesis and Pathology (See Fig 12-9.)

Perinephric abscess lies between the renal capsule and the perirenal (Gerota's) fascia. The staphylococcal type probably originates from rupture of a small renal cortical abscess, or, less commonly, from a renal carbuncle. The primary renal lesion may heal although the perinephric abscess progresses.

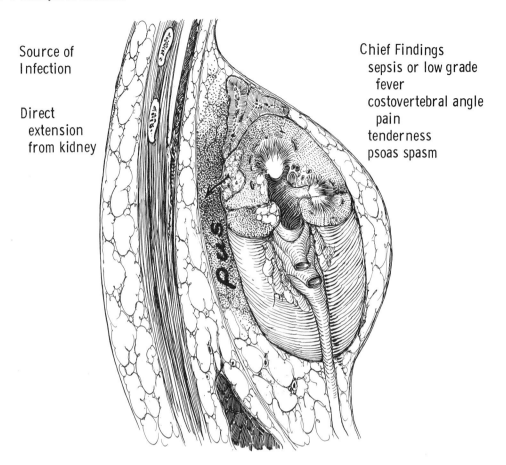

Source of
Infection

Direct
extension
from kidney

Chief Findings
sepsis or low grade
fever
costovertebral angle
pain
tenderness
psoas spasm

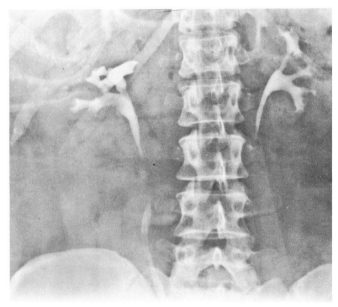

Fig 12-9. Perinephric abscess. Above: Pathogenesis. **Below:** Excretory urogram showing lateral displacement of lower pole of right kidney, scoliosis of spine, and absence of right psoas shadow. Note compression of upper right ureter by abscess.

Perinephric cellulitis and abscess, how-ever, usually complicate severe chronic renal infection such as calculous pyonephrosis or in-fected hydronephrosis. The presumption is that spontaneous extravasation of infected ma-terial occurs. In this instance, pus and bac-teria (usually gram-negative rods) are found in the urine.

Perirenal abscesses may become quite large. When advanced, they tend to point over the iliac crest (Petit's triangle) posterolateral-ly.

Clinical Findings

A. Symptoms: In the more common type (secondary to advanced chronic renal infection), a history of prolonged or recurrent urinary infection may be elicited. In the staphylococ-cal type, there is often a history of a skin in-fection a few weeks before the onset of symp-toms. Malaise may be mild or severe, de-pending upon the virulence of the invading or-ganism. Pain in the flank varies in degree. The patient may discover a tender mass in the renal area.

B. Signs: Fever may be low-grade or septic. Marked tenderness over the kidney and in the costovertebral angle is usually found. A large mass may be felt or percussed in the flank. Some rebound tenderness may be elicited. The diaphragm on the affected side may be high and fixed. Ipsilateral pleural ef-fusion is common. Scoliosis of the spine, with its concavity to the affected side, is usually seen. This is due to spasm of the psoas mus-cle, which also causes the patient to lie with the ipsilateral leg flexed on the abdomen. Edema of the skin over the abscess may be evident. Minimal edema is best demonstrated by having the patient lie on a rough towel for a few minutes.

C. Laboratory Findings: Anemia may be found. The white blood count may be markedly or only slightly elevated. The sedimentation rate is usually accelerated. The urine may be free of pus and bacteria if the renal organism is a staphylococcus. If the abscess is second-ary to other chronic renal disease, pus and bacteria (usually rods) are found. Renal func-tion tests are usually normal except in the face of chronic bilateral renal disease.

D. X-ray Findings: A plain film of the abdomen typically shows evidence of a mass in the flank. The renal and psoas shadows are obliterated because of neighboring edema. Scoliosis of the spine with its concavity to the affected side is usually seen. The presence of a calcific body in this area should suggest an abscess secondary to a calculus pyonephro-sis.

Excretory urograms may show delayed visualization due to parenchymal disease. Changes suggesting a space-occupying lesion (ie, carbuncle) may be noted, but evidence of advanced hydronephrosis or calculous pyo-nephrosis is most commonly seen. Lack of mobility of the kidney with change in position of the patient or respiration strongly suggests acute or chronic perinephritis. The entire kidney or only one pole may be displaced lat-erally by the abscess (Fig 12-9).

A barium enema may show displacement of the bowel anteriorly, laterally, or medial-ly.

A chest film may demonstrate an elevated diaphragm on the ipsilateral side, and fluoros-copy often shows fixation on respiration. Some free pleural fluid and disk atelectasis may be seen.

Retrograde urograms may be necessary if the excretory films are equivocal.

Differential Diagnosis

Chronic renal infection may cause many of the symptoms which accompany perinephric abscess: fever, localized pain, and tenderness. The urine shows evidence of infection. The plain abdominal x-ray and excretory urograms should reveal a clearly defined renal shadow; the psoas shadow should be present and the spine straight. Urographic evidence of chron-ic pyelonephritis may be seen.

Infected hydronephrosis may cause fever and localized pain and tenderness, and may ac-count for the presence of a mass in the flank. The urine is infected. Excretory urograms should make the differentiation clear.

Paranephric abscess is a collection of pus external to the perirenal fascia and is often secondary to inflammatory disease of the spine (eg, tuberculosis). Many of the signs of peri-nephric abscess may be seen on a plain x-ray film, but the finding of a bone lesion in the low thoracic area should suggest the proper diag-nosis. Urograms are normal.

Complications

Rarely, the perinephric abscess may point just above the iliac crest posterolaterally or extend downward into the iliac fossa and inguinal region. It can cross the spine within the perirenal fascia and involve the other side, but this, too, is rare.

Considerable ureteral compression from the abscess may develop, giving rise to hydro-nephrosis. Even after drainage of the abscess, ureteral stenosis may develop during the heal-ing process.

Treatment

A. Specific Measures: In the stage of perinephritis, resolution of the infection, when due to staphylococci, may be expected when proper antibiotics are used. When a frank abscess is present, surgical drainage through the flank is indicated. If the cause is primary renal disease (eg, calculus pyonephrosis, infected hydronephrosis), nephrectomy may be indicated. Whether this should be done at the time of drainage of the abscess or later depends upon the judgment of the surgeon.

B. General Measures: In the early stages, local heat may be helpful in relieving pain and muscle spasm.

C. Follow-up Care: Even though the kidney itself is normal, excretory urograms must be obtained 2 or 3 months after drainage of the abscess to be sure ureteral stenosis has not developed.

Prognosis

If the abscess is uncomplicated by primary renal disease and if proper treatment is used, prognosis is good. Removal of the kidney may be necessary if the organ is badly damaged.

Plevin, S.N., Balodimos, M.C., & R.F. Bradley: Perinephric abscess in diabetic patients. J Urol 103:539-43, 1970.

Salvatierra, O., Jr., Bucklew, W.B., & J.W. Morrow: Perinephric abscess: A report of 71 cases. J Urol 98:296-302, 1967.

NONSPECIFIC INFECTIONS OF THE URETER

Isolated infection of the ureter does not occur. Although ureteritis accompanies pyelonephritis, the former contributes few symptoms and is clinically of little importance. In the presence of chronic renal and ureteral infection, the ureteral wall may become fibrotic. This may lead to stricture formation or interfere with normal peristalsis. Except in these unusual circumstances, cure of the renal infection leads to resolution of ureteral inflammation.

NONSPECIFIC INFECTIONS OF THE BLADDER

ACUTE CYSTITIS

Etiology

Cystitis is far more common in the female than in the male. In the female, cystitis is caused by ascent of bacteria from the urethra. The symptoms of cystitis usually develop 36-48 hours after sexual intercourse. It is for this reason that the patient seldom recognizes this association. Cystitis, of course, also accompanies the rare hematogenous renal infection. Lymphogenous spread from an infected cervix seems possible but must be rare.

In man, cystitis is always secondary to some other factor: infection in the prostate or kidney or residual urine associated with the enlarged prostate. The presence of a vesical calculus or an ulcerated vesical neoplasm is often complicated by cystitis.

Infections of the bowel (eg, diverticulitis, appendiceal abscess) may involve the bladder by contiguity.

Pathogenesis and Pathology

The infected bladder, unless it is constantly insulted by an infected prostate or kidney or contains residual urine, tends to heal spontaneously. Particularly with the use of modern therapy, acute infection usually resolves without residual structural or functional injury.

In acute cystitis, the bladder either is diffusely reddened or contains multiple foci of submucosal hemorrhage. The mucosa is edematous; its surface may be covered by a purulent membrane. Superficial ulcers are occasionally seen. The muscularis is usually not involved. Microscopically, in addition to the edema, some desquamation of the mucosa can be seen. Dilatation of capillaries is striking. Leukocytic infiltration is present and may extend into the muscle. Temporary ureteral reflux through a "borderline" ureterovesical junction may occur, thus leading to secondary acute pyelonephritis.

Clinical Findings

A. Symptoms: Symptoms include burning on urination, urgency to the point of incontinence, frequency and nocturia, and often hematuria, which is usually terminal. Fever is low-grade or absent unless prostate or renal infection is present. Urinary complaints predominate; little malaise occurs. There may be mild low backache or suprapubic discomfort.

In women, the attack usually follows intercourse. In men, a quiescent prostatitis may be activated by considerable sexual excitement and alcoholic indulgence and thus cause secondary cystitis. A preceding urethral discharge (either nonspecific or gonorrheal) may imply the presence of prostatitis.

In children, most instances of cystitis really represent chronic pyelonephritis because of the high incidence of reflux at this age. There is a group of children who develop symptoms of acute hemorrhagic cystitis which has been shown to be caused by adenovirus type 2.

A history of recurrent attacks of cystitis suggests the presence of unrecognized prostatitis or residual urine, exacerbations of chronic cystitis or pyelonephritis, or, most commonly in women, ascent of bacteria in association with sexual intercourse.

B. Signs: Examination of the abdomen is usually normal. Tenderness is occasionally found over the bladder. The presence of a tender epididymis points to prostatitis as an obvious cause for the cystitis. Rectal examination may reveal a relaxed anal sphincter, suggesting neurogenic dysfunction. In men, the prostate may be enlarged, firm, and tender, even hot. (These findings are compatible with acute prostatitis.) Not until the acute phase has abated should the gland be massaged to prove the presence of infection, since the following complications can occur: bacteremia with pyelonephritis, acute epididymitis, and prostatic abscess.

Pelvic examination may reveal acute urethritis (nonspecific or gonorrheal), urethral diverticulum, vaginitis (including Trichomonas vaginitis), or cystocele (with residual urine) as causes for cystitis. The urethra may be markedly tender. Infection in Skene's glands should be sought. Vaginal discharge should be examined bacteriologically. A partially imperforate hymen or urethrohymenal fusion should be sought.

C. Laboratory Findings: The white blood count is usually elevated. Urinalysis shows pus cells and bacteria; red blood cells may be present. In acute infection, great amounts of pus are common. (In chronic disease, little or no pus is found.) Renal function is not affected.

D. X-ray Findings: Radiograms are not indicated unless stasis or renal infection is suspected. They may be needed, however, if the patient fails to respond to adequate therapy for the cystitis or if infection is recurrent; obstruction, tuberculosis, or calculus may be the cause.

E. Instrumental Examination: Cystoscopy is contraindicated during the acute phase. It should be done 7-10 days later, however, if hematuria has been noticed; an ulcerating vesical neoplasm, stone, or foreign body may be found.

Differential Diagnosis

Chronic prostatitis may cause similar symptoms, yet the urine may be normal. Prostatic massage will reveal pus in the secretion.

Allergic cystitis may have an abrupt onset. A few pus cells and monocytes are found. No bacteria are seen on the stained smear. A history of ingestion of food which has caused a similar reaction in the past may be elicited. Allergy to certain spermatocidal jellies may cause vesical irritability. A history of other allergies may be helpful.

Acute exacerbation of a chronic bladder infection may simulate a new infection, for chronic cystitis is often without symptoms. Such exacerbation usually resists routine treatment, thereby suggesting the presence of chronic disease. Cystoscopy will be of help in differentiation.

The psychosomatic cystitis syndrome may show symptoms which are similar to those of acute cystitis. However, urinalysis shows no evidence of infection. A history of recurrent attacks precipitated by anxiety or emotional upset can usually be obtained (see chapter 31).

Tuberculous cystitis may be differentiated by the finding of "sterile" pyuria on the stained smear. Tubercle bacilli usually are demonstrable on an acid-fast stain or on culture and guinea pig inoculation. There is no response to adequate therapy for a nonspecific infection. This should cause the physician to be suspicious.

Neoplasm involving the bladder may be primary or due to direct extension from the colon or cervix. With invasion and ulceration, infection is inevitable and will not respond to antibiotics. Since this is an indication for cystoscopy, the diagnosis will become obvious.

Many children, reacting to the detergents in bubble bath, may complain of symptoms suggesting cystitis. Urinalysis shows no infection.

Complications

Acute pyelonephritis is a common complication of ascending acute cystitis in little girls because of the relatively high incidence of vesicoureteral reflux in this age group. It is relatively rare in the adult.

Treatment

A. Specific Measures: Nitrofurantoin, ampicillin, penicillin G, nalidixic acid, and the tetracyclines are the most useful drugs for the treatment of acute cystitis. The sulfonamides are also efficacious and are the least expensive. If they fail to sterilize the urine within 2 weeks, a thorough urologic investigation is indicated. In those women who suffer from recurrent attacks of cystitis following intercourse, postcoital voiding and the administration of 1 gm of a sulfonamide, 100 mg of nitrofurantoin, or 400,000 units of penicillin G by mouth immediately after coitus and a similar dose the next morning will usually prevent further trouble. Landes & others have observed a marked decrease in incidence of recurrent cystitis in women following the application of povidone-iodine ointment (Betadine® ointment) to the periurethral area following the last voiding in the evening and the first voiding in the morning.

B. General Measures: The irritable bladder may be sedated by one of the following measures:

1. Alkalinization of the urine - Sixteen to 20 gm of sodium bicarbonate may be needed. Fruit juices are also helpful.

2. Antispasmodics - Many of the antispasmodics used in the treatment of gastrointestinal disorders are useful. Tincture of belladonna or atropine combined with phenobarbital may afford relief.

3. Hot sitz baths may ease severe pain and spasm. An adequate fluid intake is desired, but forcing of fluids is not necessary and only increases the patient's frequency. Further, it decreases the concentration of the antimicrobial drug in the urine.

4. Urethrohymenal fusion or incomplete hymenal perforation should be treated appropriately.

Prognosis

In the absence of stasis, acute cystitis resolves promptly with proper medical therapy. No vesical injury should result. If the infection recurs, the underlying cause must be determined.

Bass, H. N.: ''Bubble bath'' as in irritant to the urinary tract of children. Clin Pediat 7:174, 1968.

Landes, R. R., Melnick, I., & A. A. Hoffman: Recurrent urinary tract infections in women: Prevention by topical application of antimicrobial ointment to urethral meatus. J Urol 104:749-50, 1970.

Mufson, M. A., & others: Adenovirus infection in acute hemorrhagic cystitis. Am J Dis Child 121:281-5, 1971.

Reed, J. F., Jr.: Urethral-hymenal fusion: A cause of chronic adult female cystitis. J Urol 103:441-6, 1970.

Stewart, J. F.: Recurrent urinary tract infection in the female child secondary to a partial imperforate hymen. J Urol 103:353-6, 1970.

CHRONIC CYSTITIS

Etiology and Pathogenesis

Chronic infection of the bladder is often secondary to chronic infection of the upper tract. It may also be due to residual urine, ureteral reflux, or urethral stenosis. Too frequently it is the result of incomplete treatment of a simple acute cystitis. The most common cause of pyuria and bacteriuria is cystitis. The presence of these abnormal urinary constituents is not pathognomonic of pyelonephritis, which must be proved by thorough urologic examination.

Pathology

In the chronic stage, the mucosa is often pale and appears thinned. Ulceration is rare. The surface may be studded with cysts. Capacity is diminished if fibrosis of the detrusor is extensive. Pericystic fibrosis is a rare complication. A microscopic section usually shows thinning of the epithelium. The submucosa and muscle layers are infiltrated with fibroblasts, small round cells, and plasma cells.

Clinical Findings

A. Symptoms: Complaints may be those of constant or recurrent mild vesical irritability, or there may be none at all. In men, chronic cystitis may be secondary to chronic prostatitis but is more often due to obstruction distal to the bladder. In women, it may persist because of chronic urethritis or residual urine (eg, cystocele, urethral stenosis). In either male or female chronic kidney infection is often the cause. Symptoms suggesting such disease should be sought.

B. Signs: Renal tenderness (infection) or enlargement (hydronephrosis) may be noted. A distended bladder may be found. Examination of the external genitalia in the male is usually noncontributory. Rectal examination may demonstrate impaired tone of the anal sphincter, which suggests detrusor weakness related to neurogenic bladder. Prostatic enlargement or infection may be discovered. Pelvic examination may show cervicitis, vaginitis, or inflammation of Skene's or Bartholin's glands. Palpation of the urethra may reveal a mass which, when pressure is applied to it, causes pus to exude from the meatus. This finding is typical of urethral diverticulum.

C. Laboratory Findings: The blood count is usually not remarkable. If anemia is present, something other than bladder infection is the cause. In many instances few or no pus cells are found; nevertheless, the stained smear contains bacteria.

Renal function tests in simple chronic cystitis are normal. If the excretion of PSP is depressed, it means either bilateral renal damage (obstruction or infection), reflux, or vesical residual urine. In either case, such a finding is an important clue suggesting further search for the cause of chronicity.

D. X-ray Findings: A plain film of the abdomen may reveal a large kidney (hydronephrosis) or a small one (atrophic pyelonephritis). An excretory urogram shows no abnormality in uncomplicated cystitis. However, since a significant number of cases of chronic cystitis are secondary to upper urinary tract infection or vesical residual urine, this examination should always be performed. Renal calcification suggesting stone or tuberculosis may be seen.

Excretory urograms may reveal hydronephrosis due to ureteral obstruction or changes compatible with healed pyelonephritis. The cystogram may demonstrate trabeculation of the bladder wall, suggesting obstruction distal to the bladder. Ureteral reflux may be observed. The film taken after voiding may reveal residual urine. Retrograde urograms may be required.

E. Instrumental Examination: The passage of a large catheter (22 F) may reveal a urethral stricture or residual urine. Either can perpetuate chronic infection.

Cystoscopy will demonstrate the degree of a cystocele or prostatic obstruction. Ulceration of the vesical wall may be seen (tuberculosis); foreign bodies may be found. Panendoscopy may reveal the orifice of a urethral diverticulum.

Ureteral catheterization for relative renal function studies and separate urine specimens for bacteriologic survey may be needed to trace the source of the infection and determine the presence of ureteral obstruction.

Differential Diagnosis

Chronic prostatitis may cause symptoms of cystitis, but the finding of pus in the prostatic secretion makes the diagnosis.

Since chronic pyelonephritis is often without symptoms referable to the kidneys, thorough urologic investigation (including a voiding cystourethrogram) is needed to establish the cause of the infection in all cases of chronic cystitis.

Tuberculosis of the kidney and bladder is a chronic disease which may mimic chronic cystitis in every way. Certain findings should suggest the presence of tuberculosis: (1) "sterile" pyuria on a stained smear or culture of urinary sediment; (2) lack of response to the usual antibiotics; (3) evidence of a renal lesion by urography; (4) the finding of acid-fast organisms by smear, culture, or guinea pig inoculation; and (5) ulceration of the bladder wall, with biopsy positive for tuberculosis.

Emotional tension may cause chronic bladder symptoms, especially in women. This should be suspected if urinalysis is normal and emotional instability is noted. (See chapter 31.)

Senile urethritis in women past the menopause commonly causes symptoms suggesting chronic cystitis. Urinalysis is normal, and the appearance of the vaginal mucosa is typical of senile change.

Interstitial cystitis causes frequency, nocturia, and suprapubic pain when the contracted bladder becomes full. The urine is free of pus cells and bacteria. Cystoscopy reveals the typical vesical contracture, and when the bladder is overdistended the mucosa on the dome may split and bleed.

Irradiation cystitis may occur following radiotherapy of tumors in the region of the bladder (eg, cancer of the cervix). The urine may become infected if vesical ulceration develops. The history of previous x-ray or radium therapy as well as the cystoscopic finding of a pale, edematous, or telangiectatic vesical mucosa and, at times, ulceration make the differentiation. Biopsy may be indicated to rule out neoplasm.

Chronic urethritis in women may also cause long-standing symptoms suggestive of chronic cystitis. The urine, however, is negative. Panendoscopy will reveal inflammation of the urethral mucosa. Some urethral stenosis is usually found as well.

Complications

Renal infection may occur either because of an incompetent ureterovesical valve or, rarely, by the hematogenous route. Occasionally, the fibrosis of the bladder wall may cause contracture with loss of capacity. Stenosis of the intramural portion of the ureters or vesicoureteral reflux may develop, whereupon hydronephrosis follows.

Treatment

A. Specific Measures: One of the nontoxic drugs may be tried first but they usually fail to cure long-standing infections, in which case more potent antibiotics are indicated. Identification of the offending bacteria should be made if preliminary treatment fails, and sensitivity tests should be done. Antibiotic treatment must be intensive and prolonged (3-4 weeks); even under these conditions, therapy is often unsuccessful. Suppressive treatment (eg, with sulfonamides, nitrofurantoin) should then be given.

Thorough studies should be done to discover the cause of the infection (eg, urethral stenosis, prostatitis). Unless these conditions are corrected, treatment will be unsatisfactory.

B. General Measures: Since symptoms of vesical irritability are usually not as severe as those which accompany acute infection, they can usually be relieved by the measures listed on p 163.

Prognosis
Simple drug therapy often fails to eradicate the infection unless steps are taken to treat the cause (eg, enlarged prostate, chronic prostatitis, chronic urethritis in the female).

See references on p 151.

NONSPECIFIC INFECTIONS OF THE PROSTATE GLAND

ACUTE PROSTATITIS AND PROSTATIC ABSCESS

Etiology
Acute prostatic infection may be hematogenous or may occur from ascent of bacteria by way of the urethra. It is seen occasionally in childhood and has been observed in the neonatal period. A chronic quiescent prostatic infection can become acute following too vigorour prostatic massage or urethral instrumentation.

Pathogenesis and Pathology
Acute prostatic infection is usually complicated by acute cystitis and even by acute urinary retention. It may resolve (especially with proper medication), or, rarely, it may progress to abscess formation. Microscopic examination of the acutely infected gland reveals diffuse leukocytic infiltration; abscesses may be noted. Edema is marked. Similar changes are found also in the seminal vesicles, for these are usually involved when the prostate is infected.

Granulomatous prostatitis is a second form of acute prostatitis. It, too, is usually a febrile disease at onset and is usually associated with pyuria. Resolution is slow, and the gland becomes hard. It can, therefore, suggest carcinoma. Microscopically, a granulomatous reaction is noted. The stroma is infiltrated with polymorphonuclear leukocytes, lymphocytes, plasma cells, and multinucleated giant cells. The stroma shows increased fibrosis. Many of the acini have ruptured, releasing prostatic secretion into the connective tissue. It is thought that this is the cause of the severe inflammatory reaction.

Clinical Findings
A. Symptoms: Vesical irritability (burning, frequency, urgency, nocturia) may be extreme. Hematuria may be present; it is usually initial or terminal but may be total. Purulent urethral discharge may be noted. There may be perineal aching or low back pain. Moderate to high fever is usual. Cloudy urine is to be expected. Symptoms may have developed during an acute upper respiratory infection, following the extraction of infected teeth, or after urethral instrumentation. Swelling of the gland may cause urinary retention.

B. Signs: The patient ordinarily is not prostrated, but fever may be high. Urethral discharge may be present. Rectal examination reveals an exquisitely tender, enlarged, "hot" prostate. It may be quite firm. Fluctuation means abscess formation. The prostate should not be massaged while acutely inflamed. After the acute phase is over, however, massage is indicated both for diagnosis and treatment.

In the granulomatous form, the prostate may persist in its enlargement and become quite indurated, thus simulating carcinoma. Three to 6 months may be required for resolution.

C. Laboratory Findings: The white blood count is usually elevated in the range of 20,000/μl. Urinalysis shows pus and bacteria on stain and culture. Sensitivity tests should be done.

D. Instrumental Examination: Instrumentation is contraindicated during the acute stage. The only exception to this rule is to relieve acute urinary retention due to prostatic edema or abscess. If an abscess is suspected, the diagnosis may be established by perineal needle puncture.

Differential Diagnosis
Acute pyelonephritis may also be marked by severe vesical irritability. The backache

with prostatitis is usually sacral, whereas in pyelonephritis it is in the lumbar area. Rectal examination should establish the diagnosis of acute prostatitis.

Amicrobic pyuria may cause exactly the same symptoms as acute prostatitis. Urinalysis or culture, however, reveals no demonstrable organisms in amicrobic pyuria. Rectal findings also help in differentiation.

Acute congestive prostatitis due to lack of sexual intercourse may cause perineal, back, and testicular pain as well as urethral discharge. The prostate may be swollen and moderately tender. There are, however, no symptoms of vesical irritability and no fever. Massage of the prostate will produce copious secretion with prompt cessation of symptoms.

Carcinoma of the prostate may be confused with subsiding granulomatous prostatitis. Perineal needle biopsy may be indicated.

Complications

Acute urinary retention may occur from swelling of the gland. If an abscess forms, it may rupture spontaneously into the urethra, rectum, or perineum. Acute pyelonephritis may occur by the hematogenous route. This is particularly apt to happen if the prostate is massaged or if instrumentation is done during the acute stage. Acute epididymitis is not uncommon. It too is apt to occur from prostatic manipulation or instrumentation.

Treatment

A. Specific Measures: Empirically, treatment can be started with one of the tetracyclines. The results of sensitivity tests may dictate shifting to another antimicrobial. Response is usually prompt.

Instrumentation is contraindicated at first unless urinary retention occurs. After the acute phase has subsided (10-14 days), treatment of the residual prostatitis will be necessary (see below).

If a frank abscess develops, drainage by perineal needle in addition to antimicrobial medication may lead to resolution. Surgical perineal drainage or transurethral unroofing of the abscess may be necessary.

Granulomatous prostatitis may respond to corticosteroids.

B. General Measures: Perineal pain may require analgesics; sitz baths may afford some relief and may hasten resolution of the inflammation. Vesical irritability can be relieved by antispasmodics. Bed rest is essential. An adequate fluid intake is needed.

Prognosis

Prognosis is good if antibiotic therapy is instituted. If treatment is inadequate, the in-fection may become chronic and more difficult to eradicate.

See references on p 168.

CHRONIC PROSTATITIS

Etiology

Chronic prostatitis usually develops as a result of invasion of bacteria from the urethra. It may also have a hematogenous source. Inadequate treatment of acute prostatitis may lead to the chronic form. It may develop secondary to cystitis or pyelonephritis. A few cases of coccidioidomycosis granuloma of the prostate have been reported.

Pathogenesis and Pathology

An acute or subacute prostatic infection may become chronic. Chronic infection may rarely lead to contracture of the bladder neck. Function (eg, potency, fertility) is not impaired.

Chronic prostatic infection usually causes the gland to be firmer than normal due to fibrosis. The ducts may contain pus; their lining cells may degenerate. Similar changes are found in the seminal vesicles, for these are usually involved when the prostate is infected.

Clinical Findings

A. Symptoms: There are usually no symptoms. Most men with chronic prostatitis have no reason to suspect it. A few men may note an aching or ''fullness'' in the perineum, low back pain, or an unexpected low-grade fever. Urethral discomfort with ejaculation may be felt.

Symptoms accompanying a mild exacerbation may include urethral discharge (which may be the only symptom) and symptoms of cystitis. If the patient has symptoms of prostatic obstruction, these may suddenly increase as a result of swelling of the gland. Acute epididymitis may occur; this usually signifies that prostatitis exists.

Other symptoms which are often incorrectly attributed to prostatitis include infertility (uncomplicated chronic prostatitis rarely causes sterility), impotence (exceedingly rare if it occurs at all), and such psychosomatic complaints—usually associated with sexual difficulties—as nervousness, insomnia, and emotional tension.

B. Signs: Epididymitis is usually caused by prostatitis. Rectal examination may reveal a normal, boggy, or indurated prostate. There may be areas of fibrosis. Crepitation may sometimes be felt if stones are present. Massage of the prostate will produce secretion which contains pus. A few pathogens may be found on culture, but sensitivity tests have not proved helpful (Mears and Stamey). The degree of tenderness is of little help in diagnosis, since tenderness is generally determined by the pain threshold of the patient and the degree of apprehension from which he suffers.

C. Laboratory Findings: Urethral discharge should be examined both unstained (trichomonads, lecithin bodies from the prostate) and stained. The white blood count is generally normal unless an exacerbation or complication (epididymitis) is present. The urine may contain pus and bacteria. The PSP test is normal unless there is a silent bilateral renal disease (infection) or residual urine (bladder neck obstruction).

D. X-ray Findings: Plain films or excretory urograms will be normal unless there are complications (eg, prostatic or other calculi, residual urine, chronic pyelonephritis).

E. Instrumental Examination: Instrumentation is not indicated unless there is evidence of complications (eg, prostatic enlargement, urethral stricture, upper tract infection).

Differential Diagnosis

Symptoms of acute or chronic urethritis may suggest prostatitis, but the prostatic secretions in those instances will be clear.

Cystitis may be confused with prostatitis, but one must remember that cystitis in men is always secondary to renal or prostatic infection or residual urine. Again, examination of the prostatic secretion will make the differentiation.

Diseases of the anus (eg, fissure, thrombosed hemorrhoid) may cause perineal pain and, at times, urinary urgency, but proper examination of this area should make the correct diagnosis.

Complications

Acute or chronic cystitis may occur secondary to prostatic infection. Pyelonephritis by the hematogenous route may develop from exacerbation of the prostatic infection. Acute epididymitis may follow physical strain, prostatic massage, or urethral instrumentation. An exacerbation of the infection may occur spontaneously or after prostatic massage or urethral instrumentation. Contracture of the bladder neck from fibrosis of the prostatic parenchyma is occasionally seen. If so, there are symptoms of prostatism and, at times, residual urine.

Treatment

A. Specific Measures: Although the response of chronic prostatic infection to chemotherapeutic or antibiotic drugs is disappointing, they should nonetheless be employed. A complicating cystitis will usually respond rapidly. Mears & Stamey and Madsen & others, in the face of adequate serum or urinary levels, find no concentration of the various drugs tested in the prostate or its secretion. For this reason, prolonged suppressive antimicrobial therapy may be needed to keep the vesical urine sterile.

Prostatic massage is helpful. It should be done 3 or 4 times, at intervals of 7-14 days. This procedure dislodges clumps of pus cells which are obstructing prostatic ducts, thus improving drainage. Sexual intercourse should be encouraged for the same reason.

B. General Measures: Daily sitz baths may hasten resolution of the infection.

Prognosis

Although chronic prostatic infection causes little harm in itself, the complications arising from it are important. This points up the need for routine prostatic massage with microscopic examination of the secretion in all men so that silent chronic prostatitis may be discovered and treated.

Bourne, C.W., & W.A. Frishetti: Prostatic fluid analysis and prostatitis. J Urol **97**: 140-4, 1967.

Brown, H.E.: Granulomatous prostatitis: Its clinical significance. J Urol **105**:549-51, 1971.

Bush, I., Orkin, L.A., & S. Baker: Steroid therapy in non-specific granulomatous prostatitis. J Urol **92**:303-6, 1964.

Gritti, E.J., Cook, F.E., Jr., & H.B. Spencer: Coccidioidomycosis granuloma of the prostate: A rare manifestation of the disseminated disease. J Urol **89**:249-52, 1963.

Jewett, H.J., & J.A.C. Colston: Urethritis, cystitis and prostatitis: Diagnosis and treatment. M Clin North America **45**:1547-52, 1961.

Madsen, P.O., & others: The nitrofurantoin concentration in prostatic fluid of humans and dogs. J Urol **100**:54-6, 1968.

Mann, S.: Prostatic abscess in the newborn. Arch Dis Childhood **35**:396-8, 1960.

Mears, E.M., & T.A. Stamey: Bacteriologic localization patterns in bacterial prostatitis and urethritis. Invest Urol **5**:492-518, 1968.

Morrisseau, P. M., Phillips, C. A., & G. W. Leadbetter, Jr.: Viral prostatitis. J Urol **103**:767-9, 1970.

Reeves, D. S., & M. Ghilchik: Secretion of the antibacterial substance trimethoprim in the prostatic fluid of dogs. Brit J Urol **42**:66-72, 1970.

Stamey, T. A., Meares, E. M., Jr., & D. G. Winningham: Chronic bacterial prostatitis and the diffusion of drugs into prostatic fluid. J Urol **103**:187-94, 1970.

Trapnell, J., & M. Roberts: Prostatic abscess. Brit J Surg **57**:565-9, 1970.

Winningham, D. G., & T. A. Stamey: Diffusion of sulfonamides from plasma into prostatic fluid. J Urol **104**:559-63, 1970.

Youngen, R., Mahoney, S. A., & L. Persky: Prostatic abscess. Surg Gynec Obst **124**:1043-6, 1967.

NONSPECIFIC INFECTIONS OF THE SEMINAL VESICLES

Almost all infections of the prostate involve the seminal vesicles as well, but it is doubtful if seminal vesiculitis contributes any specific symptoms. Infection of the seminal vesicles without prostatitis probably does not occur. For these reasons, seminal vesiculitis is covered in the discussion of prostatic infections.

NONSPECIFIC INFECTIONS OF THE MALE URETHRA*

ACUTE URETHRITIS

Etiology

Acute urethritis is usually an ascending infection, but it can be caused by an infection descending from an infected prostate. Both gram-negative rods and gram-positive cocci are often found. Many cases appear to be caused by T-strain mycoplasmas. Often small boys develop a chemical urethritis from bubble bath preparations.

---

*See p 387 for nonspecific infection of the female urethra and p 200 for gonorrheal urethritis.

Pathogenesis and Pathology

Urethritis may ascend to the prostate and bladder. If urethritis is severe enough, a periurethral abscess may form and urethral stricture may then develop. In the acute stage of infection, the mucosa is red, edematous, and covered with a purulent exudate. It may be ulcerated. Microscopic examination shows marked edema and infiltration by leukocytes, plasma cells, and lymphocytes. Capillaries are markedly dilated. The glands of Littré may be engorged or plugged by masses of pus cells.

Acute urethritis in the female is seldom seen except in association with gonorrhea.

Clinical Findings

A. Symptoms: Urethral discharge is the leading symptom; it may be quite as profuse as that seen with gonorrhea. There may be a constant itching or burning sensation in the urethra. Burning on urination may be noted.

The onset of symptoms often seems to be related to intercourse. Symptoms may develop a few days thereafter, or the interval may be longer. A history of intercourse during menstruation, when the vaginal bacterial flora is increased, may be obtained. Usually, however, no obvious cause can be discovered.

B. Signs: The discharge may be profuse or scanty, thick and purulent, thin or mucoid. The lips of the meatus are often red, edematous, and everted.

C. Laboratory Findings: The discharge must be examined unstained and stained. Wet preparations may show trichomonads or may reveal lecithin bodies (typical of prostatic secretion). Rods and cocci may be found on the stained slide, but in many instances no bacteria are seen; this raises the question of possible infection with T-strain mycoplasmas. This step is the important one in differentiating nonspecific urethritis from gonorrheal urethritis. Cultures may be necessary in doubtful cases. Sensitivity tests are of little help in treatment.

If no discharge is available at the time of examination, the first portion of the voided urine will contain "subclinical" discharge. This should be centrifuged and the sediment treated as discharge.

The midstream specimen of urine will be free of pus and bacteria unless complications (prostatitis, cystitis) are present.

D. Instrumental Examination: Instrumentation is contraindicated during the acute stage. Later, however, the passage of a sound will rule out urethral stricture as a cause of the urethritis.

Differential Diagnosis

Gonorrheal urethritis often causes the same symptoms. The stained smear makes the differentiation.

Amicrobic pyuria may start with acute urethritis but is also associated with severe symptoms of acute cystitis. Sterile pyuria and discharge are the rule.

Trichomonas urethritis is differentiated by microscopic identification of the motile organisms.

Nonspecific prostatitis is often accompanied by urethral discharge. The absence of pus in the prostatic secretion differentiates the 2 conditions.

Complications

Prostatitis or cystitis may occur by direct extension. These complications are usually caused, however, by the passage of instruments or the use of forceful urethral irrigations.

Periurethral abscess may develop, but this also is usually a complication of injudicious urologic treatment. The abscess may rupture into the urethra or may drain through the skin. The complications of periurethral abscess are urinary fistula and urethral stricture caused by the fibrosis of the healing process.

Treatment

A. Specific Measures: Though antimicrobial therapy is not often spectacular, the combination of a sulfonamide and a tetracycline seems to afford the best result.

Prostatitis is often the cause of urethral discharge. Prostatic massage is contraindicated in the early stages of acute urethritis; if prostatitis is present, massage may exacerbate its symptoms. However, massage is indicated after a few days for differential diagnostic purposes (silent chronic prostatitis). A course of massage is indicated if prostatitis is found.

B. General Measures: Experience has shown that intercourse and the use of alcohol should be temporarily discontinued since they prolong the acute phase of the disease.

Prognosis

Acute nonspecific urethritis is at times difficult to eradicate (see Chronic Urethritis, below). Underlying causes (eg, prostatitis, urethral stricture) must be sought. Fortunately, little harm is done organically by this disease although it does cause the patient considerable anxiety.

See references on p 171.

CHRONIC URETHRITIS

Etiology

Chronic urethral infection may represent the end stage of an incompletely healed acute urethritis or may be an infection which has spread from a chronic prostatitis or has developed at the point of urethral stricture. One or more types of pyogenic organisms are usually found.

The urethral discharge may develop in men who have had no intercourse for months. Others, after a period of abstinence followed by sexual activity (frequently accompanied by moderate alcoholic intake), may develop discharge even though a condom has been used. Recurrent discharge is often a symptom of psychosexual trouble and is probably caused by psychic overstimulation of the glands of Littré.

Pathogenesis and Pathology

In chronic urethritis, the mucosa is usually granular and often appears dull but may be reddened. Microscopically, one sees lymphocytes, plasma cells, and a few leukocytes; fibroblasts are increased.

Clinical Findings

A. Symptoms: Urethral discharge is the primary symptom. It varies in amount and consistency and may appear and disappear spontaneously. The discharge may only be noticed before the first urination after waking. Some urethral irritation may be noted which is not usually related to urination. If there are symptoms of vesical irritability, prostatitis or cystitis is probably present. Psychosexual problems may be uncovered.

B. Signs: The discharge may or may not be present at the time of examination. Prostatic examination may reveal a gland which is boggy and congested or, conversely, firm, even containing fibrotic nodules. It may be normal on palpation. Many cases of chronic urethritis are secondary to chronic prostatitis.

C. Laboratory Findings: The unstained discharge should be examined for lecithin bodies and in saline for trichomonads. The former suggests a prostatic source for the urethral secretions. The discharge should be stained with methylene blue and with Gram's stain. Nonspecific organisms (rods and cocci) and gonococci should be sought. Quite often, no bacteria are seen at all; this suggests viral infection or a psychosomatic reaction. Cultures may be needed in equivocal cases.

If no discharge is present at the time of examination, the first part of the voided urine can be centrifuged, for it contains the pus cells, bacteria, and mucus which make up the discharge. It is then examined in the same manner as the discharge itself. A less preferable technic which is sometimes used is to give the patient slides on which he can place any discharge for later examination.

The midstream specimen of urine should be free of pus and bacteria unless complications are present (eg, cystitis).

D. Instrumental Examination: The passage of a sound may be arrested by a urethral stricture, which may prove to be an important factor in producing the discharge. Panendoscopy will visualize the inflamed urethral wall. It may demonstrate a urethral tumor or a diverticulum containing pus.

Differential Diagnosis

Gonorrheal urethritis develops 2-5 days following exposure. The discharge is usually profuse and purulent. The stained smear tells the story. If any doubt exists, cultures can be made.

Reiter's syndrome is characterized by iritis and arthritis as well as urethritis. The discharge is usually free of bacteria. The infective agent is not established but is thought to be a virus.

Trichomonas urethritis is difficult to diagnose because the organism is often hard to demonstrate in a wet preparation.

Complications

The urethral infection can ascend to the prostate or bladder, but this is not usual unless instrumentation is done injudiciously.

Treatment

Chemotherapeutic and antibiotic drugs do not usually cure the disease, but they should be tried. A combination of a sulfonamide and an antibiotic such as one of the tetracyclines may prove helpful.

A congested or infected prostate requires periodic massage. A urethral stricture must be dilated. Persistent urethritis sometimes responds to the daily instillation of 8 ml of 0.5% strong silver proteinate into the urethra. This solution should be retained for 5 minutes. Sexual problems should be resolved if possible. This may require psychiatric referral.

Prognosis

The disease itself is not harmful, although urinary tract complications occasionally develop from it. The psychologic effect is usually the most serious sequel to the infection.

Conger, K. B.: Gonorrhea and nonspecific urethritis. M Clin North America 48:767-72, 1964.

Csonka, G. W.: Non-gonorrheal urethritis. Brit J Ven Dis 41:1-8, 1965.
Dunlop, E. M. C., & others: Relation of TRIC agent to "non-specific" genital infection. Brit J Ven Dis 42:77-87, 1966.
Marshall, S.: The effect of bubble bath on the urinary tract. J Urol 93:112, 1965.
Shepard, M. C.: Nongonococcal urethritis associated with human strains of "T" mycoplasmas. JAMA 211:1335-40, 1970.
Symposium on non-gonococcal urethritis and human trichomoniasis. Urologia Internat 9:9-378, 1960.

NONSPECIFIC INFECTIONS OF THE EPIDIDYMIS

ACUTE EPIDIDYMITIS

Etiology

There are 3 common causes for epididymitis: (1) Preexisting prostatitis, or prostatic infection introduced by an interval or indwelling urethral catheter. (2) Prostatectomy, particularly the transurethral type, where the ejaculatory ducts are laid open in the prostatic fossa. The hydrostatic pressure with voiding or with physical strain may force urine (which contains bacteria for 8-12 weeks after the operation) down the vas. The infection may also reach the epididymis through the perivasal lymphatics. (3) Reflux of sterile urine will lead to a chemical epididymitis. Recurrent epididymitis in a young boy suggests the possibility of ureteral drainage into a seminal vesicle. Recurrent epididymitis has been described in a few patients with sarcoidosis.

Pathogenesis and Pathology

In its early stages, epididymitis is a cellular inflammation (cellulitis). It starts in the vas deferens and descends to the lower pole of the epididymis. The initial symptoms may be pain in the groin and even in the flank secondary to the vasitis.

In the acute stage, the epididymis is swollen and indurated. The infection spreads from the lower to the upper pole. On section, small abscesses may be seen. The tunica vaginalis often secretes serous fluid (inflammatory hydrocele), and this fluid may contain pus. The spermatic cord becomes thickened. The testis becomes swollen secondarily from passive congestion, but rarely becomes involved in the inflammation.

Microscopically, changes grade from edema and infiltration with leukocytes, plasma cells, and lymphocytes to actual abscess formation. The tubular epithelium may show necrosis. Resolution may be complete without residual injury, but peritubular fibrosis often develops, occluding the ducts. If bilateral, it may result in sterility.

Clinical Findings

A. Symptoms: Epididymitis often follows severe physical strain such as lifting a heavy object. It may develop after considerable sexual excitement. The trauma of urethral instrumentation may initiate the complication. It is not uncommon after prostatectomy. Prostatitis is usually the underlying cause.

Pain develops rather suddenly in the scrotum. It may radiate along the spermatic cord and even reach the flank. The pain is generally quite severe and the epididymis exquisitely sensitive. Swelling is rapid and may cause the organ to become twice the size of normal in the course of 3 or 4 hours. The temperature may reach 104°F. Urethral discharge may be noted. Symptoms of cystitis with cloudy urine may accompany the painful swelling.

B. Signs: There may be tenderness over the groin (spermatic cord) or in the lower abdominal quadrant on the affected side. The scrotum is enlarged. The overlying skin may be reddened. If abscess is present, the skin may appear dry, flaky, and thinned; it may rupture spontaneously. If seen early, the enlarged, indurated, tender epididymis may be distinguished from the testis. After a few hours, however, the testis and epididymis become one mass.

The spermatic cord is thickened by edema. Hydrocele may develop within a few days after onset, secondary to the inflammation. Urethral discharge may be seen.

Palpation of the prostate may reveal changes suggesting acute or chronic prostatitis. The gland should not be massaged during the acute phase, since the epididymitis may be made worse.

C. Laboratory Findings: The white blood count often reaches 20,000-30,000/μl. Urethral discharge, if present, should be examined both unstained and stained. Urinalysis may or may not reveal evidence of infection.

Differential Diagnosis

Tuberculous epididymitis is usually not painful. The epididymitis is usually distinguishable from the testis on palpation. "Beading" of the vas may be noted. Induration of the prostate and a thickened seminal vesicle on the ipsilateral side are compatible with tuberculosis. The finding of a "sterile" pyuria by smear and of tubercle bacilli on culture will establish the diagnosis.

Testicular tumor is almost always painless; on occasion, however, because of internal hemorrhage, there may be sudden distention of the tunica albuginea which will cause pain. The mass may be found to be separate from a normal epididymis. Prostatic examination and urinalysis will be normal. If doubt exists, urinary chorionic gonadotropins should be measured, although only 10% of testicular tumors elaborate this substance. If testicular tumor cannot be ruled out, orchiectomy should be done.

Torsion of the spermatic cord is usually an affliction of children just before puberty, although it is occasionally seen in men. Epididymitis occurs in an older age group. In the early phase of torsion, the examiner may palpate the epididymis anterior to the testis. Later, however, the testis and epididymis become one enlarged, tender mass. Prehn's sign may be helpful in differentiation: If pain is relieved when the scrotum is gently lifted onto the symphysis, the pain is due to epididymitis; if pain is increased, torsion is the more probable diagnosis. If torsion cannot be ruled out, the testis should be explored.

Torsion of the appendages of the testis or epididymis is a rare disease of prepuberal boys. These pedunculated bodies may twist, causing localized pain and swelling. If seen early, a tender nodule is felt at the upper pole of the testicle; the epididymis is normal. Later, the entire testis becomes swollen, making the differential diagnosis between epididymitis and torsion of the cord or rudimentary appendages difficult. Early surgery is necessary in this instance, for torsion of the cord must receive prompt treatment.

Testicular trauma may simulate the physical findings of acute epididymitis in every way, but the history of the injury and the absence of pyuria will help in differentiation.

Mumps orchitis is usually accompanied by parotitis. There are no urinary symptoms and the urinary sediment is free of pus cells and bacteria.

Complications

Abscess formation may occur but is rare unless urethral instrumentation or prostatic massage has been done. The abscess may drain spontaneously through the scrotum or may require surgical drainage.

Epididymal abscess may extend into and destroy the testis (epididymo-orchitis), but this is rare.

Treatment

A. Specific Measures: If the patient is seen within 24 hours after onset, the disease may be almost completely aborted by infiltrating the spermatic cord just above the testicle with 20 ml of 1% procaine hydrochloride or other local anesthetic agent, thereby obtaining complete anesthesia. Fever usually falls abruptly. Pain is decreased or may disappear almost completely. The inflammatory mass may resolve in a few days rather than the usual 2 or 3 weeks. If one injection does not afford relief, it should be repeated the next day.

Antibiotics are helpful but not curative. Secondary cystitis will usually clear quickly.

After the epididymitis has subsided (usually 2 or 3 weeks), treatment of the prostatitis is indicated.

B. General Measures: Bed rest is necessary during the acute phase (3-4 days). Support for the enlarged heavy testicle partially relieves the discomfort. Scrotal supporters are too small; the more roomy athletic supporter, lined with cotton, is best.

Analgesics should be used as necessary to combat pain. Local·heat usually affords comfort and probably hastens resolution of the inflammatory process. The sitz bath is a useful means of applying heat to the infected prostate and epididymis. If, as sometimes happens, heat increases the pain, an ice bag should be used instead.

Sexual excitement or physical strain (eg, with defecation) may exacerbate the infection and must therefore be controlled.

Prognosis

Almost all acutely inflamed epididymides resolve spontaneously, although it may take 1 or 2 weeks before all pain is gone and 4 weeks or longer for the epididymis to approach normal size and consistency. Complications are not common, although sterility is always a threat if the disease is bilateral.

See references below.

CHRONIC EPIDIDYMITIS

Chronic epididymitis is the irreversible end stage of a severe acute epididymitis which has been followed by frequent mild attacks.

In chronic epididymitis, fibroplasia has caused induration of the organ. Microscopically, the scarring is so marked that tubular occlusion is usually seen. The tissues are infiltrated with lymphocytes and plasma cells.

There are usually no symptoms except during a mild exacerbation, at which time there may be some degree of local discomfort. The patient may notice a lump in the scrotum.

The epididymis is thickened and somewhat enlarged. It may or may not be tender. It is easily distinguished from the testis on palpation. Often the spermatic cord is thickened and at times the diameter of the vas is increased. The prostate may be firm or contain areas of fibrosis. Its secretion will usually contain pus.

Urinalysis may show infection secondary to prostatitis.

Tuberculous epididymitis mimics nonspecific chronic epididymitis in every way. Beading of the vas, thickening of the ipsilateral seminal vesicle, and the finding of ''sterile'' pyuria and tubercle bacilli in the urine will make the diagnosis of tuberculous epididymitis. Cystoscopy may reveal vesical ulcers; urograms are of further help.

Testicular tumor may present with a ''lump in the testicle.'' Palpation will show either a thickened epididymis or a hard, insensitive testis (tumor).

Tumors of the epididymis are very rare. Differentiation from chronic epididymitis may ultimately be made only by the pathologist.

If chronic epididymitis is bilateral, sterility is to be expected.

Little benefit can be derived from the administration of antibiotics alone. The prostatitis which is often present must be treated. If prostatic massages cause exacerbation of the epididymal infection, vasoligation should be done in a quiescent period. The prostatitis can then be treated. Epididymectomy may at times be necessary.

Except for recurring pain and the threat of infertility in bilateral involvement, chronic epididymitis is of little consequence. Once the stage of fibrosis is reached, nothing can be done to resolve it.

Carlton, C. E., Jr., & A. J. Leader: The cystourethrographic demonstration of retrograde urinary flow in the vas deferens as a cause of epididymitis. J Urol **84**:123-5, 1960.

Gartman, E. G.: Epididymitis. Am J Surg **101**:736-41, 1961.

Miller, H. C.: Local anesthesia for acute epididymitis. J Urol **104**:735, 1970.

Smith, D. R.: Treatment of epididymitis by infiltration of the spermatic cord with procaine hydrochloride. J Urol **46**:74-6, 1941.

Winnacker, J. L., & others: Recurrent epididymitis in sarcoidosis. Ann Int Med **66**:743-8, 1967.

NONSPECIFIC INFECTIONS OF THE TESTIS

ACUTE ORCHITIS

Etiology

The testis may become inflamed from a hematogenous source. Orchitis may occur with any infectious disease (eg, Coxsackie virus infection, dengue). Patients with mumps parotitis excrete the virus in the urine. Therefore, it would appear that a complicating mumps epididymo-orchitis may also be a descending infection. The edema which develops probably leads to death of the spermatogenic cells from ischemia. Primary infection of an epididymis may involve its testis by direct extension.

Pathogenesis and Pathology

Grossly, in nonspecific orchitis, the testis is much enlarged, congested, and tense. On section, small abscesses may be noted. Microscopically, there is edema of the connective tissue with diffuse neutrophilic infiltration. The seminiferous tubules also show involvement; necrosis is present. In the healed stage, the seminiferous tubules are embedded in fibrous tissue. On histologic study they may show considerable atrophy. The interstitial cells are usually preserved.

Mumps is the most common cause of inflammation of the testis, which occurs only after puberty. It is usually unilateral but may be bilateral. Grossly, the testis is much enlarged and bluish in color. On section, because of the interstitial reaction and edema, the tubules do not extrude. Microscopically, edema and dilatation of blood vessels are noted. Neutrophils, lymphocytes, and macrophages are abundant. Tubular cells show varying degrees of degeneration. In the healed stage, the testis is small and flabby. Microscopic study in this instance shows marked tubular atrophy, although the Leydig cells are usually normal in appearance. The epididymis usually shows similar changes.

Clinical Findings

A. Symptoms: Onset is sudden, with pain and swelling of the testicle. The scrotum becomes reddened and edematous. There are no urinary symptoms, as are often seen with epididymitis. Fever may reach 40° C (104° F), and prostration may be marked.

B. Signs: The parotitis of mumps may be present or evidence of other infectious disease may be found. One or both testes may be enlarged and very tender. The epididymis cannot be distinguished from the testis on palpation. The scrotal skin may be reddened. An acute transilluminating hydrocele may develop.

C. Laboratory Findings: The white blood count is usually elevated. Urinalysis is usually normal, although some protein may be found. Abnormal renal function is found in all patients with mumps. Microhematuria and proteinuria are common. The specific virus can be found in the urine. Later, renal function and urine return to normal.

Differential Diagnosis

Acute epididymitis, when seen early, will be obvious because the involvement is solely epididymal. Later, this sign will become obscure. Urethral discharge, pyuria, and abscence of a generalized infectious disease should point to epididymitis.

Torsion of the spermatic cord may present difficulties in differentiation. In torsion, the epididymis may be felt anterior to the testis during the early stages. Absence of infectious disease tends to rule out orchitis.

Complications

In one-third to one-fourth of patients, the involved testis becomes infertile due to irreversible damage to spermatogenic cells. Androgenic function, however, is usually maintained.

Treatment

A. Specific Measures: Appropriate antibiotics are helpful in controlling some infections but are of no value in the treatment of mumps orchitis. Infiltration of the spermatic cord just above the involved testis with 20 ml of 1% procaine sometimes causes rapid resolution of the swelling and thereby relieves pain. There is evidence that this may protect spermatogenic activity as well by improving blood supply.

B. General Measures: Bed rest is necessary. Local heat is helpful and may relieve the pain. Support to the organ affords some comfort. An athletic supporter containing cotton padding is useful even when the patient is in bed.

Prophylaxis

The incidence of mumps orchitis may possibly be lessened by administering either mumps convalescent serum, 20 ml, or mumps convalescent gamma globulin, 2.5 ml, IM during the incubation period or very early in the disease. Routine administration of estrogens or corticosteroids to all postpuberal males who develop mumps has been suggested as a prophylactic against orthitis. However, there seems to be little evidence that this practice is effective.

Prognosis

Destruction of spermatogenic cells is to be feared, particularly if the disease is bilateral. This is one of the causes of infertility. The acute phase lasts about 1 week. Noticeable atrophy may be observed in 1 or 2 months.

Lyon, R.P., & H.B. Bruyn: Treatment of mumps epididymo-orchitis. JAMA **196**: 738, 1966.

Riggs, S., & J.P. Sanford: Viral orchitis. New England J Med **266**:990-3, 1962.

Utz, J.P., Houk, V.N., & D.W. Alling: Clinical and laboratory studies of mumps. IV. Viruria and abnormal renal function. New England J Med 270:1283-6, 1964.

CHEMOTHERAPEUTIC AND ANTIBIOTIC TREATMENT OF NONSPECIFIC INFECTIONS

Factors Which Influence the Choice of Drug

A. Type of Organism: To avoid relapses and chronicity, drugs or drug combinations should be employed which are capable of rapidly killing the infecting organisms. Selection of the proper drug for treating urinary tract infections depends upon (1) stained smear of sediment or discharge, (2) quantitative culture, and (3) antibiotic sensitivity tests. The stained smear differentiates cocci from bacilli, and so is of value as a nonspecific guide in the selection of a drug. Quantitative urine culture should be used as a basis for drug therapy only if a significant number of organisms are identified. Culture identification is a more accurate guide to antimicrobial therapy than a stained smear and is therefore indicated for acutely ill patients or those with symptoms of chronic infection.

B. Organ Infected: The usual acute vesical infection might be treated with a sulfonamide or nitrofurantoin, whereas a patient with acute renal infection might do better with a tetracycline.

C. Severity of Infection: The patient suffering from an overwhelming infection (eg, bacteremia) should be given the most effective antibiotic or combination of antibiotics to which the bacteria are sensitive. It is essential that the drug afford high serum and tissue levels as well.

D. Stage of Infection: Acute infections tend to be self-limiting; therefore, the less toxic drugs may suffice (eg, tetracyclines, nitrofurantoin). Chronic infections may require treatment with the most effective drug as shown by sensitivity testing (eg, kanamycin, colistin).

E. Side Reactions: The soluble sulfonamides are the least toxic of the antimicrobial agents. If circumstances warrant, side reactions must be risked (skin reaction from penicillin; bowel upset, proctitis, or vulvitis from the tetracyclines). A previous history of drug sensitivity should be taken into consideration in evaluating the drug to be used.

Sensitivity Tests

In general urologic office practice, sensitivity tests (and, therefore, cultures) are not indicated in the majority of cases. The stained smear of the urinary sediment affords some knowledge about the infecting organism. In most cases, empiric selection of drugs is effective. Exceptions include patients with chills and fever (with possible bacteremia) and those suspected of having chronic pyelonephritis.

Sensitivity tests, though not entirely reliable, are indicated in the care of those patients who are septic. Though it is now clear that the urinary concentration of the drug is of prime importance, fortunately the usual disks used in testing indicate which drug or drugs will have a bacteriostatic or bactericidal effect in the urine. (The only exception to this rule is the disk measuring sensitivity to penicillin G.) There is a reasonably good correlation between disk and tube dilution tests.

Heretofore, most authorities agreed that the efficacy of a drug was measured by its concentration in blood and tissues and the specific sensitivity of the bacteria to the drug. On this basis, the "urinary antiseptics" (ie, nitrofurantoin, nalidixic acid, and methenamine mandelate) would have no place in the treatment of parenchymal (renal) infections. Stamey, however, believes that renal infections involve the renal medulla rather than the cortex. Therefore, he postulates, the concentration of the drug in the urine is the important factor. This would account for the fact that the "urinary antiseptics" are efficacious in the treatment of pyelonephritis. His studies further show that the administration of penicillin G by mouth affords a very high concentration in the urine and that many gram-negative rod infections respond best to this drug or to nitrofurantoin.

Table 12-1. Antibiotic dosage in renal failure.*

Drug	Principal Mode of Excretion or Detoxification	Approximate Half-Life in Serum		Proposed Dosage Regimen in Renal Failure	
		Normal	Renal Failure†	Initial Dose and Route‡	Give Half the Initial Dose at Intervals Of
Penicillin G	Tubular secretion	0.5 hours	10 hours	6 gm IV	8-12 hours
Ampicillin	Tubular secretion	0.5 hours	10 hours	6 gm IV	8-12 hours
Methicillin	Tubular secretion	0.5 hours	10 hours	6 gm IV	6-8 hours
Cephalothin	Tubular secretion	0.8 hours	15 hours	8 gm IV	12 hours
Streptomycin	Glomerular filtration	2.5 hours	3-4 days	1 gm IM	3-4 days
Kanamycin	Glomerular filtration	3 hours	3-4 days	1 gm IM	3-4 days
Gentamicin	Glomerular filtration	2.5 hours	3-4 days	2 mg/kg IM	3-4 days
Vancomycin	Glomerular filtration	6 hours	8-9 days	0.5 gm IV	8-10 days
Polymyxin B	Glomerular filtration	5 hours	2-3 days	2.5 mg/kg IV	2-4 days
Colistimethate	Glomerular filtration	3 hours	2-3 days	3.5 mg/kg IM	2-4 days
Tetracyclines	Glomerular filtration and liver	8 hours	3 days	1 gm orally, or 0.5 gm IV	3 days
Chloramphenicol	Liver and glomerular filtration	3 hours	4 hours	1 gm orally or IV	8 hours
Erythromycin	Liver and glomerular filtration	1.5 hours	5 hours	1 gm orally or IV	8 hours
Lincomycin	Glomerular filtration and liver	4.5 hours	10 hours	1 gm orally or IV	12 hours

*Modified and reproduced, with permission, from Krupp & Chatton: Current Diagnosis & Treatment 1972. Lange, 1972.
†Considered here to be marked by creatinine clearance of 10 ml/minute or less.
‡For a 60 kg adult with a serious systemic infection. The "initial dose" listed is administered as an intravenous infusion over a period of 1-8 hours, or as 2 intramuscular injections during an 8-hour period, or as 2-3 oral doses during the same period.

Dosage of Drugs

Most antimicrobial drugs are excreted by the kidneys and appear in the urine in much higher concentration than in the tissues. Although small doses give sufficient concentration in the urine to suppress bacteria, such "urinary doses" are undesirable in the treatment of acute urinary infection. Antimicrobials should be given in standard therapeutic dosage or in dosage which ensures bacteriostatic or bactericidal action as determined by sensitivity tests. Since much of the effect of drugs depends upon their concentration in the urine, fluids should not be forced beyond 2000/ml day.

In the presence of renal insufficiency, care must be taken in the dosage of the drug prescribed (Table 12-1). If the patient is oliguric or has a creatinine clearance of less than 10 ml/minute, great care must be exercised. After the recommended initial dose, one half this dose should be given for (1) penicillin G, every 10 hours; (2) cephaloridine, every 24 hours; and (3) tetracyclines, kanamycin, streptomycin, polymyxin B, and colistin, every 3-4 days. Nitrofurantoin should not be used in this instance because of the risk of serious peripheral neuritis.

If the patient is uremic but the creatinine clearance is 10 ml/minute or more, possibly half the usual dose should be used. Close observation for toxicity must be pursued.

Duration of Treatment and Follow-up

Drugs should be administered for at least 14 days (often for much longer) to give the greatest chance for permanent cure of acute or chronic infections. Bacteriologic urine cultures and stained smears should be obtained at 1, 4, and 8 weeks after completion of treatment.

The Use of Antimicrobials During Pregnancy

Among the drugs ordinarily used to combat urinary tract infections, these may have a deleterious effect upon the newborn child: streptomycin (8th nerve deafness); chloramphenicol (the "gray syndrome," which is lethal); sulfonamides (kernicterus); tetracycline (inhibition of bone growth, discoloration of teeth, and hypoplastic enamel which may lead to caries). Tetracycline is most dangerous after the 4th month of pregnancy. The others are to be feared during the first trimester.

Apgar, V.: Drugs in pregnancy. JAMA **190**: 840-1, 1964.

Finegold, S. M., & others: Chemotherapy guide. California Med 111:362-87, 1969.

Kline, A. H., Blattner, R. J., & M. Lunin: Transplacental effect of tetracyclines on teeth. JAMA **188**:178-80, 1964.

Lorian, V.: The mode of action of antibiotics on gram-negative bacilli. Arch Int Med **128**:623-32, 1971.

McCracken, G. H., Jr., Eichenwald, H. F., & J. D. Nelson: Antimicrobial therapy in theory and practice. I. Clinical pharmacology. J Pediat **75**:742-57, 1969.

O'Grady, F., & W. Brumfitt: Urinary tract infection. Proceedings of the First National Symposium held in London, April, 1968. Oxford University Press, 1968.

Robinson, G. C., & K. G. Cambon: Hearing loss in infants of tuberculous mothers treated with streptomycin during pregnancy. New England J Med **271**:949-51, 1964.

Stamey, T. A., Govan, D. E., & J. M. Palmer: The localization and treatment of urinary tract infections: The role of bactericidal urine levels as opposed to serum levels. Medicine **44**:1-36, 1965.

Symposium on efficacy of antimicrobial and antifungal agents. M Clin North America **54**:1077-350, 1970.

Turck, M., Lindemeyer, R. I., & R. G. Petersdorf: Comparison of single-disc and tube-dilution techniques in determining antibiotic sensitivities of gram-negative pathogens. Ann Int Med **58**:56-65, 1963.

ANTIMICROBIAL DRUGS

Sulfonamides

The soluble sulfonamides are bacteriostatic, have a wide antibacterial spectrum, are inexpensive, and cause few significant side reactions other than skin rash and fever. They are quite useful in acute infections where toxicity is not marked. The sulfonamides which are most soluble in urine are sulfisoxazole (Gantrisin®), sulfamethizole (Thiosulfil®), and the combination of 2 or 3 different sulfonamides ("mixed sulfas"). At least 4 gm/day should be given, and treatment should be continued for 14 days or more. The long-acting sulfonamides, if used in therapeutic dosage, cause a significant incidence of skin reactions; sulfanilamide crystalluria may develop. They offer no advantage over the more soluble preparations and are contraindicated in children, in whom a number of instances of Stevens-Johnson syndrome have been reported following their use.

The sulfonamides are useful for additional therapy after an adequate course of one of the antibiotics has been given. In chronic pyelonephritis which has proved resistant to antibiotic treatment, small doses of sulfonamides (0.5 gm 2 or 3 times a day) can be given for months or years to suppress infecting bacteria.

Kass has shown that prophylactic administration of a sulfonamide (0.5 gm 2 or 3 times a day) sharply reduces the incidence of pyelonephritis in pregnancy in women who are found to have bacteriuria.

The British literature indicates that the combination of trimethoprim and a sulfonamide is superior to the latter drug alone, but trimethoprim has not yet been released for use in the USA. Only Pseudomonas aeruginosa and, to a lesser extent, Streptococcus faecalis have proved resistant. The recommended ratio of the sulfonamide to trimethoprim is 5:1. Give sulfamethoxazole, 400 mg, and trimethoprim, 80 mg, twice daily.

Penicillins

Penicillin is a bactericidal drug which has been used chiefly in coccal infections. At least 1 million units/day should be given IM. For an overwhelming infection, millions of units per day should be administered IV. Penicillinase-producing staphylococci are resistant to penicillin G but usually respond to methicillin or oxacillin, which are given parenterally, or to cloxacillin, dicloxacillin, or nafcillin, which are given by mouth. The dose of methicillin is 2-4 gm IM or IV every 6 hours. The oral preparations should be given in doses of 1-3 gm/day.

Ampicillin is a broad-spectrum penicillin which is exceedingly active against Escherichia coli and Proteus mirabilis. It is also the drug of choice for infections caused by Str faecalis. The average dose is 500 mg every 6 hours. Hetacillin is converted to ampicillin in vivo; there is no clear-cut indication for its use.

A new synthetic penicillin, carbenicillin, appears to be active against P vulgaris and E coli. The usual dose is 1-4 gm 4 times a day IV. Even larger doses are recommended for Ps aeruginosa, which seems to develop rapid resistance to the drug. When large doses are utilized, this drug is exceedingly expensive.

Stamey has found that penicillin G (800,000 units 4 times a day orally) will cure 80% of E coli infections and 90% of infections caused by P mirabilis. Massive intravenous doses of penicillin G (20-60 million units) have been suggested for severe infections caused by E coli, enterobacter, and P mirabilis. If, however, renal function is impaired, dosage at this level may cause increased concentration

Table 12-2.   Antibiotic and chemotherapeutic agents.

Drugs	Route	Adult Dose	Pediatric Dose	Minimum Rx (days)	Toxic Side Effects
Sulfonamides (sulfadiazine, sulfamerazine, sulfisoxazole; mixed*)	Oral	2 gm stat, then 4 gm/day†	50-60 mg/lb/day†	10-14	Skin rash, fever, nausea and vomiting. Rarely, hematopoietic effects and nephrotoxicity.
Penicillins Penicillin G	IV	Several million units/day	8000-200,000 units/lb/day†		
	IM	1-5 million units/day†	8000-20,000 units/lb/day†		
	Oral	2-6 million units†	0.5-2 million units†		
Procaine penicillin G	IM	1-3 million units, 1 dose	0.3-1.2 million units, 1 dose		
				7-14	Skin rashes, fever, anaphylaxis, superinfection.
Ampicillin	Oral	2-6 gm/day†	20-60 mg/lb/day†		
	IM-IV	60-150 gm/day†	60-175 mg/lb/day†		
Carbenicillin	IV	100-250 mg/lb/day†	125-250 mg/lb/day†		
Methicillin	IV-IM	8-16 gm†	80-120 mg/lb/day†		
Oxacillin Cloxacillin Dicloxacillin Nafcillin	Oral	1-3 gm/day†	20-40 mg/lb/day†		
Cephalosporins Cephalothin	IV	8-16 gm/day	20-60 mg/lb/day		
Cephaloridine	IV	4 gm/day	15-25 mg/lb/day	7-10	Anaphylaxis, fever, skin rashes, hemolytic anemia, granulocytopenia. Renal toxicity (cephaloridine).
	IM	2-4 gm/day†	15-25 mg/lb/day†		
Cephalexin	Oral	2 gm/day†	20-40 mg/lb/day†		
Tetracycline group Tetracycline	Oral	1-4 gm/day†	8-16 mg/lb/day†		
	IM-IV	0.2-2 gm/day†	4-6 mg/lb/day†		
Chlortetracycline	Oral	1-4 gm/day†	8-16 mg/lb/day†		
	IV	0.2-2 gm/day†	4-6 mg/lb/day†		
Oxytetracycline	Oral	1-4 gm/day†	8-16 mg/lb/day†	10-14	Fever, skin rash, nausea and vomiting, diarrhea. Adverse effect upon teeth of fetus and child.
	IM	1 gm/day†	4-6 mg/lb/day†		
Demecycline, methacycline, doxycycline	Oral	600 mg/day†	5 mg/lb/day†		
Minocycline	Oral	200 mg stat, then 100 mg every 12 hours	Not advised		
Chloramphenicol	Oral	1-4 gm/day†	20-40 mg/lb/day†	10-14	Nausea, vomiting, diarrhea, anemia. Aplastic anemia (rare).
	IV	1-4 gm/day	40-60 mg/lb/day		

Drug	Route	Dose	Dose per weight	Days	Side effects
Streptomycin	IM	1-3 gm/day†	8-16 mg/lb/day†	5	Skin rashes, fever, nephrotoxicity, ototoxicity (vestibular).
Neomycin	IM	1-2 gm/day†	4-6 mg/lb/day†	5-10	Nephrotoxicity, ototoxicity (auditory).
Kanamycin	IM-IV	1-2 gm/day†	6 mg/lb/day†		
Gentamicin	IM	0.5-2 mg/lb/day†	1-2 mg/lb/day†	5-10	Nephrotoxicity, ototoxicity.
Polymyxin	IV	1-2 mg/lb/day	1-2 mg/lb/day	7-10	Paresthesias, dizziness, nephrotoxicity.
Colistimethate	IM	1 mg/lb/day	2-4 mg/lb/day†		
Nitrofurantoin					
Nitrofurantoin crystals	Oral	0.4 gm/day†	2-4 mg/lb/day†	7-14	Nausea and vomiting, skin rash, pulmonary infiltration, neurotoxicity (rare).
Nitrofurantoin sodium	IV	0.18-0.36 gm/day	2-3 mg/lb/day		
Methenamine with acidifier					
Methenamine mandelate	Oral	4-6 gm/day†	20 mg/lb/day†	10-14	Vesical irritation.
Methenamine hippurate	Oral	2 gm/day†	10 mg/lb/day†		
Nalidixic acid	Oral	4 gm/day†	20 mg/lb/day†	7	Nausea and vomiting, skin rashes.

*Various combinations are in use. Most "triple sulfa" preparations contain sulfadiazine and sulfamerazine with sulfamethazine, sulfathiazole, or sulfacetamide.

†In divided doses.

Trade Names of Drugs Listed in the Table

Sulfonamides:
Various preparations by many manufacturers

Penicillins:
Ampicillin = Omnipen®, Penbritin®, Polycillin®
Carbenicillin = Geopen®
Cloxacillin sodium = Orbenin®, Tegopen®
Dicloxacillin monohydrate = Dynapen®, Veracillin®
Methicillin = Celbenin®, Democillin®, Staphcillin®
Nafcillin sodium = Unipen®
Oxacillin sodium = Prostaphlin®, Resistopen®
Penicillin G (various manufacturers)

Cephalosporins:
Cephalexin = Keforal®
Cephaloridine = Keflordin®
Cephalothin = Keflin®

Tetracyclines:
Chlortetracycline = Aureomycin®
Demecycline (demethylchlor-tetracycline) = Declomycin®
Doxycycline = Vibramycin®
Methacycline = Rondomycin®
Minocycline = Minocin®
Oxytetracycline = Terramycin®
Tetracycline (various manufacturers)

Chloramphenicol = Chloromycetin®

Streptomycin:
Various preparations by many manufacturers

Kanamycin-Neomycin Group:
Kanamycin sulfate = Kantrex®
Neomycin sulfate (various manufacturers)

Gentamicin = Garamycin®

Polymyxin Group:
Colistimethate = Coly-Mycin®
Polymyxin B sulfate = Aerosporin®

Nitrofurantoins:
Nitrofurantoin (various manufacturers)
Nitrofurantoin crystals = Macrodantin®
Nitrofurantoin sodium = Furadantin®

Methenamine With Acidifier:
Methenamine hippurate = Hyprex®
Methenamine mandelate = Mandelamine®

Nalidixic Acid = NegGram®

in the CSF, leading to neurotoxicity. It is therefore best to administer large doses of penicillin G intermittently rather than by constant drip. If penicillin is taken by mouth, it is best administered between meals and at bedtime, when the stomach is empty. Procaine penicillin maintains significant serum levels for 24 hours. The dose is 1-3 million units/day IM.

Cephalosporins

These semisynthetic drugs, while most effective in the treatment of infections caused by penicillinase-resistant coccal organisms, are bactericidal against E coli, some of the klebsiella-enterobacter group, and P mirabilis. They are usually ineffective against Ps aeruginosa and P vulgaris.

Cephalothin and cephaloridine can cause bone marrow depression and thrombocytopenia. Skin rash is not uncommon. The dose of cephalothin is 2-4 gm IV every 6 hours. Cephaloridine can be given either intravenously or intramuscularly; the dose is 0.5-1 gm every 6 hours. The claim that cephaloridine is significantly more nephrotoxic than cephalothin would seem to be justified by recent clinical experience.

Cephalexin is an effective oral cephalosporin. Its effective bacterial spectrum is similar to that of cephalothin. The dose is 1-4 gm in divided doses. It should be taken on an empty stomach. Cephaloglycine, another oral preparation, has little to recommend it.

Tetracyclines

Chlortetracycline, oxytetracycline, and tetracycline are bacteriostatic agents. All 3 may be useful in both bacillary (gram-negative) and coccal (gram-positive) infections. The dosage is 1-4 gm/day divided into 4 doses. In acute infections, treatment should be continued for 10-14 days. These drugs can be given parenterally if the patient is severely ill. Demecycline (Declomycin®) has similar properties. The oral dose is 150 mg every 6 hours. For chronic pyelonephritis, it may be necessary to give these drugs for 1 month. Even then, only suppression of the infection may be obtained. "Outdated" tetracycline may cause a syndrome typified by potassium depletion.

With renal impairment, the usual dose of the tetracyclines is apt to cause a further degree of azotemia. In such instances, the dose should be decreased. Administration of these drugs later than the 4th month of gestation may lead, in turn, to dental caries in the infant. Prolonged administration to children causes discoloration of the teeth.

Chloramphenicol (Chloromycetin®)

Chloramphenicol is a potent bacteriostatic drug, but it should be reserved for those patients suffering from serious disease due to an organism that is more likely to respond to chloramphenicol than to other drugs, as shown by sensitivity tests. It has hematopoietic toxicity which may not reveal itself until 2 months after its use. This is most apt to occur in pa-

Table 12-3. Antimicrobial spectra of chemotherapeutic and antibiotic agents in urinary tract infections.

++ Drug of choice
+ Alternative drug
± Moderate effect
C Drugs used in combination

	Sulfonamides	G, Procaine	Methicillin, Oxacillin, Etc.	Ampicillin	Carbenicillin	Cephalosporins	Tetracyclines	Chloramphenicol	Streptomycin	Neomycin, Kanamycin	Gentamicin	Polymyxin, Colistimethate	Nitrofurantoin	Methenamine With Acidifier	Nalidixic Acid
E coli	+			++	+	+	+	+	+	++	+	+	+	±	+
Klebsiella	+			++C		++C	+		+	++	+	+		±	+
Enterobacter (aerobacter)	±					±	+C	+	+C	++	+			±	+
Serratia					+					+	++				
P mirabilis	±	++		++		+	±	+	±	+	+		±	±	±
P vulgaris and others					+	+	+	+	+	++	+	++	+	±	
Ps aeruginosa					+	+	+	+	±	+	++	++	±		
Str hemolyticus	+	++	±	±		++	+		++C	++C				±	
Str faecalis (enterococcus)	±	+C		++C		++	+		+C						
S aureus	±	++C	±	+		++	+	+							
Penicillinase-producing			++			+		+							

Table 12-4. Antimicrobial spectra of antimicrobial agents in gram-negative rod infections based on concentration of drugs in urine (Stamey). *

++ Drug of choice + Alternative drug	Penicillin G (Orally)	Nitrofurantoin	Colistin	Oxytetracycline	Streptomycin	Nalidixic Acid
E coli	++	++	++	+		
Klebsiella-enterobacter			++	+	+	++
P morganii		+		++	+	
P mirabilis	++				++	
Ps aeruginosa			++	++	+	

*Neomycin is effective against 85-100% of all above bacteria.

tients with hepatic or renal insufficiency. Serial reticulocyte counts should be done. Optic neuritis has been reported as a complication in a few children. Two to 4 gm/day are given in divided doses. Chloramphenicol should not be used during the first 2 months of life.

Streptomycin

This is a bactericidal drug, and in the presence of susceptible organisms it may sterilize the urine rapidly. One-half to 1 gm should be administered IM every 6-12 hours. Since the bacteria rapidly becomes resistant to streptomycin, therapy should be discontinued after 5 days and treatment continued with another drug. Eighth nerve toxicity is rare with such a short treatment schedule. Streptomycin is quite effective against P mirabilis and P morganii and has some effect on infection caused by Pseudomonas (Stamey). Dihydrostreptomycin, because of its severe toxic effect upon auditory function, should not be used.

Neomycin and Kanamycin (Kantrex®)

These bactericidal drugs are similar in action and toxicity, although kanamycin is both less active and less toxic than neomycin. They are effective in the treatment of infections caused by gram-negative rods (excluding Ps aeruginosa) and staphylococci.

Because these drugs are nephrotoxic and cause deafness and skin rashes, they should be employed only to combat the most serious infections. They are poorly absorbed from the intestinal tract; parenteral administration is therefore necessary.

Gentamicin (Garamycin®)

This drug is somewhat similar to kanamycin but shows some differences in antibac-

terial activity. It is particularly useful in severe infections caused by E coli, pseudomonas, proteus, serratia, and klebsiella-enterobacter. The dose is 1-3 mg/kg/day IM in 3 equal doses for 7-10 days. Evidence of toxicity involving the kidneys and the eighth nerve must be sought.

Polymyxin B and Colistimethate (Polymyxin E, Coly-Mycin®)

These closely related bactericidal drugs have some nephrotoxic effect, but nephrotoxicity does not commonly occur when renal function is normal (though a few instances of acute tubular necrosis due to a hypersensitivity reaction have been reported). Few other drugs are effective against Ps aeruginosa. They are not effective in the treatment of P vulgaris infections. If renal function is impaired, the usual dose should be reduced by one-half. If urinalysis reveals hematuria, casts, or protein, these signs will disappear when the drug is withdrawn. Both drugs are administered intramuscularly. The average dose for both is 1-2 mg/lb/day in divided doses. The injection of polymyxin is painful. Colistimethate, which contains a local anesthetic, is the drug of choice. For intravenous therapy, polymyxin B sulfate, 1-2 mg/kg/day, is preferable. Toxic effects include renal impairment, paresthesias, and dizziness. These disappear on cessation of the drug.

URINARY ANTISEPTICS

Nitrofurantoin (Furadantin®, Macrodantin®)

The usual disk sensitivity test is useful even though this drug causes no measurable serum or tissue level for it does reflect sensitivity to its concentration in the urine, which is of paramount importance in the cure of most infections of the urinary tract. Since blood and tissue levels of the drug are insignificant, it should not be used for serious infections. The dose is 100 mg 4 times a day. To suppress chronic infection, 50 mg can be given 2 or 3 times a day. Nitrofurantoin is not effective against Ps aeruginosa infections. Sodium nitrofurantoin can be injected intravenously if the patient is unable to take it by mouth. This produces adequate levels in the urine. The intravenous dose is 180-360 mg/day in divided doses. The chronic use of this drug in the uremic patient is contraindicated; it may cause a severe and progressive polyneuritis. Instances of allergic pneumonitis associated with fever and cough have been reported. Resolution occurs when the drug is stopped.

Methenamine With Organic Acid (Mandelamine®, Hiprex®)

Methenamine is one of the oldest drugs used in the treatment of urinary tract infections. The addition of mandelic or hippuric acid affords an acid urine which in itself is bacteriostatic. In order to be efficacious, methenamine mandelate must be given in a dose of 3-6 gm/day in divided doses. The recommended dose of methenamine hippurate is 1 gm twice a day. The pH of the urine should be 5.5 or lower, and the urinary output should be limited to 1000 ml/day in order to afford adequate concentration of formaldehyde. The pH can be checked by the patient with nitrazine paper; additional acidification may be necessary. Ascorbic acid, 1 gm 4 times a day, is an efficient acidifier. Formaldehyde, the active bacteriostatic agent liberated in the urine, may cause vesical irritability or even hematuria. Use of the acidified methenamines is contraindicated in the face of renal insufficiency; acidosis may occur.

Methenamine is a useful drug for prolonged suppressive therapy, but the full dosage should be prescribed. Should the dose be cut in half, not only is there less methenamine available but less urinary acidification as well, thus negating its effect.

Nalidixic Acid (NegGram®)

Nalidixic acid is a naphthyridine derivative which is effective against gram-negative rods with the exception of Ps aeruginosa. It is ineffective against enterococci. It has been shown that the bacteria develop resistance rather rapidly, so it does not seem to lend itself to chronic suppressive therapy. The recommended dose is 4 gm/day in divided doses. Toxic symptoms include skin rash,

nausea, drowsiness, and, rarely, convulsions. False-positive tests for urinary 17-ketosteroids and glucose occur when this drug is present in the urine.

Abramowicz, M., & C. M. Edelmann, Jr.: Nephrotoxicity of anti-infective drugs. Clin Pediat 7:389-90, 1968.

Adler, S., & D. P. Segal: Nonoliguric renal failure secondary to sodium colistimethate: A report of four cases. Am J Med Sc 261: 109-14, 1971.

Atlas, E., & others: Nalidixic acid and oxolinic acid in the treatment of chronic bacteriuria. Ann Int Med 70:713-21, 1969.

Axline, S. G., Yaffe, S. J., & H. J. Simon: Clinical pharmacology of antimicrobials in premature infants. II. Ampicillin, methicillin, oxacillin, neomycin, and colistin. Pediatrics 39:97-107, 1967.

Bailey, A., & others: Cephalexin—a new oral antibiotic. Postgrad MJ 46:157-8, 1970.

Beirne, G. J., & others: Acute renal failure caused by hypersensitivity to polymyxin B sulfate. JAMA 202:62-4, 1967.

Bulger, R. J., & U. Roosen-Runge: Bactericidal activity of the ampicillin/kanamycin combination against Escherichia coli, enterobacter-klebsiella and proteus. Am J Med Sc 258:7-13, 1969.

Chang, N., Giles, C. L., & R. H. Gregg: Optic neuritis and chloramphenicol. Am J Dis Child 112:46-8, 1966.

Cothier, A. J., Jr., & E. E. Anderson: Tetracycline-induced azotemia. J Urol 95:16-18, 1966.

Cox, C. E., O'Connor, F. J., & S. S. Lacy: Clinical effectiveness of intramuscular sodium nitrofurantoin against urinary tract infections. J Urol 105:113-8, 1971.

Davies, W.: Treatment of urinary tract infections in children with nalidixic acid. Brit J Urol 39:138-42, 1967.

Dillon, M. L., & R. W. Postlewait: Cephaloridine in patients with impaired renal function. JAMA 218:250-1, 1971.

Dorfman, L. E., & J. P. Smith: Sulfonamide crystalluria: A forgotten disease. J Urol 104:482-3, 1970.

Ellis, F. G.: Acute polyneuritis after nitrofurantoin therapy. Lancet 2:1136-8, 1962.

Elwood, C. M., Lucas, G. D., & R. C. Muehrcke: Acute renal failure associated with sodium colistimethate treatment. Arch Int Med 118:326-34, 1966.

Eykyn, S.: Use and control of cephalosporins. J Clin Path 24:419-29, 1971.

Fass, R. J., Perkins, R. L., & S. Saslaw: Cephalexin—a new oral cephalosporin: Clinical evaluation in sixty-three patients. Am J Med Sc 259:187-200, 1970.

Fulop, M., & A. Drapkin: Potassium-depletion syndrome secondary to nephropathy apparently caused by "outdated tetracycline." New England J Med **272**:986-9, 1965.

Gerstein, A. R., & others: The prolonged use of methenamine hippurate in the treatment of chronic urinary tract infection. J Urol **100**:767-71, 1968.

Grossman, E. R., & others: Tetracyclines and permanent teeth: The relation between dose and tooth color. Pediatrics **47**:567-70, 1971.

Harris, M. J., Wise, G., & J. Beveridge: The Stevens-Johnson syndrome and long-acting sulfonamides. Australian Paediat J **2**:101-9, 1966.

Harrison, L. H., & C. E. Cox: Bacteriologic and pharmacodynamic aspects of nalidixic acid. J Urol **104**:908-13, 1970.

Hunter, I. J.: In vitro sensitivity of 368 urinary organisms to trimethoprim-sulfamethoxazole and other antibacterials. MJ Australia **2**:317-20, 1970.

Kabins, S. A.: Interactions among antibiotics and other drugs. JAMA **219**:206-12, 1972.

Katul, M. J., & I. N. Frank: Antibacterial activity of methenamine hippurate. J Urol **104**:320-4, 1970.

Koch-Weser, J., & others: Adverse reactions to sulfisoxazole, sulfamethoxazole, and nitrofurantoin. Arch Int Med **128**:399-404, 1971.

Kunin, C. M.: A guide to use of antibiotics in patients with renal disease. A table of recommended doses and factors governing serum levels. Ann Int Med **67**:151-8, 1967.

Kunin, C. M.: A ten-year study of bacteriuria in schoolgirls: Final report of bacteriologic, urologic, and epidemiologic findings. J Infect Dis **122**:382-93, 1970.

Lerner, P. I., Smith, H., & L. Weinstein: Penicillin neurotoxicity. Ann New York Acad Sc **145**:310-7, 1967.

Levin, H. S., & B. M. Kagan: Antimicrobial agents: Pediatric dosages, routes of administration and preparation procedures for parenteral therapy. P Clin North America **15**:275-90, 1968.

Llerna, O., & O. H. Pearson: Interference of nalidixic acid in urinary 17-ketosteroid determinations. New England J Med **279**:983-4, 1968.

Marks, M. I., & T. C. Eickhoff: Carbenicillin: A clinical and laboratory evaluation. Ann Int Med **73**:179-87, 1970.

McCracken, G. H., Jr., & L. G. Jones: Gentamicin in the neonatal period. Am J Dis Child **120**:524-33, 1970.

McHenry, M. C., & others: Gentamicin dosages for renal insufficiency. Ann Int Med **74**:192-7, 1971.

Merrill, S. L., & others: Cephalothin in serious bacterial infection. Ann Int Med **64**:1-12, 1966.

Meuwissen, H. J., & G. C. Robinson: The ototoxic antibiotics. Clin Pediat **6**:262-9, 1967.

Meyers, B. R., Sabbaj, J., & L. Weinstein: Bacteriological, pharmacological, and clinical studies of carbenicillin. Arch Int Med **125**:282-6, 1970.

Miller, H., & E. Phillips: Antibacterial correlates of urine drug levels of hexamethylenetetramine and formaldehyde. Invest Urol **8**:21-33, 1970.

Möhring, K., Genster, H. G., & P. O. Madsen: Treatment of urinary tract infections with cephalexin. J Urol **106**:757-60, 1971.

Murphy, F. J., & S. Zelman: Ascorbic acid as a urinary acidifying agent: 1. Comparison with the ketogenic effect of fasting. J Urol **94**:297-9, 1965.

Nelson, J. D.: Carbenicillin—a major new antibiotic. Am J Dis Child **120**:382-3, 1970.

Neuvonen, P. J., & others: Interference of iron with the absorption of tetracyclines in men. Brit MJ **4**:532-4, 1970.

Ngan, H., & others: Nitrofurantoin lung. Brit J Radiol **44**:21-3, 1971.

Reeves, D. S.: Sulfamethoxazole/trimethoprim: The first two years. J Clin Path **24**:430-7, 1971.

Ronald, A. R., Turck, M., & R. G. Petersdorf: A critical evaluation of nalidixic acid in urinary-tract infections. New England J Med **275**:1081-9, 1966.

Ross, R. R., Jr., & G. F. Conway: Hemorrhagic cystitis following accidental overdose of methenamine mandelate. Am J Dis Child **119**:86-7, 1970.

Sachs, J., & others: Effect of renal function on urinary recovery of orally administered nitrofurantoin. New England J Med **278**:1032-5, 1968.

Shapiro, S., & others: Drug rash with ampicillin and other penicillins. Lancet **2**:969-72, 1969.

Smith, E. K., & J. D. Williams: The use of cephalexin monohydrate in chronic bacteriuria and acute urinary tract infection. Brit J Urol **42**:522-8, 1970.

Stamey, T. A., Govan, D. E., & J. M. Palmer: The localization and treatment of urinary tract infections: The role of bactericidal urine levels as opposed to serum levels. Medicine **44**:1-36, 1965.

Steinhauer, B. W., & others: The klebsiella-enterobacter-serratia division. Clinical and epidemiologic characteristics. Ann Int Med **65**:1180-94, 1966.

Symposium: The synergy of trimethoprim and sulfonamides. Postgrad MJ **45**(Suppl), 1969.

Tallgren, L.G., & C.H. von Bonsdorff: The effect of varying the pH level upon the sensitivity of urinary bacteria to antibiotics. Acta med scandinav **178**:543-51, 1965.

Turck, M.: Broad-spectrum penicillin and other antibiotics in the treatment of urinary tract infections. Ann New York Acad Sc **145**:344-53, 1967.

Turck, M., & others: Sodium ampicillin given parenterally. Arch Int Med **117**:242-9, 1966.

Wallerstein, R.O., & others: Statewide study of chloramphenicol therapy and fatal aplastic anemia. JAMA **208**:2045-50, 1969.

Weinstein, L., & K. Kaplan: The cephalosporins. Ann Int Med **72**:729-39, 1970.

Weinstein, L., Lerner, P.I., & W.H. Chew: Clinical and bacteriologic studies of the effect of "massive" doses of penicillin G on infections caused by gram-negative bacilli. New England J Med **271**:525-33, 1964.

Weinstein, L., Madoff, M.A., & C.M. Samet: The sulfonamides. New England J Med **263**:793-800, 842-9, 1960.

Whalley, P.J., & others: Disposition of tetracycline by pregnant women with acute pyelonephritis. Obst Gynec **36**:821-6, 1970.

Wilkowske, C.J., & others: Serratia marcescens. JAMA **214**:2157-62, 1970.

Zangwill, D.P., & others: Antibacterial organic acids and chronic urinary tract infection. Arch Int Med **117**:801, 1962.

•   •   •

13 . . .

Specific Infections
of the Urinary Tract

TUBERCULOSIS

Tubercle bacilli may invade one or more
(or even all) of the organs of the genitourinary
tract and cause a chronic granulomatous infection which shows the same characteristics as
tuberculosis in other organs. Urinary tuberculosis is a disease of young adults (60% of
the patients are between the ages of 20-40)
and is a little more common in males than in
females.

Etiology

The infecting organism is Mycobacterium
tuberculosis, which reaches the genitourinary
organs by the hematogenous route from another
part of the body. Primary foci of tuberculous
infection include the lungs, lymph nodes, tonsils, intestines, bones, and joints. Commonly the primary focus is not symptomatic or
apparent.

The kidney and possibly the prostate are
the primary sites of tuberculous infection in
the genitourinary tract. All other genitourinary organs become involved either by ascent
(prostate to bladder) or descent (kidney to
bladder, prostate to epididymis). The testis
may become involved by direct extension from
epididymal infection.

Pathogenesis (See Fig 13-1.)

A. Kidney and Ureter: When a shower of
tubercle bacilli hits the renal cortex, the organisms may be destroyed by normal tissue
resistance. Evidence of this is commonly seen
in autopsies of persons who have died of tuberculosis; only scars are found in the kidneys.
However, if enough bacteria of sufficient virulence become lodged in the kidney and are not
overcome, a clinical infection is established.
The initial focus in the kidney is usually in the
cortex.

Tuberculosis of the kidney progresses
slowly; it may take 15-20 years to destroy a
kidney in a patient having good resistance to
the infection. As a rule, therefore, there is
no renal pain and little or no clinical disturb-
ance of any type until the lesion has involved

the calyces or the pelvis, at which time pus
and organisms may be discharged into the
urine. It is only at this stage that symptoms
(of cystitis) are manifested. The infection
then proceeds to the pelvic mucosa and the
ureter, particularly its upper and vesical ends.
This may lead to stricture and back pressure
(hydronephrosis).

As the disease progresses, a caseous
breakdown of tissue occurs until the entire kidney is replaced by cheesy material. Calcium
may be laid down in the reparative process.
The ureter undergoes fibrosis and tends to be
shortened and therefore straightened. This
change leads to a "golf hole" (gaping) ureteral
orifice, typical of an incompetent valve.

B. Bladder: Vesical irritability develops
as an early clinical manifestation of the disease as the bladder is bathed by infected material. Tubercles form later, usually in the
region of the involved ureteral orifice, and
finally coalesce and ulcerate. These ulcers
may bleed. With severe involvement, the bladder becomes fibrosed and contracted; this
leads to marked frequency. Ureteral reflux
or stenosis and, therefore, hydronephrosis
may develop. If contralateral renal involvement develops later, it is probably a separate
hematogenous infection.

C. Prostate and Seminal Vesicles: The
passage of infected urine through the prostatic
urethra will ultimately lead to invasion of the
prostate and one or both seminal vesicles.
There is no local pain.

On occasion, the primary hematogenous
lesion in the genitourinary tract is in the prostate. Prostatic infection can extend to the
bladder and descend to the epididymis.

D. Epididymis and Testis: Tuberculosis
of the prostate can extend along the vas or
through the perivasal lymphatics and affect
the epididymis. This is a slow process, and
there is therefore usually no pain. If the epididymal infection is extensive and abscess
forms, it may rupture through the scrotal skin,
thus establishing a permanent sinus, or it may
extend into the testicle.

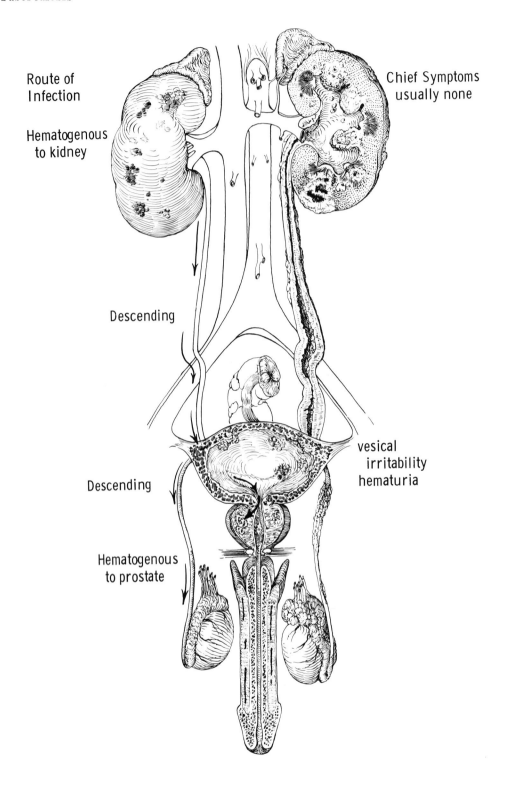

Route of
Infection

Hematogenous
to kidney

Chief Symptoms
usually none

Descending

Descending

Hematogenous
to prostate

vesical
irritability
hematuria

Fig 13-1. Pathogenesis of tuberculosis of the urinary tract.

Pathology

A. Kidney and Ureter: The gross appearance of the kidney with moderately advanced tuberculosis is often normal on its outer surface, although it is usually surrounded by marked perinephritis. Usually, however, there is a soft, yellowish localized bulge. On section, the involved area is seen to be filled with cheesy material (caseation). Widespread destruction of parenchyma is evident. In otherwise normal tissue, small abscesses may be seen. The walls of the pelvis, calyces, and ureter may be thickened, and ulceration appears frequently in the region of the calyces at the point at which the abscess drains. Ureteral stenosis may be complete, causing "autonephrectomy." Such a kidney is fibrosed and functionless. Under these circumstances, the bladder urine may be normal and symptoms absent.

Microscopically, the caseous material is seen as an amorphous mass. The surrounding parenchyma shows fibrosis with tissue destruction, small round cell and plasma cell infiltration, and epithelial and giant cells typical of tuberculosis. Acid-fast stains will usually demonstrate the organisms in the tissue. Similar changes can be demonstrated in the wall of the pelvis and ureter.

In both the kidney and ureter, calcification is common. It may be macroscopic or microscopic. Such a finding is strongly suggestive of tuberculosis. Secondary renal stones occur in 10% of patients.

In the most advanced stage of renal tuberculosis the parenchyma may be completely replaced by caseous substance or fibrous tissue. Perinephric abscess may develop, but this is rare.

B. Bladder: In the early stages, the mucosa may be inflamed, but this not a specific change. The bladder is quite resistant to actual invasion. Later, tubercles form and can be seen easily, especially through the cystoscope, as white or yellow raised nodules surrounded by a halo of hyperemia. With severe vesical contracture, reflux may occur.

Microscopically, the nodules are typical tubercles. These break down to form deep, ragged ulcers. At this stage the bladder is quite irritable. With healing, fibrosis develops which involves the muscle wall.

C. Prostate and Seminal Vesicles: Grossly, the exterior surface of these organs may show nodules and areas of induration from fibrosis. Areas of necrosis are common. On rare occasion healing may end in calcification. Large calcifications in the prostate should suggest tuberculous involvement.

D. Spermatic Cord, Epididymis, and Testis: The vas deferens is often grossly involved; fusiform swellings represent tubercles. The epididymis is enlarged and quite firm. It is usually separate from the testis, although occasionally it may adhere to it. Microscopically, the changes typical of tuberculosis are seen. Tubular degeneration may be marked.

The testis is usually not involved except by direct extension of an abscess in the epididymis.

Clinical Findings

Tuberculosis of the genitourinary tract should be considered in the presence of any of the following situations: (1) chronic cystitis which refuses to respond to adequate therapy, (2) the finding of pus without bacteria in a methylene blue stain or culture of the urinary sediment, (3) gross or microscopic hematuria, (4) a nontender, enlarged epididymis with a beaded or thickened vas, (5) a chronic draining scrotal sinus, or (6) induration or nodulation of the prostate and thickening of one or both seminal vesicles (especially in a young man). A history of present or past tuberculosis elsewhere in the body should cause the physician to suspect tuberculosis in the genitourinary tract when signs or symptoms are present.

The diagnosis rests upon the demonstration of tubercle bacilli in the urine (acid-fast stain, culture, guinea pig inoculations). The extent of the infection is determined by (1) the palpable findings in the epididymides, vasa deferentia, prostate, and seminal vesicles; (2) the renal and ureteral lesions as revealed by excretory urograms; (3) involvement of the bladder as seen through the cystoscope; (4) the degree of renal damage as measured by loss of function; and (5) the presence of tubercle bacilli in one or both kidneys.

A. Symptoms: There is no classical clinical picture of renal tuberculosis. Most symptoms of this disease, even in the most advanced stage, are vesical in origin (cystitis). Vague generalized malaise, fatigability, low-grade but persistent fever, and night sweats are some of the nonspecific complaints. Even vesical irritability may be absent, in which case only proper collection and examination of the urine will afford the clue. Active tuberculosis elsewhere in the body is found in less than half of patients with genitourinary tuberculosis.

1. Kidney and ureter - Because of the slow progression of the disease, the affected kidney is usually completely asymptomatic. On occasion, however, there may be a dull ache in the flank. The passage of a blood clot, secondary calculi, or a mass of debris may cause renal and ureteral colic. Rarely, the

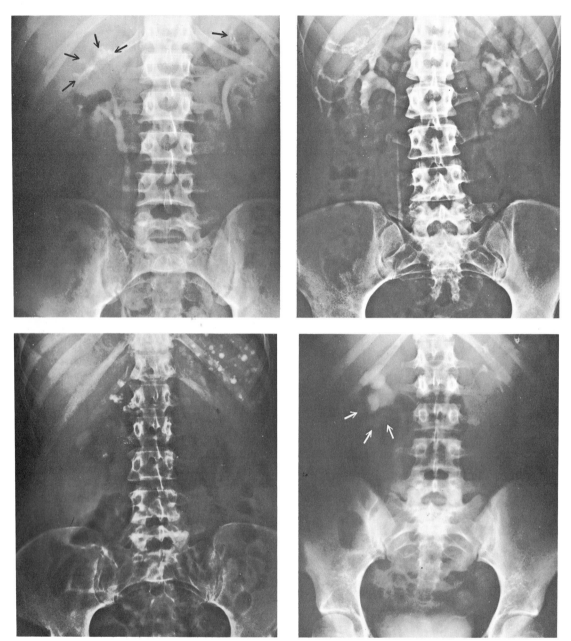

Fig 13-2. Radiologic evidence of tuberculosis. Above left: Excretory urogram showing ''moth-eaten'' calyces in upper renal poles. Calcifications in upper calyces; right upper ureter is straight and dilated. **Below left:** Plain film showing calcifications in right kidney, adrenals, and spleen (tuberculosis of right kidney and Addison's disease). **Above right:** Excretory urogram showing ulcerated and dilated calyces on the left. **Below right:** Excretory urogram. Dilatation of calyces, upper right ureter dilated and straight. Arrows point to poorly defined parenchymal abscesses.

presenting symptom may be a painless mass in the abdomen.

2. Bladder - The earliest symptoms of renal tuberculosis may arise from secondary vesical involvement. These include burning, frequency, and nocturia. Hematuria is occasionally found and is of either renal or vesical origin. At times, particularly in a late stage of the disease, the vesical irritability may become extreme. If ulceration occurs, suprapubic pain may be noted when the bladder becomes full.

3. Genital tract - Tuberculosis of the prostate and seminal vesicles usually causes no symptoms. The first clue to the presence of tuberculous infection of these organs is the onset of a tuberculous epididymitis.

Tuberculosis of the epididymis usually presents as a painless or only mildly painful swelling. An abscess may drain spontaneously through the scrotal wall. A chronic draining sinus should be regarded as tuberculous until proved otherwise. In rare cases the onset is quite acute and may simulate an acute nonspecific epididymitis.

B. Signs: Evidence of extragenital tuberculosis may be found (lungs, bone, lymph nodes, tonsils, intestines).

1. Kidney - There is usually no enlargement or tenderness of the involved kidney.

2. External genitalia - A thickened, nontender or only slightly tender epididymis may be discovered. The vas deferens often is thickened and beaded. A chronic draining sinus through the scrotal skin is almost pathognomonic of tuberculous epididymitis. In the more advanced stages, the epididymis cannot be differentiated from the testis upon palpation. This may mean that the testis has been directly invaded by the epididymal abscess.

Hydrocele occasionally accompanies tuberculous epididymitis. The "idiopathic" hydrocele should be tapped so that underlying pathologic changes, if present, can be evaluated (epididymitis, testicular tumor).

3. Prostate and seminal vesicles - These organs may be normal to palpation. Ordinarily, however, the tuberculous prostate shows areas of induration, even nodulation. The involved vesicle is usually indurated, enlarged, and fixed. If epididymitis is present, the ipsilateral vesicle usually shows changes as well.

C. Laboratory Findings: Proper urinalysis affords the most important clue to the diagnosis of genitourinary tuberculosis. If all 3 methods described below are used, errors in bacteriologic diagnosis will be rare.

1. Persistent pyuria without organisms on culture or on the smear stained with methy-

lene blue means tuberculosis until proved otherwise. Acid-fast stains done on the concentrated sediment from a 24-hour specimen are positive in at least 60% of cases. This must be corroborated by a positive culture or, preferably, guinea pig inoculation.

About 15-20% of patients with tuberculosis have secondary pyogenic infection; the clue ("sterile" pyuria) is thereby obscured. If clinical response to adequate treatment fails and pyuria persists, tuberculosis must be ruled out by bacteriologic and roentgenologic means.

2. Cultures for tubercle bacilli from urine are positive in a high percentage of cases of tuberculous infection. In the face of strong presumptive evidence of tuberculosis, negative cultures should be repeated.

3. Inoculation of guinea pigs with the suspected urine usually demonstrates tuberculous lesions in these animals. Four to 6 weeks are necessary, however, for a definite answer. This is the most conclusive test, for it fulfills Koch's postulates.

The blood count may be normal or may show anemia in advanced disease. The sedimentation rate is usually accelerated.

Tubercle bacilli may often be demonstrated in the secretions from an infected prostate. Renal function will be normal unless there is bilateral damage: As one kidney is slowly injured, compensatory hypertrophy of the normal kidney develops. It can also be infected with tubercle bacilli, or may become hydronephrotic from fibrosis of the bladder wall (ureterovesical stenosis) or vesicoureteral reflux.

If tuberculosis is suspected, perform the tuberculin test. A positive test, particularly in an adult, is hardly diagnostic; but a negative test in an otherwise healthy patient speaks against a diagnosis of tuberculosis.

D. X-ray Findings (Fig 13-2): A chest film which shows evidence of tuberculosis should cause the physician to suspect tuberculosis of the urogenital tract in the presence of urinary signs and symptoms. A plain film of the abdomen may show enlargement of one kidney or obliteration of the renal and psoas shadows due to perinephric abscess. Punctate calcification in the renal parenchyma may be due to tuberculosis. Renal stones are found in 10% of cases. Calcification of the ureter may be noted, but this is rare (Fig 7-2). Small prostatic stones the size of grape-seeds in the region of the symphysis pubis are ordinarily not due to tuberculosis, but large calcific bodies may be.

Excretory urograms can be diagnostic if the lesion is moderately advanced. The typical changes include (1) a "moth-eaten" appearance of the involved ulcerated calyces, (2) obliteration of one or more calyces, (3) dilatation of the calyces due to ureteral stenosis from fibrosis, (4) abscess cavities which connect with calyces, (5) single or multiple ureteral strictures, with secondary dilatation, with shortening and therefore straightening of the ureter, and (6) absence of function of the kidney, due to complete ureteral occlusion and renal destruction (autonephrectomy).

If the excretory urograms demonstrate gross tuberculosis in one kidney, there is no need to do a retrograde pyelogram on that side. In fact, there is at least a theoretical danger of hematogenous or lymphogenous dissemination resulting from the increased intrapelvic pressure. Retrograde urography should, however, be carried out on the unsuspected side as a verification of its normality. This is further substantiated if the urine from that side is free of both pus cells and tubercle bacilli.

E. Instrumental Examination: Thorough cystoscopic study is indicated even when the offending organism has been found in the urine and excretory urograms show the typical renal lesion. This will clearly demonstrate the extent of the disease. Cystoscopy may reveal the typical tubercles or ulcers of tuberculosis. Biopsy can be done if necessary. Severe contracture of the bladder may be noted. A cystogram may reveal ureteral reflux. A sterile specimen of urine should also be obtained for further study. Ureteral catheters are then passed to the renal pelves. This will afford urine specimens from each kidney for bacteriologic examination. Relative function of each kidney can be determined with the PSP test. Considerable destruction is necessary, however, before this test shows impairment.

Differential Diagnosis

Chronic nonspecific cystitis or pyelonephritis may mimic tuberculosis perfectly, especially since 15-20% of cases of tuberculosis are secondarily invaded by pyogenic organisms. If nonspecific infections do not respond to adequate therapy, a search for tubercle bacilli should be made. Painless epididymitis points to tuberculosis. Cystoscopic demonstration of tubercles and ulceration of the bladder wall means tuberculosis. Urograms are usually definitive.

Acute or chronic nonspecific epididymitis may be confused with tuberculosis since the onset of tuberculosis is occasionally quite painful. It is rare to have palpatory changes in the seminal vesicles with nonspecific epididymitis, but these are almost routine findings in tuberculosis of the epididymis. The presence of tubercle bacilli in the urine is diagnostic.

On occasion only the pathologist can make the diagnosis by microscopic study of the surgically removed epididymis.

Amicrobic cystitis usually has an acute onset and is often preceded by a urethral discharge. "Sterile" pyuria is found, but tubercle bacilli are absent. Cystoscopy may reveal ulcerations, but these are acute and superficial. Although urograms show mild hydroureter and even hydronephrosis, there is no ulceration of the calyces, as seen in renal tuberculosis.

Interstitial cystitis is typically characterized by frequency, nocturia, and suprapubic pain with vesical filling. The urine is usually free of pus. Tubercle bacilli are absent.

Multiple small renal stones or nephrocalcinosis seen by x-ray may suggest the type of calcification seen in the tuberculous kidney. In renal tuberculosis the calcium is in the parenchyma, although secondary stones are occasionally seen.

Necrotizing papillitis, which may involve all of the calyces of one or both kidneys or, rarely, a solitary calyx, shows calyceal lesions (including calcifications) which simulate those of tuberculosis. Careful bacteriologic studies will fail to demonstrate tubercle bacilli.

Medullary sponge kidneys may show small calcifications just distal to the calyces. The calyces, however, are sharp and no other stigmas of tuberculosis can be demonstrated.

Complications

A. Renal Tuberculosis: Perinephric abscess may cause an enlarging mass in the flank. A plain film of the abdomen will show obliteration of the renal and psoas shadows. Renal stones may develop if secondary nonspecific infection is present. Uremia is the end stage if both kidneys are involved.

B. Ureteral Tuberculosis: Scarring with stricture formation is one of the typical lesions of tuberculosis and most commonly affects the juxtavesical portion. This may cause progressive hydronephrosis. Complete ureteral obstruction may cause complete nonfunction of the kidney.

C. Vesical Tuberculosis: When severely damaged, the bladder wall becomes fibrosed and contracted. Stenosis of the ureters or reflux occurs, causing hydronephrotic atrophy.

D. Genital Tuberculosis: The ducts of the involved epididymis become occluded. If this is bilateral, sterility results. Abscess of the epididymis may rupture into the testis, through the scrotal wall, or both, in which case the spermatogenic tubules may slough out.

Treatment

Tuberculosis must be treated as a generalized disease. Even when it can be demonstrated only in the urogenital tract, one must
assume activity elsewhere. (It is theoretically possible, however, for the primary focus
to have healed spontaneously.) This means
that basically the treatment is medical, ie,
rest and antimicrobial drugs. Surgical excision of an infected organ, when indicated,
is merely an adjunct to overall therapy.

A. Renal Tuberculosis: If bacteriologic
study reveals unilateral involvement and pyelography shows no gross evidence of necrosis,
a strict medical regimen should be established.
Complete bed rest is essential at first, and
physical activity must be limited for 18-24
months (depending on response). The following drugs are given for at least 2 years.
  1. Cycloserine, 250 mg twice a day by
mouth.
  2. Sodium aminosalicylic acid (PAS),
15 gm/day orally in divided doses.
  3. Isoniazid (INH), 5 mg/kg in divided
doses.
  4. Pyridoxine, 100 mg/day in divided
doses, will counteract the vitamin B_6 depletion effect of isoniazid.

If bacteriologic study reveals tuberculosis
and the urogram shows a deformity (necrosis)
typical of tuberculosis in one kidney only, combined medical and surgical treatment (nephrectomy) may be indicated. Medical treatment by itself may not heal such a lesion: Bed
rest and antibiotic therapy as described above
should be instituted for 1-3 months. If culture
for tubercle bacilli is positive after 3 months
of medical therapy, nephrectomy should be
done. After nephrectomy, medical treatment
is continued in the dosages outlined above.

If bacteriologic and radiographic studies
demonstrate bilateral disease, only medical
treatment can be considered. The only exceptions are (1) severe sepsis, pain, or bleeding
from one kidney (may require nephrectomy as
a palliative or life-saving measure) and (2)
marked advance of the disease on one side and
minimal damage on the other (consider removal of the badly damaged organ).

B. Vesical Tuberculosis: Tuberculosis
of the bladder is always secondary to renal or
prostatic tuberculosis; it tends to heal promptly when definitive treatment for the "primary"
genitourinary infection is given. Vesical
ulcers which fail to respond to this regimen
may require transurethral electrocoagulation.
Vesical instillations of 0.2% monoxychlorosene
(Clorpactin®) may also stimulate healing.

Should extreme contracture of the bladder
develop, it may be necessary to divert the
urine from the bladder or perform subtotal
cystectomy and anastomose a segment of ileum
or sigmoid to the remainder (ileocystoplasty,
sigmoidocystoplasty) in order to afford comfort.

C. Tuberculosis of the Epididymis: This
is never an isolated lesion; the prostate is
always involved and usually the kidney as well.
Only rarely does the epididymal infection break
through into the testis. Treatment is medical.
If after months of treatment an abscess or a
draining sinus exists, epididymectomy is indicated.

D. Tuberculosis of the Prostate and Seminal Vesicles: Although a few urologists advocate the removal of the entire prostate and the
vesicles when they become involved by tuberculosis, the majority opinion is that only medical therapy is indicated. Control can be
checked by culture of the semen for tubercle
bacilli.

E. General Measures for All Types:
Physical and mental rest and optimum nutrition are no less important in treating tuberculosis of the genitourinary tract than in the
treatment of tuberculosis elsewhere. Bladder
sedatives may be given for the irritable bladder.

F. Treatment of Complications: Perinephric abscess usually occurs when the kidney is destroyed. The abscess must be drained,
and nephrectomy should be done either then
or later to prevent development of a chronic
draining sinus. Prolonged antimicrobial therapy is indicated. If ureterovesical stricture
or reflux develops and causes progressive
hydronephrosis of the uninvolved kidney, diversion of the urine by cutaneous ureterostomy,
nephrostomy, or replacement of the diseased
ureter with a segment of ileum may have to
be done to prevent death from uremia. For
this reason, serial excretory urograms are
necessary even under medical treatment.

Prognosis

Prognosis varies with the extent of the
disease and the organs involved, but has been
greatly improved since tuberculosis of the
genitourinary tract has come to be treated as
a systemic disease (bed rest, antituberculo-
sis chemotherapy). If the infection is limited
to one kidney only and the bladder is uninvolved
with tubercles or ulcers, the prognosis should
be good to excellent. The urine must be carefully examined every 6 months for at least 5
years. If the tuberculosis is limited to one kidney but the bladder is involved, the prognosis is
fair to good. The bladder may become fibrotic

and obstruct the ureter to the normal kidney. In tuberculosis of the genital tract, the prognosis is poor to fair. Medical therapy will cure a few but in most cases will merely slow the progression of the disease. Advanced bilateral renal tuberculosis is incurable and has a poor prognosis. In order to postpone uremia, care must be taken to divert the urinary stream if ureteral strictures or vesicoureteral reflux cause changes due to back pressure.

Beck, A. D., & V. F. Marshall: Is nephrectomy obsolete for unilateral renal tuberculosis? J Urol **98**:65-70, 1967.

Björn-Hansen, R., & T. Aakhus: Angiography in renal tuberculosis. Acta radiol (diag) **11**:167-76, 1971.

Bloom, S., Wechsler, H., & J. K. Lattimer: Results of a long-term study of non-functioning tuberculous kidneys. J Urol **104**:654-7, 1970.

Borthwick, W. M.: Present position of urinary tuberculosis. Brit J Urol **42**:642-6, 1970.

Ehrlich, R. M., & J. K. Lattimer: Urogenital tuberculosis in children. J Urol **105**:461-5, 1971.

Friedenberg, R. M., Ney, C., & R. A. Stachenfield: Roentgenographic manifestations of tuberculosis of ureter. J Urol **99**:25-9, 1968.

Hanley, H. G.: Cavernotomy and partial nephrectomy in renal tuberculosis. Brit J Urol **42**:661-6, 1970.

Kerr, W. K., Gale, G. L., & K. S. S. Peterson: Reconstructive surgery for genitourinary tuberculosis. J Urol **101**:254-66, 1969.

Küss, R., & others: Indications and early and late results of intestino-cystoplasty: A review of 185 cases. J Urol **103**:53-63, 1970.

Lattimer, J. K., & others: Current treatment for renal tuberculosis. J Urol **102**:2-6, 1969.

Lattimer, J. K., Reilly, R. J., & A. Segawa: The significance of the isolated positive urine culture in genitourinary tuberculosis. J Urol **102**:610-3, 1969.

Malament, M., Auerbach, O., & J. T. Harris: Limitation of chemotherapy on advanced cavitary tuberculosis of the kidney. J Urol **99**:700-6, 1968.

Mangelson, N. L., Saunders, J. C., & S. A. Brosman: Urogenital tuberculosis. J Urol **104**:309-14, 1970.

Roylance, J., & others: Radiology in the management of urinary tract tuberculosis. Brit J Urol **42**:679-87, 1970.

St. Hill, C. A., & J. G. Gow: Investigation into the isolation of ''M. tuberculosis'' from urine. Brit J Urol **38**:163-70, 1966.

Walker, D., & W. P. Jordan, Jr.: Tuberculous ulcer of the penis. J Urol **100**:36-7, 1968.

AMICROBIC (ABACTERIAL) CYSTITIS

Amicrobic cystitis is a rare disease of abrupt onset with a marked local vesical reaction. Although it acts like an infectious disease, bacterial search for the usual urinary pathogens is negative. It affects adult men and occasionally children, usually boys. It may be a form of Reiter's disease.

Etiology

Men usually give a history of recent sexual exposure. Leptospira, pleuropneumonia-like organisms, and viruses have been isolated or suspected, but have not been proved to be the etiologic agent. Recently, adenovirus type 2 has been isolated from the urine of children suffering from acute hemorrhagic cystitis.

Pathogenesis and Pathology

Whatever the source and identity of the invader, the disease is primarily manifested as an acute inflammation of the bladder. Vesical irritability is severe and is often associated with terminal hematuria. The mucosa is red and edematous, and superficial ulceration is occasionally seen. A thin membrane of fibrin often lies upon the wall. Similar changes may be noted in the posterior urethra. The renal parenchyma is not involved, although the pelvic and ureteral mucosa may show mild inflammatory changes. Some dilatation of the lower ureters is apt to develop. This may be due to an inflammatory reaction about the ureteral orifices, for these changes regress after successful treatment.

Microscopically, there is nothing specific about the reaction. The mucosa and submucosa are infiltrated with neutrophils, plasma cells, and eosinophils. Submucosal hemorrhages are common; superficial ulceration of the mucosa may be noted.

Clinical Findings

A. Symptoms: All symptoms are local. Urethral discharge, which is usually clear and mucoid but which may be purulent, may be the initial symptom in men. Symptoms of acute cystitis come on abruptly. Urgency, frequency, and burning may be severe. Terminal hematuria is not uncommon. Suprapubic discomfort or even pain may be noted; it is most apt to be present as the bladder fills, and is relieved somewhat by voiding. There is no fever or malaise.

B. Signs: Some suprapubic tenderness may be found. Urethral discharge may be profuse or scanty, and purulent or thin and mucoid. The prostate is usually normal to palpation. Massage is contraindicated during the acute stage of urinary tract infection. When done later, infection is usually found to be absent.

C. Laboratory Findings: Some leukocytosis may develop. The urine is grossly purulent and may contain blood as well. Stained smears reveal an absence of bacteria. Routine cultures are uniformly negative. In a few cases, pleuropneumonia-like organisms and spirochetes have been identified, but the significance of this is not yet clear. Search for tubercle bacilli is not successful.

Urethral discharge reveals no bacteria. Renal function is not impaired.

D. X-ray Findings: Excretory urograms may demonstrate some dilatation of the lower ureters, but these changes regress completely when the disease is cured. The bladder shadow is small because of its markedly diminished capacity. Cystograms may reveal reflux.

E. Instrumental Examination: Cystoscopy is not indicated in the face of acute inflammation of the bladder. It has been done, however, when the diagnosis was obscure and tuberculosis suspected. In such cases it reveals redness and edema of the mucosa. Superficial ulceration may be noted. Bladder capacity is markedly diminished. Biopsy of the wall shows nonspecific changes.

Differential Diagnosis

Tuberculosis causes symptoms of cystitis, which, however, usually come on gradually and become severe only in the stage of ulceration. A painless, nontender enlargement of an epididymis suggests tuberculosis. Although both tuberculosis and amicrobic cystitis produce pus without bacteria, thorough laboratory study will demonstrate tubercle bacilli only in the former. On cystoscopy the tuberculous bladder may be studded with tubercles. The ulcers in this disease are deep and of a chronic type. The changes in amicrobic cystitis are more acute; ulceration, if present, is superficial. Excretory urograms in tuberculosis may show "moth-eaten" calyces typical of infection with acid-fast organisms.

Nonspecific (pyogenic) cystitis may mimic amicrobic cystitis perfectly, but pathogenic organisms are easily found on a smear stained with methylene blue or on culture.

Cystitis secondary to chronic nonspecific prostatitis occasionally produces pus without bacteria. The findings on rectal examination, the pus in the prostatic secretion, and the response to sulfonamides point to the proper diagnosis.

Vesical neoplasm may ulcerate, become infected, and bleed; hence it may mimic amicrobic cystitis. Bacteriuria, however, will be found. In case of doubt, cystoscopy is indicated.

Interstitial cystitis may be accompanied by severe symptoms of vesical irritability. However, it usually affects women past the menopause, and urinalysis is entirely negative except for a few red cells. Cystoscopy should be diagnostic.

Complications

Amicrobic cystitis is usually self-limited. Rarely, secondary contracture of the bladder develops. Under these circumstances, vesicoureteral reflux may be noted.

Treatment

A. Specific Measures: One of the tetracyclines or chloramphenicol, 1 gm/day orally in divided doses for 3-4 days, is said to be curative in 75% of cases. Streptomycin, 1-2 gm/day IM for 3-4 days, may be tried. Neoarsphenamine is also effective and may still be the drug of choice. The first dose is 0.3 gm IV; subsequent dosage is 0.45 gm IV every 3-5 days for a total of 3-4 injections.

Penicillin and the sulfonamides are without effect.

In the cases reported in children, cure occurred spontaneously.

B. General Measures: Bladder sedatives are usually of little help if symptoms are severe. Analgesics or narcotics may prove necessary to combat pain. Hot sitz baths may relieve spasm.

Prognosis

The prognosis is excellent.

Moore, T., Parker, C., & E. C. Edwards: Sterile non-tuberculous pyuria. Brit J Urol 43:47-51, 1971.
Numazaki, Y., & others: Acute hemorrhagic cystitis in children. Isolation of adenovirus type 2. New England J Med 278:700-4, 1968.

CANDIDIASIS

Candida (Monilia) albicans is a yeast-like fungus that is a normal inhabitant of the respiratory and gastrointestinal tracts and the vagina. The intensive use of potent modern antibiotics is apt to disturb the normal balance between normal and abnormal organisms, thus allowing fungi such as candida to overwhelm an otherwise healthy organ. The bladder and, to a lesser extent, the kidneys have proved vulnerable; candidemia has been observed.

The patient may present with vesical irritability or symptoms and signs of pyelonephritis. Fungus balls may be passed spontaneously. The diagnosis is made by observing mycelial or yeast forms of the fungus microscopically in a properly collected urine specimen. The diagnosis may be confirmed by culture. Excretory urograms may show calyceal defects and ureteral obstruction (fungus masses).

Vesical candidiasis usually responds to alkalinization of the urine with sodium bicarbonate. A urinary pH of 7.5 is desired; the dose is regulated by the patient, who checks the urine with indicator paper. Should this fail, amphotericin B should be instilled via catheter 3 times a day. Dissolve 100 mg of the drug in 500 ml of 5% dextrose solution.

If there is renal involvement, irrigations of the renal pelvis with a similar concentration of amphotericin B is efficacious. In the presence of systemic manifestations or candidemia, intravenous amphotericin B is indicated though it is quite toxic. Give 1-5 mg/day in divided doses in 5% dextrose. The concentration of the solution should be 0.1 mg/ml.

Clark, R.E., Minagi, H., & A.J. Palubinskas: Renal candidiasis. Radiology **101**: 567-72, 1971.

Harbach, L.B., Burkholder, G.V., & W.E. Goodwin. Renal candidiasis. Brit J Urol **42**:258-64, 1970.

Schönebeck, J., & B. Winblad: Primary renal candida infection. Scandinav J Urol Nephrol **5**:281-4, 1971.

Tennant, F.S., Remmers, A.R., Jr., & J.E. Perry: Primary renal candidiasis. Arch Int Med **122**:435-40, 1968.

Williams, R.J., Chandler, J.G., & M.J. Orloff: Candida septicemia. Arch Surg **103**:8-11, 1971.

ACTINOMYCOSIS

Actinomycosis is a chronic granulomatous disease in which fibrosis tends to become marked and spontaneous fistulas are the rule. On rare occasions the disease involves the kidney, bladder, or testis by hematogenous invasion from a primary site of infection. The skin of the penis or scrotum may become involved through a local abrasion. The bladder may also become diseased by direct extension from the appendix, bowel, or fallopian tube.

Etiology
Actinomyces israelii (A bovis).

Clinical Findings
There is nothing specifically pathognomonic about the symptoms or signs in actinomycosis. The microscopic demonstration of the organisms, which are visible as yellow bodies called "sulfur granules," makes the diagnosis. If persistently sought for, these may be found in the discharge from sinuses or in the urine. Definitive diagnosis is established by culture.

Urographically, the lesion in the kidney may resemble tuberculosis (eroded calyces) or tumor (space-occupying lesion).

Treatment
Penicillin is the drug of choice. The dosage is 1-6 million units a day for 3 months. The sulfonamides and tetracyclines also appear to be helpful. Surgical removal of the infected organ is usually indicated.

Prognosis
Removal of the involved organ (eg, kidney or testis) may be promptly curative. Drainage of a granulomatous abscess may cause the development of a chronic draining sinus. Chemotherapy is helpful.

Anhalt, M., & R. Scott, Jr.: Primary unilateral actinomycosis: Case report. J Urol **103**:126-9, 1970.

Grobert, M.J., & A.J. Bischoff: Actinomycosis of the testicle: Case report. J Urol **87**:567-72, 1962.

McPartland, N., Grove, J.S., & B. Chomet: Actinomycosis of penis. J Urol **86**:95-7, 1961.

PARASITIC INFECTIONS OF THE GENITOURINARY TRACT

TRICHOMONIASIS IN THE MALE

Etiology
Trichomonas vaginalis is the most common cause of vaginitis; about 15% of women harbor the organism. It is found not infrequently in the urethra and prostate in men and in the bladder in both sexes. It is transmitted to men by sexual intercourse. The sexual partners of all women with trichomoniasis should be examined for trichomonads.

Clinical Findings
A. Symptoms and Signs: Men harboring the organism may suffer from some degree of

urethral itching and discharge which may be thin or purulent, scanty or profuse; at times there is frequency and burning on urination. There are usually, however, no symptoms at all.

B. Laboratory Findings:

1. Urethral discharge, wet preparation - The discharge should be mixed immediately with 1-2 ml of saline or Trichomonas® solution and studied microscopically. In about 10% of those whose wives harbor the protozoon, motile trichomonads (about the size of pus cells) are seen. A dried smear should be stained with methylene blue to study the bacterial flora as well, since secondary infection with pyogenic bacteria is common.

2. Urethral scrapings will reveal the organisms microscopically in 75% of cases. Dark-field examination may prove helpful.

3. Urine, wet preparation - The sediment of a centrifuged specimen of urine should be studied for the motile organisms. This is successful in 25% of patients.

4. Prostatic secretion - Motile trichomonads may be discovered in the secretion obtained by prostatic massage.

5. Culture of semen, prostatic secretion, or urethral discharge - If the wet preparations are negative, a suitable culture medium should be inoculated, incubated for 48 hours at 37° C, and examined microscopically. With this technic, 90% of men whose wives are infested by Trichomonas vaginalis will have a positive culture.

Treatment

Once the diagnosis has been made, a condom should be used during intercourse until treatment has been successful.

A. Systemic: Metronidazole (Flagyl®), 400 mg twice a day, should be administered by mouth for 7 days. It is curative in 90% of cases in both men and women. Similar results can be obtained with nitrimidazine, 250 mg twice a day for 6 days.

B. Local (if chemotherapy fails):
1. For urethritis -
a. Silver nitrate, 1:8000, urethral irrigations daily for 1-3 weeks, depending upon response.
b. Strong silver proteinate (Protargol®), 0.5%, 8 ml, urethral instillations twice a day for 2 weeks. The solution should be retained for 5 minutes.
c. If secondary nonspecific infection is present, antibiotics are indicated.
2. For prostatitis - Prostatic massage every 7-10 days; the organisms usually disappear promptly from the secretion.

3. For cystitis - If the urethroprostatitis responds to treatment, the trichomonad cystitis usually clears spontaneously. If it does not, daily urethrovesical irrigations with silver nitrate, 1:8000, should be given for 10 days.

Prognosis

Most trichomonad infections respond promptly to metronidazole or nitrimidazine. Vigorous treatment of the man's sexual partner is imperative.

Cohen, L.: Nitrimidazine in the treatment of trichomonas vaginalis vaginitis. Brit J Ven Dis **47**:177-8, 1971.
Keighley, E. E.: Trichomoniasis in a closed community: Efficacy of metronidazole. Brit MJ **1**:207-9, 1971.
Lumsden, W. H. R., Robertson, D. H. H., & G. J. C. McNeillage: Isolation, cultivation, low temperature preservation, and infectivity titration of trichomonas vaginalis. Brit J Ven Dis **42**:145-54, 1966.
McClean, A. N.: Treatment of trichomoniasis in the female with a 5-day course of metronidazole (Flagyl). Brit J Ven Dis **47**:36-7, 1970.
Moffett, M., & others: Nitrimidazine in the treatment of trichomoniasis. Brit J Ven Dis **47**:173-6, 1971.
Weston, T. E. T., & C. S. Nicol: Natural history of trichomonal infection in males. Brit J Ven Dis **39**:251-7, 1964.

SCHISTOSOMIASIS
(Bilharziasis)

Schistosoma haematobium, a blood fluke, invades primarily the bladder. Schistosomiasis is endemic and very common in most of Africa and in Madagascar, Southern Portugal, Greece, and the Near and Middle East. In some areas 25-50% of the population are affected. Its manifestations are severe in Egypt but mild in central Africa.

Etiology

The adult female S haematobium is a threadlike white worm. The male is about 1 cm and the female 2 cm long. They lodge in the venous plexus of the bladder wall, where the female lays myriads of eggs which occlude the smaller vessels. The eggs are extruded into the bladder and voided with the urine. These eggs are oval and possess a terminal spine. If they are passed into warm fresh water, they hatch and the larvae (miracidia) are freed. If within a few hours they enter a

particular fresh-water snail, they reach the
sporozoite stage, multiplying rapidly and
emerging from their host as cercariae (fork-
tailed larvae).

If these cercariae find a human host, they
penetrate the skin and enter the vascular system. Only those reaching the portal vein sur-
vive. In the liver the larvae develop into the
adult stage. They then migrate against the
blood stream to the veins of the bladder, and
mate. The female lays eggs, and the cycle is
repeated. The adult flukes live for many years;
untreated, the disease is progressive.

Pathogenesis and Pathology

The eggs with their terminal spines penetrate the wall of the vein with the assistance of
muscular contraction. This allows the eggs to
be extruded into the vesical cavity. Healing is
by scar formation and the bladder gradually
becomes thickened and contracted. The appearance of calcification of the bladder wall is
caused by calcium deposition in the shells of
the ova. The intramural portions of the ureters may become stenotic, with consequent
hydronephrosis. Ureteral reflux is common.
With the advent of secondary infection, peri-
cystitis may occur. Ulcerations and papillomatous lesions develop on the vesical mucosa. The incidence of bulky squamous cell
carcinomas in patients suffering from schistosomiasis is very high.

The major lesion is in the trigonal area.
Mucosal congestion and edema is at first the
only finding, but, as the eggs approach the
mucosa, "tubercles" are noted which are
quite similar to the lesion of tuberculosis.
The small yellow nodule represents the egg
and the specific cellular reaction around it.
The egg is surrounded by a zone of hyperemia.
Larger nodular and polypoid masses develop
later and then break down and ulcerate. At
this stage the eggs are easily found in the
urine. In the later stages, fibrosis may be
extreme.

Microscopic examination of the bladder
wall reveals many eggs surrounded by neutrophils, eosinophils, and foreign body giant cells.
Calcified eggs are seen in the submucosa and
muscle layer. Later, fibroplastic proliferation dominates the picture.

Clinical Findings

A. Symptoms: Intense itching may be
present when the parasites are invading the
skin. Generalized symptoms develop in about
1-3 months, when the adult flukes begin to lay
eggs. The patient may develop headache,
backache, chills, fever, and profuse sweats.

Symptoms of cystitis appear when the
bladder wall has become involved. Terminal
hematuria is common. If untreated, the bladder symptoms gradually increase in severity.
As ulcerations develop, these symptoms may
be extreme. Secondary infection exacerbates
the symptoms. Calcific incrustation and even
stones may form. Markedly contracted bladders are sometimes seen. Renal pain may be
experienced as ureteral stenosis or reflux
leads to hydronephrosis. Death may occur as
a result of uremia or general sepsis.

B. Signs: In the early stages the physical
examination is noncontributory. Later, urethral stricture and perineal fistulas may be
found. A mass in the flank may be discovered
if hydronephrosis is present. Rectal examination may reveal fibrosis of the prostate and
base of the bladder. Elephantiasis of the external genitalia may occur as a result of
lymphatic obstruction, but this is rare.

C. Laboratory Findings: During the egg-
laying stage, leukocytosis is present; eosinophils often outnumber neutrophils. Anemia
may be due to blood destruction by the flukes
or may be secondary to nonspecific infection
or uremia. The urine contains pus, red blood
cells, and the eggs of S haematobium. These
findings establish the diagnosis. Nonspecific
pyogenic organisms may also be found. Renal
function may be impaired in the presence of
ureteral stenosis or vesicoureteral reflux.

D. X-ray Findings: Calcifications in the
bladder wall or lower ureters may be demonstrated on a plain film of the abdomen. Excretory urograms may show hydroureters and
hydronephroses due to vesicoureteral reflux
or stenosis. Cystograms may demonstrate
a contracted bladder, vesical tumor, or reflux.

E. Instrumental Examination: Urethral
strictures may be discovered on attempting
the passage of a catheter or other instrument.
Cystoscopy may show varying stages of the
disease: tubercle formation, nodulation with
tubercle formation, widespread ulceration,
papillomatous reaction, carcinoma, vesical
stones or calcium deposits, and evidence of
severe fibrosis and contracture of the bladder
wall. Biopsy of the lesions will show the eggs.

Differential Diagnosis

Nonspecific cystitis may be differentiated
from schistosomiasis in the early stages since,
although no bacteria will be found on a stained
smear, eggs will probably be discovered.
Nonspecific cystitis will ordinarily respond to
antibiotics; schistosomiasis will not.

Tuberculosis cystitis may be confused
with schistosomiasis since the history in both
may be the same, neither responds to the usual
antibiotics, and, superficially at least, the

cystoscopic appearance may be similar (tubercles). Careful urinalysis should demonstrate the eggs in one and tubercle bacilli in the other. Excretory urograms may show the typical renal lesion of tuberculosis. Cystoscopic biopsy gives a positive differentiation.

Amicrobic cystitis has a more abrupt onset than schistosomiasis. In neither disease are bacteria found on stained smear unless secondary infection has occurred. In the early stages (hyperemia and edema), cystoscopy may not be helpful, but the changes associated with schistosomiasis later become obvious. Again, the finding of eggs in the urine or on cystoscopic biopsy establishes the diagnosis.

Vesical neoplasm may be differentiated by proper urinalysis (eggs) and cystoscopic biopsy. It must be remembered, however, that the incidence of squamous cell carcinoma is high in schistosomiasis.

Complications

Complications of schistosomiasis may include vesical fibrosis and contracture, bladder neck obstruction, perineal or suprapubic fistulas, vesical calculus, squamous cell carcinoma of the bladder, ureteral obstruction with hydronephrosis, vesicoureteral reflux, secondary infection with perivesical abscess, pyelonephritis, and general sepsis.

Treatment

Treatment is quite satisfactory if the diagnosis is made before complications develop.

A. Specific Measures:
1. Stibophen (Fuadin®) is the drug of choice; it is less toxic than tartar emetic and is given IM rather than IV. The first dose is 1.5 ml; the second, 3.5 ml. Subsequent doses are 5 ml given on alternate days until a total of 75-100 ml have been administered. If relapse should occur (rarely), the course should be repeated.
2. Antimony and potassium tartrate (tartar emetic) is given IV. The total dose is 1.6 gm. The drug can be given on alternate days. The first dose is 60 mg; the second, 90 mg; subsequent doses, 120 mg.
3. Other useful drugs include sodium antimony dimercaptosuccinate (Astiban®), lucanthone hydrochloride (Miracil D®, Nilodin®), and niridazole (Ambilhar®).

B. General Measures: Secondary infection can be combated with the sulfonamides and antibiotics. Supportive treatment may be indicated (eg, transfusions for anemia).

C. Treatment of Complications: If vesical fibrosis is of such a degree that urinary frequency is a problem, colocystoplasty or ileocystoplasty is indicated. Urethral fistulas or strictures will require plastic repair. Vesicoureteral obstruction (or reflux) indicates the need for ureterovesical reimplantation.

Control

Sanitary measures can do a great deal to reduce the incidence of schistosomiasis in endemic areas. Attempts at control have been made by draining ponds and canals, thus decreasing the population of fresh water snails. Little, however, has been accomplished. Chemicals may be added to water to minimize snail infestation. Intensive chemotherapy of infected persons has so far failed to decrease the incidence of the disease.

Prognosis

If the diagnosis is made early (at the time of initial vesical symptoms), medical treatment is almost always curative. Reinfection may occur in endemic areas.

In the later stages of the disease (fibrosis, secondary infection), prognosis is only fair. Specific therapy, even if it eradicates the fluke and kills the eggs, cannot reverse the disabling secondary changes. In many endemic areas schistosomiasis ranks high on the list of fatal diseases.

Al-Ghorab, M.M., El-Badawi, & H. Effat: Vesico-ureteric reflux in urinary bilharziasis. A clinico-radiological study. Clin Radiol 17:41-7, 1966.

Farid, Z., & others: Symptomatic, radiological, and functional improvement following treatment of urinary schistosomiasis. Lancet 2:1110-3, 1967.

Farid, Z., & others: Urinary schistosomiasis treated with sodium antimony tartrate—a quantitative evaluation. Brit MJ 3:713-4, 1968.

Forsyth, D.M., & C. Rashid: Treatment of urinary schistosomiasis. Lancet 1:130-3, 1967.

Ghoneim, M.A., Ashamallah, A., & M.A. Khalik: Bilharzial strictures of the ureter presenting with anuria. Brit J Urol 43: 439-43, 1971.

Lucas, A.O., & others: Radiological changes after medical treatment of vesical schistosomiasis. Lancet 1:631-3, 1966.

Marks, C.: Schistosomiasis and its surgical sequelae. Am J Surg 111:805-12, 1966.

Talib, H.: The problem of carcinoma of bilharzial bladder in Iraq. Brit J Urol 42: 571-9, 1970.

Zaher, M.F., & A.A. El-Deeb: Bilharziasis of the prostate: Its relation to bladder neck obstruction and its management. J Urol 106:257-61, 1971.

FILARIASIS

Filariasis is endemic in the countries bordering the Mediterranean, in South China and Japan, the West Indies, and the South Pacific islands, particularly Samoa. Limited infection, as seen in US soldiers during World War II, gives an entirely different clinical picture than the frequent reinfections usually encountered among the native population.

Etiology

Wuchereria bancrofti is a thread-like nematode about 0.5 cm or more in length which lives in the human lymphatics. The female, in the lymphatics, gives off microfilariae, which are found, particularly at night, in the peripheral blood. The intermediate host (usually a mosquito), biting an infected person, becomes infested with microfilariae which develop into larvae. These are in turn transferred to another human being, in whom they reach maturity. Mating occurs, and microfilariae are again produced.

Pathogenesis and Pathology

The adult nematode in the human host invades and obstructs the lymphatics; this leads to lymphangitis and lymphadenitis. In longstanding cases the lymphatic vessels become thickened and fibrous; there is a marked reticuloendothelial reaction.

Clinical Findings

A. Symptoms: In mild cases (few exposures), the patient suffers recurrent lymphadenitis and lymphangitis with fever and malaise. Not infrequently, inflammation of the epididymis, testis, scrotum, and spermatic cord occurs. These structures then become edematous, boggy, and at times tender. Hydrocele is common. In advanced cases (many exposures), obstruction of major lymph channels may cause chyluria and elephantiasis.

B. Signs: Varying degrees of painless elephantiasis of the scrotum and extremities develop as obstruction to lymphatics progresses.

C. Laboratory Findings: Chylous urine may look normal if minimal amounts of fat are present, but, in an advanced case or following a fatty meal, it is milky. In the presence of chyluria, large amounts of protein are to be expected. Hypoproteinemia is found, and the albumin/globulin ratio is reversed. Both white and red cells are found. The fat will be dissolved by chloroform; the urine will therefore become clear.

Marked eosinophilia is the rule in the early stages. Microfilariae may be demonstrated in the blood, which should preferably be drawn at night. The adult worm may be found by biopsy. Skin and complement fixation tests are highly successful in diagnosis.

D. X-ray Findings: Retrograde urography and lymphangiography may reveal the renolymphatic connections in patients with chyluria.

Treatment

A. Specific Measures: Diethylcarbamazine (Hetrazan®) is the drug of choice. The dose is 3 mg/kg orally 3 times daily for 21 days. This drug kills the microfilariae but not the adult worms. Several courses of the drug may be necessary.

B. General Measures: Prompt removal of recently infected patients from the endemic area almost always results in regression of the symptoms and signs in early cases.

C. Surgical Measures: Elephantiasis of the scrotum may require surgical excision.

D. Treatment of Chyluria: Mild cases require no therapy. If nutrition is impaired, the lymphatic channels may be sealed off by irrigating the renal pelvis with 2% silver nitrate solution. Should this fail, renal decapsulation and resection of the renal lymphatics should be performed.

Prophylaxis

In endemic areas, mosquito abatement programs must be intensively pursued.

Prognosis

If exposure has been limited, resolution of the disease is spontaneous and the prognosis is excellent. Frequent reinfection may lead to elephantiasis of the scrotum or chyluria.

Akisada, M., & S. Tani: Filarial chyluria in Japan. Lymphangiography, etiology and treatment in 30 cases. Radiology 90:311-7, 1968.

Cahill, K.M.: Filarial chyluria: A biochemical and radiologic study of five patients. J Trop Med 68:27-31, 1965.

Campbell, B.L., Wilson, J.D., & P.J. Scott: Studies of the anatomy, physiology and clinical variability of chyluria. Australian Ann Med 15:336-45, 1966.

Harder, H.I., & D. Watson: Human filariasis. Am J Path 42:333-9, 1964.

Koehler, P.R., & others: Lymphography in chyluria. Am J Roentgen 102:455-65, 1968.

Lloyd-Davies, R.W., Edwards, J.M., & J.B. Kinmonth: Chyluria: A report of five cases with particular reference to lymphography and direct surgery. Brit J Urol 39:560-7, 1967.

ECHINOCOCCOSIS
(Hydatid Disease)

Involvement of the urogenital organs by hydatid disease is relatively rare in the USA. It is common in Australia, New Zealand, South America, Africa, Asia, and Europe, especially where sheep are raised.

Etiology

The adult tapeworm (Echinococcus granulosus) inhabits the intestinal tracts of carnivorous animals, especially dogs. Their eggs pass out with the feces and may be ingested by such animals as sheep, cattle, pigs, and occasionally men. Larvae from these eggs pass through the intestinal wall of the various intermediate hosts and are disseminated throughout the body. In man, the liver is principally involved, but about 3% of infected humans develop echinococcosis of the kidney.

If a cyst of the liver should rupture into the peritoneal cavity, the scolices (tapeworm heads) may directly invade the retrovesical tissues, thus leading to the development of cysts in this area.

Clinical Findings

If renal hydatid disease is closed (not communicating with the pelvis), there may be no symptoms until a mass is found. If communicating, there may be symptoms of cystitis, and renal colic may occur as cysts are passed from the kidney. Eosinophilia is the rule. X-ray films may show calcification in the wall of the cyst (Fig 13-3), and urograms often reveal changes typical of a space-occupying lesion. The finding of scolices and hooklets in the urine is pathognomonic. A positive skin sensitivity test (Casoni) is suggestive. Complement fixation tests are positive in 90% of cases.

Retroperitoneal (perivesical) cysts may cause symptoms of cystitis, or acute urinary retention may develop secondary to pressure. The presence of a suprapubic mass may be the only finding. It may rupture into the bladder and cause hydatiduria, which establishes the diagnosis.

Treatment

Nephrectomy is generally the treatment of choice of renal hydatid disease, although

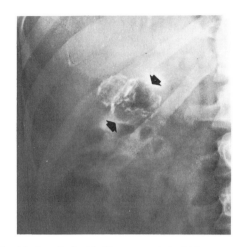

Fig 13-3. Hydatid disease, right kidney.
Plain film showing 2 calcified hydatid cysts.

aspiration and marsupialization have also been recommended. Retroperitoneal cysts are best treated by marsupialization and curettage.

Prognosis

Echinococcosis of the kidney usually has a good prognosis. The problem presented by perivesical cysts is more troublesome. After surgical intervention, drainage may be prolonged. It must be remembered, too, that involvement of other organs, especially the liver, is usually present.

Baltaxe, H. A., & R. J. Fleming: The angiographic appearance of hydatid disease. Radiology **97**:599-604, 1970.

Deliveliotis, A., Kehayas, P., & M. Varkarakis: The diagnostic problem of the hydatid disease of the kidney. J Urol **99**:139-47, 1968.

Henry, J. D., & others: Echinococcal disease of the kidney: Report of case. J Urol **96**: 431-5, 1966.

Kirkland, K.: Urological aspects of hydatid disease. Brit J Urol **38**:241-54, 1966.

Makki, H.: Renal hydatid disease. Brit J Surg **54**:265-9, 1967.

Raffii, P., & W. Dutz: Hydatid cysts of the kidney. J Urol **97**:815-17, 1967.

•   •   •

14...
Urologic Aspects of Venereal Diseases in the Male

GONORRHEA

Gonorrhea is primarily a urethritis. Untreated, it usually is a self-limited disease, the bacteria dying out as a rule within 6 months. Complications, however, can be severe. Infection affords no immunity to subsequent attack.

Antibiotics have diminished the incidence of gonorrhea, but it is still the most common reportable infectious disease in the USA. Fortunately, disabling complications (prostatitis, epididymitis, urethral stricture, endocarditis, and arthritis) are now relatively rare.

Neisseria gonorrhoeae, the specific organism of gonorrhea, is almost without exception transmitted through sexual contact. The organisms are kidney-shaped and arranged as diplococci with their relatively flat surfaces apposed. They are gram-negative and are typically located within the neutrophils, although they are frequently found extracellularly as well. On occasion other pyogenic cocci (staphylococci) are also located intracellularly, but these can usually be differentiated morphologically from gonococci.

The pathologic findings consist mainly of diffuse infiltration of the tissues by neutrophils, lymphocytes, and plasma cells.

Clinical Findings

A. Symptoms: The first symptom of gonorrhea is a purulent urethral discharge, which usually appears 4-10 days after sexual exposure. There is usually some burning on urination, and urethral itching is common. Frequency, urgency, and nocturia do not occur unless the posterior urethra and prostate become involved (rare with antibiotic therapy).

B. Signs: The purulent urethral discharge is yellow or brown. The meatus is red and edematous, and its lips are everted. The urethra may be thickened and tender. The inflammation is mucosal and submucosal.

Prostatic massage and urethral instrumentation are contraindicated during the acute phase of the disease. If severe urinary symptoms are present and urinary obstruction supervenes, palpation of the prostate gland may reveal it to be swollen, hot, and tender (acute prostatitis).

C. Laboratory Findings: The urethral discharge should first be examined, unstained and in saline, for trichomonads. Both Gram's and methylene blue stains should be done in order to establish a bacteriologic diagnosis. If microscopic study reveals the typical intracellular gram-negative diplococci, cultures are not necessary. If discharge is unobtainable, the first part of the urine should be centrifuged and the sediment treated as urethral discharge.

When the infection is limited to the anterior urethra, only the first portion of the urine is cloudy. If posterior urethritis develops, the entire stream becomes purulent. Gonococci are then found in the stained sediment of the midstream specimen.

In equivocal cases, cultures of the purulent discharge are necessary. Because gonococci die rapidly on drying, specimens must be cultured very promptly on special media (chocolate blood agar) in an atmosphere of 10% carbon dioxide.

Differential Diagnosis

Nonspecific and trichomonad urethritis cause the same symptoms as gonorrhea, although the discharge in the latter is usually more purulent and profuse. Study of the discharge, both fresh and stained, demonstrates the etiologic organisms.

Complications

Most complications are local (periurethral) and prostatic. They are rare, but may still occur if the diagnosis is missed or if improper treatment (without antibiotics) is instituted. Periurethritis may develop and may lead to abscess formation; in the healing process, periurethral fibrosis will cause stricture. Posterior urethritis and prostatitis occur if the disease process extends beyond the external sphincter. Symptoms of cystitis may occur at this stage, and all of the urine passed is purulent. The infection may then descend to the epididymis, causing a very painful swelling of that organ.

Gonorrheal arthritis is occasionally observed as a complication of bacteremia, which may be manifested by typical cutaneous lesions. Acute polyarthritis may develop, and monoarticular disease with effusion may be seen. These usually respond promptly with definitive antibiotic therapy. Meningitis and endocarditis are quite rare.

Treatment

The gonococcus is very sensitive to most antibiotics, although there is some evidence that it is becoming increasingly resistant to penicillin. At least 90% of patients respond promptly to the proper drug given in adequate dosage. The discharge usually disappears in 12 hours, and complications seldom develop. In about 10-15% of patients, a scanty, thin discharge will remain following treatment. This usually disappears within a few days, particularly when treated with tetracycline.

Proof of cure rests on the absence of gonococci in whatever discharge remains or in the washings from the urethra (the first portion of the voided urine). If gonococci are absent, culture of the prostatic secretion should then be done. If this is negative for gonococci, cure has been established. If the infective bacteria have not been eradicated by one antibiotic, another drug or combination of drugs should be used. Since syphilis may also have been contracted simultaneously the blood serology must be checked in 3 weeks and then after 3, 6, 12, and 24 months.

A. Specific Measures: Repository penicillin, 2.4-4.8 million units IM, cures over 90% of cases. This effect may be enhanced by giving 2.5 gm of probenecid. Oral penicillins are also effective. A single dose of ampicillin, 3.5 gm orally, plus probenecid, also results in a high cure rate. The tetracyclines also cure 90% of infected persons. It has recently been reported that the gonococci in the Far East are showing increasing resistance to penicillin whereas they are quite sensitive to the tetracyclines. Since we can expect this strain in other parts of the world, the combination of penicillin and a tetracycline seems indicated. A total of 10 gm can be administered in doses of 0.5 gm every 6 hours. Streptomycin, 2 gm IM in divided doses, or kanamycin, 2 gm IM in a single injection, is also effective. Sulfonamides fail to eradicate the disease in about 1/2 of patients since many strains of gonococci are sulfonamide-resistant.

B. General Measures: Response to the antibiotics is so prompt that general measures are not necessary. Sexual intercourse should be avoided until cure has been established.

C. Treatment of Complications: Complications are exceedingly rare. If any of the following develop, more extensive antibiotic therapy is indicated: acute prostatitis, acute epididymitis, periurethral abscess, cystitis, and arthritis. Urethral stricture requires urethral dilatations.

Prevention

A single and almost foolproof method of prophylaxis against gonorrhea is the proper use of antibiotics in the first few hours before or after exposure (does not prevent syphilis): (1) penicillin, 1 million units orally or 300,000 units IM; (2) chlortetracycline, chloramphenicol, oxytetracycline, tetracycline, or erythromycin, 1 gm orally as one dose; or (3) streptomycin, 1 gm IM.

Local prophylaxis (for both syphilis and gonorrhea), although less effective than antibiotic prophylaxis, is often successful if used within 1 hour of exposure. It consists of thorough washing of the genitalia and hands with soap and water, the generous application of 30% mild mercurous chloride (calomel) ointment over the penis, scrotum, and adjacent skin (antisyphilis), and the instillation of 8 ml of 1% strong silver proteinate or 10% mild silver proteinate solution into the urethra (antigonorrhea); this should be held in for 5 minutes. Since local prophylaxis is neither as reliable nor as convenient as antibiotics, it should be reserved for areas where antibiotics are not available for this purpose.

Prognosis

The prognosis is excellent if gonorrhea is diagnosed early and treated properly.

Brewer, G. F., Davis, J. R., & M. Grossman: Gonococcal arthritis in an adolescent girl. Am J Dis Child **122**:253-4, 1971.

Cooke, C. L., & others: Gonococcal arthritis. A survey of 54 cases. JAMA **217**:204-5, 1971.

Ellner, P. D.: Diagnosis of gonococcal infection. Clin Med **78**:16-20, June 1971.

Glaser, S., Boxerbaum, B., & J. H. Kennell: Gonococcal arthritis in the newborn. Am J Dis Child **112**:185-8, 1966.

Holmes, K. K., Counts, G. W., & H. N. Beaty: Disseminated gonococcal infection. Ann Int Med **74**:979-93, 1971.

Kvale, P. A., & others: Single oral dose ampicillin-probenecid treatment of gonorrhea in the male. JAMA **215**:1449-53, 1971.

Schroeter, A. L. , & G. J. Pazin: Gonorrhea.
Ann Int Med **72**:553-9, 1970.

Smithurst, B. A. : Treatment of acute gonorrheal urethritis with three drug regimes.
Brit J Ven Dis **46**:398-400, 1970.

Wheeler, J. K. , Heffron, W. A. , & R. C.
Williams, Jr. : Migratory arthralgias and
cutaneous lesions as confusing initial manifestations of gonorrhea. Am J Med Sc **260**:
150-9, 1970.

THE PRIMARY PENILE LESION
OF SYPHILIS

Syphilis is caused by infection with Treponema pallidum, a distinctive spirochete. It
makes its appearance about 2-4 weeks after
sexual exposure. A painless papule or pustule
develops on the glans, corona, foreskin, shaft,
or even the pubic area or on the scrotum and
breaks down to form an indurated, punched-
out ulcer. The lesion may be so small and
transient that it may be missed.

Microscopically the tissues are heavily
infiltrated with small round cells and plasma
cells. Some proliferation of the intimal linings
of the blood vessels develops. Neutrophils may
be numerous if secondary infection occurs.

Clinical Findings

A. Symptoms and Signs: The patient usually presents himself because of the appearance
of a painless penile sore 2-4 weeks after sexual
contact. The ulcer is relatively deep, has indurated edges, a clean base, and is not painful on pressure. If untreated, spontaneous
healing is slow. Discrete, enlarged inguinal
lymph nodes may be palpable. They are not
tender unless the primary lesion has become
infected by pyogenic organisms, which occurs
very rarely.

B. Laboratory Findings: The diagnosis is
made by finding the pathogenic spirochetes in
the serous discharge from the ulcer on dark
field examination. Serologic tests for syphilis
may remain negative for 1-3 weeks after the
appearance of the chancre.

Differential Diagnosis (See Table 14-1.)

The primary penile lesions of chancroid,
lymphogranuloma venereum, granuloma inguinale, gangrenous and erosive balanitis,
and herpes may resemble the chancre of
syphilis. All penile ulcers must be considered
luetic until proved otherwise. Borrelia vincenti may be present and is most difficult to
distinguish from Treponema pallidum in the
dark field.

Erythroplasia of Queyrat (see p 293) may
resemble a chancre. Dark field examination
and biopsy will clarify the diagnosis.

Complications

Urologic complications of syphilis are
rare. They include gummas of the testis and
neurosyphilis reflected as a neurogenic bladder.

Treatment

Give 2.4 million units of procaine penicillin G with 2% aluminum monostearate into the
buttocks and then 1.2 million units IM every
other day for a total dose of 4.8 million units.
Other satisfactory regimens include (1) benzathine penicillin G, 1.2 million units in each
gluteal muscle, or (2) procaine penicillin G,
600,000 units IM daily for 8 days.

Prevention

Give benzathine penicillin G, 2.4 million
units IM in one dose.

Prognosis

The prognosis is excellent. Relapse is
rare and requires more intensive penicillin
therapy. The blood serology of the patient
should, however, be rechecked every 6 months
for 3 years after treatment. The spinal fluid
should be examined to rule out central nervous
system syphilis, which requires more intensive treatment.

The patient should be cautioned not to have
sexual intercourse until cure has been obtained.

Desmond, F. B. : The diagnosis of infectious
syphilis. New Zealand MJ **73**:135-8, 1971.

Youmans, J. B. : Syphilis and other venereal
diseases. M Clin North America **48**:573-
814, 1964.

CHANCROID
(Soft Chancre)

Chancroid is a common venereal disease
whose primary ulcer may simulate the chancre
of syphilis or lymphogranuloma venereum. It
is usually accompanied by inguinal adenitis.
The highest incidence occurs in men with long
foreskins who practice poor hygiene.

The infecting organism is Hemophilus
ducreyi, a short, nonmotile, gram-negative
streptobacillus which usually occurs in chains.
It is found with difficulty on stained smear;
cultures are more successful. The incubation
period is 3-5 days.

Macroscopically, one or several small
penile ulcers are present. Biopsy of chancroid
shows endothelial proliferation without much

fibroplasia in the midzone; the deeper tissues are diffusely infiltrated with small round cells and plasma cells. These findings are considered to be diagnostic.

Inguinal adenitis, usually unilateral, develops in about 50% of cases. Progression is rapid, although the lesion may resolve spontaneously or go on to suppuration and spontaneous evacuation.

Clinical Findings

A. Symptoms: A few days after sexual exposure, one or more painful, dirty-appearing ulcers may be noted. They enlarge gradually. In 2 or 3 weeks, large, tender inguinal lymph nodes appear. These may suppurate and drain spontaneously. About 50% of patients have fever to 39° C (102.2° F), malaise, and headache.

B. Signs: The ulcer is rarely more than 1-2 cm in diameter. It is usually shallow and has irregular edges. The base is friable and bleeds easily. On occasion it may become very extensive and destructive.

C. Laboratory Findings: Diligent search of a smear stained with Gram's stain shows Hemophilus ducreyi in 50% of cases. Culture, if available, is more successful. Skin tests (Ducrey test) are positive in about 75% of patients. Biopsy is diagnostic in all cases. Tests for other venereal ulcers should be done to establish or rule out the possibility of double infections: (1) dark field examination for spirochetes (syphilis and erosive balanitis), (2) complement fixation or Frei test (lymphogranuloma venereum), (3) search for Donovan bodies (granuloma inguinale), and (4) serologic tests for syphilis.

Differential Diagnosis (See Table 14-1.)

Chancroid must be differentiated from other ulcerative lesions of the external genitalia.

Complications

Secondary infection with spirochetes (Vincent's) and fusiform bacilli may cause marked destruction of tissue, but this is not common. Phimosis or paraphimosis may develop during the healing stage.

Treatment

A. Specific Measures: Even in the bubo stage, response to the tetracyclines is excellent. The optimum dose is 0.5 gm every 6 hours for 7 days. The sulfonamides, 4 gm/day for 10 days, are only slightly less effective. Penicillin is without effect.

B. General Measures: Cleanliness is of the greatest importance. The parts should be washed regularly with bland soap and water. Oils and greases are contraindicated.

C. Treatment of Complications: If the symbiotic infection of fusiform bacilli and spirochetes complicates the picture, penicillin should be used in addition, although the antibiotics which are administered for the chancroidal infection will probably overcome these infections also. If phimosis or paraphimosis develops, surgical correction may be necessary. During the acute stage, only a dorsal slit is indicated. Later, circumcision can be done. Aspiration of fluctuant inguinal nodes may be necessary.

Prevention

Thorough washing of the genitalia with soap and water after sexual intercourse, or any of the antibiotics which are useful in treatment, will prevent the disease.

Prognosis

With proper antibiotic therapy, the prognosis for immediate cure is excellent.

LYMPHOGRANULOMA VENEREUM
(Lymphopathia Venereum)

Lymphogranuloma venereum is an infectious venereal disease caused by a specific, large organism of the psittacosis-LGV-trachoma (Chlamydia) group. The disease is characterized by a transient genital lesion followed by lymphadenitis and at times, in the female, rectal stricture. In men, because of the anatomy of the lymphatics, the inguinal and subinguinal nodes become matted, and, although many resolve, the majority undergo suppuration and form multiple sinuses.

Microscopically the lesion shows acute and subacute inflammation. There is nothing specific or diagnostic in its appearance. The lymph nodes show abscesses and a heavy infiltration of neutrophils. Hyperplasia of lymphoid elements then takes place and plasma cells appear. In the late stages the capsular areas become fibrotic; the centers are necrotic.

Clinical Findings

A. Symptoms and Signs: The penile lesion develops 7-21 days after sexual exposure; it heals spontaneously and rapidly and thus is often not seen. This lesion may be papular or vesicular, although only a superficial erosion may occur. A few days or weeks later, painful enlargement of inguinal nodes develops; because the primary lesion is so often missed, this may be the initial symptom. Later the matted nodes usually break down, whereupon multiple sinuses develop. At the stage of bubo formation, constitutional symptoms are present. These include chills, fever, headache, generalized joint pains, and nausea and vomiting. Skin rashes are frequent.

Rectal stricture is a late manifestation of the disease in females. If present, it can usually be palpated. It tends to be annular in type and may almost close the lumen. When this has developed, a change in bowel habits is evident.

B. Laboratory Findings: The white blood cell count may reach 20,000/μl during the stage of lymph node invasion. Anemia may also develop. The sedimentation rate is accelerated. Serum proteins (globulin) are increased. The Frei test (intradermal) is positive in about two-thirds of those who have or have had the disease. Complement fixation tests, if positive, are almost pathognomonic for present or past lymphogranuloma venereum. These tests cannot differentiate reliably between infection caused by any member of the chlamydia group of organisms. The serologic test for syphilis may give a weak false-positive reaction. This is usually transient, however.

Differential Diagnosis (See Table 14-1.)

All penile ulcers should be regarded as of syphilitic origin until proved otherwise; dark field examinations for T pallidum and serologic studies are essential. Lymphogranuloma venereum must be suspected in any rectal stricture in a female.

Complications

Untreated or late cases may develop multiple sinuses from involved lymph nodes. Elephantiasis of the genitalia can occur if lymphatic drainage is severely obstructed. Occasionally in women (rarely in men), proctitis and rectal stricture may occur. Stricture sometimes becomes manifest years after the initial infection.

Treatment

A. Specific Measures: Chloramphenicol and the tetracyclines are effective even in the stage of bubo formation. The usual dose for each is 0.5-1 gm every 6 hours for a total dose of 15-30 gm. These antibiotics are also reported to be moderately effective in relieving the anorectal stricture. They do not affect the fibrous tissue, however; their value probably lies in controlling viral activity and suppressing secondary infection, thus reducing edema associated with the inflammation.

Sulfonamides, 4 gm/day for 3-4 weeks, although they probably have no effect upon the virus, control secondary bacterial infection.

Streptomycin and penicillin are not effective.

B. Treatment of Complications: Aspiration of fluctuant inguinal nodes is indicated. Draining sinuses may have to be excised. Rectal stenosis may require surgical measures.

Prevention

Washing the genitals with soap and water immediately after sexual exposure is a successful preventive measure. One of the tetracycline group of antibiotics given for 1-2 days immediately after exposure may be a useful means of prophylaxis.

Prognosis

The prognosis is excellent. Only the late complications seen in old cases present difficulties (genital elephantiasis and rectal stricture).

Abrams, A.J.: Lymphogranuloma venereum. JAMA 205:199-202, 1968.
Stewart, D.B.: The gynecologic lesions of lymphogranuloma venereum and granuloma inguinale. M Clin North America 48:773-86, 1964.

GRANULOMA INGUINALE

Granuloma inguinale is a chronic venereal infection of the skin and subcutaneous tissues of the genitalia, perineum, or inguinal regions. The incubation period is 2-3 months.

The infective agent is Donovania granulomatis, a bacterium related to Klebsiella pneumoniae (Friedländer's bacillus). It grows with difficulty on artificial media containing egg yolk, or in the yolk sac of the chick embryo.

The ulcer does not excite a constitutional reaction and does not involve the lymph nodes or lymphatics.

The microscopic picture shows nonspecific infection, with necrosis of the skin and small abscesses. In the deeper portions there is an infiltration of plasma cells, giant cells, neutrophils, and large monocytes; the cytoplasm of the monocytes contains numerous Donovan bodies, the intracellular stage of the etiologic organism.

Clinical Findings

A. Symptoms and Signs: The first sign of the disease is an elevation on the skin of the genitals or adjacent skin (commonly the groin), which finally breaks down. This moderately painful superficial ulcer gradually spreads and can become quite extensive. The base of the ulcer is covered by pink granulation tissue which bleeds easily. There is a more or less purulent discharge, particularly if secondary infection develops.

B. Laboratory Findings: Identification of the Donovan body in large monocytes on a stained smear makes the diagnosis. Scrapings from the base of the lesion are placed on a slide, fixed in air, and stained. Wright's and Giemsa's staining technics are both adequate.

In case of doubt, biopsy may be done. The Donovan bodies take up hematoxylin as well as silver salts.

Complement fixation and skin sensitivity tests are not dependable and not readily available.

Differential Diagnosis

See Table 14-1.

Complications

Secondary infection may cause deep ulceration and tissue destruction. Sinuses may result. Marked phimosis may occur in advanced cases, even to the point of urinary obstruction. Other venereal diseases may be present at the same time.

Treatment

A. Specific Measures: The tetracyclines and chloramphenicol have proved curative in a high percentage of cases. Dosage is 1 gm/day in divided doses for 7-14 days.

Streptomycin is also effective. The dose is 1 gm/day IM for 10 days.

B. Treatment of Complications: Secondary infection is effectively combated in most instances by the drug used to cure the primary disease. If fusiform bacilli and spirochetes (Borrelia vincenti) are present, penicillin may be used also.

Prevention

The use of a condom does not prevent perigenital inoculation. Thorough washing with soap immediately after contact will often prevent infection. The tetracycline antibiotics given for several days following contact may afford protection.

Prognosis

There are no serious complications, and antibiotics are quite efficient in treatment. The prognosis is excellent.

Davis, C.M.: Granuloma inguinale. JAMA 211:632-6, 1970.

Lal, S., & C. Nicholas: Epidemiological and clinical features in 165 cases of granuloma inguinale. Brit J Ven Dis 46:461-3, 1970.

Stewart, D.B.: The gynecologic lesions of lymphogranuloma venereum and granuloma inguinale. M Clin North America 48:773-86, 1964.

EROSIVE AND GANGRENOUS BALANITIS

This is one of the less common penile lesions, presumably of venereal origin. A long foreskin is almost a necessary prerequisite to the development of the lesion since the infecting organisms are anaerobic. Lack of local hygiene also contributes to the establishment of the disease. The lesion ulcerates progressively and proceeds to gangrene of the glans and at times even of the shaft of the penis. The incubation period is 3-7 days.

The infecting organisms are a spirochete (Borrelia vincenti) and a gram-positive bacillus (vibrio) acting in symbiosis. Both organisms are stained by the common dyes.

Microscopic examination of a biopsy shows nothing specific; the picture is one of acute inflammation. Neutrophilic and small round cell infiltration is extensive. The offending organisms are numerous.

Clinical Findings

A. Symptoms: The patient complains of local pain, a profuse, foul discharge, and, if the foreskin can be retracted, a progressive ulcerative lesion of the glans, foreskin, or shaft of the penis. In acute cases, chills, fever, and marked malaise may develop. Burning on urination is common, and is caused by the inflammatory reaction in and about the urinary meatus.

B. Signs: The ulceration usually starts in the region of the corona under a tight, unclean prepuce. The ulcer gradually spreads and produces a foul, often profuse discharge. The accompanying edema may prevent retraction of the foreskin; a dorsal slit may be necessary before the lesion can be observed. As the disease progresses, the invasion of the penile tissue goes deeper, and, if it is not treated by appropriate means, portions of the penis may become gangrenous. In extreme cases the entire penis and even the scrotum may be destroyed.

C. Laboratory Findings: The finding of many spirochetes and fusiform bacilli in a smear is strongly suggestive, but it must be remembered that other ulcerative venereal lesions can be secondarily invaded by these organisms.

Table 14-1. Differential diagnosis of genital ulcers.

	Syphilitic Chancre	Chancroid	Lymphogranuloma Venereum	Granuloma Inguinale	Erosive and Gangrenous Balanitis	Herpes Progenitalis	Epithelioma
Etiology	T pallidum	H ducreyi (Ducrey's bacillus)	Bedsonia bacterium	Donovania granulomatis	Vibrio and spirochete (Bor vincenti)	Virus	-
Incubation time	2-4 weeks	3-10 days	3-21 days	2-3 months	3-7 days	Unknown (often recurrent)	-
Early lesion	Enlarging papule which finally ulcerates.	Macule → papule, then formation of ulcer.	Transient, usually not seen. Papule or macule heals rapidly.	Superficial ulcer of skin.	Single or multiple ulcerations which fuse and spread.	Multiple superficial vesicles on the foreskin or glans.	May appear as small ulcer.
Advanced local lesion	Ulcer becomes deep and edges indurated. Heals spontaneously.	Ulcer gradually spreads. May become extensive. Multiple lesions.	None	Becomes serpiginous and may spread widely.	Ulcers become deep and painful. May spread rapidly. Profuse foul discharge.	Vesicles may coalesce and form superficial ulcer which heals spontaneously.	May become large and destructive.
Local pain	Absent unless secondarily infected.	Very painful.	None	Little	Very painful.	Slight local burning or itching.	None unless secondarily infected.
Involvement of inguinal lymph nodes	Discrete, rubbery, nontender.	In 50% of cases, nodes are enlarged and tender. May suppurate.	In almost all cases in 2-8 weeks after primary sore. Matted, tend to break down. Multiple sinuses.	None	Discrete, only mildly tender.	None	Metases usually unilateral. Painless.
Definitive diagnosis	T pallidum on dark field examination. Serology.	Skin test, stained smear or culture, biopsy.	Frei test, complement fixation test.	Stained organisms in scrapings from ulcer or biopsy.	Spirochetes and fusiform bacilli on dark field examination or stained smear.	Isolation of virus.	Biopsy

Differential Diagnosis

See Table 14-1.

Complications

If the disease is untreated, severe damage may occur to the penis and adjacent structures. If the infection is mild or is aborted by appropriate means, some fibrosis of the foreskin may occur. Contracture of this tissue leads to phimosis.

In elderly men the fulminating form of this disease is to be feared, as overwhelming sepsis is often rapidly fatal.

Treatment

A. Specific Measures: Penicillin is the drug of choice; 600,000-1,200,000 units/day for 5-7 days usually suffices. The tetracyclines are also effective; the dosage is 2 gm/day in divided doses for 5-7 days.

B. General Measures: If response to antibiotics is not prompt, dorsal slit of the prepuce may be indicated for purposes of hygiene and because aerobic conditions discourage the organisms. Mild soap and water or hydrogen peroxide soaks are helpful and will combat the malodorous discharge.

C. Treatment of Complications: Plastic procedures on a badly damaged organ may be necessary. Circumcision is indicated if phimosis develops.

Prevention

Proper hygienic care of the redundant foreskin will prevent the disease, but circumcision is definitive. This is a disease of filth and neglect.

Prognosis

If diagnosed and treated early, the prognosis is excellent. Superficial loss of skin is replaced spontaneously with surprisingly little scar. Neglected patients may, however, suffer severe local tissue destruction.

•　　•　　•

General References

Catterall, R.D.: The advance of the venereal diseases. Lancet 2:103-8, 1963.

King, A., & C. Nicol: Venereal Diseases. Davis, 1964.

15...

Urinary Stones

Urinary lithiasis is one of the most common diseases of the urinary tract. It occurs more frequently in men than in women, but is rare in children and in blacks; a familial predisposition is often encountered.

If a stone is not obstructive, it is not apt to cause injury or symptoms. If it blocks a urinary passage (eg, the ureteropelvic junction), it leads to severe symptoms and renal damage. Since stones tend to recur, a patient with a nonobstructive stone may later form a stone which will cause obstruction; for this reason, investigation of the cause of the first stone is of importance in the prevention of later renal injury.

RENAL STONE

Etiology

All the causes of renal stone formation are not known, but in most cases multiple factors are involved. At least 90% of stones contain calcium (or magnesium) in combination with phosphate or oxalate. The remainder are of organic composition (cystine, uric acid).

The following factors are known to influence the formation of uroliths:

A. Hyperexcretion of Relatively Insoluble Urinary Constituents:

1. Calcium - (Normal urinary excretion of calcium on a low-calcium diet [no milk or cheese for 4 days] is 100-175 mg/24 hours.) The major calcium foods are milk and cheese. Marked hypercalciuria may be seen in the adult who drinks a quart or more of milk per day. It has been shown that the lactose in milk causes increased absorption of calcium from the gut. The amount of calcium contained in hard water has also been said to cause hypercalciuria.

Prolonged immobilization (spinal cord injury, fractures, poliomyelitis) and certain bone diseases (eg, metastatic cancer, myeloma, Paget's disease) cause hypercalciuria.

Under these circumstances calcium excretion may reach 450 mg/day.

Primary hyperparathyroidism causes hypercalciuria and hyperphosphaturia as well as hypercalcemia and hypophosphatemia. Two-thirds of these patients have renal stones.

Idiopathic hypercalciuria is almost exclusively seen in males. Serum calcium is normal, serum phosphorus is decreased. Even on a low-calcium intake these patients may excrete as much as 500 mg in 24 hours. This may reflect increased absorption of calcium from the gut.

Hypervitaminosis D may so increase absorption of calcium from the intestine that urinary excretion of this ion may reach pathologically high levels.

Renal tubular acidosis causes excretion of calcium since the formation of ammonia and titratable acidity are defective.

2. Oxalate - At least 50% of renal stones are composed of calcium oxalate. Cabbage, rhubarb, spinach, tomatoes, celery, and cocoa contain considerable oxalate, but limitation of these foods has little effect in prophylaxis because the major source of oxalate is endogenous.

Hyperoxaluria is a genetic disorder affecting the metabolism of glyoxylic acid, which forms oxalate rather than glycine. It is a rare phenomenon, but it is one of the common causes of nephrolithiasis and nephrocalcinosis in children. It is often lethal.

3. Cystine - Cystinuria is a hereditary disease. It is somewhat uncommon, and only a small percentage of these patients form stones. Other amino acids (ornithine, lysine, and arginine) are also lost simultaneously; however, these are quite soluble and do not form stones. The loss of these amino acids is due to a defect in renal tubular reabsorption.

4. Uric acid - Uric acid stones may form when there is rapid tissue breakdown, ie, in the chemotherapeutic treatment of leukemia, polycythemia, and carcinoma; for this reason it is important to maintain an alkaline urine when treating these diseases. The administration of allopurinol (Zyloprim®) should also

be considered. Uric acid formers have a consistently low urinary pH. This may be caused by decreased tubular formation of ammonia. Most of these patients are Italians or Jews. Elevated serum uric acid is often observed secondary to thiazide diuretic therapy, but this can be controlled by giving probenecid. Many patients with gout form uric acid calculi, particularly when under treatment for their arthritis; most of these patients have elevated blood uric acid levels and increased urinary uric acid excretion. Gout is not a necessary condition for the formation of uric acid stones, however.

5. Silicon dioxide - Long-term use of magnesium trisilicate in the treatment of peptic ulcer may lead to the formation of radiopaque silicon stones.

B. Physical Changes Which Occur in the Urine:

1. Increased concentration of salts and organic compounds - This may be due to low fluid intake; excessive water losses in febrile diseases, in hot climates, or in occupations causing excessive perspiration; or excessive water losses due to vomiting and diarrhea.

2. Urinary magnesium/calcium ratio - This appears to have some influence on stone formation. Acetazolamide (Diamox®) causes a decrease in the ratio and is related to an increased incidence of stone formation. The thiazides, which appear to contribute to the prevention of recurrence of stone, cause an increase in the ratio.

3. Urinary pH - The mean urinary pH is 5.85. It is influenced by diet and is altered by ingestion of acid or alkaline medication (eg, treatment of peptic ulcer) and carbonic anhydrase inhibitors (ie, acetazolamide) used in the treatment of glaucoma. The latter cause an increase in urinary pH. Urea-splitting bacteria (by liberating ammonia) make the urine strongly alkaline (pH 7.5+). The inorganic salts are less soluble in an alkaline medium (calcium phosphate forms at a pH of 6.6+ and magnesium ammonium phosphate precipitates at pH of 7.2+). Organic substances (eg, cystine, uric acid) are least soluble at a pH below 7.0 (maximum insolubility, pH 5.5).

4. Colloid content - It has long been claimed that the colloids in the urine allow the inorganic salts to be held in a supersaturated state. Recent work has tended to negate this theory.

5. "Good" and "evil" urine - Howard finds that some types of urine promote while others prevent stone formation. When rachitic rat cartilage is placed in "good" urine, calcification does not occur. In "evil" urine the cartilage becomes calcified. "Evil" urine, however, becomes "good" urine on the ad-

ministration of 3-6 gm/day of phosphate. The use of aluminum hydroxide gels which absorb phosphate in the gut is therefore probably contraindicated if an attempt is being made to prevent calcium stone formation.

C. A Nidus (Core or "Nucleus") Upon Which Precipitation Occurs: Randall observed that calcific plaques ("Randall's plaques") are commonly seen on the renal papillae. He believed they develop as a result of injury to cells of the collecting tubule secondary to infection elsewhere. Randall postulated that when the overlying mucosa finally ulcerates, the calcification acts as a nidus to which the insoluble substances in the urine can adhere. Vermeulen has recently verified this observation.

Garvey and Boyce have shown that most stones develop by precipitation of crystals (ie, calcium oxalate, etc) on an organic matrix formed of amino acids and carbohydrates. Other masses that can act as nidi include blood clots, clumps of epithelial or pus cells, or even bacteria.

Necrotic ischemic tissue and foreign bodies may encourage the precipitation of relatively insoluble substances. Tissues of this sort may be caused by neoplasms, retained necrotic papillae, or ulceration of mucous membranes by infection.

D. Medullary Sponge Kidney: This disorder may be complicated by stones which form secondary to stasis or infection of urine in the dilated collecting tubules.

Pathology

The size and position of the stone govern the development of secondary pathologic changes in the urinary tract. The obstruction caused by a small stone lodged in the ureteropelvic junction or in the ureter may slowly destroy a kidney (Fig 10-4), whereas a relatively large stone may be so placed as to cause little renal damage.

Infection is a common complication of an obstructing renal stone because of the stasis which it causes. The very presence of such a foreign body seems to decrease the local resistance to hematogenous infection. The parenchymal ischemia caused by local pressure from an enlarging staghorn stone may progressively damage a kidney.

The Physical Characteristics of Urinary Calculi (See Fig 15-1.)

(1) Calcium phosphate stones (often mixed with magnesium ammonium phosphate) may be soft or hard; they are usually yellow or brown (sometimes dark), often form staghorn masses, and are frequently laminated. They are read-

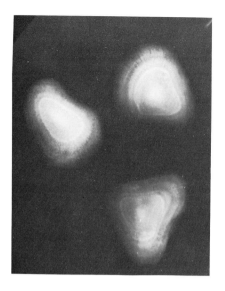
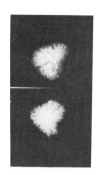
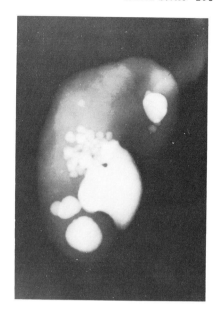

Fig 15-1. **X-ray appearance of stones.** **Left:** Calcium phosphate, laminated. **Center:** Calcium oxalate, spiculated. **Right:** Cystine, homogeneous. (Reproduced, with permission, from Albright & Reifenstein: Parathyroid Glands and Metabolic Bone Disease. Williams & Wilkins, 1948.)

ily seen on x-ray films; the lamination, if present, is clearly visible.

(2) Magnesium ammonium phosphate stones are usually yellow and somewhat friable. Staghorn formation is common. On radiograms their density lies between that of calcium oxalate and cystine. Lamination may be noted if calcium oxalate or phosphate is also present.

(3) Calcium oxalate stones ("jackstones," "mulberry stones") are usually small, rough, and hard. Staghorn formation is rare. Spicules radiating from a central core can often been seen on x-rays.

(4) Cystine stones are smooth and light yellow or yellow-brown. They have a "waxy" appearance, and are usually multiple and bilateral. They may enlarge quite rapidly, sometimes coalescing to form staghorn calculi. Although their density is relatively low, they can be identified on a roentgenogram as homo-

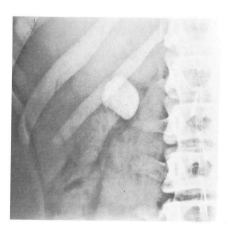
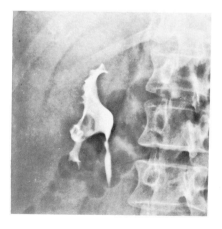

Fig 15-2. **Cystine and uric acid stones.** **Left:** Plain film showing homogeneous, mildly opaque stone, typically cystine. **Right:** Excretory urogram showing uric acid stone as "negative" shadow because radiopaque medium is more dense than the stone.

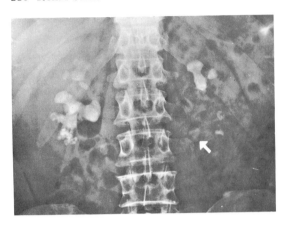 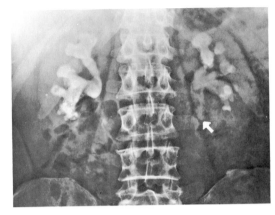

Fig 15-3. **Bilateral staghorn calculi and left upper ureteral stone.** **Left:** Plain film. Arrow points to ureteral stone. **Right:** Excretory urogram showing bilateral impaired function.

geneous, slightly opaque, smoothly rounded bodies (Fig 15-2). On occasion they contain some calcium salts, in which case the stone may show some lamination.

(5) Uric acid crystals can precipitate in the renal parenchyma. The stones formed from these crystals in the renal pelvis are usually small and hard, varying in color from yellow to reddish-brown. They may be multiple. If they are composed of pure uric acid crystals, they cannot be seen on plain x-ray films. On excretory urograms they are present as "negative" shadows (Fig 15-2).

Radiopacity

Radiopacity is directly related to the density of the stone compared to that of water:

	Density	Degree of Radiopacity
Calcium phosphate	22.0	Very opaque
Calcium oxalate	10.8	Opaque
Magnesium ammonium phosphate	4.1	Moderately opaque
Cystine	3.7	Slightly opaque
Uric acid	1.4	Nonopaque

Clinical Findings

A. Symptoms: The history should include a survey of fluid intake, diet (amount of milk, cheese), drugs (alkalies, analgesics, acetazolamide, vitamin D), periods of immobilization, previous passage of stones, and the presence of gout. There may be a family history of stone formation due to hereditary hyperoxaluria, cystinuria, hyperuricemia, or renal acidosis.

If the stone is still submucosal (Randall's plaque) or adherent to the parenchyma, there are no symptoms. The same is usually true of a small stone trapped in a minor calyx.

If the stone is free and obstructs a calyx or the ureteropelvic junction, there will be dull flank pain from parenchymal and capsular distention, colic from hyperperistalsis and smooth muscle spasm of calyces and pelvis; total hematuria; nausea, vomiting, and abdominal distention from paralytic ileus. Chills, high fever, and vesical irritability are due to infection.

Staghorn calculus may be asymptomatic even if infection is present. Symptoms which occur are most apt to be gastrointestinal and simulate gallbladder disease, peptic ulcer, or less specific enteric syndromes. Urologic symptoms may include mild back or flank pain, hematuria, and those due to infection (chills, fever, increased renal pain, and symptoms of cystitis).

B. Signs: Tenderness in the costovertebral angle or over the kidney may or may not be present. Acute renal infection may cause more definite findings. If marked hydronephrotic atrophy has occurred as a result of prolonged ureteral obstruction, a mass in the flank may be seen, felt, or percussed. Some muscle rigidity over the kidney may be found, and rebound tenderness may be elicited, particularly if acute infection is present. Abdominal distention and diminished peristalsis usually accompany acute renal colic.

C. Laboratory Findings:

1. Blood count - The white blood count may be increased as a result of pain or complicating infection. If renal function is not adequate, anemia may be found.

2. Urinalysis - Protein may be noted because of the presence of red blood cells. Pus cells and bacteria may be seen. Oxalate bodies are often observed in hyperparathy-

roidism, renal tubular acidosis, and hyper-oxaluria. Calcium phosphate casts suggest hypercalciuria.

If the pH of the urine is higher than 7.6, urea-splitting organisms must be present, for the kidneys cannot produce urine in this range of alkalinity. Such a finding strongly suggests that the stones are composed of magnesium ammonium phosphate. Fixation of the pH at 6.5 is compatible with renal tubular acidosis. Consistently low pH is a common cause of the formation of uric acid calculi.

A search should be made for crystals in the sediment; the type may afford a clue to the type of stone (Fig 5-1). Cystine and uric acid crystals may be precipitated by adding a few drops of glacial acetic acid (which lowers the pH to about 4.0) to a test tube of urine which is then refrigerated. Cystine crystals resemble benzene rings; uric acid crystals are typically amber-brown in color.

A simple chemical screening test for cys-tine: To 5 ml of urine made alkaline with am-monium hydroxide, add 2 ml of 5% sodium cyanide and let stand for 5 minutes. Add a few drops of fresh 5% sodium nitroprusside. A deep purplish-red color means hypercys-tinuria. The definitive diagnosis and proper treatment rest upon quantitative estimation of the amount of alpha-aminonitrogen and of cystine (and cysteine) excreted in 24 hours. Normal people excrete about 1 mg/lb (up to 150 mg/24 hours) of alpha-aminonitrogen and 50-180 mg of cystine (and cysteine) in a like period. Mild cystinurics excrete 200-400 mg of cystine (and cysteine); moderate cystinurics excrete 400-1000 mg, whereas those with a severe tubular defect may excrete up to 3600 mg/day.

The Sulkowitch test should be done, in conjunction with specific gravity determination, on all patients with urinary stone. If strongly positive (especially if the urine is dilute), hypercalciuria is present. A positive test should be repeated after milk and cheese have been withdrawn for 4 days. If the test is still strongly positive, blood chemistry studies should be done (see below) since hyperpara-thyroidism may be the cause.

After 4 days on a diet free of milk and cheese, the amount of calcium excreted in the urine in 24 hours should be determined. More than 175 mg calcium/24 hours suggests hyper-parathyroidism or idiopathic hypercalciuria unless some obvious cause for calcium excess is found (eg, immobilization). The finding of hyperphosphaturia is compatible with a renal phosphate leak and strongly suggests hyper-parathyroidism when hypercalcemia and hyper-calciuria are found.

A 24-hour urine specimen should be sub-jected to a quantitative test for oxalate. The upper limit of normal is 50 mg. Levels as high as 200-300 mg/24 hours may be encoun-tered. There may be so much oxalate in the urine that all calcium may be precipitated by it, thus causing a negative Sulkowitch test. The normal uric acid excretion is 300-600 mg/24 hours.

Test for presence of urea-splitting bac-teria: Incubate noninfected acid urine with a few drops of the infected urine overnight. If pH increases, urea-splitting organisms are present.

3. Renal function tests - The PSP may be normal even in the presence of bilateral stag-horn stones or in chronic unilateral obstruc-tion due to stone. Acute obstruction at the ureteropelvic junction may suddenly depress the PSP to 2/3 of normal. The complication of renal infection may also interfere with renal function.

NPN, blood creatinine, or urea nitrogen determination is indicated if the PSP is less than 30% in one-half hour. Unless the patient is dehydrated, elevation of any one of these indicates decreased renal function.

4. Blood chemistry studies - Fasting se-rum calcium and phosphorus should be deter-mined on 3 occasions. Serum proteins should also be estimated, since almost half of the calcium is normally un-ionized and bound to protein. If serum proteins are decreased but total calcium is normal, an increase in ionized calcium is indicated. (See Fig 15-4, left.) Hypercalcemia with hypophosphatemia strongly suggests primary hyperparathyroidism, but normal serum phosphate is found in 60% of these patients. Estimation of serum chloride concentration may prove helpful in the differ-ential diagnosis of hypercalcemia. It is above 102 mEq/liter in hyperparathyroidism and be-low this figure in other conditions (eg, cancer of the breast).

Hypercalcemia is most commonly seen in association with osteolytic or disseminated malignant disease, especially cancers of the breast and lung, multiple myeloma, leukemia, and sarcoidosis.

Determination of the tubular reabsorption of phosphate (TRP) may prove helpful in the diagnosis of hyperparathyroidism when mini-mum hypercalcemia and normal blood phosphate levels are obtained. The normal range of tubular reabsorption of phosphate is about 90-95% with low phosphate intake and 85% with high phosphate intake. In hyperparathyroidism the values range from 40-80%, demonstrating the typical phosphate leak.

Serum alkaline phosphatase (normal is 2-4.5 Bodansky units) is increased in hyper-parathyroidism only if bone disease (eg, oste-itis fibrosa cystica) is present.

Elevated serum uric acid (normal is 2-6 mg/100 ml) is found in 50% of uric acid stone formers.

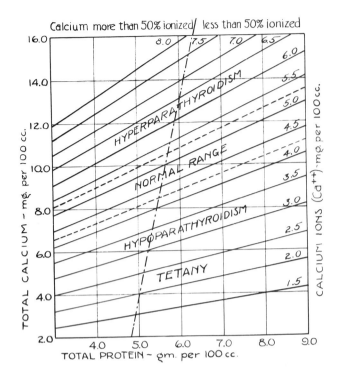

Calcium more than 50% ionized / less than 50% ionized

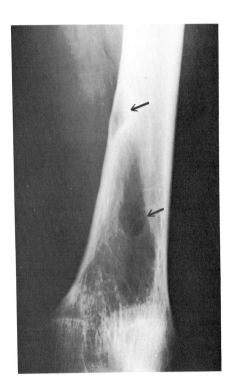

Fig 15-4. Left: Nomogram showing relation of calcium level to total proteins. (Reproduced, with permission, from McLean & Hastings: Am J Med Sc **189:**601, 1935.) **Right:** Osteitis fibrosa cystica with hyperparathyroidism. Note cystic changes in femur (arrows).

If CO_2 combining power of the plasma or serum is decreased, acidosis is present. Such a finding might be the clue to the cause of hypercalciuria and stone formation, because when renal tubular damage is advanced, calcium is excreted as fixed base rather than sodium and ammonium. Low CO_2 combining power in the presence of high serum chloride is compatible with renal tubular acidosis or severe chronic renal insufficiency. Electrophoretic analysis of the serum will point to sarcoidosis or myeloma as the cause of hypercalcemia.

D. X-Ray Findings: At least 90% of renal stones are radiopaque and are readily visible on a plain film of the abdomen unless they are small or overlie bone. It is necessary to differentiate renal stone from calcified mesenteric lymph nodes, calcium in rib cartilage, gallstones, and solid medication (pills) present in the intestinal tract. Because the plain film is two-dimensional, it has only presumptive value except in the case of a staghorn stone, which is never confused with other findings (Fig 15-3).

The morphology of the stone may give a clue to its chemical nature (Fig 15-1).

Bone disease may be discovered in the ribs, spine, pelvis, or femoral heads. This may afford a clue to the etiology of hypercalciuria (eg, hyperparathyroidism, metastatic carcinoma, Paget's disease). X-rays of the long bones and skull may also show changes typical of these disorders (Fig 15-4, right). Early signs of hyperparathyroidism are cortical resorption in the phalanges and absence of the lamina dura of the teeth.

Excretory urograms are necessary because they accurately localize the calcific shadow unless the kidney is without function or unless it is acutely blocked by a stone (Fig 15-3). Oblique views may also be helpful. If a urogram is not obtained but the kidney shadow becomes dense (nephrogram, Fig 15-8), acute obstruction of a good kidney has probably occurred. If the stone is nonopaque, the films will demonstrate obstruction (dilatation), and the stone may appear as a darker area ("negative" shadow) in the renal pelvis (Fig 15-2). Excretory urograms also measure renal function, which is helpful in judging definitive treatment.

If function is poor, retrograde urograms may be needed.

E. Renal Scan: If the excretory urograms imply poor renal function, isotope studies may prove helpful in further assessing this factor (see chapter 8). If the damage is irreversible, the ^{203}Hg scan will show little uptake by the tubules while the scintillations afforded by ^{131}I will be minimal. ^{99m}Tc will reveal poor vascularity. Such findings might indicate the need for nephrectomy rather than nephrolithotomy.

F. Instrumental Examination: Cystoscopy for diagnostic purposes is seldom necessary if the excretory urograms are satisfactory. Ureteral catheterization may prove helpful in localizing infection and measuring renal function. Such studies in conjunction with retrograde urograms may be the deciding factor in the choice of treatment (pyelolithotomy vs nephrectomy).

G. Examination of Stone: Examination of previously passed stones and chemical examination of stones removed or passed is useful in establishing the etiology of stone formation, especially in differentiating "primary" (metabolic) stones from "secondary" stones (eg, stones formed due to infection).

Differential Diagnosis

Acute pyelonephritis may start with acute and severe renal pain, thus mimicking a renal stone lodged at the ureteropelvic junction. Pus and bacteria are found in the urine, although it must be remembered that infection may be a complication of renal stone. Urograms will decide the issue. Chronic infection may be associated with little or no back pain and few if any vesical symptoms. Urinalysis and radiographic study will settle the diagnosis.

Renal tumor may sometimes simulate stone, particularly if a blood clot causes obstruction (pain, hematuria). Urography will establish the diagnosis.

Tumor of the renal pelvis or calyx can cause renal colic and hematuria. The urogram, showing a space-occupying lesion, may be confused with a nonopaque stone (Figs 15-2 and 17-7). Urinary cytology is helpful in differential diagnosis, but at times the diagnosis is made at the operating table.

Renal tuberculosis may be painful and, if associated with bleeding, may mimic renal stone. A plain abdominal x-ray may show calcium deposits in the renal shadow. Stone complicates tuberculosis in 10% of cases. A "sterile" pyuria and a suspicion of tuberculosis on urography suggests the diagnosis. Demonstration of acid-fast bacilli is diagnostic.

Papillary necrosis may be confused with renal stone because if sloughed papillae are not passed they tend to undergo peripheral calcification, thus giving the radiographic appearance of uric acid stone containing an outer shell of calcium. The history, diminished renal function, pyuria, and the typical radiographic appearance of papillitis should make the diagnosis (Fig 12-4).

Infarction of the kidney, commonly secondary to a cardiac lesion, usually occurs without pain or gross hematuria; if the infarction is massive, however, renal pain and microscopic or even gross hematuria may be produced. Evidence of a cardiac lesion (eg, subacute bacterial endocarditis, atrial fibrillation) should suggest the possibility of infarction.

Complications

The presence of a stone lowers resistance to bacterial invasion. This is particularly true if the stone is obstructive. Calculi complicated by infection may cause pyonephrosis and ultimate complete destruction of the kidney, which becomes a cavity containing stones and purulent material only.

Obstruction of the ureter at the ureteropelvic junction leads to hydronephrosis. If this progresses, the parenchyma of the kidney is ultimately destroyed. Obstruction of a calyx causes hydrocalycosis and focal renal damage. Complicating infection contributes to further injury.

Gradual enlargement of a stone in the renal pelvis exerts pressure upon the parenchyma, leading to ischemia and necrosis.

The rare epidermoid carcinoma of the renal pelvis is almost always associated with an infected kidney containing a stone.

Treatment

A. Conservative Measures:

1. No surgery is necessary in the following cases -

a. Randall's plaque requires no treatment as long as it remains submucosal. Later, however, it may become free and pass down the ureter and cause obstruction.

b. A small stone trapped in a minor calyx and causing few if any symptoms and no renal damage is best ignored.

c. A conservative approach is usually indicated for coralliform stones, particularly in the elderly, as long as the symptoms remain minimal or absent, since extensive incisions into the renal parenchyma are necessary for their removal.

d. Stones due to renal tubular acidosis should be treated conservatively even if multiple since they may pass spontaneously with adequate medical treatment (alkalies).

2. Combat infection - This is of particular importance if the bacteria are urea-splitting, for they encourage the progression of calcium phosphate or magnesium stone

formation. Unfortunately this is often not successful.

3. Attempts at dissolution - Chemical dissolution of renal stones requires indwelling ureteral catheters for constant "through-and-through" irrigation with G (or M) solution, and is usually mechanically impracticable. Sand and stone fragments occlude the catheters and cause acute obstruction. This may lead to exacerbation of pyelonephritis, and bacteremia and renal cortical abscesses may result.

Some uric acid stones may dissolve on allopurinol (Zyloprim®) therapy. Cystine stones may likewise disappear when D-penicillamine is administered.

B. Surgical Measures: Removal of the stone is indicated if the stone is obstructive and causes undue pain or progressive renal damage, or if the infection complicating a stone cannot be eradicated. Nephrectomy may be necessary if obstruction and infection have markedly impaired renal function.

Prevention

Patients who have formed stones should be managed prophylactically in an attempt to prevent recurrences. The measures indicated depend upon the type of stone formed in the past. If a stone is not available for chemical analysis, its composition may be surmised from the following data: (1) x-ray density and morphology of stones in the urinary tract, (2) types of crystals in the urine, (3) positive test for urinary alpha-aminonitrogen and cystine, and (4) abnormalities in blood chemistry (calcium, phosphorus, uric acid).

A. General Measures: Stone-formers must maintain a high urine volume to keep solutes well diluted. Combat infection by use of appropriate antibiotics. Eliminate obstruction and stasis by surgical means. Avoid recumbency.

Ask the patient if he is a "vitamin addict." He may be taking vitamin D, as well as minerals which may include considerable calcium. Calcium stone formers should maintain an acid urine. Indiscriminate use of alkalies for gastric distress should be questioned.

B. Specific Measures: Prophylactic treatment specific for the various types of stones is as follows:
1. Calcium and magnesium ammonium phosphate stones - If caused by primary hyperparathyroidism, the parathyroid glands should be explored.
a. Diet - Eliminate milk and cheese (dairy products) if hypercalciuria is discovered.
b. Urinary pH - Calcium phosphate and magnesium ammonium phosphate stones form most readily in neutral or alkaline urine. The

pH of the urine should be kept below 6.0. It may be tested by the patient with Nitrazine® paper. Cranberry juice, 200 ml 4 times a day; ascorbic acid, 1 gm 4 times a day; and sodium or potassium acid phosphate are the most efficient acidifiers. In renal tubular acidosis, alkali should be given in the form of sodium and potassium citrate; this will dramatically reduce the output of urinary calcium.
c. Converting stone-forming urine to nonstone-forming urine - According to Howard, stone formers manufacture "evil" urine. This effect can be negated by the administration of 2.5 gm of neutral sodium (or potassium) phosphate (Na_2HPO_4) daily in divided doses. Sodium (or potassium) acid phosphate, 4-6 gm/day, is also effective. The potassium salts are preferable.
d. Diuretics - Yendt has observed that the administration of a benzothiadiazine diuretic (eg, hydrochlorothiazide [Hydro-Diuril®], 50 mg twice a day) decreases the amount of calcium in the urine by one-half in patients with idiopathic hypercalciuria. Magnesium is increased.
2. Oxalate stones (calcium oxalate) - Prescribe phosphate and limit calcium intake (see above). There is no effective method for decreasing the amount of oxalate in the urine even in hyperoxaluria. Foods high in oxalate should be deleted from the diet, though the effect of this is questionable.

The administration of magnesium oxide, 150 mg 3 times a day, may control recurrence of oxalate stones. It does not diminish the level of urinary excretion; the magnesium may combine with oxalate, thus forming a more soluble complex.
3. Metabolic stones (uric acid, cystine) - Keep the pH at 7.0 or higher, thereby increasing the solubility of these substances (up to 100%). This can sometimes be done with an alkaline-ash diet (high in vegetable and fruit content, low in protein), but added alkalies are usually needed (give 50% sodium citrate solution, 1-2 tsp 4 times daily or oftener as needed). The patient can follow his urine pH with paper indicators. A low-purine diet (one weekly serving of meat, poultry, or fish) should be prescribed for the uric acid stone-former. Allopurinol (Zyloprim®), a xanthine oxidase inhibitor, by decreasing the endogenous production of uric acid, has proved very effective in preventing recurrence of uric acid calculi. The dose is 300 mg every 12 hours.

In severe cystinurics (over 1200 mg/24 hours), a low-methionine diet may be necessary in order to decrease the amount of endogenous cystine, but this diet is not very palatable. If the above measures fail to decrease the urinary cystine to safe levels, penicillamine (Cuprimine®) should be added to the regimen. This preparation (30 mg/kg/day in divided doses) usually reduces the amount of cystine in the urine to 100 mg or less per day. Pyridoxine, 50 mg/day, should also be given. Stone formation ceases; some stones may dissolve. Skin rashes are not uncommon but can be controlled by corticosteroids, which are given for a few weeks and then withdrawn. The nephrotic syndrome has been observed as a complication of the drug. It subsides when the drug is withdrawn.

Recently, a new drug, N-acetylpenicillamine, has received a trial. It appears to be as effective as penicillamine but is less toxic.

C. Mixed Stones: If the patient forms more than one type of stone and the prophylactic regimens interfere with each other, it is best to determine which is the primary stone and direct prophylactic measures against that type of stone in an effort to prevent recurrence.

Prognosis

The recurrence rate of renal stone is significant, and prognosis must therefore be guarded. The patient must be carefully followed for months or even years. The real danger from renal stone is not the pain but the kidney destruction caused by obstruction and infection.

Bass, H. N., & B. Emanuel: Nephrolithiasis in childhood. J Urol 95:749-53, 1966.

Blackman, J. E., & others: Urinary calculi and the consumption of analgesics. Brit MJ 2:800-2, 1967.

Bower, B. F., & G. S. Gordan: Hormonal effects of nonendocrine tumors. In: Annual Review of Medicine, Annual Reviews 16: 83-118, 1965.

Cochran, M., & others: Hyperoxaluria in adults. Brit J Surg 55:121-8, 1968.

DeConti, R. C., & P. Calabresi: Use of allopurinol for prevention and control of hyperuricemia in patients with neoplastic disease. New England J Med 274:481-6, 1966.

Drach, G. W., Smith, M. J. V., & W. H. Boyce: Medical therapy of renal calculi. J Urol 104:635-9, 1970.

Dudzinski, P. J., Painter, M. R., & E. L. Lewis: Operations on the intrarenal collecting system: Report of 4 cases. J Urol 102:285-8, 1969.

Elliott, J. S.: Calcium stones: The difference between oxalate and phosphate types. J Urol 100:687-93, 1968.

Ettinger, B., & F. O. Kolb: Factors involved in crystal formation in cystinuria. In vivo and in vitro crystallization dynamics and a simple, quantitative colorimetric assay for cystine. J Urol 106:106-10, 1971.

Frimpter, G. W.: Medical management of cystinuria. Am J Med Sc 255:348-57, 1968.

Gleason, D. C., & E. J. Potchen: The diagnosis of hyperparathyroidism. Radiol Clin North America 5:277-87, 1967.

Gordan, G. S., & B. S. Roof: Laboratory tests for hyperparathyroidism. JAMA 206:2729-31, 1968.

Herrin, J. T.: The child with urolithiasis. Practical considerations in diagnosis and management. Clin Pediat 10:306-8, 1971.

Howard, J. E.: Tried, true, and new ways to treat and prevent kidney stones. Resident and Staff 16:67-79, 1970.

Jennis F., & others: Staghorn calculi of the kidney: Clinical, bacteriological and biochemical features. Brit J Urol 42:511-8, 1970.

Kerr, W. S., Jr.: Surgical management of renal stones with emphasis on infundibulotomy. J Urol 103:130-3, 1970.

Knisley, R. E.: Hypercalcemia associated with leukemia. Arch Int Med 118:14-6, 1966.

Lagergren, C.: Development of silica calculi after oral administration of magnesium trisilicate. J Urol 87:994-6, 1962.

Lloyd, H. M.: Primary hyperparathyroidism: An analysis of the role of the parathyroid tumor. Medicine 47:53-71, 1968.

Marsden, P., & others: Familial hyperparathyroidism. Brit MJ 3:87-90, 1971.

Massry, S. G., & others: Inorganic phosphate treatment of hypercalcemia. Arch Int Med 121:307-12, 1968.

Nemoy, N. J., & T. A. Stamey: Surgical, bacteriological, and biochemical management of "infection stones." JAMA 215:1470-6, 1971.

Oreopoulos, D. G., Soyanno, M. A. O., & M. G. McGeown: Magnesium/calcium ratio in urine of patients with renal stones. Lancet 2:420-2, 1968.

Prien, E. L., Jr.: The riddle of urinary stone disease. JAMA 216:503-7, 1971.

Raisz, L. G.: The diagnosis of hyperparathyroidism (or what to do until the immunoassay comes). New England J Med 285: 1006-10, 1971.

Silver, S. & H. Brendler: Use of magnesium oxide in management of familial hyperoxaluria. J Urol 106:274-9, 1971.

Smith, M. J. V., & W. H. Boyce: Allopurinol and urolithiasis. J Urol 102:750-3, 1969.

Smith, M. J. V., & others: Uricemia and urolithiasis. J Urol 101:637-42, 1969.

Stein, J., & H. A. Smythe: Nephrotic syndrome induced by penicillamine. Canad MAJ 98:505-7, 1968.

Stephens, A. D., & R. W. E. Watts: The treatment of cystinuria with N-acetyl-D-penicillamine, a comparison with the results of D-penicillamine treatment. Quart J Med 40:355-70, 1971.

Symposium on urinary stone. Am J Med 45: 654-783, 1968.

Ts'ai-Fan, Y., & A. B. Gutman: Uric acid nephrolithiasis in gout. Ann Int Med **67**: 1133-48, 1967.

Uhlír, K.: The peroral dissolution of renal calculi. J Urol **104**:239-47, 1970.

Vermeulen, C. W., Ellis, J. E., & Te-C. Hsu: Experimental observations on the pathogenesis of urinary calculi. J Urol **95**:681-90, 1966.

Vermeulen, C. W., & F. A. Fried: Observations on dissolution of uric acid calculi. J Urol **94**:293-6, 1965.

Vermeulen, C. W., & others: Renal papilla and calculogenesis. J Urol **97**:573-82, 1967.

Walls, J., Morley, A. R., & D. N. S. Kerr: Primary hyperoxaluria in adult siblings: With some observations on the role of regular haemodialysis therapy. Brit J Urol **41**: 546-53, 1969.

Weber, A. L.: Primary hyperoxaluria. Am J Roentgenol **100**:155-61, 1967.

Wenzl, J. E., & others: Nephrolithiasis and nephrocalcinosis in children. Pediatrics **41**:57-61, 1968.

Wills, M. R., & others: Normocalcemic primary hyperparathyroidism. Am J Med **47**: 384-91, 1969.

Wills, M. R.: Value of plasma chloride and acid-base status in the differential diagnosis of hyperparathyroidism from other causes of hypercalcaemia. J Clin Path **24**: 219-27, 1971.

Yendt, E. R., Guay, G. F., & D. A. Garcia: The use of thiazides in the prevention of renal calculi. Canad MAJ **102**:614-20, 1970.

Yendt, E. R.: Renal calculi. Canad MAJ **102**: 479-89, 1970.

Yendt, E. R., & R. J. A. Gagne: Detection of primary hyperparathyroidism, with special reference to its occurrence in hypercalciuric females with "normal" or borderline serum calcium. Canad MAJ **98**:331-6, 1968.

URETERAL STONE

Ureteral stones originate in the kidney. Gravity and peristalsis both contribute to spontaneous passage into and down the ureter.

Ureteral stones are seldom completely obstructive; they are usually spiculated, so that urine can flow around them. Occasionally a stone will remain lodged in a ureter for many months without harming the kidney. Partial obstruction is usually present, however; this causes dilatation of the ureter and renal pelvis proximal to the stone. In the early phase, this dilatation is due more to distention than to "hydronephrosis," which implies definite renal damage. If the stone passes within

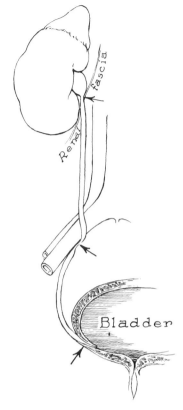

Fig 15-5. Points of ureteral narrowing. The ureter is narrow at 3 points: (1) at the ureteropelvic junction, (2) at the point where the ureter crosses over the iliac vessels, and (3) in the ureterovesical zone. A stone which passes the ureteropelvic junction has an excellent chance, therefore, of continuing the whole distance. If it becomes arrested, it is usually in the lower 5 cm of the ureter.

a few days, no evidence of renal injury can be shown. However, if the stone is definitely obstructive and is allowed to remain for weeks or months, irreparable damage to the renal parenchyma can occur (see Fig 10-4). A stone is apt to be arrested in the narrowest points in the ureter (Fig 15-5). If infection should complicate the urinary stasis, further renal damage results.

Clinical Findings

A. Symptoms: (See Fig 15-6.) Pain is usually abrupt in onset and becomes severe within a matter of minutes. There are 2 types of pain: (1) the radiating, colicky, agonizing pain (from hyperperistalsis of the smooth muscle of the calyces, pelvis, and ureter), and (2) the rather constant ache in the costovertebral area and flank (from obstruction and capsular tension). The radiation of the pain at

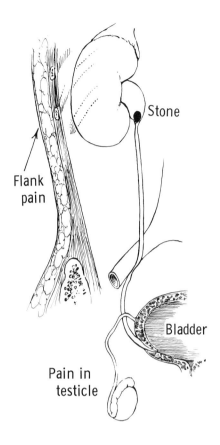

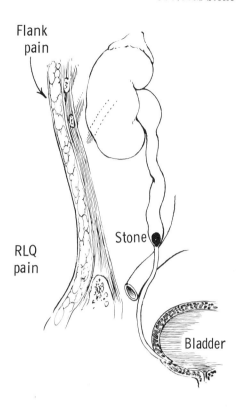

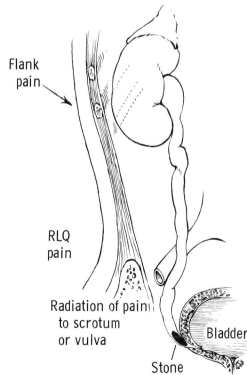

Fig 15-6. **Radiation of pain with various types of ureteral stone. Above left:** Ureteropelvic stone. Severe costovertebral angle pain from capsular and pelvic distention; acute renal and ureteral pain from hyperperistalsis of smooth muscle of calyces, pelvis, and ureter, with pain radiating along the course of the ureter (and into the testicle, since the nerve supply to the kidney and testis is the same). The testis is hypersensitive. **Above right:** Midureteral stone. Same as above but with more pain in the lower abdominal quadrant. **Left:** Low ureteral stone. Same as above with pain radiating into bladder, vulva, or scrotum. The scrotal wall is hyperesthetic. Testicular sensitivity is absent. When the stone approaches the bladder, urgency and frequency with burning on urination develop as a result of inflammation of the bladder wall around the ureteral orifice.

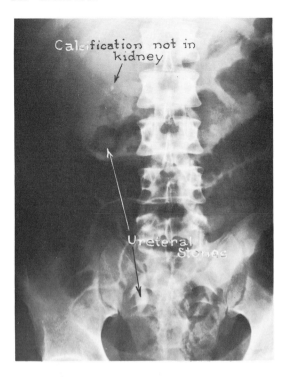

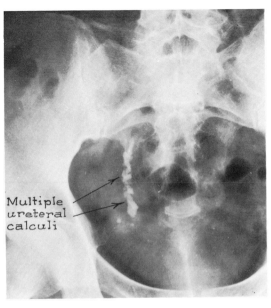

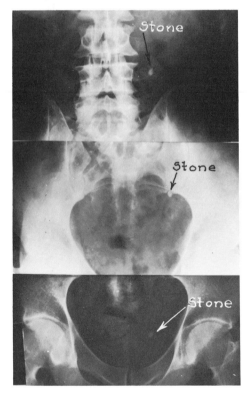

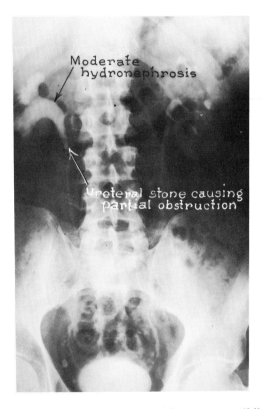

Fig 15-7. **Radiograms showing ureteral stones. Above left:** Two stones in right ureter, mildly radiopaque; cystine. **Above right:** Multiple stones, right ureter. **Below left:** Plain films showing progress of stone down ureter. **Below right:** Stone in upper right ureter causing moderate obstruction.

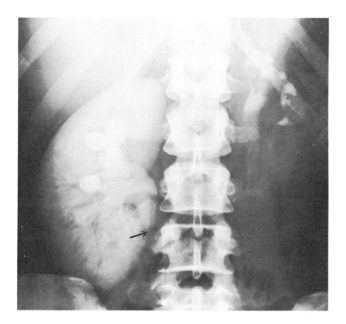

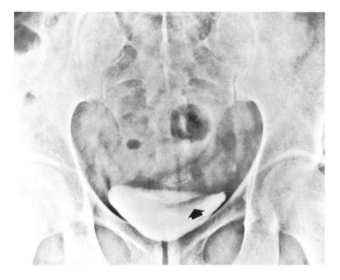

Fig 15-8. Ureteral stone. Above: "Nephrogram" caused by acute ureteral obstruction. Marked density of renal parenchyma with moderate hydronephrosis. Arrow points to nonopaque (uric acid) stone. Left kidney is contracted and scarred from previous infections. **Below:** Patient has just passed left ureteral calculus. Note secondary edema of left intravesical ureter as depicted by arrow and a second stone in the left ureter just above the bladder.

times suggests the position of the stone. If high in the ureter, the colic may radiate to the testicle. As the stone nears the bladder the pain may spread to the scrotum or appear in the vulva. This is due to the common innervation of these organs and the lower ureter. At times the pain comes on more slowly and may be felt more anteriorly. It may occasionally be quite mild. In these instances, the diagnosis may not at first be obvious.

Gastrointestinal symptoms are commonly associated with stone in the ureter. Nausea and vomiting almost always occur, and abdominal distention due to paralytic ileus is always present. These symptoms may be so severe that the renal and ureteral pain may be overshadowed and an intraperitoneal lesion sought (eg, bowel obstruction, ruptured peptic ulcer, cholelithiasis, or acute appendicitis.

Gross hematuria is observed in about one-third of cases; small clots may be passed.

Even in the absence of infection, symptoms of urgency and frequency may develop when the stone approaches the bladder.

Existing chronic renal infection may be exacerbated by the ureteral obstruction. Chills and fever with increased back pain may be noted. It is not common for stone to be complicated by acute (new) infection unless it is introduced by instrumentation. If this does occur, chills, fever, and sepsis are to be expected.

B. Signs: The patient is usually in agony, pacing the floor rather than lying quietly in bed (as a patient with peritoneal irritation is apt to do). Nothing he does affords relief. His skin may be cold and clammy, and he may exhibit other signs of mild shock. There is marked tenderness in the costovertebral angle and flank. Fist percussion posteriorly causes severe pain. Spasm of the abdominal muscles on the affected side is to be expected.

Fever indicates that infection complicates the picture. The abdomen is distended, tympanitic, and quiet on auscultation. The ipsilateral testis may be hypersensitive if the stone is in the upper ureter. It may be retracted. The scrotal skin may be hyperesthetic if the stone lies low. At times a juxtavesical ureteral stone may be felt vaginally.

C. Laboratory Findings: Same as for renal stone.

D. X-Ray Findings: A plain film of the abdomen may show a calcific body in the region of the ureter. This constitutes merely presumptive grounds for the diagnosis, however, for the observed shadow may be a phlebolith or other intra-abdominal calification.

Excretory urograms are invaluable (Fig 15-7). The ureterogram places the calcification in the ureter and usually demonstrates dilatation of the ureter above the stone. It also reveals what is happening to the kidney (degree of obstruction). On occasion, no "dye" may enter the renal pelvis or ureter because of the obstruction, but a marked denseness of the renal shadow occurs (Fig 15-8). This is evidence of good kidney function and acute ureteral obstruction. The acute ureteral obstruction may cause extravasation of the radiopaque fluid in the region of the renal hilum. This finding in itself is of no consequence.

In the case of a nonopaque stone, a "negative" gray or black shadow is seen within the white area of the ureter. This may be difficult to differentiate from ureteral tumor or blood clot.

The diagnosis of ureteral stone may be established by demonstrating that the suspicious shadow hugs the cystoscopically placed ureteral catheter in both the anteroposterior and oblique views.

E. Instrumental Examination: Cystoscopy and ureteral catheterization are seldom needed for the diagnosis of ureteral stone. Instrumental examination should be avoided unless a proper conclusion cannot be drawn otherwise. No matter how careful one is, instrumentation always carries bacteria from the urethra into the urinary tract. Infection introduced in this way unnecessarily complicates the problem.

Differential Diagnosis

Passage of crystals down the ureter may occur during treatment or an exacerbation of gout or in oxaluria after excessive ingestion of high-oxalate foods. Symptoms and signs are the same as those seen in stone, and hematuria is just as common. X-ray examination is usually normal, however. The presence of many crystals in the urine may suggest the etiology of the colic.

A tumor of the kidney or renal pelvis may bleed, and a clot or piece of necrotic tumor tissue may pass down the ureter. This will simulate ureteral stone perfectly. Excretory urograms should demonstrate a space-occupying lesion in the kidney and a "negative" shadow in the ureter. Retrograde urograms may then be indicated for more definitive diagnosis.

Ureteral tumor is often obstructive and may cause colic. Hematuria is common. X-ray visualization of the urinary tract should make the diagnosis.

Obstructive chronic lesions of the ureter may cause severe recurrent pain. These include congenital ureteral stenosis and extraureteral obstructions such as may be caused by lymph nodes containing cancer. A careful history and physical examination and excretory urograms should lead to the correct diagnosis.

Acute pyelonephritis may start so abruptly and the pain may be so acute as to suggest stone. The finding of pyuria and bacteriuria with normal urograms should establish the diagnosis.

Acute gallbladder disease (stone or infection) may be confused with ureteral stone if severe pain is referred to the back. A previous history of dyspepsia or jaundice is helpful. It is true, however, that renal and ureteral stones also cause gastrointestinal symptoms. Red cells in the urine suggest urinary stone. Cholecystograms and urography should settle the matter.

An aneurysm of the abdominal aorta may cause pain suggestive of left renal colic. Palpation of the aneurysm, absence of hematuria, and normal excretory urograms will differentiate the two. Aortography is definitive.

A sloughed papilla passing down the ureter may simulate ureteral stone. Urinalysis shows evidence of infection. Excretory urograms will reveal the typical changes of papillary necrosis.

Complications

The major complication of ureteral stone is obstruction, usually only partial. Permanent renal damage is rare except in the case which remains undiagnosed or is inadequately treated. Bilateral ureteral calculi may cause anuria. Drainage of the kidney by ureteral catheters or removal of the stones must be accomplished.

Infection may gain a foothold in the presence of the obstruction, but it is usually introduced by the cystoscopist in his attempts to remove the stone. Drainage either by catheter or surgical attack is indicated in addition to appropriate antibiotic therapy.

Treatment

A. Specific Measures: About 80% of stones which reach the ureter can pass spontaneously and should always be allowed to do so as long as complications do not develop. Antispasmodics may be helpful. Physical activity should be encouraged and adequate fluid intake maintained to increase ureteral peristalsis. A stone small enough to pass down the ureter will have no difficulty traversing the urethra.

Cystoscopic manipulation or surgical intervention (ureterolithotomy) is necessary if the stone is too large to pass the ureteral lumen spontaneously. Stones up to 0.5 cm in diameter and even a few up to 1 cm in diameter may pass without surgical or cystoscopic assistance. The onset of infection may require removal of the obstructing agent before sepsis can be controlled. If periodic excretory urograms show progressive hydronephrosis or if pain remains intense and incapacitating, removal of the stone is indicated.

B. General Measures: Morphine or a similar opiate is necessary to control pain. It should be given intravenously. Morphine sulfate, 8 mg, or a comparable drug in the same relative strength, should be given immediately and repeated in 5 minutes if relief has not been obtained. Pain can usually be controlled thereafter by subcutaneous injection. Initial subcutaneous morphine, even in doses of 30 mg, is disappointing for relief of pain of this degree.

Atropine, 0.8 mg subcut, is the antispasmodic of choice. Methantheline bromide (Banthine®), 0.1 gm IV, will usually relieve the pain; unfortunately, it may paralyze bladder action for some hours as well. Other antispasmodics can be given by mouth, but their efficacy is questionable.

Heat to the flank or a hot bath is often helpful as an adjunct to drug analgesia.

Prevention

See p 214.

Prognosis

About 80% of stones which enter the ureter will pass spontaneously in a few days or weeks. If the effect of the stone upon the kidney is checked at intervals with excretory urograms, the physician is in a position to protect the function of the kidney by judicious intervention if necessary.

Arnaldsson, Ö., & D. Holmlund: Defects in the urographic contrast medium above and below a ureteric calculus. Acta radiol (diag) 11:26-32, 1971.

Constantian, H. M.: Use of the Davis nylon loop extractor for removal of low ureteral calculi. J Urol 97:248-50, 1967.

Evans, A. T., Hoodin, A. O., & A. J. Farrell: Another look at the looped catheter. Am J Surg 109:247-52, 1965.

Fox, M., Pyrah, L. N., & F. P. Raper: Management of ureteric stone: A review of 292 cases. Brit J Urol 37:660-70, 1965.

Green, L. F., & S. N. Rous: Manipulative treatment of ureteral calculi. GP 27:141-7, March 1963.

Harrow, B. R.: Unusual renal peripelvic extravasation requiring operative drainage. J Urol 102:564-6, 1969.

Smulewicz, J. J., & others: Spontaneous rupture of the collecting system of the kidney: An evaluation. J Urol 104:507-11, 1970.

Wisoff, C. P., & R. Parsavand: Edema of the interureteric ridge - a useful Roentgen sign. Am J Roentgenol 86:1123-6, 1961.

VESICAL STONE

Primary vesical stones are rare in this country but occur commonly in northwest India, the Middle East, and parts of China. The cause is not known, but it appears to be dietary; the calculi may be secondary to vitamin B_6 deficiency. Once removed, these vesical stones rarely recur.

Secondary vesical stone develops as a complication of other urologic disease; 95% occur in men. The most common cause of secondary vesical stone is infection of residual urine with urea-splitting organisms (eg, proteus). This partial urinary retention may be due to prostatic or bladder neck obstruction, cystocele, or neurogenic bladder. Stagnation is particularly marked in vesical diverticula; stones are often found when diverticula are present (Fig 15-10).

A stone passed through the ureter usually passes on through the urethra. In obstruction or stasis, it may remain in the bladder and act as the nucleus for precipitation of more urinary salts.

A markedly inflamed or ulcerated bladder may predispose to stone formation. This is seen in vesical schistosomiasis and following irradiation of the bladder.

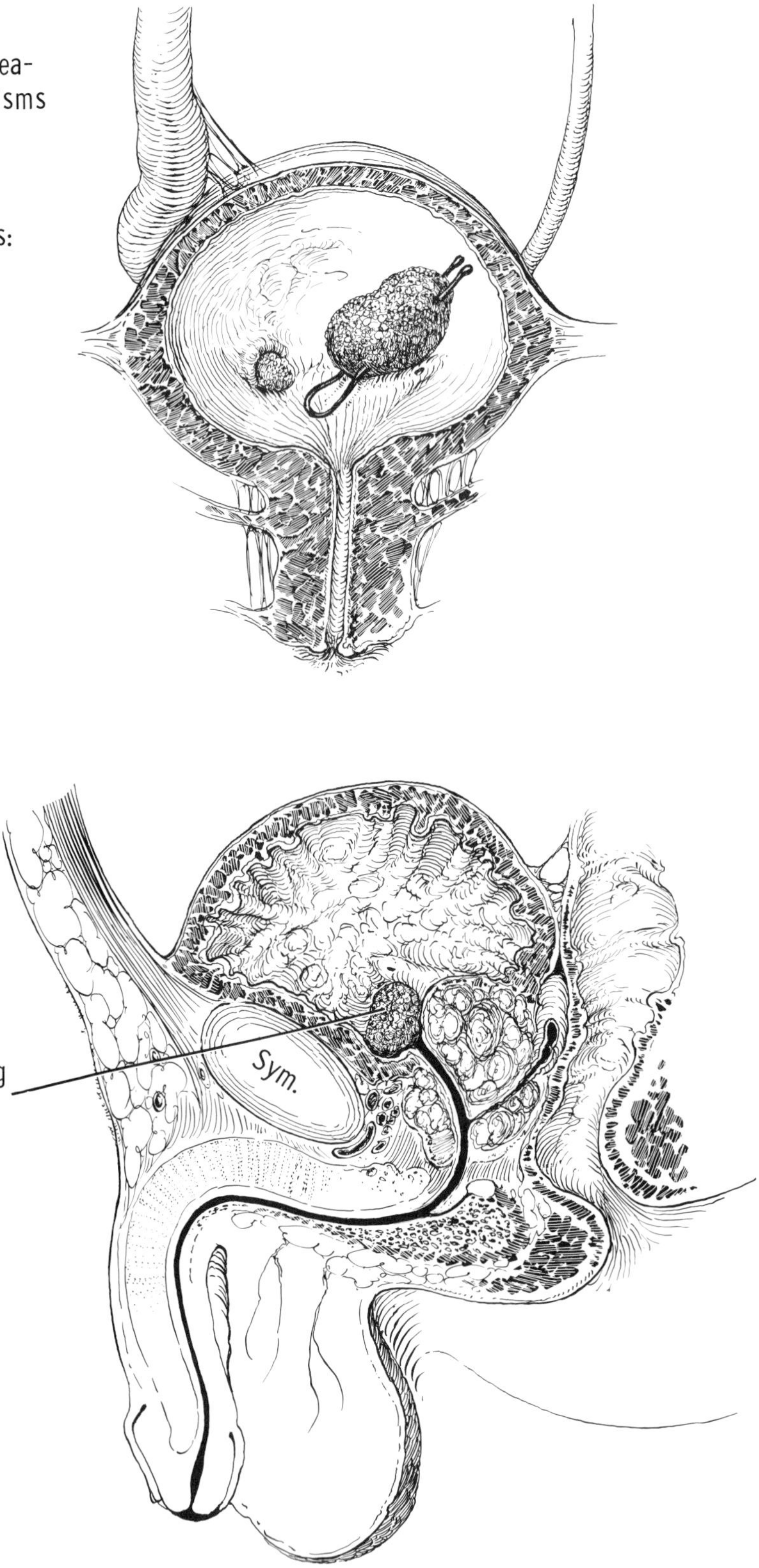

Obstruction with
  infection by urea-
    splitting organisms

Other less
  common causes:
    renal stone
    foreign body
    parasites

Symptoms and signs
  sudden interruption of
    urinary stream with
    radiation of pain
    down urethra
  also urinary
    symptoms of under-
    lying disease (e.g.,
    prostatism,
    secondary cystitis)

Stone occluding
  vesical neck

Sym.

Fig 15-9. Genesis and symptoms and signs of vesical calculus.

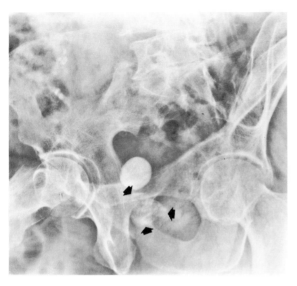 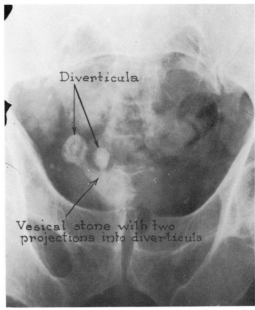

Fig 15-10. **Vesical stones. Left:** Oblique plain film showing smooth, round bladder stone and an irregular stone in the prostatic urethra; post-prostatectomy. **Right:** Plain film showing dumbbell-shaped stone in bladder with projections into diverticula.

Foreign bodies occasionally are introduced into the bladder, particularly in women. These include nonabsorbable sutures, candles, nail files, chewing gum, and even crochet hooks. They may act as nidi for the precipitation of calcific deposits (Fig 15-9). Infection complicates the picture and quickens calculus formation particularly if the bacteria are urea-splitters.

Pathology

Vesical stones may be single or multiple. If single, they are ovoid; if multiple, they often are faceted. In addition to the infection which is uniformly present with secondary stones, their presence further increases the inflammation of the bladder.

Most vesical stones are radiopaque (calcium phosphate, calcium oxalate, or ammonium magnesium phosphate), but some are radiolucent (uric acid). At times even calcium stones are invisible on a plain film. This may be due to the presence of large amounts of matrix.

Clinical Findings

A. Symptoms: Symptoms of chronic urinary obstruction or stasis and infection occur in most cases, for these are the common causes of vesical stone. There may be a history of the introduction of a foreign body into the bladder. The patient may complain of sudden interruption of his urinary stream associated with pain radiating down the penis when the stone rolls over the bladder neck. He may be unable to void except in certain positions which cause the stone to move off the bladder neck. Considerable hematuria may be noted, although this can occur also with pure obstruction or infection.

B. Signs: Only giant calculi can be felt suprapubically. The bladder may be visible, palpable, or percussible if there is a great deal of residual urine. Palpation of the urethra may reveal a thickening compatible with stricture. Rectal examination may demonstrate a relaxed anal sphincter (neurogenic bladder) or an enlarged or hard (cancerous) prostate. Cystocele may be noted.

C. Laboratory Findings: The urine is almost always infected. Blood cells are commonly found. Excretion of PSP may be depressed because of chronic obstruction. A flattened curve (first and second half-hour specimens about equal in amount) suggests residual urine.

D. X-Ray Findings: Vesical stones are usually visible on a plain film (Fig 15-10). They must be differentiated from calcified ovaries and fibroids. Oblique films are usually helpful. Excretory urograms may show back pressure changes in the kidneys, and a film taken after voiding may reveal residual urine. Diverticula may be noted. Stones will be localized in the excretory or retrograde cystograms.

E. Instrumental Examination: The attempt to pass a catheter or sound may lead to the diagnosis of urethral stricture. Successful passage of a catheter after urination allows estimation of the degree of obstruction and stasis by recovering residual urine. The positive diagnostic step of "sounding" for stone may be accomplished by passing a sound into the bladder. The definitive "click" of the instrument on the stone can readily be heard or felt. Cystoscopy usually visualizes the stone or stones and the obstructive lesion with its secondary vesical changes (Fig 10-1).

Differential Diagnosis

A pedunculated tumor of the bladder can suddenly occlude the vesical orifice, thereby simulating vesical stone. Cystoscopy will make the differentiation.

Extravesical calcifications on x-rays of the vesical region may appear to be in the bladder but are actually in the veins, omental fat pads, ovaries, or fibroids of the uterus. Cystoscopy will help in differentiating these.

Complications

A primary stone will lead eventually to infection. If infection is present, it will be worsened by the presence of a calculus, which in turn will defeat attempts to sterilize the urine.

Vesicoureteral reflux is commonly associated with vesical calculi. Removal of the calculi may cause spontaneous cessation of the reflux.

A small vesical concretion may pass down the urethra and become lodged there. This may cause complete urinary obstruction.

Prevention

Stasis and infection, whether primary or secondary, must be eradicated.

Treatment

A. Specific Measures:

1. Cystoscopy and surgical removal -
a. Transurethral route - Small stones can be removed by cystoscopic manipulation; large ones can be crushed (litholapaxy) and the fragments washed out. If the patient has an obstructing prostate which can be removed by transurethral resection, both procedures may be undertaken at the same time.

b. Suprapubic route - This route must be used for removal of stones which are too large for transurethral removal or crushing. Suprapubic prostatectomy may also be indicated.

2. Chemical dissolution - This is usually successful but it fails to treat the cause of the stone formation. It may be indicated if the patient is considered to be an unwarranted surgical risk or if he refuses surgery or cystoscopic removal.

In the dissolution of calcium and magnesium ammonium phosphate calculi, excellent results are obtained with hemiacidrin (Renacidin®). Thirty ml of 10% solution are instilled; the catheter is clamped for 30-60 minutes. This is repeated 4-6 times a day. A continuous drip through a 3-way Foley catheter may also be used.

Calcium salts and magnesium ammonium phosphate are highly soluble in citric acid. Suby and Albright have evolved buffered solutions of this compound.

"Solution G" (pH 4.0)

Citric acid (monohydrated)	32.25
Magnesium oxide (anhydrous)	3.84
Sodium carbonate (anhydrous)	4.37
Water, qs ad	1000.0

If this solution proves irritating, the amount of sodium carbonate can be increased to 8.84 gm ("solution M," which has a pH of 4.5).

In order to dissolve organic matrix, 0.05% pepsin should be added to the solution. The resulting mixture can be sterilized by passing it through a millipore filter.

Through an indwelling catheter, 60-100 ml of solution G (or M) are introduced into the bladder. The fluid is retained for one-half hour, and the bladder is then drained. This procedure is repeated at frequent intervals (every 1-2 hours).

These solutions may fail with markedly radiopaque (hard) stones. They have no effect on uric acid or cystine.

B. General Measures: Analgesics for pain and antibiotics for control of infection are used for relief of distressing symptoms until the stone can be removed and its cause eliminated.

C. Treatment of Complications: Infection cannot be eradicated until the stone and the cause of the obstruction are removed. Urethral stone may be extracted transurethrally or pushed back into the bladder and then extracted or crushed.

Prognosis

The rate of recurrence of vesical stone is low if the primary cause (obstruction) is successfully treated.

Andersen, D. A.: The nutritional significance of primary bladder stones. Brit J Urol **34**: 160-77, 1962.

Aurora, A. L., Taneja, O. P., & D. N. Gupta: Bladder stone disease of childhood. I. An epidemiological study. Acta paediat scandinav **59**:177-84, 1970. II. A clinico-pathological study. 385-98, 1970.

Mulvaney, W. P., & D. C. Henning: Solvent treatment of urinary calculi: Refinements in technique. J Urol **88**:145-9, 1962.

Reuter, H. J.: Electronic lithotripsy: Transurethral treatment of bladder stones in 50 cases. J Urol **104**:834-8, 1970.

PROSTATIC CALCULI

Prostatic calculi are seldom of clinical importance. They are commonly seen in association with benign prostatic hyperplasia, although in rare cases in younger persons they may be secondary to an advanced but healing tuberculous prostatitis.

Prostatic calculi are formed of desquamated epithelial cells which finally acquire a shell of calcium. They average about 1-2 mm in diameter and are brown to black in color. They are situated between the hypertrophied adenoma and the surgical capsule. Therefore, on enucleation of the enlarged prostate or complete transurethral prostatectomy, they tend to be extruded.

On a plain film they are situated in the region of the pubic symphysis (Fig 15-11).

The importance of prostatic calculi lies in the fact that they cause indurated areas in the prostate which may be mistaken for carcinomas.

Fox, M.: The natural history and significance of stone formation in the prostate gland. J Urol **89**:716-27, 1963.

NEPHROCALCINOSIS

Nephrocalcinosis is a precipitation of calcium in the tubules, parenchyma, and, occasionally, in the glomeruli of the kidney. The presence of nephrocalcinosis means that primary or secondary impairment of renal function has occurred. It is therefore a more serious disease than calculus. Nephrocalcinosis and calculus formation may exist together.

Etiology and Pathogenesis

The common causes of nephrocalcinosis are hypercalcemia and hyperparathyroidism. Hypercalciuria with hypercalcemia may be due to hyperparathyroidism (nephrocalcinosis or calculi are found in about 75% of hyperparathyroid patients); hypervitaminosis D, particularly when accompanied by a high calcium intake; acute osteoporosis due to immobilization, especially in children; or metastatic malignancy involving bone.

Hypercalciuria without hypercalcemia may be caused by chronic renal insufficiency, particularly that due to chronic pyelonephritis, glomerulonephritis, or polycystic kidney disease, all of which are sometimes accompanied by calcific deposits in the kidneys. Phosphate retention leads to compensatory hypocalcemia,

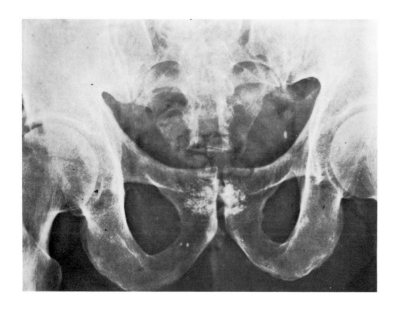

Fig 15-11. Prostatic calculi seen in typical locations behind the symphysis pubis.

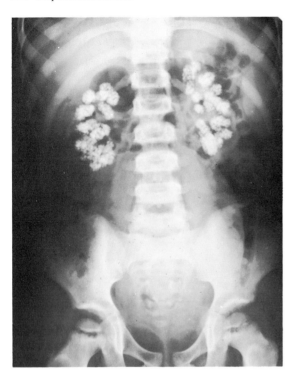

Fig 15-12. Nephrocalcinosis. Plain film showing parenchymal calcification in both kidneys. Large globular soft tissue shadow (greatly distended bladder) in midline extending from pelvis to level of lower poles of kidneys. It has displaced the bowel to the flanks.

which in turn results in secondary hyperparathyroidism and increased calcium excretion. Hyperchloremic acidosis resulting from the loss of the power of the tubules to elaborate ammonia leads to excretion of calcium as well as potassium and sodium. The hypercalciuria contributes to the precipitation of calcium salts.

Nephrocalcinosis without hypercalciuria is most commonly due to excessive intake of milk and soluble alkalies, particularly in the treatment of peptic ulcer. It is also observed in hyperoxaluria.

Pathology

The kidneys may be grossly normal or there may be obvious changes suggesting advanced renal disease (eg, hydronephrosis, chronic pyelonephritis). Calcific deposits in the tubules are seen microscopically. Primary tubular or glomerular lesions may also be noted.

Metastatic calcification is not uncommonly found in many other organs, including the skin, lungs, stomach, spleen, pancreas, cornea, thyroid, and around the joints.

Clinical Findings

A. Symptoms: There are no symptoms which suggest nephrocalcinosis, although these patients at times pass stones and sand. The complaints are those of the primary disease

(eg, primary hyperparathyroidism or renal insufficiency). In childhood there may be lack of normal growth, and bone changes suggestive of rickets.

B. Signs: The physical examination is usually negative. Signs of the primary cause may be found, as follows: (1) parathryoid adenoma or hyperplasia, (2) metastatic calcifications around the joints or in the cornea ("band keratopathy") as viewed with a slit-lamp, (3) punched-out lesions in the fingertips (sarcoidosis), (4) pseudofractures (osteomalacia), (5) bilateral renal masses (polycystic kidneys, (6) dwarfism, or (7) pseudorickets.

C. Laboratory Findings: Anemia may be noted in advanced renal disease. The urinary pH is fixed between 6.0-7.0 in renal tubular acidosis. Pus and bacteria will be found in the urine in association with chronic renal infection. Casts and protein are constant findings in glomerulonephritis. Calcium phosphate casts may be seen. The Sulkowitch test is strongly positive in primary hyperparathyroidism with hypercalciuria; it may be positive with secondary parathyroid hyperplasia as well.

Renal function tests will demonstrate some impairment of function whether the primary cause of the calcification is renal or not. Nitrogen retention is common.

Hypercalcemia and hypophosphatemia are to be expected in primary hyperparathyroidism. In chronic renal disease (with secondary hyperparathyroidism), the serum calcium may be low or normal and the phosphate normal or elevated.

Hyperchloremic acidosis (low blood pH) and hypokalemia accompany renal tubular acidosis.

Serum alkaline phosphatase will be elevated if nephrocalcinosis is accompanied by bone disease (osteitis, osteomalacia, etc).

D. X-Ray Findings: A plain film of the abdomen will show the pathognomonic parenchymal calcifications (Fig 15-12). These consist of minute calcific densities with a linear arrangement in the region of the renal papillae and radiating outward from the calyces. If renal function is not seriously impaired, excretory urograms will show that the calcium is in the renal parenchyma and not in the calyces although true stones may be present as well. These films may reveal changes compatible with atrophic pyelonephritis or hydronephrosis. X-rays of bones may show osteitis fibrosa generalisata and a soft tissue calcification of "renal rickets" (osteonephropathy).

Differential Diagnosis

Renal stones are usually discrete and lie in the calyces or pelvis.

In renal tuberculosis renal calcification is also parenchymal but tends to be related to the pericalyceal zones. Furthermore, the calcification is punctate rather than striated. Pus cells and tubercle bacilli are present, and excretory urograms will usually show the mucosal ulcerations or abscess cavities of tuberculosis.

Medullary sponge kidneys may develop multiple small calculi in their dilated cystic collecting tubules. Renal function is usually normal. Excretory urograms help in the differentiation.

Complications

Calcification secondary to extrarenal disease (eg, hyperparathyroidism) causes impairment of renal function. The calcium deposits secondary to preexisting renal disease cause more damage. If stones form and cause obstruction, particularly if secondary infection ensues, further renal injury occurs.

Treatment

A. Specific Measures: Treat the primary cause of the disease (eg, remove the parathyroid adenoma, relieve obstruction, and treat urologic infection).

B. General Measures: Discontinue vitamin D and give a low-calcium diet (delete dairy products, especially milk and cheese), encourage mobilization, and force fluids. If osteomalacia is present vitamin D and calcium may have to be given in spite of nephrocalcinosis.

If renal function is poor and hyperphosphatemia and hyperchloremic (renal tubular) acidosis exist, replace base to decrease hypercalciuria: give a 50% solution of sodium or potassium citrate (or a combination of both), 4-8 ml 4 times daily. Sodium bicarbonate, 4 gm 4 times daily, can be given in orange juice or water. The goal is alkalinization (pH of 7.0-7.5) of the urine. Additional potassium is also indicated.

Prognosis

If the nephrocalcinosis is secondary to primary renal disease, the prognosis is poor although life can be prolonged significantly with adequate treatment. If the renal calcification has developed because of extrarenal disease and if renal function is fairly good, correction of the underlying disease may terminate the progression of kidney damage. Frequently, however, the outlook is poor even in these instances.

Dretler, S. P., & others: The physiologic approach to renal tubular acidosis. J Urol 102:665-9, 1969.

Editorial: Renal tubular acidosis. Ann Int Med 54:1290-5, 1961.

Fletcher, R. F., Jones, J. H., & D. B. Morgan: Bone disease in chronic renal failure. Quart J Med 32:321-39, 1963.

Haquani, A. H., & M. M. Ram: Renal tubular insufficiency. J Pediat 61:242-55, 1962.

Punsar, S., & T. Somer: The milk-alkali syndrome. Acta med scandinav 173:435-49, 1963.

Pyrah, L. N., & A. Hodgkinson: Nephrocalcinosis. Brit J Urol 32:361-73, 1960.

Stanbury, S. W., & G. A. Lumb: Parathyroid function in chronic renal failure. Quart J Med 35:1-23, 1966.

•   •   •

16...

Injuries to the Genitourinary Tract

EMERGENCY MANAGEMENT

Orkin has evolved a method of examining the severely injured patient from the urologic point of view. These steps are never contra-indicated and contribute greatly to the early diagnosis of urologic injuries, thus materially decreasing mortality and morbidity.

If possible, after shock and hemorrhage have been treated, a complete description of the accident should be obtained from the patient or from an observer. The site of injury and the principal location of the pain should be ascertained. Hematuria, oliguria, or anuria require careful attention. Blood from the urethra, unassociated with urination, suggests urethral injury distal to the external urinary sphincter.

Evidence of trauma to the kidneys, ureters, bladder, or urethra must be sought. Significant signs of injury include ecchymoses over the various organs, local tenderness, masses (from bleeding or urinary extravasation), blood from the urethra, and the passage of bloody urine. Injuries to the external genitalia should be obvious. Abdominal paracentesis should be performed if intraperitoneal hemorrhage is suspected. Frequent careful examinations are essential to discover rapidly-enlarging masses, which may represent profuse bleeding (as from a lacerated kidney).

Rectal examination must be made and repeated. It may reveal upward displacement of the prostate if the gland has been torn from the membranous urethra. Swelling and bogginess of the tissues about the urethra suggest extravasation.

X-rays should be made when the patient can be moved. A plain film of the abdomen is invaluable. A fractured pelvis is often associated with urethral or vesical injury; fracture of the lower ribs or transverse processes of the upper lumbar vertebrae is often seen with injury to the kidney. Extravasation of blood or urine from an injured kidney will be revealed by a large area of grayness in the vicinity of the kidney and obliteration of the renal and psoas shadows.

Special Examinations

Instrumental examination should be made as symptoms indicate and the patient's condition warrants. No inflexible rules can be made about when these should be performed; the physician must carefully evaluate each patient.

A. Catheterization and X-ray Examinations: The following steps should be performed in the sequence given.

1. Catheterization - An attempt should be made to confirm the continuity of the urethra by passing a urethral catheter. Microscopic blood found in the urine is of no significance (catheter trauma), but grossly bloody urine means injury to the urinary tract. If the catheter cannot be passed into the bladder, urethrograms should be made.

2. Excretory urograms - The catheter should then be clamped and excretory urograms taken unless significant hypotension is present, in which case renal blood flow is impaired and visualization of the kidneys poor or absent. Infusion urography may, however, improve the quality of the films. These may reveal lack of excretion by one kidney or extravasation of the opaque fluid from a tear in any of the urinary organs. They may also show blood clots if there is hemorrhage into the hollow excretory passages.

3. Retrograde cystograms - Retrograde filling of the bladder should then be done by instilling at least 350 ml of radiopaque fluid through the catheter. An x-ray film of the bladder area is then taken. The catheter is opened and the fluid allowed to drain. Films taken at this time will reveal extravasation posterior to the bladder.

4. Urethrograms - The catheter should then be withdrawn into the urethra and 20-30 ml of opaque material again instilled. Appropriate x-ray films may reveal periurethral extravasation or a collection of fluid about the prostate or anterior to the bladder. If a catheter cannot be successfully passed, a urethrogram should be made as the catheter is withdrawn from the point of obstruction.

B. Cystoscopy and Retrograde Urography: These examinations are seldom needed but should be done when more information is needed and if the condition of the patient warrants it.

C. Indwelling Catheter: An indwelling catheter should be left in the bladder. A small tear in the urethra or bladder, if missed on the above examinations, may heal without complications.

Baker, W.N.W., Mackie, D.B., & J.F. Newcombe: Diagnostic paracentesis in the acute abdomen. Brit MJ **3**:146-9, 1967.

Currie, D.J.: Early management of the critically injured. Canad MAJ **95**:862-70, 1966.

Fox, J.A.: A diagnostic sign of extraperitoneal hemorrhage. Brit J Surg **53**:193-5, 1966.

Holland, M.E., Hurwitz, L.M., & C.M. Nice, Jr.: Traumatic lesions of the urinary tract. Radiol Clin North America **4**:433-50, 1966.

Orkin, L.A.: The diagnosis of urological trauma in the presence of other injuries. S Clin North America **33**:1473-94, 1953.

Rieser, C.: Diagnostic evaluation of suspected genitourinary tract injury. JAMA **199**:714-9, 1967.

INJURIES TO THE KIDNEY

Traumatic injuries to the kidney are not common, but they are potentially serious and may be complicated by injuries to other organs or structures. They occur most commonly during athletic activities or in industrial or traffic accidents. Ninety percent occur in men. Mild trauma may rupture an abnormal kidney (eg, hydronephrosis, Wilms's tumor).

Etiology (See Fig 16-2.)
The most common mode of injury is direct trauma to the abdomen, flank, or back. Indirect ("contrecoup") injury, caused by falling from a height and landing on the feet or buttocks, is less common. On rare occasion, acute abdominal muscle contractions have caused a hydronephrotic kidney to burst. Penetrating wounds caused by knives or bullets are rarely seen in peacetime.

Pathogenesis
The mechanics of renal lacerations are explained by the fact that the kidney contains a large amount of fluid, ie, urine and blood. The force of a sudden blow to the kidney is therefore transmitted equally throughout its tissues. The fibrous capsule which surrounds the kidney does to some extent protect the parenchyma from splitting.

The relative rarity of serious renal injury is due to the fact that the kidneys are protected by the rib cage and by the heavy muscles of the back. Furthermore, the kidneys are mobile in their adipose beds and are thus able to absorb the shock of a blow.

Pathology and Classification (See Fig 16-1.)
A. Early Pathology: Lacerations usually occur transverse to the long axis of the kidney or tend to radiate from the hilus. Renal injuries are classified pathologically as follows:

1. Simple bruising and ecchymosis - Contusion or bruising of the renal parenchyma is the most common lesion.

2. Hematoma - If, in association with contusion, the renal capsule is ruptured, a small perirenal hematoma may form.

3. Fissures - Incomplete fissures of the parenchyma may occur. If they involve the renal pelvis only, hematuria without perinephric hematoma occurs. If the renal capsule is torn, a large perirenal hematoma may develop. Hematuria is usually microscopic.

4. Lacerations - If the laceration extends through capsule and pelvis, extravasation of both blood and urine occurs. Hematuria may be marked. Tears in the renal pelvis or ureter lead to urinary extravasation with only slight bleeding. This is rare as an isolated lesion.

5. Rupture of the renal vascular pedicle - This causes massive bleeding which may prove rapidly fatal. Thrombosis of the renal artery has been reported.

6. Other pathologic lesions associated with renal lacerations include peritoneal tears with intraperitoneal bleeding, other visceral injuries, and fractures of the spine or ribs.

If bleeding stops spontaneously, the hematoma may absorb, become infected, or liquefy. The blood in the latter case is then absorbed and a collection of clear amber fluid remains (ie, perirenal cyst).

B. Late Pathology: (See Fig 16-3.)
1. Hydronephrosis and infection - At times the perirenal tissues will undergo fibrosis following extravasation of blood or urine, and ureteral obstruction may develop; this leads to hydronephrosis. Renal infection may then follow.

2. Atrophy or fibrosis - If the blood supply to the organ is impaired (rupture, thrombosis), atrophy is to be expected. Renovascular hypertension may develop. Renal lacerations heal by fibrosis; scar formation may be extensive if vascular damage was great or bleeding extensive.

Clinical Findings
Gross hematuria following any injury means trauma to the urinary tract. Signs and

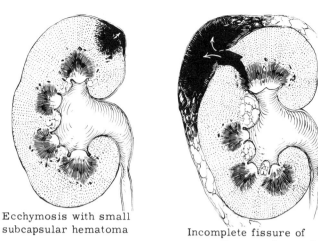

Ecchymosis

Ecchymosis with small
subcapsular hematoma

Incomplete fissure of
parenchyma and capsule
with perirenal hematoma

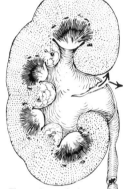

Incomplete fissure of
parenchyma and pel-
vis; gross hematuria

Tear in pelvis or
ureter; urinary
extravasation

Fig 16-1. Types and degrees of
renal injury.

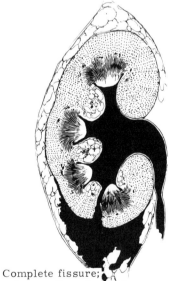

Complete fissure;
extravasation of
blood and urine;
gross hematuria

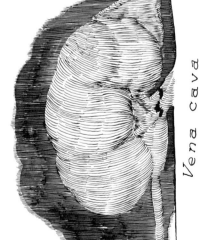

Laceration of renal
vascular pedicle with
severe perirenal
hemorrhage

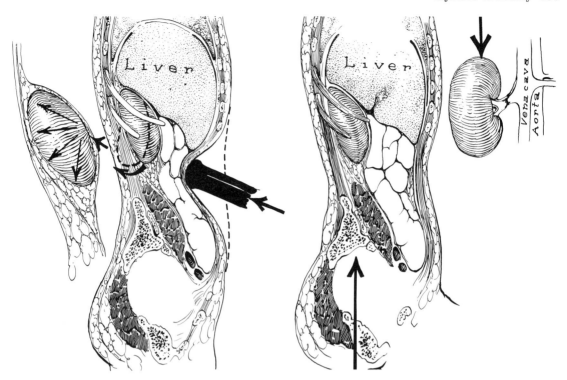

Fig 16-2. **Mechanisms of renal injury.** **Left:** Direct blow to abdomen. Inset shows force of blow radiating from the renal hilum. **Right:** Falling on buttocks from a height (contrecoup of kidney). Inset shows direction of force exerted upon the kidney from above. Tear of renal pedicle.

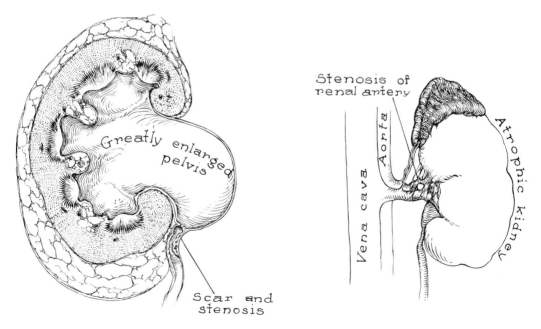

Fig 16-3. **Late pathology.** **Left:** Ureteropelvic stenosis with hydronephrosis secondary to fibrosis from extravasation of blood and urine. **Right:** Atrophy of kidney caused by injury (stenosis) of arterial blood supply.

symptoms localized to one flank and the finding of impaired function of that kidney are strongly suggestive. Extravasation of opaque medium, as shown on x-ray films, is diagnostic.

A. Symptoms: A history or evidence of physical injury is usually present. Pain in the renal area may be obscured by the severity of other injuries (ie, fractures or injury to other viscera). Gross hematuria, not necessarily proportionate to the severity of the injury, is usually noted with the first voiding. It may be intermittent or continuous. Nausea, vomiting, and abdominal distention due to intestinal ileus are common in the presence of retroperitoneal bleeding. Urinary retention may occur from clots in the bladder. Oliguria may accompany the hypotensive phase of shock. There may be symptoms of injuries to other organs.

B. Signs: Shock or signs of hemorrhage may be found with severe renal injury or in the presence of multiple injuries. Ecchymosis may be noted over the flank or back. Local tenderness is present. A mass in the flank may be caused by extravasation of blood or urine but if the overlying peritoneum has been torn these fluids may leak into the peritoneal cavity; hence, no flank mass develops. If local tenderness precludes careful palpation, percussion is invaluable. Rigidity of the abdominal muscles on the affected side and rebound

tenderness are common. Abdominal distention and hypoperistalsis are to be expected. The testicle on the ipsilateral side may be hypersensitive. The possibility of injuries to organs of the chest or of the abdomen should be explored. Fracture of the pelvis should cause one to suspect injury to the bladder or urethra.

C. Laboratory Findings: The hematocrit, especially when followed serially, is of the greatest importance; progressive anemia means progressive hemorrhage which may require heroic surgical intervention. Hematuria is present in almost all cases. It is usually marked at first. Infection may be found later if ureteral obstruction develops.

D. X-Ray Findings: A plain film of the abdomen may prove quite helpful. It may show increased grayness of the renal area, loss of renal and psoas shadows, scoliosis of the spine with concavity on the affected side; fractures of the transverse processes, spine, lower ribs, or pelvis; and changes in the bowel pattern compatible with paralytic ileus.

An upright film, if it can be taken, may reveal gas under the diaphragm because of rupture of the intestinal tract.

In the face of hypotension, infusion urography is the method of choice for visualizing the upper urinary tract. Excretory urograms should be obtained as soon as practicable (Fig

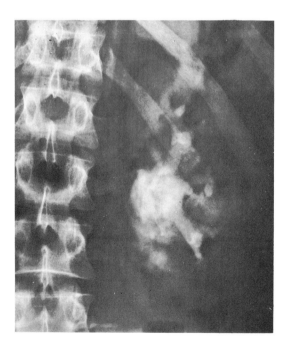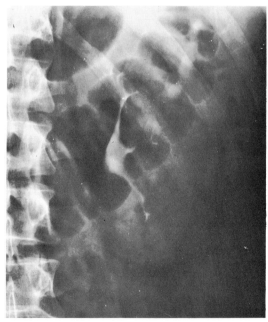

Fig 16-4. Renal injury. Left: Excretory urogram showing extravasation of radiopaque fluid. Conservative treatment. Right: Excretory urogram, same patient, 10 days later; normal urogram.

16-4). They may show a normal kidney on the opposite side (on more than one occasion a solitary kidney has been removed because of injury); normal function and configuration, if injury is minimal; delayed visualization, if injury (or hypotension) is present; deformed renal pelvis or calyces, if lacerations (or blood clots) have occurred; extravasation of dye within the renal shadow or into the perirenal space; and displacement or deformity of the pelvis or ureter from extrarenal extravasation of blood or urine. Nonvisualization does not necessarily mean severe damage. Lack of function may be secondary to shock or reflex in origin, even though damage is minimal.

Retrograde urograms delineate the degree of injury quite clearly, but they are seldom needed. In case of doubt as to the degree of injury, particularly of the major renal arteries, angiography should be considered. This procedure may reveal splenic or hepatic trauma as well.

E. Renal Scanning: Rectilinear scanning of the kidneys with ^{203}Hg has proved helpful in judging renal blood flow and tubular function. Lack of uptake implies injury or laceration of the renal artery. Areas of decreased activity are compatible with renal contusion. Absence of uptake in one renal pole suggests its amputation. The gamma camera affords more information, however. In addition to the changes observed with mercury, the hippurate shows areas of decreased or absent function as well as perirenal extravasation of the radioactive urine. Technetium study reveals absence of perfusion of blood into the kidney with injury to the renal artery or localized absence of activity if the kidney is fragmented (Fig 8-7).

F. Instrumental Examination: Cystoscopy and ureteral catheterization may be necessary. If excretory urography shows the contralateral kidney to be normal, there is no need to catheterize that side.

Differential Diagnosis

Trauma to the lumbar muscles or fractures of ribs, spine, or transverse processes may cause local symptoms suggesting renal injury. Hematuria is absent and urograms normal.

Complications

A. Early: The immediate complication of importance is perirenal hemorrhage, which may cause rapid exsanguination. The patient with an injured kidney must be observed closely. Blood pressure, pulse, and hematocrit should be taken frequently. Evidence of an enlarging mass must be sought. It is often helpful to outline a mass with ink on the skin so its progress can be followed. It must be remembered, however, that serious renal

trauma may be accompanied by a peritoneal tear which may allow the escape of blood and urine into the peritoneal cavity. Hence, the expected mass will not develop. In 70-80% of cases bleeding will stop spontaneously. If the kidney has been badly fractured, the degree of bleeding will warrant early surgery. Secondary bleeding and its accompanying shock may develop as late as a week or 2 following the injury.

Even though the extravasation of urine and the bleeding cease, secondary perirenal infection may supervene. Perirenal blood will cause fever to 37.5-38.3° C (100-101° F). Higher temperatures suggest infection. Increased pain and tenderness are to be expected. Abdominal muscle rigidity may become marked; rebound tenderness may develop. Edema of the skin over the back may be observed.

B. Later: The patient should be reexamined (including excretory urograms) after an interval of 3-6 months to determine the presence of progressive hydronephrosis from periureteral fibrosis, which may occur in the healing process; renal atrophy, if the blood supply has been impaired; and perirenal cyst, if complete absorption of the hematoma (or urinary extravasation) does not occur.

If thrombosis of the renal artery develops, hypertension secondary to the renal ischemia may supervene.

Treatment

A. Emergency Measures: Treat shock and hemorrhage.

B. Surgical Measures: Since two-thirds of injured kidneys are merely contused, bleeding will cease spontaneously. Even some of the ruptured organs will heal without surgical care (Fig 16-4). Ten to 20% of cases may require early surgical intervention because of alarming hemorrhage. Drainage of the perirenal space, suture of the renal laceration, partial nephrectomy, or nephrectomy may be necessary.

C. General Measures: Opiates for pain should be withheld until the completion of the diagnostic steps; they may mask accompanying intra-abdominal or pulmonary lesions. Bed rest is indicated until hematuria has ceased and local signs of injury have largely subsided.

D. Treatment of Complications: Perinephric infection requires surgical drainage. Late complications may require nephrectomy or repair of secondary ureteral obstruction.

Prognosis

In contusions of the kidney, the prognosis is excellent; they heal spontaneously and leave no demonstrable renal lesion. When rupture occurs, serious complications may supervene. It is important to follow these cases by periodic urography and blood pressure determinations for many months.

Evans, A., & R. A. Mogg: Renal artery thrombosis due to closed trauma. J Urol **105**: 330-4, 1971.

Halpern, M.: Angiography in renal trauma. S Clin North America **48**:1221-33, 1968.

Joachim, G. R., & E. L. Becker: Spontaneous rupture of the kidney. Arch Int Med **115**: 176-83, 1965.

Lang, E. K., & others: Arteriographic assessment of injury resulting from renal trauma. An analysis of 74 patients. J Urol **106**:1-8, 1971.

Mahoney, S. A., & L. Persky: Intravenous drip nephrotomography as an adjunct in the evaluation of renal injury. J Urol **99**:513-6, 1968.

Morrow, J. W., & R. Mendez: Renal trauma. J Urol **104**:649-53, 1970.

Morse, T. S., & others: Kidney injuries in children. J Urol **98**:539-47, 1967.

Prince, J. C., & C. K. Pearlman: Thrombosis of the renal artery secondary to trauma. J Urol **102**:670-4, 1969.

Redman, H. C., Reuter, S. R., & J. J. Bookstein: Angiography in abdominal trauma. Ann Surg **169**:57-66, 1969.

Scott, R., Jr., Carlton, C. E., Jr., & M. Goldman: Penetrating injuries of the kidney: An analysis of 181 patients. J Urol **101**:247-53, 1969.

Smith, M. J. V., Seidel, R. F., & A. F. Bonacarti: Accident trauma to the kidneys in children. J Urol **96**:845-7, 1966.

Vermillion, C. D., McLaughlin, A. P., & R. C. Pfister: Management of blunt renal trauma. J Urol **106**:478-84, 1971.

Woodruff, J. H., Jr., & others: Radiologic aspects of renal trauma with the emphasis on arteriography and renal isotope scanning. J Urol **97**:184-8, 1967.

INJURIES TO THE URETER

Injuries to the ureter from external violence or penetrating wounds are relatively rare. They usually occur accidentally during difficult and extensive gynecologic operations or during abdominoperineal resection of the rectum. They may also occur from cystoscopic ureteral manipulation.

Etiology

A large pelvic tumor may displace a ureter far from its usual site. In this instance the surgeon may inadvertently cut it. Marked inflammatory adhesions may make the ureter hard to identify, in which case it may be easily injured during surgery. If a ureter is invaded by tumor of the rectum, colon, or ovary, it may have to be resected with the tumor. Extensive lymph node dissection or x-ray therapy to the area may impair ureteral blood supply, and necrosis may follow.

A ureter may be injured by a penetrating object (eg, a bullet), causing urinary extravasation. Injury to neighboring viscera must be sought. The ureter may be perforated by the cystoscopist, particularly if the ureteral wall is diseased. This occurs most commonly in association with manipulation of a ureteral stone.

Pathogenesis and Pathology

If the ureter is completely or partially divided during surgery but the surgeon is unaware of the accident, urinary extravasation will occur. Extravasation may be intraperitoneal or extraperitoneal. A urinary fistula may form between the severed ureter and the surgical wound or the vagina, or an enlarging collection of urine at the site of the injury will become evident. If the urine becomes infected, signs of peritonitis or cellulitis will develop. If uninfected, urine in the free peritoneal cavity may cause few symptoms other than gradual abdominal distention from the urine itself. Some degree of ureteral compression or stenosis is to be expected with ureteral injury; this leads to hydronephrosis.

Should the ureter be inadvertently sutured or ligated, progressive hydronephrosis will develop. Renal infection may then occur. Because of ischemia, the ureter may slough at the site of ligation. Delayed extravasation or fistula formation may then be observed.

Clinical Findings

A. Symptoms: If the accident is not recognized at the time of surgery, the patient usually complains of pain in the flank and lower abdominal quadrant. Vomiting may be severe. Paralytic ileus is often marked. The patient will become quite ill if pyelonephritis or peritonitis complicates the picture. Urine may suddenly begin to drain through the abdominal or perirenal wound or through the vagina, which may relieve all the foregoing symptoms. Anuria following pelvic surgery suggests bilateral ureteral injury or occlusion.

B. Signs: Abdominal distention and lack of peristalsis are evident if ileus is marked. Signs of peritonitis (rebound tenderness) may be noted if there is leakage of urine into the free peritoneal cavity. Urine may be seen draining from the surgical wound or vagina. If there is any question about whether the fluid is actually urine, the patient can be given 0.2 gm of methylene blue by mouth or 5 ml of indigo carmine IV. The injection of the latter causes transient hypertension. Both are excreted by the kidney and stain the urine. Vaginal examination may reveal the site of the urinary fistula.

C. Laboratory Findings: Blood count and urinalysis contribute little to the diagnosis. The PSP may be slightly depressed if one ureter is occluded. The serum creatinine will rise quickly if bilateral ureteral obstruction is present.

D. X-Ray Findings: A plain film of the abdomen may reveal a large area of increased density in the region of the injured ureter due to a large collection of extravasated urine. Excretory urograms may demonstrate extravasation of the radiopaque fluid at the site of injury (Fig 16-5). When the injury is near the bladder, however, it may be confused with a vesicovaginal fistula. Ureteral injuries are usually associated with some degree of ureteral obstruction; thus, hydronephrosis and hydroureter down to the point of trauma are to be expected.

If the ureter is completely occluded as a result of recent injury, no radiopaque material will collect in the renal pelvis, but progressive increase in density of the renal parenchyma may be observed on the later films.

Retrograde ureterograms will show the site and degree of the injury.

E. Isotope Scanning: (See chapter 8.) If one ureter has been ligated, the radioisotope renogram will show a further increase of counts, rather than a drop off after the secretory phase due to accumulation of urine in the renal pelvis (Fig 8-8). The scintillation camera, using ^{131}I, will show slow transport of the isotope to the pelvis where the photon activity will become intense because of stasis.

F. Instrumental Examination: Cystoscopy and ureteral catheterization demonstrate patency or obstruction and afford ureterograms and pyelograms (Fig 16-5).

Differential Diagnosis

Postoperative peritonitis may be mimicked by ureteral injury if there is leakage of infected urine into the peritoneal cavity. Ureteral

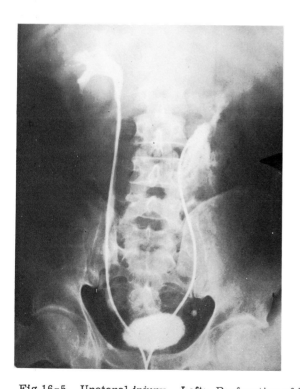 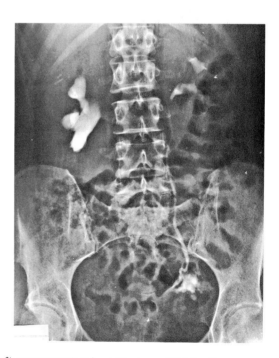

Fig 16-5. Ureteral injury. Left: Perforation of left upper ureter by catheter. **Right:** Carcinoma of cervix; preoperative irradiation therapy and Wertheim operation. Partial ureteral obstruction on right (hydronephrosis), ureterovaginal fistula on left. Site of ureteral fistula demonstrated.

catheterization or excretory urograms should make the differentiation clear.

Oliguria may be due to dehydration or bilateral but incomplete ureteral injury. A survey of fluid and electrolyte intake and output (urinary, gastrointestinal, and invisible losses), body weight, PSP test, hematocrit, and the urinary specific gravity should establish the diagnosis with regard to dehydration. Immediate total anuria means bilateral obstruction. The isotope renogram or the camera scan should contribute useful information.

Acute renal failure, due to shock or transfusion with incompatible blood, also causes oliguria. It may be differentiated from surgical ureteral injury by finding no more than a trace of PSP excretion in 1 hour, and fixation of the urinary chloride concentration at 30-40 mEq/liter. In case of doubt, ureteral catheterization will be definitive. Isotope studies are also helpful.

Evisceration may be confused with ureteral injury since the early sign of eventration is the onset of profuse drainage of clear, odorless transudate from the wound which may be mistaken for urine. In case of doubt, the skin should be opened widely and the peritoneal rent sought.

Vesicovaginal and ureterovaginal fistulas both present with urinary drainage from the vagina. Methylene blue solution instilled into the bladder will be found in the vagina only if vesicovaginal fistula is present. Cystoscopy should visualize the defect in the base of the bladder.

Complications

Complications of ureteral injury include urinary fistula, ureteral stenosis with hydronephrosis, renal infection; peritonitis, if urine drains into the peritoneal cavity; and uremia, if the injury is bilateral.

Treatment

Reparative surgery should be undertaken as soon as the injury is recognized. In simple perforation from a ureteral catheter or other instrument, surgical drainage is not necessary. The ureteral wall will heal spontaneously.

A. Immediate: The ureter should not be tied off. The ureteral tip usually undergoes necrosis, and fistula results. If the tie holds, progressive hydronephrosis is inevitable.

The following surgical methods are available if the injury is recognized when it occurs:

1. Anastomosis of the 2 ends over a catheter or ''T'' tube.

2. Implantation of the proximal end of the ureter into the bladder (ureteroneocystostomy), or into a tube formed from a bladder flap if a segment of the ureter has been resected. The injured ureter can also be anastomosed into the side of the contralateral ureter.

3. If a bladder flap tube cannot be made long enough, the defect can be replaced with an isolated section of ileum.

4. Temporary ureterostomy or nephrostomy, if the patient's condition does not permit primary anastomosis, preserves kidney function and permits elective repair later.

B. Late: If the injury is discovered during the postoperative period, early intervention is indicated before the inflammatory reaction becomes severe or fibrosis occurs. If delayed ureteral repair is attempted, the methods available are end-to-end anastomosis, implantation of the ureter into the bladder or into a bladder flap, transureteroureterostomy, and replacement of the damaged ureter with an isolated ileal segment. Autotransplantation of the kidney into the iliac fossa has been accomplished for high ureteral injury. Nephrectomy may be indicated if the other kidney is normal.

Prevention

The surgeon must be careful to identify the ureters when extensive pelvic surgery is done. In case of doubt, the surgeon should perform a high longitudinal ureterotomy and pass a catheter down the ureter. This area should be drained extraperitoneally. In difficult cases, preliminary to surgery, indwelling ureteral catheters should be placed so that the ureters may be easily felt. The insignificant risks in such a maneuver are greatly outweighed by the advantages.

Prognosis

Prognosis is best in those injuries repaired at the time they are sustained. Patients operated upon within the first week following injury usually achieve good ureteral repair. After marked fibrosis has developed the results are not very good; nephrectomy may be required.

Calame, R. J., & J. H. Nelson, Jr.: Ureterovaginal fistula as a complication of radical pelvic surgery. Arch Surg 94:876-80, 1967.

Carlton, C. E., Jr., Scott, R., Jr., & A. G. Guthrie: The initial management of ureteral injuries: A report of 78 cases. J Urol 105: 335-40, 1971.

Goldstein, A. G., & K. B. Conger: Perforation of the ureter during retrograde pyelography. J Urol 94:658-64, 1965.

Gross, M., Peng, B., & K. Waterhouse: Use of the mobilized bladder to replace the pelvic ureter. J Urol 101:40-4, 1969.

Hardy, J. D.: High ureteral injuries. Management by autotransplantation of the kidney. JAMA 184:97-101, 1963.

Hulse, C. A., & others: Conservative management of ureterovaginal fistula. J Urol **99**: 42-9, 1968.

Lee, R. A., & R. E. Symmonds: Ureterovaginal fistula. Am J Obst Gynec **109**:1032-5, 1971.

Walker, J. A.: Injuries of the ureter due to external violence. J Urol **102**:410-3, 1969.

Wesolowsky, S.: Bilateral ureteral injuries in gynecology. Brit J Urol **41**:666-75, 1969.

Williams, J. L., & R. W. Porter: The Boari bladder flap in lower ureteric injuries. Brit J Urol **38**:528-33, 1966.

INJURIES TO THE BLADDER

The urinary bladder may be injured by external forces; during surgery, including accidental incision in pelvic surgery or in the repair of hernia; and in transurethral manipulations.

Rupture of the bladder caused by a direct blow presupposes a bladder distended with urine. It can also be perforated by bony spicules from a fractured pelvis.

Pathogenesis and Pathology

A sudden blow to the full bladder causes a sharp rise in intravesical pressure; this may either contuse the wall or split it (Fig 16-6). With such an injury, the extravasation of urine is usually intraperitoneal. If the vesical contents are infected, death from peritonitis will occur unless the laceration is closed surgically or seals itself spontaneously. If the urine is sterile, few symptoms may develop immediately although anuria with uremia becomes obvious and "ascites" develops as the urine progressively fills the peritoneal cavity. If this urine becomes infected (following catheterization or cystoscopy or from bacteria carried there by the blood stream), true peritonitis supervenes. A few cases of spontaneous rupture have been reported. This presupposes obstruction distal to the bladder.

Vesical lacerations secondary to fracture of the pelvis cause extraperitoneal extravasation of urine. If this urine is infected or later becomes so, a spreading cellulitis develops and death occurs unless adequate drainage is afforded. Rupture and perforation of the bladder, then, are fatal injuries unless treated promptly.

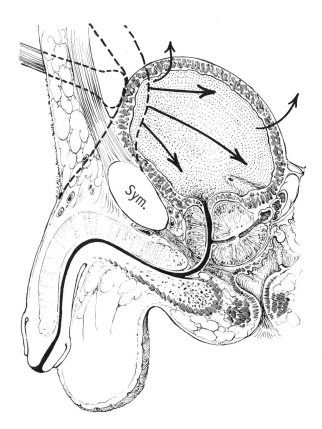

Fig 16-6. Mechanism of vesical injury. A direct blow over the full bladder causes increased intravesical pressure. If the bladder ruptures it will usually rupture into the peritoneal cavity.

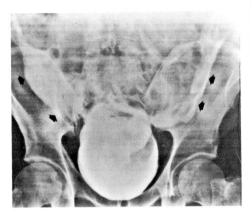
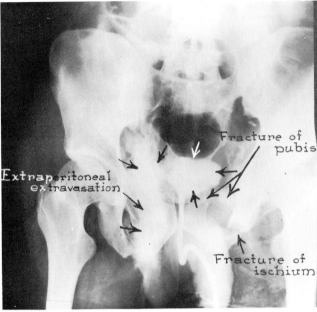

Fig 16-7. Vesical injuries. Left: Retrograde cystogram showing intraperitoneal extravasation. Note radiopaque material in both lumbar gutters. **Right:** Retrograde cystogram showing extraperitoneal rupture of the bladder secondary to fracture of the pelvis.

Clinical Findings

A history of an injury or blow to the lower abdomen followed by low abdominal pain and hematuria is strongly suggestive of vesical injury. Fracture of the pelvis is commonly accompanied by injury to the bladder. The finding of suprapubic tenderness or a mass is suggestive; signs of peritonitis may be elicited. Cystography is the most dependable test. If, however, clinical judgment suggests the presence of vesical trauma, even a normal cystogram should be ignored.

A. Symptoms: There is usually a history of injury. If the patient can urinate, hematuria is to be expected, but he may not be able to urinate at all. Pain is present low in the abdomen. Pain in the shoulder may be noted if there is urine in the peritoneal cavity. High fever suggests infection.

B. Signs: Shock may be profound, especially if multiple injuries have been suffered. There may be evidence of local trauma, eg, a bullet or knife wound, or ecchymosis. Marked tenderness in the suprapubic area is to be expected. There may be rebound tenderness if the laceration involves the peritoneum. Spasm of the muscles of the lower abdomen occurs even though the extravasation is perivesical. A board-like abdomen suggests intraperitoneal rupture. The skin over the symphysis commonly becomes quite cool immediately after

rupture occurs. A large suprapubic mass may be felt or percussed as the perivesical collection of fluid develops. This will contain blood, urine, and sometimes pus. Rectal examination may reveal a large boggy mass obliterating the normal landmarks. Evidence of other injuries is usually present.

C. Laboratory Findings: The hematocrit may demonstrate anemia from loss of blood or hemoconcentration from shock. The white blood count and neutrophils are increased. Urinalysis reveals hematuria, either gross or microscopic. The presence of bacteria means infection, either preexisting or new. If a significant amount of urine escapes into the peritoneal cavity, the serum BUN/creatinine ratio is significantly increased.

D. X-Ray Findings: A plain film may reveal fractures of the pelvic bones. About 15% of patients with a fractured pelvis will have a vesical injury (Fig 16-7). Increased grayness from a perivesical collection of urine and blood may be seen. Excretory urograms will be helpful in surveying the kidneys for damage. Extravasation of the opaque material may be noted in the perivesical tissues. The bladder may be displaced by extravesical blood or urine.

A cystogram is the most dependable test for vesical injury (Fig 16-7). Instill 350-400 ml of radiopaque fluid and take anteroposterior and oblique films. Then drain the vesical contents and take another film. This may reveal small amounts of extravasated fluid lying behind the bladder or in the cul-de-sac.

E. Instrumental Examination: The passage of a catheter will detect possible injury to the urethra. If an injured person cannot void, he should be catheterized. The presence of bloody urine must be investigated.

If 350-500 ml of sterile solution is instilled into the bladder and the full amount is recovered, the bladder is probably intact. On occasion, however, this may afford erroneous information; omentum or blood clot may temporarily plug the laceration.

Cystoscopy is usually not very helpful. Bleeding and clots may obscure vision, and a laceration may be missed.

Differential Diagnosis

Hematuria and signs of injury to abdominal organs can also arise from an injured kidney. A mass and tenderness in the flank and evidence of fractures in the renal area are suggestive of renal injury. Changes on a plain film of the abdomen or on excretory urograms should establish the diagnosis. A normal cystogram will relieve any lingering doubt.

Urethral injury may accompany fractures of the pelvis. Exploration of the urethra with a catheter is helpful, and a urethrogram will show extravasation through the injured wall.

Complications

In extraperitoneal rupture the extravasation of large amounts of blood and urine is often complicated by infection. If untreated, a necrotizing phlegmon ensues; the mortality rate in this instance is high. Abdominal or peritoneal fistulas may develop.

In intraperitoneal rupture, if the urine becomes infected generalized peritonitis occurs. If this is untreated, death is to be expected.

Treatment

A. Emergency Measures: Treat shock and hemorrhage.

B. Specific Measures:
1. Extraperitoneal rupture - If the rupture is extraperitoneal, the site of the injury should be drained surgically. Urologists as a rule favor suprapubic cystostomy as a more reliable method than catheterization for keeping the bladder empty and at rest. The peritoneum should be opened and intraperitoneal organs explored for associated injury.
2. Intraperitoneal rupture - When the tear is intraperitoneal, it should be closed transperitoneally. If the point of rupture is inaccessible, suprapubic cystostomy permits

healing without complications. Extravasated fluid in the peritoneal cavity should be aspirated. Injury to other organs should be sought.

Prognosis

If the diagnosis is made and proper treatment instituted within 6-12 hours after the injury, morbidity and mortality will be minimal. If treatment is delayed for a few days, perivesical infection or peritonitis may develop and may not be controllable; the number of deaths under these circumstances will be significant.

Dhall, G.I., Dhall, K., & I.C. Pathak: Massive hematuria after obstructed labor. Obst Gynec 28:360-2, 1966.

Flaherty, J.J., & others: Relationship of pelvic bone fracture patterns to injuries of urethra and bladder. J Urol 99:297-300, 1968.

Graber, E.A., O'Rourke, J.J., & T. McElrath: Iatrogenic bladder injury during hysterectomy. Obst Gynec 23:267-73, 1964.

Kamat, M.H., Corgan, F.J., & J.J. Seebode: Spontaneous rupture of the bladder. Arch Surg 100:735-7, 1970.

Ko, K.W., Randolph, J., & F.X. Fellers: Peritoneal self-dialysis following traumatic rupture of the bladder. J Urol 91:343-6, 1964.

Reid, R.E., & J.R. Herman: Rupture of the bladder and urethra: Diagnosis and treatment. New York J Med 65:2685-96, 1965.

Thompson, I.M., Johnson, E.L., & G. Ross, Jr.: The acute abdomen of unrecognized bladder rupture. Arch Surg 90:371-4, 1965.

INJURIES TO THE URETHRA

The various parts of the urethra can be contused, lacerated, or avulsed. Injuries to the deep urethra are the most serious and are often associated with fracture of the pelvis. Urethral stricture is a common complication.

Because treatment and sequelae vary with the nature and site of the trauma, these injuries are discussed as injuries to the membranous urethra, the bulbous urethra, and the pendulous urethra.

1. INJURIES TO THE MEMBRANOUS URETHRA

Etiology

The urogenital diaphragm (ie, triangular ligament) encloses the membranous urethra, Cowper's glands, and the external urinary

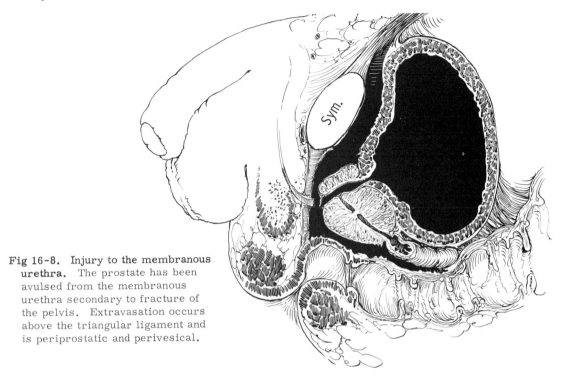

Fig 16-8. Injury to the membranous urethra. The prostate has been avulsed from the membranous urethra secondary to fracture of the pelvis. Extravasation occurs above the triangular ligament and is periprostatic and perivesical.

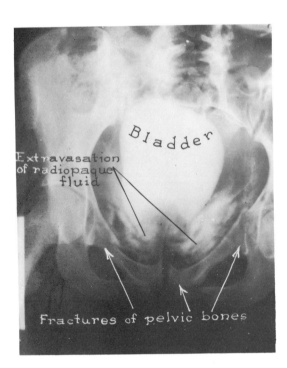

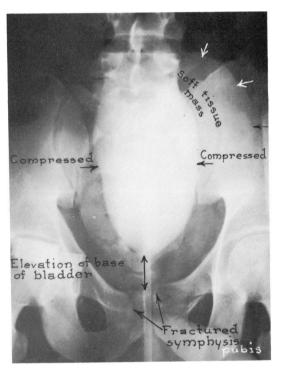

Fig 16-9. Injury to the membranous urethra. Left: Retrograde cystogram showing periprostatic extravasation; laceration of membranous urethra with fracture of pelvis. **Right:** Retrograde cystogram showing elevation and lateral compression of bladder due to periprostatic and perivesical extravasation of blood and urine; laceration of membranous urethra from fracture of pelvis.

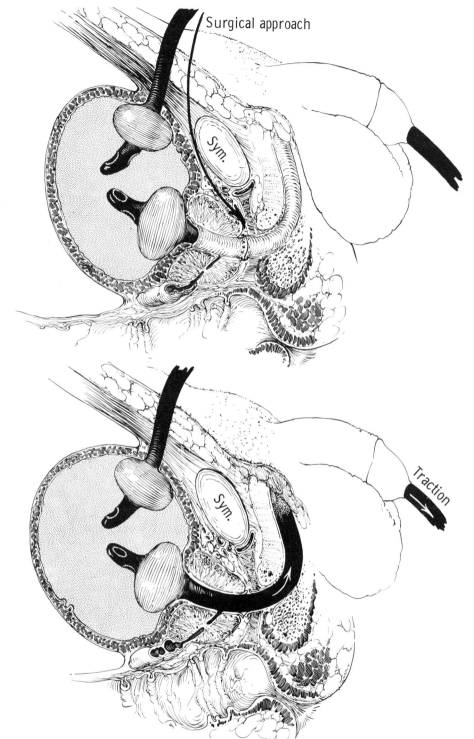

Fig 16-10. Methods of repair of injuries of the membranous urethra. Above: Retropubic exposure and suture of membranous urethra over an indwelling catheter; suprapubic cystostomy. **Below:** If suture of the urethra is not feasible, a Foley (self-retaining) catheter should be placed and traction exerted on the catheter in order to appose the ends of the divided urethra. Tying the ends of the 2 catheters together with braided silk will guard against dislodgment of the urethral catheter should its bag deflate.

sphincter. It is firmly attached to the pubic bone. In pelvic fractures, this fascia may be torn, shearing off the prostate from the membranous urethra. Bony spicules may perforate the urethra, and the bladder also may be lacerated.

Pathogenesis and Pathology (See Fig 16-8.)

These injuries usually occur in association with trauma to other organs or structures. They occur just above the urogenital diaphragm. This causes extravasation of blood and urine into the periprostatic and perivesical tissues. Only if the triangular ligament is badly damaged will the extravasation present in the perineum. The extravasated urine leads to a necrotizing phlegmon which may become infected. If this is not properly treated, early death may ensue from sepsis.

Clinical Findings

A. Symptoms: Urethral bleeding may be noted. A history of injury, usually severe, is always obtained. Pain is present in the perineum or low in the abdomen. The patient may be unable to void.

B. Signs: Urethral bleeding or hematuria is present. There may be a mass in the suprapubic area. The area may be dull to percussion. Suprapubic tenderness may be marked. This may be due to extravasation or to a fracture of the pelvis with associated hematoma. Rectal examination may reveal a large boggy mass of extravasated blood and urine. The prostate may be dislodged upward if it has been avulsed from the membranous urethra (Fig 16-8).

C. Laboratory Findings: There may be anemia from hemorrhage or hemoconcentration from shock. The white blood cell count is elevated, especially if infection has supervened. The urine usually is grossly bloody. In the case of minor contusions, hematuria may be only microscopic.

D. X-Ray Findings: A fracture of the pelvis may be shown on a plain x-ray film. Twenty to 30 ml of radiopaque fluid should be instilled into the catheter passed to the point of arrest. An x-ray will show the site of extravasation (Fig 16-9). If the catheter passes to the bladder, a cystogram should be taken to demonstrate vesical injury.

E. Instrumental Examination: If a catheter can be passed to the bladder, the urethral lesion is minor. In more extensive injuries, the catheter may be arrested at the site of injury.

Differential Diagnosis

Vesical and urethral injuries are apt to occur following severe trauma and fracture of the pelvis. Rectal examination may reveal that the prostate is riding free from the membranous urethra. In the latter instance a catheter will not pass. The instillation of radiopaque fluid and the taking of appropriate x-rays will reveal the true site of injury.

In injury to the bulbous urethra there is perineal swelling due to blood, urine, or both. A urethrogram is diagnostic.

Complications

Hemorrhage about the prostate and bladder may be marked in the early stages. Urinary extravasation may occur if the patient is unable to urinate. This may lead to severe sepsis if diagnosis is late.

Urethral stricture is a common late complication. This is particularly true if proper treatment is not instituted early. Sexual impotence (loss of erection) may develop in one-third of men, probably as a result of nerve injury. Impaired control of urination occasionally results. This may be due to direct injury to the external sphincter or may be secondary to nerve damage.

Treatment

A. Emergency Measures: Treat shock and hemorrhage.

B. Specific Measures: If a urethral catheter of adequate size (22-24 F) can be successfully passed to the bladder, it should be left in place for 14-21 days. Simple lacerations usually heal well with only this simple splinting. If a catheter cannot be passed to the bladder, surgical intervention is imperative. The principles of treatment include the following:

1. Suture the injured urethra if possible and then place a splinting urethral catheter (24-28 F) in the bladder (Fig 16-10). The catheter should be left in place for 3 weeks.

2. If repair by suture cannot be done, an indwelling catheter of the self-retaining type should be placed under vision; 1 pound of traction upon the external end of the catheter will bring about apposition of the ruptured urethra (Fig 16-10). The catheter should be left in place for 3 weeks.

3. Drains should be placed down to the site of injury and left in place for 7-10 days.

C. General Measures: If treatment has been instituted late and sepsis is already present, broad-spectrum antibiotics should be used as a life-saving measure as well as to minimize fibrous reaction. Analgesics and sedation should be used as indicated.

D. Treatment of Complications: It must be assumed that all patients suffering from deep urethral injuries will develop strictures. It is therefore necessary to get urethrograms or pass urethral sounds periodically for as long as 6-12 months in order to discover the development of a stricture. If stricture does occur, definitive treatment is required.

There is no treatment that will correct loss of erections. Little can be done for the patient with impaired sphincteric function.

Prognosis

Unless other serious injuries have been sustained, the mortality rate for injury to the membranous urethra is quite low; this is true even though perivesical phlegmon has developed because of delayed treatment. The antibiotics are successful in combating this.

The most troublesome complication is urethral stricture, which may require the periodic passage of a sound for the rest of the patient's life. Surgical correction of the stricture may be necessary. If this is not done, chronic infection of the bladder and even of the kidneys may develop; vesical and renal stones may form because of stasis and complicating infection.

Cullum, P. A.: Rupture of the male bladder and posterior urethra following external violence. Brit J Surg ,54:258-65, 1967.

Gibson, G. R.: Impotence following fractured pelvis and ruptured urethra. Brit J Urol **42**:86-8, 1970.

Kaiser, T. F., & F. C. Farrow: Injury of the bladder and prostatomembranous urethra associated with fracture of the bony pelvis. Surg Gynec Obst **120**:97-112, 1965.

Ragde, H., & G. F. McInnes: Transpubic repair of severed prostatomembranous urethra. J Urol **101**:335-7, 1969.

Reid, R. E., & J. R. Herman: Rupture of the bladder and urethra; diagnosis and treatment. New York J Med **65**:2685-96, 1965.

2. INJURIES TO THE BULBOUS URETHRA

Etiology

Injuries to the bulbous urethra, which lies just inferior to the urogenital diaphragm, may result from instrumentation but are most commonly caused by forcibly falling astride an object. The urethra is apt to be contused or lacerated (Fig 16-11).

Pathogenesis and Pathology

A. Contusion: If the urethra is only contused, some evidence of perineal hematoma may be noted. In all probability, this will resolve without sequelae. A large hematoma might require drainage. Mild stricture, caused by healing, may result from the fibrosis.

B. If laceration occurs, blood and urine extravasate into the perineum; if extravasation is extensive it spreads to the scrotum and penis, then up the abdominal wall. It is limited by Colles' fascia (Figs 1-9 and 16-11). Serious infection ensues if diagnosis is late. If the laceration is untreated, stricture formation is inevitable.

Clinical Findings

A. Symptoms: A history of perineal injury, either external or by a urethral instrument, can usually be obtained. There is local pain and some bleeding from the external meatus. If a urethral tear is present, an attempt at urination may cause sudden perineal swelling from extravasation. If the patient is seen a few days after the accident there may be symptoms of severe sepsis (eg, fever, prostration).

B. Signs: Some urethral bleeding may be seen. Its degree is not necessarily a measure of the severity of the injury. Local tenderness is present in the perineum. A large mass may be found locally. This may represent blood, urine, or both. If seen late, swelling and discoloration of the skin of the scrotum, penis, and lower abdominal wall may be noted. This represents extensive extravasation and at times inflammation.

C. Laboratory Findings: Anemia is not common, for blood loss is usually not excessive. The WBC may be markedly elevated, particularly if secondary infection of the perineum, genitalia, and abdominal wall has developed. Blood is present in the urine if the patient is able to void.

D. X-Ray Findings: The instillation of 20-30 ml of radiopaque fluid into the urethra will demonstrate the site and degree of the injury (Fig 16-12).

E. Instrumental Examination: A catheter may pass to the bladder if the urethra is merely contused or lacerated on one side. If the catheter is arrested, the injury is more serious.

Differential Diagnosis

Laceration or avulsion of the membranous urethra often accompanies fracture of the pelvis. The extravasation of blood and urine in this type is almost always above the urogenital diaphragm, whereas that from the bulb is into

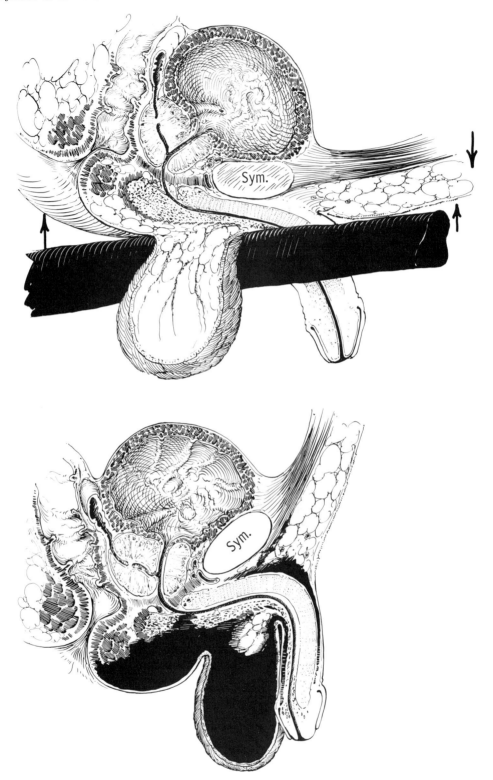

Fig 16-11. **Injury to the bulbous urethra.** **Above:** Mechanism: Usually a perineal blow or fall astride an object; crushing of urethra against inferior edge of symphysis pubis. **Below:** Extravasation of blood and urine enclosed within Colles' fascia (Fig 1-9).

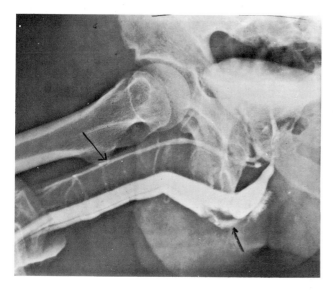

Fig 16-12. **Urethral injury.** Oblique urethrogram showing extravasation in region of bulbous urethra. Pressure injection caused radiopaque solution to enter venous system. (This is the mechanism for emboli if oily lubricants are injected into the urethra.)

the perineum and external genitalia. A urethrogram will solve the problem.

Complications

Considerable bleeding from injury to the corpus spongiosum may occur early. If the urethra is ruptured, urinary extravasation occurs when the patient attempts to urinate.

Stricture at the site of trauma is a common late complication, particularly in the more severe injuries.

Treatment

A. Specific Measures:

1. Nonobstructed urethra - If the patient can void well and the perineal hematoma is not extensive, the injury should be left alone. The blood will almost surely be absorbed, and the contused urethra will heal. If the hematoma becomes infected, it should be drained. Later, urethral sounds must be passed or urethrograms done to be sure that stricture does not develop. If stricture should occur, periodic dilation or even surgical repair will be required (see p 383).

2. Severe injuries - If there is urinary extravasation, or if urination is impossible, an attempt should be made to pass a catheter to the bladder. If this is successful the catheter should be left in place for 3 weeks. If it is not successful (due to more severe urethral injury), surgical exploration and repair are required. A splinting catheter should be left in the urethra for 3 weeks.

3. Extensive extravasation - If urinary extravasation is extensive, these areas (perineum, scrotum, lower abdominal wall) must also be drained. It is questionable, however,

whether the radical drainage formerly prescribed is still necessary now that potent antibiotics are available.

The urethral caliber must be observed during the next few months. If stenosis develops, the stricture must be treated (see p 383).

4. Very severe injuries - If the patient has been badly hurt, suprapubic cystostomy and drainage of the perineum may be all that can be accomplished initially; later it may be necessary to resect the stenotic portion of the urethra and anastomose its healthy ends. Postoperative stricture must be sought and, if present, treated.

B. General Measures: When the urethral injury is adjudged minor and no specific treatment is indicated, antimicrobial drugs are not warranted. If urinary extravasation has occurred, antimicrobials should be administered.

Prognosis

Mortality is low unless there are more severe injuries to other structures. Antibiotics will almost always save the patient with urinary extravasation, even if it has been initially neglected.

Urethral stricture is the only serious complication. If this is not treated, urinary tract infection and its complications (stone, renal damage) may ensue.

Ezell, W.W., & others: Mechanical traumatic injury to the genitalia in children. J Urol **102**:788-92, 1969.

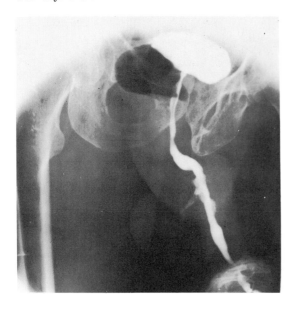

Fig 16-13. Urethral injury. Urethrogram showing extravasation of a radiopaque material from lacerated pendulous urethra at penoscrotal junction.

3. INJURIES TO THE PENDULOUS URETHRA

Etiology

Injuries to the penile urethra from direct blows are not common since the penis, except during erection, tends to "ride" with a blow. The erect organ may, however, be fractured and the urethra become torn.

The urethra is most often injured by injudicious instrumentation. The most common injury of this sort is the perforating injury that may result when a metal sound of small caliber is being passed to dilate a stricture. The pendulous urethra may also sustain injury from penetrating wounds.

Pathogenesis and Pathology

These injuries are usually mild and little more than contusions. Some periurethral bleeding may develop, but this is usually quickly absorbed. The urethra may be injured by the passage of the resectoscope (size 28 F) used for transurethral prostatectomy. Postoperative stricture may ensue.

Clinical Findings

A. Symptoms and Signs: Some urethral bleeding is to be expected. Swelling of the pendulous portion of the penis is common.

B. Laboratory Findings: If the patient can urinate, red cells are found in the urine.

C. X-Ray Findings: A urethrogram may reveal the site of injury, although extravasation is rare with these injuries (Fig 16-13).

D. Instrumental Examination: Attempts to pass a catheter may fail if the laceration is extensive.

Differential Diagnosis

Swellings from lesions of the bulb are in the perineum; swellings from injuries to the distal urethra are local. In case of doubt, a urethrogram will demonstrate the site of the injury.

Complications

Large hematomas and urinary extravasation are not common unless the urethra has been badly torn. Urethral stenosis may develop as the urethra heals.

Treatment

A. Specific Measures: If urination proceeds normally, an indwelling catheter is not needed. Small hematomas will be absorbed. Large ones may require drainage. If bleeding is profuse, a catheter can be passed and the penis then tightly bandaged to prevent further bleeding. If a small amount of urine should pass into the tissues, it will be absorbed; if it is extensive, surgical drainage is indicated. When extravasation of urine occurs, a catheter should be passed to the bladder and left in place for 10 days. If the injury is severe and if passage of a catheter is unsuccessful, surgical repair of the injured urethra is indicated. A splinting catheter should be left in place for 14 days.

B. General Measures: Antibacterial drugs are not needed unless infection has occurred.

Prognosis

These injuries are usually not serious. The only sequel of note is urethral stricture, the complications of which can be serious. These include chronic infection of the urinary tract and urolithiasis.

Blumberg, N.: Anterior urethral injuries. J Urol **102**:210-3, 1969.

INJURIES TO THE PENIS

The penis may be injured by a penetrating object (eg, knife, bullet) or by a blow when the organ is erect. The placement of a constricting band about the shaft (eg, metal washer, string, rubber band) can also cause injury from ischemia which may lead to gangrene.

The skin may be lacerated or even avulsed if caught in machinery. One or more of the corpora can be ruptured, in which case profuse bleeding may occur beneath Colles' fascia; this may spread over the scrotum, perineum, and up over the lower abdomen. Pressure from swelling may lead to gangrene. Associated urethral injury is not uncommon.

The history of injury is usually obtainable. The skin may be lacerated or avulsed. Great swelling from bleeding may be evident. Edema distal to a constricting band may be marked. The bleeding from laceration or contusion will usually cease spontaneously. Large hematomas may require evacuation.

Constricting bodies must of course be removed. Immediate or late urethral injury should be sought. Extensive loss of skin will require skin grafting.

Fleming, J. P.: Reconstruction of the penis. J Urol **104**:213-8, 1970.
Kendall, A. R., & L. Karafin: Repair of the denuded penis. J Urol **98**:484-6, 1967.
Meares, E. M., Jr.: Traumatic rupture of the corpus cavernosum. J Urol **105**:407-8, 1971.
Shiraki, I. W., & B. E. Trichel: Traumatic dislocation of the penis. J Urol **101**:186-8, 1969.

INJURIES TO THE SCROTUM

Local injuries or blows may cause ecchymosis or hematoma. They are not serious and heal spontaneously. Lacerations may need suture; avulsion will require skin grafts.

Millard, R., Jr.: Scrotal construction and reconstruction. Plast Reconstr Surg **33**: 10-5, 1966.

INJURIES TO THE TESTIS

Because of their mobility, the testes are seldom injured. If traumatized, the patient experiences severe pain. Nausea and vomiting are common, and shock may result. The injury may be a mild contusion or the testis may be lacerated, in which case bleeding into the tunica vaginalis (hematocele) may be profuse. Only in the latter case is surgical intervention required; suture of the tear is imperative.

On rare occasion a severe local injury may dislocate the testicle into the abdomen, penis, perineum, or adjacent areas. Replacement in the scrotum requires surgical intervention.

Even mild wounds may result in thrombosis of blood vessels which leads to atrophy of the testis. Penetrating wounds will require closure of the scrotal and testicular incisions.

Gross, M.: Rupture of the testicle: The importance of early surgical treatment. J Urol **101**:196-7, 1969.
McCormack, J. L., Kretz, A. W., & R. Tocantins: Traumatic rupture of the testicle. J Urol **96**:80-2, 1966.
Merricks, J. W., & F. B. Papierniak: Traumatic rupture of the testicle. J Urol **103**: 77-9, 1970.
Sethi, R. S., & W. Singh: Traumatic dislocation of testes. J Urol **98**:501-2, 1967.

OBSTETRIC INJURIES TO THE URETHRA AND BLADDER

If there is disproportion between the circumference of the baby's head and the mother's pelvis and if labor is therefore prolonged, urethral ischemia may occur. Necrosis may cause a urethrovaginal (or vesicovaginal) fistula. Improperly placed forceps may tear these urologic structures. Surgical repair is required.

Because of attenuation of supporting tissues of the urethra and base of the bladder during delivery, weakness of these structures develops. Thus the urethra and bladder sag into the vagina (urethrocele, cystocele), and stress incontinence results. Operations to improve the support of the urethra and vesical base or to elevate and fix the bladder neck usually relieve this distressing symptom.

•   •   •

17 . . .

*Tumors of the Genitourinary Tract**

Neoplasms of the prostate gland, bladder, and kidney are among the most common abnormal growths which afflict the human body. They are often silent, so that diagnosis may not be possible until quite late. Tumors of the testis are highly malignant and afflict young men. Neoplasms of the ureter, penis, scrotum, epididymis, and seminal vesicle are rare.

MANIFESTATIONS OF UROGENITAL TRACT NEOPLASMS

Hematuria

Gross or microscopic hematuria is common when ulceration of a vesical, ureteral or renal pelvic neoplasm occurs or when a renal parenchymal tumor breaks through the pelvic lining. It is seen often with benign prostatic hypertrophy, in which case bleeding is usually from dilated veins in the region of the bladder neck. Symptoms of prostatism plus hematuria do not, therefore, necessarily mean prostatic cancer; in fact, bleeding from the malignant prostate does not occur until the tumor grows through the mucosa of the base of the bladder or urethra.

Pain

A. Renal Pain: Renal carcinoma can incite pain in the costovertebral angle (from renal capsular distention) if the tumor bleeds into its own substance. Renal and ureteral colic may occur if a blood clot or a mass of cells passes down the ureter. This type of pain is due to hyperperistalsis of the pelvis or ureter.

B. Ureteral Pain: Ureteral tumors (rare) usually cause ureteral obstruction and occasionally colic.

C. Vesical Pain: Ulceration of a vesical tumor predisposes to midtract (bladder) infection, which causes painful urination. With extravesical extension, constant suprapubic pain which increases with urination may be experienced.

D. Low Back Pain: Pain low in the back with radiation down one or both legs in an elderly man strongly suggests metastases to the pelvis and lumbar spine from cancer of the prostate. Local (perineal) pain is seldom a symptom of neoplasia of the prostate.

E. Testicular Pain: Testicular neoplasm typically causes little or no pain, but if spontaneous bleeding occurs into the tumor it can mimic painful lesions (eg, torsion of the spermatic cord, acute epididymitis).

Dysuria

Hesitancy, impaired caliber and force of the urinary stream, and terminal dribbling are most commonly caused by benign prostatic hypertrophy, but cancer of the prostate can produce the same difficulties. A tumor of the bladder on or near the internal vesical orifice may cause similar symptoms. Cystoscopy is therefore necessary in all cases of bladder neck obstruction.

Tumor of the urethra causes progressive diminution of the urinary stream. A palpable urethral mass suggests tumor or stricture. Biopsy may be needed for positive differentiation.

Skin Lesions

Tumors or ulcers of the penile and scrotal skin may be benign or malignant but can be caused by infection. If there is the slightest doubt, a specimen should be obtained for biopsy.

Palpable Mass

A. Renal Mass: Renal tumors frequently present no symptoms other than the discovery of a tumor mass by the patient or the doctor. Neoplasms can be confused with simple renal cysts, polycystic kidney, hydronephrosis, cyst of the pancreas, or an enlarged spleen.

---

*Adrenal tumors and retroperitoneal extrarenal tumors are discussed in chapter 20.

B. Abdominal Mass: An intra-abdominal mass near the umbilical region should suggest metastases to the preaortic lymph nodes from tumor of the testis. A suprapubic midline mass may represent a dilated (obstructed) bladder or may be caused by gastrointestinal or gynecologic tumor. It is not common for a vesical neoplasm to be palpable suprapubically except on bimanual (abdominorectal or abdominovaginal) examination under anesthesia.

C. Prostatic Mass: When the prostate is diffusely stony-hard and fixed it is almost certainly cancerous, but a hard area in the gland may pose a problem in differential diagnosis. The possibilities include early cancer, fibrosis from chronic infection, prostatic calculi, granulomatous prostatitis, and tuberculosis. At times the differentiation can only be made by biopsy.

D. Testicular Mass: A painless, firm testis should be regarded as neoplastic until proved otherwise. Gummas may cause induration, but they are rare; serology will be helpful in differentiation.

Fever
Tumors of the kidney may excite no symptoms other than fever. Tumors of the urinary organs may also cause obstruction and be complicated by sepsis.

Erythrocytosis
Erythrocytosis occurs in association with 4% of renal cancers, including Wilms's tumor. It may also be noted with certain benign renal lesions.

Urinalysis
In most individuals with vesical neoplasms and transitional cell tumors of the ureter or renal pelvis, the urinary sediment stained with methylene blue will reveal round (transitional) epithelial cells; therefore the presence of these cells should always arouse suspicion of tumor. Cytologic examination of urine sediment using Papanicolaou technics is discussed in chapter 5.

Urinary Lactic Acid Dehydrogenase
The urinary level of this enzyme is apt to be increased in patients with carcinoma of the kidney, bladder, and prostate. It is also elevated in serious medical renal disease and is, therefore, rather nonspecific.

SYMPTOMS AND SIGNS OF METASTASES

Tumors of the genitourinary tract often cause no local symptoms or definite signs. Clinical manifestations may arise only from metastases.

A. Central Nervous System: Tumors of the kidney or prostate may metastasize to the central nervous system. The first symptoms may therefore be neurologic.

B. Lungs: Tumors of the kidney, prostate, and testis often spread to the lungs. Pleuritic pain may suggest secondary pleural involvement.

C. Liver: Renal tumors frequently metastasize to the liver, which then becomes enlarged and nodular. If compression of the common duct occurs, jaundice will be noted.

D. Lymph Nodes: Enlargement of the left supraclavicular lymph nodes may be the only finding in cancer of the kidney or testis. Palpable para-aortic abdominal masses in a young man may mean tumor of the testis. Edema of one or both legs may develop from compression of the iliac vessels by masses of lymph nodes containing tumor cells from cancer of the prostate or bladder.

E. Bones: Metastasis to the skeletal system is most common from cancer of the prostate and kidney. This may cause pain in the bone, spontaneous fracture, or neurologic manifestations due to metastasis to the spine.

TUMORS OF THE RENAL PARENCHYMA

BENIGN TUMORS

From the clinical standpoint, benign tumors of the kidney are rare. However, small adenomas are often seen at autopsy. Their cells resemble those of the adult renal tubule. There is evidence that these adenomas are the source of the carcinomas of the renal parenchyma which are seen quite frequently in the adult.

Benign tumors of the renal parenchyma include adenomas, hemangiomas, fibromas, endometriosis, lipomas, myomas, angiomyolipomas, and neurofibromas. Most of these

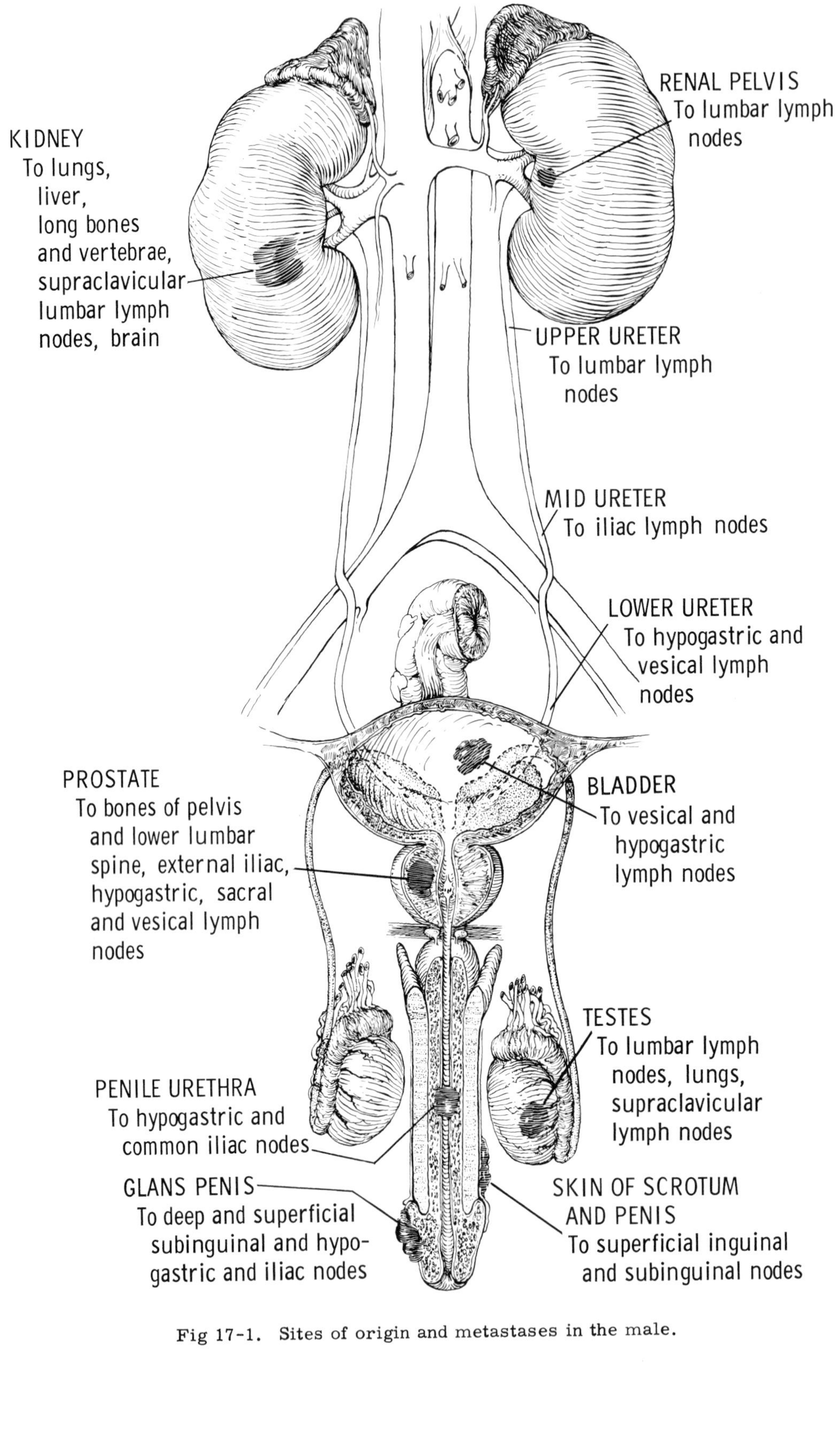

KIDNEY
 To lungs,
 liver,
 long bones
 and vertebrae,
 supraclavicular
 lumbar lymph
 nodes, brain

RENAL PELVIS
 To lumbar lymph
 nodes

UPPER URETER
 To lumbar lymph
 nodes

MID URETER
 To iliac lymph nodes

LOWER URETER
 To hypogastric and
 vesical lymph
 nodes

PROSTATE
 To bones of pelvis
 and lower lumbar
 spine, external iliac,
 hypogastric, sacral
 and vesical lymph
 nodes

BLADDER
 To vesical and
 hypogastric
 lymph nodes

TESTES
 To lumbar lymph
 nodes, lungs,
 supraclavicular
 lymph nodes

PENILE URETHRA
 To hypogastric and
 common iliac nodes

GLANS PENIS
 To deep and superficial
 subinguinal and hypo-
 gastric and iliac nodes

SKIN OF SCROTUM
AND PENIS
 To superficial inguinal
 and subinguinal nodes

Fig 17-1. Sites of origin and metastases in the male.

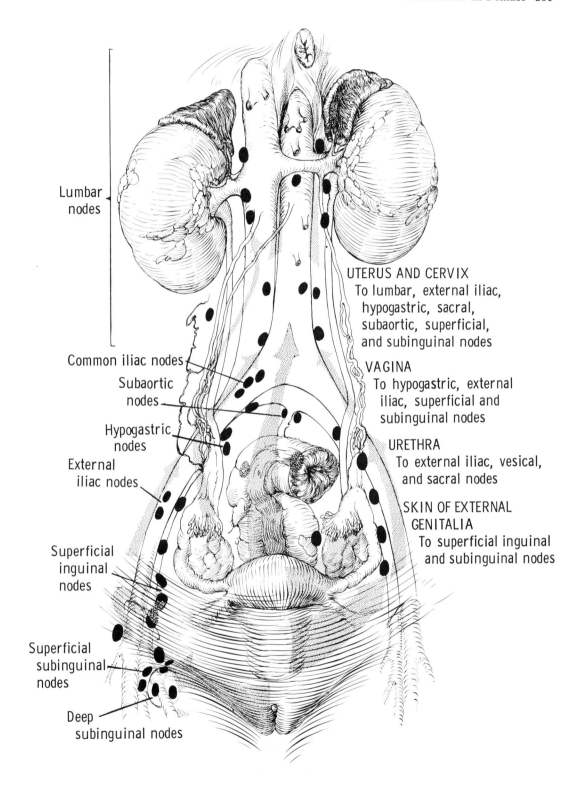

Lumbar nodes

Common iliac nodes

Subaortic nodes

Hypogastric nodes

External iliac nodes

Superficial inguinal nodes

Superficial subinguinal nodes

Deep subinguinal nodes

UTERUS AND CERVIX
To lumbar, external iliac, hypogastric, sacral, subaortic, superficial, and subinguinal nodes

VAGINA
To hypogastric, external iliac, superficial and subinguinal nodes

URETHRA
To external iliac, vesical, and sacral nodes

SKIN OF EXTERNAL GENITALIA
To superficial inguinal and subinguinal nodes

Fig 17-2. Sites and routes of metastases in the female.

are small, little more than 1-2 cm in diameter. Mixed connective tissue tumors (hamartoma, angiomyolipoma) are occasionally found in association with tuberous sclerosis. They are often multiple and bilateral.

Large tumors of this type do occur and present signs and symptoms similar to those described under carcinoma; it is almost impossible to differentiate these from the malignant variety by urographic means. The kidney must, therefore, be removed.

Burkholder, G.V., Beach, P.D., & R. Hall: Fetal renal hamartoma. J Urol 104:330-6, 1970.

Hajdu, S.I., & L.G. Koss: Endometriosis of the kidney. Am J Obst Gynec 106:314-5, 1970.

McCullough, D.L., Scott, R., Jr., & H.M. Seybold: Renal angiomyolipoma (hamartoma): Review of the literature and report of 7 cases. J Urol 105:32-44, 1971.

Murphy, G.P., & F.K. Mostofi: Histologic assessment and clinical prognosis of renal adenoma. J Urol 103:31-6, 1970.

Olurin, E.O., Ajayi, O.O., & B.O. Osunkoya: Tuberous sclerosis: A report of two renal presentations. Brit J Urol 43:432-8, 1971.

Peterson, N.E., & H.T. Thompson: Renal hemangioma. J Urol 105:27-31, 1971.

Silbiger, M.L., & C.C. Peterson, Jr.: Renal angiomyolipoma: Its distinctive angiographic characteristics. J Urol 106:363-5, 1971.

Teplick, J.G.: Tuberous sclerosis. Extensive roentgen findings without the usual clinical picture: A case report. Radiology 93:53-5, 1969.

Waldbaum, R.S., & others: Tuberous sclerosis with bilateral angiomyolipomas of the kidney: Case report with 8-year followup. J Urol 106:180-3, 1971.

Wigger, H.J.: Fetal hamartoma of kidney. A benign, symptomatic, congenital tumor, not a form of Wilms' tumor. Am J Clin Path 51:323-37, 1969.

ADENOCARCINOMA
(Grawitz's Tumor; Hypernephroma)

About four-fifths of renal neoplasms are adenocarcinomas, and two-thirds of these occur in men. A few are observed in childhood. Because adenocarcinomas produce symptoms relatively late, prognosis is poor.

Etiology

There has been considerable disagreement over the origin of adenocarcinomas. Grawitz thought they arose from intrarenal adrenal rests, and the term "hypernephroma" was coined to describe them. The leading opinion now, however, is that they arise from the cells of the renal tubules or from the benign adenomas. This theory is based on the histologic findings. Most tumors of true adrenal tissues are "functioning," whereas adenocarcinomas are not. Smoking has been suspected as a cause of adenocarcinoma of the kidney.

Pathogenesis and Pathology

Adenocarcinoma usually arises in one of the renal poles. As the neoplasm expands, it compresses adjacent renal tissue and displaces calyces, blood vessels, and the pelvis, which then become distorted and tend to surround the mass. It is this characteristic which leads to urographic diagnosis. Multiple adenocarcinomas are often found in patients suffering from Lindau's disease.

The renal veins and even the vena cava are frequently invaded. This may be associated with the nephrotic syndrome or hepatic dysfunction. At times a column of tumor extends into the right heart. Occlusion of the renal vein may cause marked dilatation of the perirenal vessels and varicocele. As enlargement increases, intraperitoneal organs may be displaced (eg, stomach, intestines, spleen) or the diaphragm elevated. The tumor may invade adjacent muscle or organs (eg, duodenum, diaphragm).

Adenocarcinoma usually has a well-defined fibrous capsule. On section, the tumor is yellow and often contains zones of hemorrhage or necrosis. It produces a definite expansion of the kidney. Calcification may develop and may be visible on x-ray film.

Microscopically, varying patterns of cells may be seen even in the same tumor. In general, the cells resemble renal tubule cells and have small eccentric nuclei and an abundant clear cytoplasm. At times the cytoplasm may be more opaque and granular. A papillary or even anaplastic pattern may be seen. Tumors with well differentiated clear cells seem to offer the best prognosis.

Most visceral metastases occur by way of the blood stream. The liver, lungs, and long bones (and occasionally the brain and adrenal glands) may be affected. Lumbar lymph nodes about the renal pedicle may become involved, and enlarged left supraclavicular nodes are occasionally seen. The kidney is involved secondarily by metastases from other organs in 7.6% of autopsies. The bronchus is the most common primary site.

Clinical Findings

A. Symptoms: Gross total hematuria is the most common symptom and is usually not accompanied by pain. It occurs in two-thirds of patients. Pain may be the initial symptom

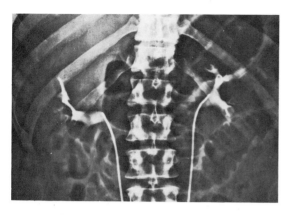
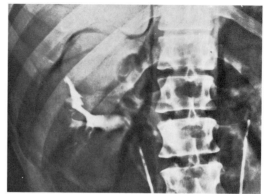
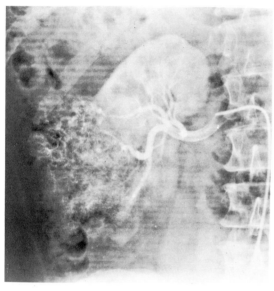
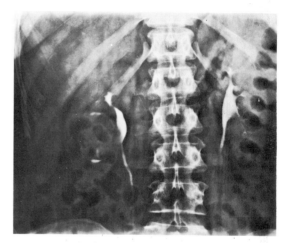

Fig 17-3. Adenocarcinoma of the kidney. Above left: Retrograde urogram showing lateral displacement of upper pole of right kidney and elongation and distortion of upper calyces (carcinoma). Left urogram normal. **Above right:** Same patient. Retrograde urogram combined with pneumogram shows extent of mass and its relation to calyces. Normal right adrenal. **Below left:** Selective renal angiogram showing marked vascularity of mass in lower portion of right kidney typical of malignant tumor. **Below right:** Excretory urogram. Distortion of the pelvis, middle and lower calyces of right kidney. Space-occupying lesion (adenocarcinoma). The left kidney is normal.

but is usually a late manifestation. It may be of the dull type felt in the back, resulting from back pressure from ureteral compression, perirenal extension, or hemorrhage into the substance of the kidney; or it may be colicky if a clot or mass of tumor cells passes down the ureter.

Occasionally a patient may discover a mass in the flank in the absence of other symptoms. Gastrointestinal complaints resembling the syndromes of peptic ulcer or gallbladder disease may be the only subjective manifestations. These are caused by reflex action or by displacement or invasion of intraperitoneal organs. Unexplained low-grade fever may be the only symptom.

Symptoms from metastases may also occur as the first manifestations of renal tumor. These include unexplained loss of weight, increasing weakness, and anemia. Bone pain, spontaneous fracture, pulmonary difficulties, or a mass in the left side of the neck (Virchow's nodes) may be the presenting complaint.

B. Signs: A mass is often discovered in the flank. It must be pointed out, however, that the kidneys lie rather high, particularly on the left side. In an obese or muscular per-

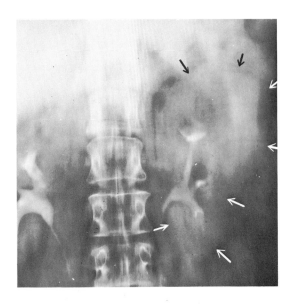

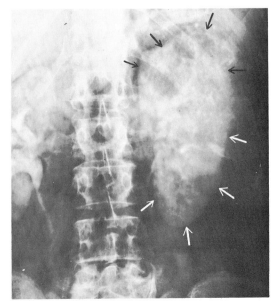

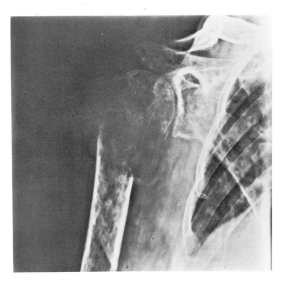

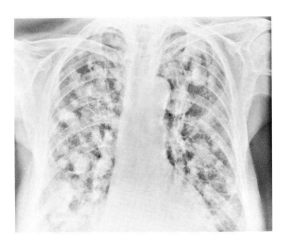

Fig 17-4. Adenocarcinoma of the kidney. **Above left:** Excretory urogram with tomography showing marked expansion of upper pole and elongated upper calyx, left kidney. **Above right:** Angionephrotomogram, same patient, showing pooling of radiopaque fluid in cancer of upper pole,
left kidney. **Below left:** Osteolytic metastases to humerus. **Below right:** Metastases to lung.
Note typical ''cannonball'' lesions.

son, considerable enlargement can be present
and still defy detection. Fixation may mean
local invasion. Involvement of the vena cava
by tumor or thrombosis may cause the development of dilated veins on the abdominal wall.
An acute hydrocele or varicocele may develop
as a rare and late sign if the spermatic vein
is occluded. This is most apt to occur on the
left side because this vein drains into the left
renal vein.

Arteriovenous fistulas are occasionally
observed in association with renal adenocarcinoma. This is suggested in the presence of
cardiomegaly, diastolic hypertension, and a
systolic murmur and bruit over the mass.
The diagnosis is made on angiography.

Metastatic signs are varied and may be
the presenting manifestations of the illness.
A palpable mass in the left supraclavicular
region may mean metastases to lymph nodes.

Physical examination of the lung fields may reveal no pathologic changes even though metastases are present. Tenderness or even a palpable mass may be found over bone involved by tumor. Edema of the legs may be secondary to neoplastic involvement of the vena cava. The liver is a common site of metastases, in which case it may be enlarged and nodular. Ascites may be found. Loss of weight may be marked.

C. Laboratory Findings: Gross or microscopic hematuria is the cardinal finding, and even a few red cells must be explained. Erythrocytosis with an increased plasma erythropoietin level occurs in 3-4% of patients. Anemia may be present in advanced disease. Total renal function is usually not impaired, for even the involved kidney retains some function and bilateral renal cancer is rare. The sedimentation rate is usually accelerated. Hypercalcemia with secondary effects on muscle, heart, and brain may be noted; a parathyroid-like hormone can be extracted from the tumor in these patients. Urinary lactic dehydrogenase activity is increased with most cancers of the kidney and bladder. A few false positives may occur.

The presence of a hypernephroma may cause hepatic insufficiency as shown by tests of liver function. Removal of the tumor causes the test results to return to normal.

D. X-Ray Findings (Simple Technics): A plain film of the abdomen often shows an enlarged kidney; a definite bulge of its contour is significant. The incidence of cystic or curvilinear calcification is 7%. The psoas margin may be obscured if a solid tumor overlies the muscle. If the tumor is a cyst, the psoas margin may be visible through it (Fig 7-12). The renal shadow may be displaced in any direction, depending upon the location of the tumor. A low left kidney in particular must not be ignored. Osteolytic metastases may be noted (Fig 17-4) on bone x-rays.

Excretory urograms usually show a filling defect caused by a space-occupying lesion (Fig 17-3). Calyces are bent, elongated, or otherwise distorted by the enlarging tumor. On rare occasion the ureter may be compressed, and hydronephrosis may develop. If considerable renal tissue is destroyed by tumor, visualization may be poor. If the renal vein is involved, no excretion of dye may be seen; this is a bad prognostic sign.

If excretory urograms do not afford the necessary information for diagnosis, ureteral catheterization and retrograde urograms must be done (Fig 17-3). Oblique and lateral views should also be taken in order to depict minor deformities of the calyces and pelvis.

A chest film may show the typical nodular metastases, usually multiple (Fig 17-4). A gastrointestinal series or barium enema will show displacement of the stomach or bowel if the renal mass is large.

E. Special Radiographic Studies: Nephrotomography almost always reveals increased opacification of a tumor because of its increased vascularity (Fig 17-4). Aortography, particularly the selective type, produces a dense renal shadow (due to the presence of contrast material in the renal vessels and tubules) and may thereby reveal a bulge of the renal outline, indicating a tumor. Further, because of the great vascularity of the tumor (Fig 17-3), pooling of the opaque material will occur within it on the late films (5 seconds after injection). A cyst will cast no shadow at all.

Venacavagraphy or selective renal phlebography may reveal the presence of tumor in the renal vein or vena cava.

F. Isotope Scanning: A rectilinear scan, using ^{203}Hg, will reveal a "cold" area because functioning parenchyma has been displaced by the tumor. The scan will be similar to that seen with simple renal cyst (Fig 21-3). The gamma camera will show a negative shadow with both ^{203}Hg and ^{131}I; but with ^{99m}Tc, which reveals the vasculature of the kidney, the tumor area will show normal or increased perfusion (Fig 8-3).

G. Instrumental Examination: If the patient has gross hematuria when seen, immediate cystoscopy will demonstrate its source. Postponing cystoscopy almost guarantees that this valuable information will be lost, for renal tumors bleed intermittently.

H. Cytology: The Papanicolaou technic has been applied to the urinary sediment but rarely proves helpful.

Differential Diagnosis

Hydronephrotic kidney may be accompanied by pain, tumor, and hematuria. Gross bleeding, however, is rare. Urography will establish the diagnosis.

Polycystic kidney disease may also present with hematuria and a renal mass, but total renal function is usually impaired even though only one kidney is large enough to be felt. Hypertension is common with polycystic disease. Renal angiography or a technetium scan should differentiate the 2 lesions.

Simple cyst of the kidney may cause flank pain and may be palpable, but gross or even microscopic hematuria is unusual. Tumors are often associated with an increased sedimentation rate and an elevated urinary LDH level; cysts are not. Tumor and cyst both occupy space in the kidney, and so urograms of both may be similar. Cysts tend to be more extrinsic; solid tumors are prone to occupy the deeper renal tissues. If the renal mass overlies the psoas, the muscle is apt to be obliterated by a solid tumor but may be visible through a cyst (Fig 7-12). Nephrotomograms (Fig 7-5) or angiograms (Fig 17-3) will usually make the differentiation: A cyst fails to opacify; a tumor becomes unusually dense.

If the radiographic diagnosis is cyst, this can be further confirmed by passing a needle into the mass. The fluid recovered should be analyzed for fat, whose presence confirms the diagnosis of cyst, and subjected to cytologic examination. Radiopaque fluid is then introduced and appropriate films taken (Fig 21-5). Differentiation may be possible only at surgery.

Renal tuberculosis can cause renal pain, a palpable mass, and gross hematuria, but symptoms of vesical irritability and pyuria are usually present. Acid-fast bacteria can almost always be demonstrated. Cystoscopy may reveal tuberculous cystitis, and urograms should make an unequivocal differentiation.

A stone in the kidney or ureter can cause renal pain and hematuria, but the pain is often more acute. Roentgenograms should differentiate between stone and tumor.

Ureteral or renal pelvic tumor may mimic renal tumor, causing renal pain and often a palpable hydronephrotic kidney. Gross hematuria may also be present. Urography will clearly differentiate the two.

Adrenal or other extrarenal tumor (pancreatic pseudocyst) may present a palpable mass (either the tumor or a displaced kidney), but hematuria and pain are unusual. Most adrenal tumors are functional and cause definite signs and symptoms (eg, hirsutism, amenorrhea, obesity). Adenomas and carcinomas of the adrenal cortex cause increased levels of urinary LDH. Pheochromocytoma and neuroblastoma elaborate increased amounts of vanilmandelic acid in the urine. Urography and other studies will show a mass displacing the kidney whose calyces are normal.

Chronic pyelonephritis often causes renal pain and hematuria, but such kidneys are not enlarged. Symptoms of cystitis are often noted. The finding of pus and bacteria in the urine is suggestive. Urography should establish the diagnosis.

The xanthogranulomatous pyelonephritic kidney usually does not show function on excretory urograms, but retrograde urograms reveal a distorted calyceal system not unlike that seen with tumor. The differentiation is often made only at surgery, but angiography may prove helpful.

Tumors of the bladder usually cause hematuria. Excretory urograms will reveal an absence of calyceal distortion, although hydronephrosis may be present if a ureteral orifice

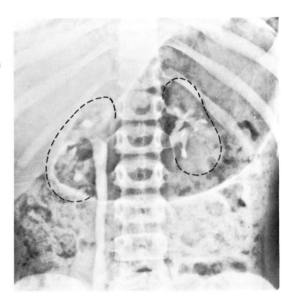

Fig 17-5. Renal pseudotumor. Bilateral healed pyelonephritis secondary to vesicoureteral reflux. Localized compensatory hypertrophy in lower pole of left kidney displaces calyces suggesting presence of space-occupying lesion.

is occluded. The cystogram may reveal a defect consistent with tumor (Fig 17-9). Cystoscopy will reveal the growth.

A kidney deformed by scarring due to infarction or multiple attacks of acute pyelonephritis may develop focal areas of renal compensatory hypertrophy which, with expansion, may deform the calyces, thus simulating tumor (Fig 17-5). Renal angiography will establish the proper diagnosis.

Renal lymphoma or Hodgkin's disease leads to deformity of the calyces. The tumors are usually bilateral and multiple. Evidence of lymphoma elsewhere is helpful in differential diagnosis. Angiography may be helpful, but Hodgkin's tumor may be very vascular.

Complications

The complications of adenocarcinomas are largely related to local invasion or distant metastases. A few patients develop hydronephrosis from ureteral compression, hypertension from interference with the blood supply to the organ, or arteriovenous fistula. Occlusion of the renal vein by tumor may cause findings compatible with the nephrotic syndrome. Rarely, hematuria may be severe enough to threaten to cause death from exsanguination.

Treatment

A. Nephrectomy: If there are no demonstrable metastases, radical nephrectomy, including removal of the perinephric fat, should be performed. If hemorrhage is intractable, nephrectomy may be necessary even though metastases are demonstrated. Erythrocytosis, if present, subsides after nephrectomy. Urinary LDH will react in kind. The red blood cell count and LDH may rise again if metastases occur.

Partial nephrectomy for cancer in a solitary kidney should be considered.

B. X-Ray Therapy: Adenocarcinomas of the kidney and their metastases are usually radioresistant. Most authorities feel that x-ray therapy is therefore not indicated either preoperatively or postoperatively, but a few authors disagree.

C. Chemotherapy: Chemotherapy has been disappointing. The administration of medroxyprogesterone (Provera®) or testosterone has had some palliative effect in a few cases.

Prognosis

About 35% of patients suffering from cancer of the kidney are alive 5 years after nephrectomy. The outlook is poor if the renal vein or vena cava has been invaded by tumor. Metastases may develop even 10-15 years after removal of the primary growth. The percentage of cures can only be increased by subjecting all patients suffering from hematuria—microscopic or gross; persistent, transient, or intermittent—to complete urologic study. The prognosis in children is more promising.

Adolfsson, G.: Regression of hypernephroma. Urol Internat 21:365-74, 1966.

Arner, O., Blank, C., & T. von Schreeb: Renal adenocarcinoma: Morphology, grading of malignancy, prognosis. A study of 197 cases. Acta chir scandinav Supp 346: 1965.

Aron, B.S., & M. Gross: Renal adenocarcinoma in infancy and childhood: Evaluation of therapy and prognosis. J Urol 102:497-503, 1969.

Bennington, J.L., & F.A. Laubscher: Epidemiologic studies on carcinoma of the kidney. I. Association of renal adenocarcinoma with smoking. Cancer 21:1069-71, 1968.

Bosniak, M.A., O'Connor, J.F., & L.H. Caplan: Renal arteriography in patients with metastatic renal cell carcinoma. JAMA 203:249-54, 1968.

Bosniak, M.A., & others: Metastatic neoplasm to the kidney. A report of four cases studied with angiography and nephrotomography. Radiology 92:989-93, 1969.

Cox, C.E., & others: Renal adenocarcinoma: 28-year review, with emphasis on rationale and feasibility of preoperative radiotherapy. J Urol 104:53-61, 1970.

Dehner, L.P., Leestma, J.E., & E.B. Price, Jr.: Renal cell carcinoma in children: A clinicopathologic study of 15 cases and review of the literature. J Pediat 76:358-68, 1970.

Donati, R.M., & others: Erythrocythemia and neoplastic tumors. Ann Int Med 58:47-55, 1963.

Felson, B., & M. Moskowitz: Renal pseudotumors: The regenerated nodule and other lumps, bumps, and dromedary humps. Am J Roentgenol 107:720-9, 1969.

Fenlon, J.W., Silber, I., & P.R. Koehler: Perirenal masses simulating renal tumors. J Urol 106:448-50, 1971.

Folin, J.: Angiography in renal tumors. Its value in diagnosis and differential diagnosis as a complement to conventional methods. Acta radiol Supp 267, 1967.

Friedenberg, M.J., & H.J. Spjut: Xanthogranulomatous pyelonephritis. Am J Roentgenol 90:97-108, 1963.

Ghosh, S.K., & W.L. Donegan: Partial nephrectomy for carcinoma in a congenital solitary kidney. J Urol 104:380-3, 1970.

Gorder, J.L., & F.L. Stargardter: Pancreatic pseudocysts simulating intrarenal masses. Am J Roentgenol 107:65-8, 1969.

Gross, M., & S. Minkowitz: Ureteral metastasis from renal adenocarcinoma. J Urol 106:23-6, 1971.

Kiely, J.M., Wagoner, R.D., & K.E. Holley: Renal complications of lymphoma. Ann Int Med 71:1159-75, 1969.

Kikkawa, K., & E.C. Lasser: ''Ring-like'' or ''rim-like'' calcification in renal cell carcinoma. Am J Roentgenol 107:737-42, 1969.

King, M.C., & others: Normal renal parenchyma simulating tumor. Radiology 91: 217-22, 1968.

Kölln, C.P., & others: Bilateral partial nephrectomy for bilateral renal cell carcinoma: A case report. J Urol 105:45-8, 1971.

Lytton, B., Rosof, B., & J.S. Evans: Parathyroid hormone-like activity in a renal carcinoma producing hypercalcemia. J Urol 93:127-31, 1965.

Marshall, V.F., & others: Surgery for renal cell carcinoma in the vena cava. J Urol 103:414-20, 1970.

McCoy, R.M., Klatte, E.C., & R.K. Rhamy: Use of inferior venacavography in the evaluation of renal neoplasms. J Urol 102:556-9, 1969.

Meaney, T.F.: Errors in angiographic diagnosis of renal masses. Radiology 93:361-6, 1969.

Morris, J.G., & others: The diagnosis of renal tumors by radioisotope scanning. J Urol 97:40-54, 1967.

Olsson, C.A., Moyer, J.D., & R.O. Laferte: Pulmonary cancer metastatic to the kidney—

a common renal neoplasm. J Urol **105**:492-6, 1971.

Paine, C. H., Wright, F. W., & F. Ellis: The use of progestogen in the treatment of metastatic carcinoma of the kidney and uterine body. Brit J Cancer **24**:277-82, 1970.

Peeling, W. B., Mantell, B. S., & B. G. F. Shepheard: Post-operative irradiation in the treatment of renal cell carcinoma. Brit J Urol **41**:23-30, 1969.

Rafla, S.: Renal cell carcinoma. Natural history and results of treatment. Cancer **25**:26-40, 1970.

Ram, M. D., & G. D. Chisholm: Hypertension due to hypernephroma. Brit MJ **4**:87-8, 1969.

Rho, Yong-Myun: Von Hippel-Lindau's disease. Canad MAJ **101**:135-42, 1969.

Riding, G. R.: Renal adenocarcinoma: Regression of pulmonary metastases following irradiation of primary tumor. Cancer **27**: 936-8, 1971.

Robson, C. J.: Radical nephrectomy for renal cell carcinoma. J Urol **89**:37-42, 1963.

Samuels, M. L., Sullivan, P., & C. D. Howe: Medroxyprogesterone acetate in the treatment of renal cell carcinoma (hypernephroma). Cancer **22**:525-32, 1968.

Schoenfeld, M. R., & R. Bernstein: Hypernephroma, marked renal vein dilatation and the Bernoulli phenomenon. Am J Med **50**: 845-8, 1971.

Seabury, J. C., Jr.: Renal rhabdomyosarcoma. JAMA **201**:1043-4, 1967.

Seltzer, R. A., & D. E. Wenlund: Renal lymphoma. Arteriographic studies. Am J Roentgenol **101**:692-5, 1967.

Small, M. P., Anderson, E. E., & W. H. Atwill: Simultaneous bilateral renal cell carcinoma: Case report and review of literature. J Urol **100**:8-14, 1968.

Svane, S.: Tumor thrombus of the inferior vena cava resulting from renal carcinoma. A report on 12 autopsied cases. Scandinav J Urol Nephrol **3**:245-56, 1969.

Wagle, D. G., & G. P. Murphy: Hormonal therapy in advanced renal cell carcinoma. Cancer **28**:318-21, 1971.

Warren, M. M., Kelalis, P. P., & D. C. Utz: The changing concept of hypernephroma. J Urol **104**:376-9, 1970.

Weigensberg, I. J.: The many faces of metastatic renal carcinoma. Radiology **98**:353-8, 1971.

White, A. A., & A. J. Palubinskas: Renal Hodgkin's disease. Angiographic demonstration. Radiology **96**:551-2, 1970.

Wise, G. J., Bosniak, M. A., & P. B. Hudson: Arteriovenous fistula associated with renal cell carcinoma of the kidney. Brit J Urol **39**:170-7, 1967.

Yates-Bell, A. J., & B. S. Cardell: Adenocarcinoma of the kidney in children. Brit J Urol **43**:399-402, 1971.

EMBRYOMA
(Wilms's Tumor;
Adenomyosarcoma, Nephroblastoma)

Embryoma of the kidney is a highly malignant mixed tumor. It is almost exclusively a disease of children under the age of 6 years; in this age group it is second in incidence only to tumors of the orbit, and is the most common abdominal tumor in children. Five percent are bilateral.

Etiology

Wilms's tumor is considered by most investigators to be congenital and to arise from embryonal cells trapped in the kidney. About 6% are clinically present at birth, and these, if large, may cause dystocia.

Pathogenesis and Pathology

Wilms's tumor may arise in any portion of the kidney. It usually becomes quite large before it is discovered. Pain is not common. Hematuria is rare and late, for this tumor seldom breaks through the renal pelvis.

The tumor is usually large, pale, and lobulated. The surface of the kidney is usually covered by large, thin-walled veins. Little viable renal tissue may be left. On cut section, the tissue is usually yellow or white and heterogeneous; hemorrhagic and cystic areas are often found. Microscopically the major tissues are of connective tissue origin: muscle, cartilage, and myxomatous or lipomatous tissue. The epithelial structures may be undifferentiated or may resemble renal tubules or even glomeruli. The term "adenomyosarcoma" has therefore been used to describe these tumors. Possibly half of these tumors will show abnormal chromosome sets.

If preoperative x-ray treatment has been given, the tumor may be small; in fact, the kidney may be only slightly enlarged. The entire tumor may be necrotic and hemorrhagic, although viable sarcoma and carcinoma cells are usually found microscopically. These primitive cells are quite radiosensitive.

The usual route of metastasis is through the blood stream; the lungs, liver, and brain are most commonly involved. Regional lumbar lymph nodes may be affected.

Clinical Findings

A. Symptoms: The most common symptom is a palpable mass in the flank, usually

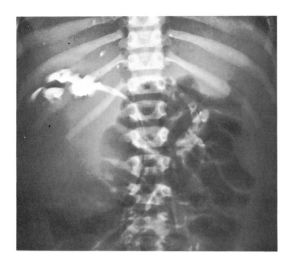

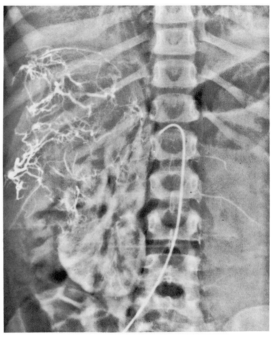

Fig 17-6. **Wilms's tumor. Left:** Excretory urogram showing large globular mass in right upper quadrant with displacement and distortion of calyces. Upper right ureter displaced over spine. **Below:** Bilateral embryomas as shown on angiography. **Left:** Early phase of left selective angiogram showing arcing of major renal arteries, vascular pooling, and typical tumor vessels. **Right:** Late phase of right selective angiogram showing vascular mass in upper pole.

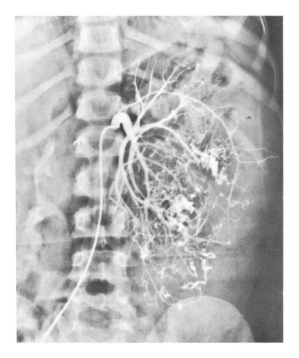

discovered by the child's parents. Rarely, pain may be experienced from local invasion or ureteral compression (hydronephrosis). Other symptoms include loss of weight, anorexia or vomiting from displacement or invasion of the enteric tract, and hematuria (unusual).

B. Signs: A palpable mass in the flank of a child under age 6 must be regarded as Wilms's tumor (or neuroblastoma of the adrenal) until proved otherwise. The mass does not transilluminate. An enlarged nodular liver strongly suggests that metastasis from the renal tumor has occurred. The lungs usually reveal no abnormal physical signs even though they contain metastases. Hypertension is common in children with embryoma of the kidney; it is often relieved by removal of the involved organ. Weight loss is a prominent feature of the late stage of the disease. In 1-2% of cases congenital aniridia has been observed. This is often associated with microencephaly, cataracts, glaucoma, and mental retardation.

C. Laboratory Findings: Anemia may be found. Urinalysis is usually normal; the finding of red cells is unusual. Tests of total renal function are usually normal, for even the involved kidney usually retains some function. Urinary LDH may be increased, particularly if metastasis has occurred.

D. X-Ray Findings:

1. Simple technics - A greatly enlarged renal shadow is usually evident on a plain film of the abdomen. There may be a rim of calcification around the periphery of the tumor. The bowel, as demonstrated by the gas pattern, may be displaced. There may be evidence of enlargement of the liver.

Excretory urograms usually show great distortion of the pelvis and calyces on the involved side (Fig 17-6), although lack of excretion may occur. Retrograde urograms will reveal in more detail the intrarenal distortion caused by a space-occupying lesion. Oblique and lateral views add a useful third dimension to the survey.

A chest film may disclose metastases to the lungs.

Gastrointestinal series and barium enema usually reveal marked displacement of the stomach and bowel by the tumor.

2. Special radiographic studies - Renal angiography (Fig 17-6) will show the size of the renal mass, the typical pooling of radiopaque material in the tumor, and neovascularity. It is rarely necessary, however, and its inherent dangers must be remembered.

E. Instrumental Examination: Cystoscopy and ureteral catheterization are indicated for the purpose of obtaining retrograde urograms if excretory urograms are inadequate.

F. Cytology: Papanicolaou studies will seldom be of help for the tumor rarely breaks through the pelvic lining.

Differential Diagnosis

Neuroblastoma of the adrenal medulla is an exceedingly malignant tumor which, for the most part, afflicts children under age 3. It usually presents as a mass in the flank, but since it metastasizes early and widely and by both lymphatics and blood vessels, the first symptoms may be caused by metastases. Neuroblastoma tends to invade the muscles of the back; it may therefore present a visible bulge in the costovertebral angle. Urography, either excretory or retrograde, should permit differentiation. Neuroblastoma tends to displace the kidney; Wilms's tumors are intrinsic renal lesions and therefore distort the calyces. Neuroblastomas frequently contain stippled calcification on the plain film. The osseous metastases are frequently bilateral and almost symmetrical, involving many bones. The urinary vanillylmandelic acid level is increased with neuroblastoma but is normal with Wilms's tumor. LDH is increased in Wilms's tumor but is normal with neuroblastoma.

Eight instances of congenital mesoblastic nephroma have been reported. This is a benign tumor and would not respond to radiation therapy. Angiography should make the diagnosis, but this may clarify itself only at the operating table.

Hydronephrosis may also cause a mass in the flank. It is usually softer than a tumor. It may transilluminate. If secondarily infected, pyuria will be found. Urography is diagnostic.

Multicystic kidney seen in the newborn presents as a nodular mass in one flank and may, therefore, be confused with Wilms's tumor. This cystic kidney fails to secrete radiopaque material. The ureter is usually not connected to the mass; therefore retrograde urography will not afford a urogram. Angiography may be required to settle the matter, but the diagnosis may be made only at the operating table.

Polycystic kidney disease may cause a palpable mass, although enlargement is usually bilateral. Renal function tests are depressed, and urograms show bilateral calyceal distortion. It must be remembered, however, that 5% of Wilms's tumors are bilateral. Renal angiography may be needed in case of doubt.

Treatment

A. Specific Measures:

1. Radiation therapy - If it is judged that the tumor is too large to allow nephrectomy readily, preoperative irradiation should be administered. If the diagnosis is accurate, dramatic shrinkage of the mass should be observed.

Following nephrectomy, radiotherapy to the tumor bed should be considered, although some authorities fear damage to the spine.

2. Nephrectomy - If the mass can be removed easily, preliminary x-ray therapy is not necessary; nephrectomy should be performed promptly. A few patients with bilateral Wilms's tumors have been subjected to bilateral nephrectomy followed by renal transplantation.

3. Chemotherapy - This tumor has proved to be quite sensitive to dactinomycin (Cosmegen®), which should be started a few days before surgery and continued daily for 1 week and then at weekly intervals. Other dosage schedules have also been suggested.

B. Palliative Measures: If metastases are widespread—and particularly if they are discovered in bone or the brain—the prognosis appears to be hopeless, though radiotherapy and chemotherapy should not be withheld. Vincristine has been found useful under these circumstances. Instances have been reported in which resection of pulmonary and even hepatic metastases has led to cure.

Prognosis

In the absence of demonstrable metastases, about 80-90% of these children will be cured by nephrectomy, radiation therapy and chemotherapy. Even in the presence of pulmonary lesions, combined therapy offers cure in about 50% of cases. The younger the child, the better the outlook. Since it seems probable that the tumor has its inception at the time of conception, cure may be assumed if the child lives for a period equal to nine months plus its age at the time of surgery. Thus, a patient operated upon at the age of 20 months may be considered cured if he is free of disease 29 months after surgical intervention (Collins). The prognosis is improved if the capsule has not been invaded.

Anderson, E. E., & others: Bilateral diffuse Wilms' tumor: a 5-year survival. J Urol 99:707-9, 1968.

Balsaver, A. M., Gibley, C. W., Jr., & C. F. Tessmer: Ultrastructural studies in Wilms's tumor. Cancer 22:417-27, 1968.

Bannayan, G. A., Huvos, A. G., & G. J. D'Angio: Effect of irradiation on the maturation of Wilms' tumor. Cancer 27:812-8, 1971.

Bolande, R. P., Brough, A. J., & R. J. Izant, Jr.: Congenital mesoblastic nephroma of infancy. Pediatrics 40:272-8, 1967.

Cox, D.: Chromosome constitution of nephroblastomas. Cancer 19:1217-24, 1966.

DeLorimier, A. A., & others: Treatment of bilateral Wilms' tumor. Am J Surg 122:275-80, 1971.

Farah, J., & J. E. Lofstrom: Angiography of Wilms's tumor. Radiology 90:775-7, 1968.

Fleming, I. D., & W. W. Johnson: Clinical and pathologic staging as a guide in the management of Wilms' tumor. Cancer 26:660-5, 1970.

Fraumeni, J. F., & A. G. Glass: Wilms' tumor and congenital aniridia. JAMA 206:825-8, 1968.

Jagasia, K. H., & W. G. Thurman: Congenital anomalies of the kidney in association with Wilms' tumor. Pediatrics 35:338-40, 1965.

Kenny, G. M., & others: Erythropoietin levels in Wilms' tumor patients. J Urol 104:758-61, 1970.

Leen, R. L. S., & I. G. Williams: Bilateral Wilms' tumor. Seven personal cases with observations. Cancer 28:802-6, 1971.

Meng, C. H., & M. Elkin: Angiographic manifestations of Wilms' tumor. Am J Roentgenol 105:95-104, 1969.

Newman, D., & F. Vellios: Adult carcinosarcoma (adult Wilms' tumor) of the kidney. Clin Path 42:45-54, 1964.

Schneider, B., & others: Wilms' tumor: The evolution of a treatment program. Am J Roentgenol 108:92-7, 1970.

Stein, J. J., & W. E. Goodwin: Bilateral Wilms' tumor, including report of a patient surviving ten years after treatment. Am J Roentgenol 96:626-34, 1966.

Symposium. Cancer of the urogenital tract. Wilms' tumor. JAMA 204:981-90, 1968.

Uson, A. C., Wolff, J. A., & P. Tretter: Current treatment of Wilms' tumor. J Urol 103:217-21, 1970.

Vietti, T. J., & others: Vincristine sulfate and radiation therapy in metastatic Wilms' tumor. Cancer 25:12-20, 1970.

Wagget, J., & C. E. Koop: Wilms' tumor: Preoperative radiotherapy and chemotherapy in the management of massive tumors. Cancer 26:338-40, 1970.

Wedemeyer, P. P., & others: Resection of metastases in Wilms' tumor: A report of three cases cured of pulmonary and hepatic metastases. Pediatrics 41:446-51, 1968.

Woodard, J. R., & M. K. Levine: Nephroblastoma (Wilms' tumor) and congenital aniridia. J Urol 101:140-3, 1969.

SARCOMA

Sarcomas of the kidney are rare. They may be made up of smooth or striated muscle, fibroplastic tissue, or fat. They may become quite large and fill the flank. Spread is usually by way of the blood stream; the lungs and bones are commonly involved.

The signs and symptoms are usually the presence of a mass and local pain. Hematuria is not common. Spontaneous perirenal hemorrhage may cause the first symptoms (pain, shock).

The diagnosis rests on urographic evidence of a space-occupying lesion. Preoperative differentiation from all other types of renal tumor is impossible.

In the absence of metastases, nephrectomy is indicated unless lymphoblastoma is suspected, in which case radiation therapy should be used. The prognosis is quite poor for the entire group. The incidence of distant metastases and local recurrence after surgical extirpation is high.

Gupta, O. P., & M. K. Dube: Rare primary renal sarcoma. Brit J Urol **43**:546-51, 1971.

Jenkins, J. D., Anderson, C. K., & R. E. Williams: Renal sarcoma. Brit J Urol **43**:263-7, 1971.

TUMORS OF THE RENAL PELVIS AND URETER

Histologically, the epithelial tumors of the renal pelvis and ureter resemble the tumors of the bladder. They may be benign or malignant.

Although malignant tumors of the ureter arising from mesenchymal tissues have been described, they are rare and will therefore not be discussed here. Suffice it to say that clinically they mimic the more common epithelial growths and benign polyps.

TUMORS OF THE RENAL PELVIS

Most tumors arising from the calyceal or pelvic mucosa are papillary in type. They comprise about 10% of tumors of the kidney. Hematuria is usually the earliest symptom.

Etiology

The cause of the papillary growths is not known. Their tendency to ''seed'' in the ureter and bladder suggests that the mucosa generally is susceptible to such change. The rare epidermoid carcinoma is usually associated with chronic infection or stone; chronic inflammation may therefore play a part in its genesis.

The metabolites of tryptophan (alpha-aminophenols) are at present suspect as carcinogenic agents. For a discussion of this subject, see p 265.

Pathogenesis and Pathology

These tumors may cause obstruction to calyces or even the ureteropelvic junction, thereby causing renal pain and the changes associated with back pressure. The more malignant types tend to invade the parenchyma. Hematuria occurs earlier than in adenocarcinomas of the parenchyma. Similar tumors may also be found in the ureter and bladder, particularly in the region of the ipsilateral ureteral orifice. It is therefore necessary to remove the kidney, ureter, and adjacent bladder wall when dealing with these growths. Most papillary tumors of the renal pelvis are

malignant. Metastases are usually not widespread. The regional lumbar nodes may be involved.

Microscopically, these tumors show a central core of connective tissue which is covered by transitional epithelium. Invasion of the supporting stroma or mucosa or the finding of many cells in mitosis is evidence of malignancy, but at times it is difficult to draw the line between the malignant and benign types. Epidermoid cancers are invasive and highly malignant, and survival is rare. They are usually associated with severe chronic infection or lithiasis. They also spread to the regional lymphatics. Microscopic examination reveals the typical picture presented by squamous cell tumors seen elsewhere in the body.

Clinical Findings

A. Symptoms: Gross painless hematuria is the most common complaint of patients with renal pelvic tumor. Bleeding is at times quite profuse. Flank pain may be due to ureteral obstruction from the tumor; there may be ureteral colic from passage of clots.

B. Signs: Tenderness may be found over the kidney, particularly if ureteral obstruction has occurred or if infection has supervened. A palpably enlarged kidney is not common.

C. Laboratory Findings: Anemia can be marked if bleeding is profuse. Gross or microscopic hematuria is to be expected, but at intervals the urine may be free of red cells. Renal infection can result from obstruction or can be primary with epidermoid tumors, in which case pus and bacteria will be found in the urine. Renal function tests will be of little help; although the kidney may be gradually destroyed by the tumor, the other kidney will assume the lost function.

D. X-Ray Findings: A plain film of the abdomen will probably not be of much value, for the kidney is ordinarily not grossly enlarged. Excretory urograms, if good filling occurs, will show a space-occupying lesion in the pelvis (Fig 17-7) or a calyx. A chest film should be taken routinely, although metastases to the lungs are not common.

Retrograde urography should reveal the filling defect. Secondary ureteral growths may also be demonstrated. Selective renal angiography may reveal an unusually large ureteropelvic artery or even tumor blush.

E. Instrumental Examination: Cystoscopy must be done immediately if and when gross bleeding is present; blood may be seen spurting from one ureteral orifice. During cystoscopy, search must be made for ''satellite'' tumors on the bladder wall.

F. Cytology: The Papanicolaou technic or methylene blue smear of the urinary sediment is usually positive.

Differential Diagnosis

Adenocarcinoma of the kidney will cause hematuria. Such a tumor is apt to be palpable or may be visible on a plain film of the abdomen as an expansion of a portion of the kidney. Urograms will show the intrarenal nature of the growth. However, blood clots in the renal pelvis can mimic pelvic tumor.

A nonopaque renal stone may cause hematuria and renal pain. A mass may be palpable if hydronephrosis develops. Urograms will show a space-occupying lesion of the pelvis, but the outline of the negative (black) shadow (representing the stone) tends to be smoothly round or oval with stone and irregular (papillary) with tumor (Fig 15-2). With tumor, cytology may be positive.

An opaque renal stone may be associated with an epidermoid carcinoma of the renal pelvis. Diagnosis under these circumstances may be difficult and may be possible only at the time of surgical exploration for the treatment of the calculus.

Renal tuberculosis may mimic pelvic neoplasm. The urogram may show irregularity of the pelvic outline due to ulceration. This might suggest tumor. The patient with urinary tract tuberculosis usually complains of vesical irritability and has a "sterile" pyuria. Acid-fast organisms can be demonstrated in the urine.

Complications

On rare occasion, hemorrhage may be so severe that emergency nephrectomy is necessary.

Hydronephrosis or hydrocalycosis may arise from progressive obstruction. Secondary infection may then develop.

Treatment

A. Specific Measures: Once the diagnosis has been made and evidence of metastasis ruled out, the kidney, ureter, and the periureteral portion of the bladder must be removed. This radical procedure is necessary because secondary ureteral and vesical tumors may be present or may develop later in the ureteral stump or bladder.

B. Palliative Measures: Even though metastases are demonstrated it may be advisable to remove the affected kidney if pain or infec-

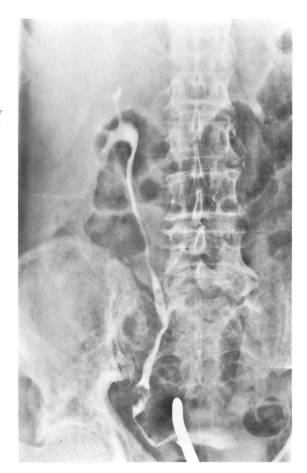
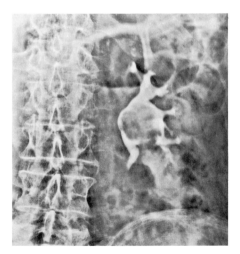

Fig 17-7. Left: Excretory urogram showing space occupying lesion of left renal pelvis. Transitional cell carcinoma. **Right:** Retrograde urogram showing "negative" shadow caused by transitional cell carcinoma of the lower right ureter without evidence of obstruction.

tion from obstruction is severe or if bleeding is profuse.

Tumors of the renal pelvis are radioresistant. Little can be expected from radiotherapy.

Prognosis

The prognosis for the patient suffering from benign tumor is excellent. With low-grade malignancies the outlook is good (75% are alive after 5 years); it is fair to poor if the papillary tumor is undifferentiated (25% are alive after 5 years). Epidermoid carcinoma is almost always fatal within 1 year.

Grabstald, H., Whitmore, W. F., & M. R. Melamed: Renal pelvic tumors. JAMA **218**:845-54, 1971.

Lagergren, C., & A. Ljungqvist: The arterial vasculature of renal pelvic carcinomas. Acta chir scandinav **130**:321-30, 1965.

Magri, J., & E. A. Atkinson: Primary amyloidosis of the ureter. Brit J Urol **42**:37-42, 1970.

Mitty, H. A., Baron, M. G., & M. Feller: Infiltrating carcinoma of the renal pelvis. Angiographic features. Radiology **92**:994-8, 1969.

Poole-Wilson, D. S.: Occupational tumours of the renal pelvis and ureter arising in dye-making industry. Proc Roy Soc Med **62**:93-4, 1969.

Schapira, H. E., & H. A. Mitty: Tumors of the renal pelvis: Clinical review with emphasis on selective angiography. J Urol **106**:642-5, 1971.

Sherwood, T.: Upper urinary tract tumours following on bladder carcinoma: Natural history of urothelial neoplastic disease. Brit J Radiol **44**:137-41, 1971.

TUMORS OF THE URETER

Tumors of the ureter are rare; the majority are malignant and papillary in type. A little more than half of them occur in men.

Etiology

Although the cause of these tumors is not known, there is increasing evidence that carcinogens are involved.

Pathogenesis and Pathology

Ureteral tumors may be primary or may be associated with similar tumors of the renal pelvis or bladder. Although they usually bleed, many of the symptoms are caused by ureteral obstruction (eg, renal and ureteral pain).

These neoplasms are similar in all respects to those of the renal pelvis and bladder. Most are papillary; a few are sessile. Squamous cell carcinoma is rare. Fibrous polyps are occasionally seen.

Transitional cell carcinomas range from a low to a high grade of malignancy. The most malignant show invasion of the stroma and ureteral wall by pleomorphic cells which have a marked tendency to metastasize to regional lymph nodes, lungs, and liver.

Clinical Findings

A. Symptoms: The most common symptom is hematuria, usually intermittent and sometimes quite profuse. There may be a dull pain over the kidney, caused by ureteral obstruction. Acute renal colic can occur from the passage of clots down the ureter. There may be symptoms of urinary tract infection (secondary to obstruction). These include fever, back pain, and vesical irritability.

B. Signs: Physical findings are usually absent. If the kidney has become hydronephrotic from ureteral obstruction, it may be palpable. If it is infected, it may be tender. An enlarged liver or a mass of lymph nodes (metastatic involvement) may be felt.

C. Laboratory Findings: Anemia may be found if bleeding is prolonged or severe. Gross or microscopic hematuria is usually present. Evidence of infection may be found on urinalysis. Renal function will ordinarily not be impaired unless the other kidney is also diseased.

D. X-Ray Findings: A plain film of the abdomen may show an enlarged renal shadow (hydronephrosis) secondary to ureteral obstruction. Excretory urograms will usually make the diagnosis (Fig 17-7). There is often dilatation of the urinary passages proximal to the obstructive tumor, and an intraureteral space-occupying lesion may be noted as the cause for the obstruction. An x-ray of the chest should be taken as soon as the diagnosis of ureteral tumor is made since metastases may be found in the lungs.

A ureteral catheter passed up the ureter for urography often forms a loop at the site of the tumor. Radiograms may demonstrate the lesion. Oblique views are often helpful.

E. Instrumental Examination: Cystoscopy should be done immediately if the patient is actively bleeding in order to locate the source of the hemorrhage. It must be done also to observe for "seeding" of secondary growths on the bladder wall. Occasionally the tumor can be seen protruding from the ureteral orifice.

Ureteral catheterization may cause considerable blood to drain from the catheter when it passes by the tumor. When its tip reaches the renal pelvis, the urine becomes clear: this may therefore be of diagnostic significance.

F. Cytology: Papanicolaou studies or a methylene blue smear of the urinary sediment may prove helpful if the diagnosis cannot be established by urography.

Differential Diagnosis

Ureteral calculus, if it is radiolucent, may cause the same symptoms and signs as ureteral tumor. The urogram in each case will show a ''negative'' or black shadow in the ureter with dilatation of the tract above it. Stone is suggested if a ''grating'' feeling is noted as the catheter is passed by it. The correct diagnosis may be possible only at surgery.

Ureteral stenosis, often secondary to compression by masses of lymph nodes involved by cancer (eg, cervix), can mimic ureteral tumor. The discovery of a primary tumor will make the diagnosis.

Complications

Hydronephrosis is often found with ureteral tumor.

Because obstruction is usually present, infection is a common complication of ureteral tumor. The pyuria usually fails to clear despite appropriate medication; this should indicate the need for urography, which will demonstrate the tumor.

Treatment

A. Specific Measures: In the absence of demonstrable metastases, ureteronephrectomy and the resection of the periureteral bladder wall are necessary.

B. Palliative Measures: Little can be accomplished if metastases are present, since these tumors are usually radioresistant. Ureteronephrectomy may be necessary to relieve pain due to the obstruction or to control otherwise intractable bleeding. It may also be indicated because of severe and persistent infection of the kidney.

Prognosis

The prognosis in the benign type is excellent; with the malignant transitional cell carcinomas, it is only fair. Patients with squamous cell tumors or tumors which have involved the ureteral muscle and regional lymph nodes are rarely cured.

Bloom, N. A., Vidone, R. A., & B. Lytton: Primary carcinoma of the ureter: A report of 102 new cases. J Urol 103:590-8, 1970.

Crum, P. M., & others: Benign ureteral polyps. J Urol 102:679-82, 1969.

Hawtrey, C. E.: Fifty-two cases of primary ureteral carcinoma: A clinical-pathologic study. J Urol 105:188-93, 1971.

Lang, E. K., & M. Nourse: The roentgenographic diagnosis of obstructive lesions of the ureter. J Urol 101:812-20, 1969.

Meyer, P. C.: The histologic grading of primary epithelial neoplasms of the ureter. J Urol 102:30-6, 1969.

Takaha, M., Nagata, H., & T. Sonoda: Localized amyloid tumor of the ureter: Report of a case. J Urol 105:502-4, 1971.

Watts, H. G.: Primary tumors of the ureteral stump: Report of 2 cases and review of literature. J Urol 104:258-61, 1970.

TUMORS OF THE BLADDER

Tumors of the bladder are the second most common of all genitourinary neoplasms. (Only prostatic tumors occur more frequently.) Seventy-five percent are found in men. Most are seen after age 50. Papillomatous growths submit readily to transurethral treatment if diagnosed early. Infiltrating (transitional cell) types constitute one of the most difficult of all urologic problems.

Etiology

It has long been established that prolonged exposure to certain industrial aromatic amines (eg, 2-naphthylamine, benzidine, 4-aminodiphenyl) may be associated with a high incidence of vesical neoplasm. Recent work suggests that the multiple transitional cell tumors involving the urinary tract (eg, renal pelvis, ureter, bladder) probably are caused by carcinogens, particularly tryptophan. This substance and the industrial amines listed above are metabolized to ortho-aminophenols by the liver, conjugated with sulfate or glucuronic acid, and excreted through the kidneys. These materials are attacked by hydrolytic enzymes (beta-glucuronides), thus liberating orthophenols, some of which have been proved to be carcinogenic in dogs and mice. These carcinogens are found in increased concentration in the urines of those patients harboring vesical tumors (Boyland). Price finds increased urinary levels in about one-half of his subjects. Lewis and others could not corroborate these findings. It is thought that many years of exposure to these carcinogens are necessary to stimulate the growth of these tumors.

There is evidence that the activity of urinary beta-glucuronidase is increased mere-

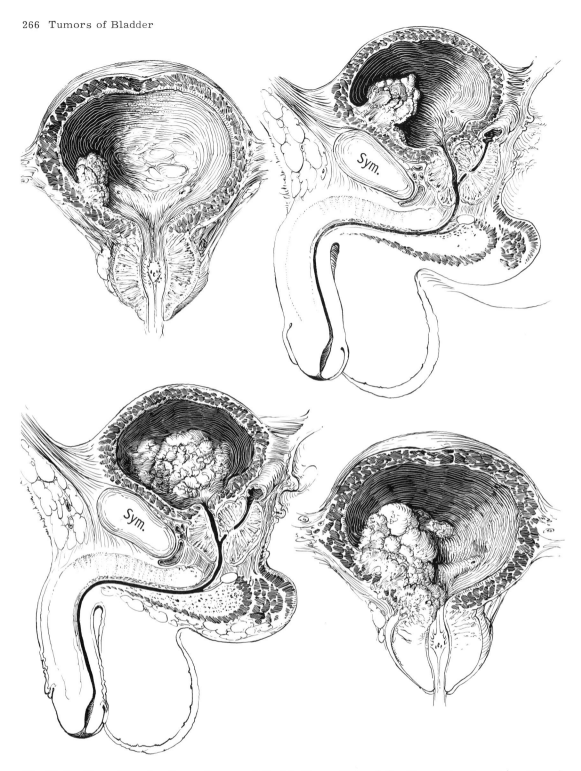

Fig 17-8. Transitional cell carcinomas of the bladder. **Above left:** Transitional cell (papillary) carcinoma with minimal invasion of the bladder wall. This is compatible with a grade II, stage A tumor. **Above right:** Larger, more invasive transitional cell carcinoma, probably grade II-III, stage B_1. **Below left:** More extensive transitional cell carcinoma involving the right ureteral orifice, compatible with grade III, stage B_2. **Below right:** Advanced large, invasive carcinoma of the bladder; occlusion of right ureteral orifice with extension into the bladder neck and prostate (grade IV, stage C).

ly by forcing fluids and by the presence of vesical infection, even schistosomiasis. This substance is also found in increased amounts in the presence of other cancers, benign enlargement of the prostate, renal infection, renal cyst, and urolithiasis. Kallet and Lapcol claim that this enzyme is elaborated by urologic epithelial cells which have been damaged; therefore, increases in urinary levels of beta-glucuronidase are of no diagnostic significance.

Smoking has been cited as a cause of the increased incidence of vesical neoplasm in Denmark. It has recently been shown that smokers experience a 50% increase in carcinogenic metabolites of tryptophan excreted in the urine. On cessation of smoking, the levels return to normal. The high incidence of cancer of the bladder in patients with severe vesical schistosomiasis is well known.

Pathogenesis and Pathology

It is customary to judge transitional cell vesical carcinomas in 2 ways: (1) The degree of differentiation of the cells, and (2) the depth of penetration of the tumor into the vesical wall.

A. The Grade and Stage of the Tumor:
1. Grade - The degree of cell differentiation.

Grade I tumors are quite well differentiated. The lamina propria is usually not involved. Most are relatively small, are papillary in type, and have a narrow base. These are curable by transurethral means but are radio-resistant.

Grade II tumors are papillary in type, show less differentiation of their cells, and are apt to invade the lamina propria if not the detrusor muscle itself. They tend to be larger than the grade I tumors and have a wider connection with the bladder wall. They are often curable by transurethral resection. They do not respond too well to radiotherapy.

Grade III and IV neoplasms are poorly differentiated, even anaplastic. They tend to be nodular rather than papillary, and as a rule are quite invasive. They respond poorly to transurethral removal as well as cystectomy but are sensitive to radiotherapy.

2. Stage - The degree of invasion.
Stage O represents a papillary tumor which has not invaded the lamina propria.

Stage A tumors have invaded the lamina propria but not the muscle of the vesical wall.

Stage B$_1$ neoplasms have extended into the superficial half of the detrusor muscle.

Stage B$_2$ tumors are found in the deep muscle layers.

Stage C tumors have extended into the perivesical fat or have involved overlying peritoneum.

Stage D tumors have demonstrable metastases (eg, lymph nodes, liver).

B. Type and Location: Since 80% of vesical tumors arise on the base of the bladder, they may involve one or both ureteral orifices or the vesical neck. Hydroureteronephrosis and pyelonephritis are common complications. When tumors ulcerate, they bleed and often become infected.

Most growths are papillary in type and are malignant. They may be single or multiple; generalized papillomatosis is not uncommon. Generally speaking, the larger the tumor and the broader its base, the more malignant it is, and nodular tumors are more malignant than the papillary types.

Lamb has noted that aberrations in chromosome count and structural abnormality are apt to be seen in the undifferentiated tumors.

After successful treatment of even the grade I and II types that are superficial (stages O and A), there is a definite tendency for new tumors to develop elsewhere in the bladder. This suggests that the appearance of these tumors is in some way related to a generally increased susceptibility of the mucosa to neoplastic proliferation, perhaps in response to carcinogens. This is true also of the renal pelvic and ureteral transitional cell tumors.

Vesical neoplasms most commonly metastasize to the vesical, hypogastric, common iliac, and lumbar nodes. The bones, liver, and lungs are at times affected.

Rarely, other types of vesical neoplasms may be encountered:

(1) Epidermoid carcinoma: About 5% of vesical neoplasms are of the squamous cell variety. These are ordinarily highly malignant (anaplastic), deeply invasive, and metastasize early. With a few exceptions, they are incurable.

(2) Adenocarcinoma is very rare. It often arises in a urachal remnant.

(3) Rhabdomyosarcomas are quite rare. They occur most frequently in male children and adolescents. They infiltrate widely, metastasize early, and are usually fatal.

(4) Primary malignant lymphomas, neurofibromas, hemangiomas, and pheochromocytomas are rare. The latter may be associated with attacks of hypertension during voiding.

(5) Cancers of the skin (melanoma), stomach, lung, and breast may metastasize to the bladder. Vesical invasion by endometriosis may occur.

Clinical Findings

A. Symptoms: Gross hematuria is the most common symptom. As with all tumors of the urinary tract, hematuria is usually intermittent. All bleeding, severe or mild, prolonged or transient, must be accounted for.

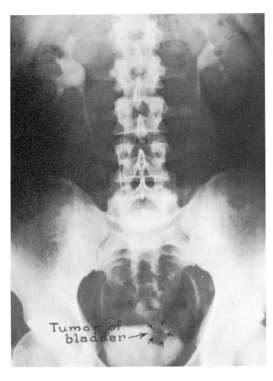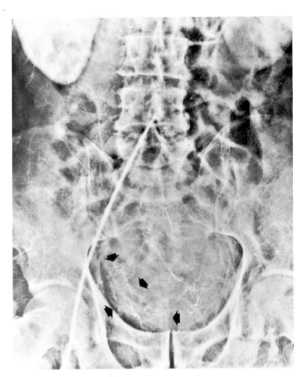

Fig 17-9. Tumors of the bladder. Left: Excretory urogram showing space-occupying lesion (transitional cell carcinoma) on the left side of the bladder; the upper tracts are normal. **Right:** Vesical angiogram, delayed film, showing increased vascularity of a deeply invasive transitional carcinoma grade IV, stage C, right vesical wall. Some of these vessels are presumed to be typical of tumor.

If infection supervenes, symptoms of cystitis will usually be present. These include burning on urination, urgency, frequency, and nocturia. Symptoms of bladder neck obstruction may develop if the tumor encroaches on the internal orifice. These include hesitancy and decrease in force and caliber of the urinary stream. If there is perivesical extension, suprapubic pain may be constant and severe. Pain in the flank may be noted if the growth obstructs a ureteral orifice and produces hydronephrosis. This may be complicated by renal infection, which may cause increased pain and high fever. If metastases are present, if infection is severe, or if anemia has developed, the patient may complain of weakness and loss of weight.

B. Signs: In most cases nothing abnormal can be found on physical examination. Renal tenderness or enlargement may be present due to ureteral obstruction and infection. A suprapubic mass may be noted on rare occasion. This might be due either to a large cancer or to urinary retention caused by clots or invasion of the bladder neck by tumor. On vaginal examination a mass at the base of the bladder may be noted. Less often, rectal examination may reveal an invasive mass in the trigonal area. Bimanual palpation (abdominorectal or abdominovaginal) is of the greatest importance in feeling and estimating the size and extent of the growth. This is best done under anesthesia. Signs of metastases may be noted. These include palpable abdominal masses (involved lymph nodes along the iliac vessels) and edema of one or both legs from occlusion of the iliacs.

C. Laboratory Findings: Anemia is not uncommon and may be from loss of blood, severe infection, or uremia caused by occlusion of both ureteral orifices by the growth. The urine may be very bloody, but between bouts of bleeding few if any red cells may be found. Pus and bacteria may also be noted. Renal function tests are usually normal unless there is bladder neck obstruction with residual urine or obstruction of both ureteral orifices. The level of LDH in the urine is often elevated.

D. X-Ray Findings: Excretory urograms are usually normal but may show the tumor itself (Fig 17-9), evidence of ureteral obstruction or a primary tumor of the renal pelvis or ureter as a cause of the "primary" vesical growth. Retrograde cystograms may show the tumor if it is large enough. A "fractionated" cystogram may afford evidence of invasion of the tumor into the vesical wall. First, the vesical capacity is determined. This amount of diluted radiopaque medium is then prepared. One-fourth of this amount is then instilled into the bladder and an x-ray exposure made. The other three-fourths are successively instilled, and an x-ray exposure is then made on the same film. If the tumor is superficial, the vesical wall will fill symmetrically; in the presence of invasion, that portion of the wall will not expand. Vesical angiography may afford information concerning depth of infiltration of the tumor. It is quite accurate in revealing stage C and stage D tumors (Fig 17-9). Lymphangiography will reveal evidence of lymph node metastases.

E. Instrumental Examination: Cystoscopy almost always reveals the tumor. Biopsy of the lesion should be routine. A few tumors may be missed by this means, but these can be visualized if the patient is given tetracycline for a few days before cystoscopy, using ultraviolet illumination. The tetracycline causes fluorescence of the tumor.

F. Cytology: Papanicolaou preparations or, preferably, the simpler methylene blue stain of fresh urinary sediment will almost always reveal transitional cells shed from the tumor. Well-differentiated tumors shed round cells of rather uniform size with large nuclei. When anaplastic tumors are present the urinary sediment usually reveals large epithelial cells (often in clumps) with very large dark staining nuclei.

This procedure is also useful in the follow-up of these patients and as a screening test for those exposed to chemical carcinogens. Suspicious cells (carcinoma in situ) may be noted months before a tumor can be discovered cystoscopically.

Differential Diagnosis

Renal or ureteral tumors also cause hematuria. Urograms will demonstrate the renal or ureteral lesion. Palpation or a plain abdominal film may reveal an enlarged kidney. It must be remembered that tumors of the renal pelvis or ureter may "seed" to the bladder wall, and the "primary" vesical neoplasm may really be "secondary."

Endometriosis occasionally involves the bladder. Bleeding and vesical irritability may be most marked at the time of the menses. Cystoscopically, the lesion is bluish in color and looks like a vascular tumor. Pelvic examination usually reveals evidence of other sites of involvement.

Acute nonspecific infections of the bladder or prostate may cause hematuria, but bleeding is usually terminal and associated with symptoms of cystitis. A tumor often becomes infected, however. Differentiation depends upon cystoscopy.

Benign prostatic hypertrophy commonly causes hematuria, often initial or terminal. Cystoscopy is necessary in the differential diagnosis.

Tuberculosis of the urinary tract often causes bleeding. A "sterile" pyuria is usually found, and tubercle bacilli can be demonstrated by special technics. Excretory urograms will be negative for tumor but may show evidence of calyceal ulceration. Again, cystoscopy will establish the diagnosis.

Renal, ureteral, or vesical stones may mimic tumor, but a plain film or excretory urogram will usually demonstrate them.

Acute hemorrhagic nephritis in an adult may require differentiation from tumor. The urinary findings (casts), hypertension, and edema should lead to the proper diagnosis. In case of doubt, cystoscopy is indicated.

Tumors of the cervix or bowel may invade the bladder. Demonstration of the primary tumor and a biopsy of the vesical lesion should settle the diagnosis.

Complications

Secondary infection of the bladder is common when the tumor ulcerates. It may be severe. Renal infection is not uncommon when ureteral obstruction ensues. Urinary retention may develop if the tumor invades the bladder neck.

Hydronephrosis due to ureteral occlusion is common. If bilateral, uremia supervenes. This is the most common cause of death.

Hemorrhage may become a problem.

Treatment

There is still considerable disagreement about the proper treatment of vesical neoplasms. Certainly the low-grade superficial tumors lend themselves well to transurethral resection. For the more malignant and invasive tumors, the physician must choose between radiotherapy and radical surgery or a combination thereof.

A. Surgical Measures: Most single or multiple papillomas are best treated by transurethral resection, care being taken to "saucerize" deeply into the wall of the bladder in order to remove the base of the tumor completely. This procedure will cure many of the papillary carcinomas (eg, stage O, A, B_1, grade I, II). However, if the tumor has invaded deeply into the vesical muscle (stage

B_2, C), this method will usually fail.

Partial (segmental) cystectomy is feasible if the malignant tumor does not lie on the base of the bladder, for in this case one or both ureteral orifices might have to be sacrificed. Unfortunately, fewer than 20% of vesical tumors are restricted to areas far removed from the trigone.

Total cystectomy (with removal of the prostate) is often practiced for the treatment of papillomatosis and many of the more undifferentiated invasive tumors. Diversion of the urinary stream presents a problem. Ureterosigmoidostomy results in urinary continence but frequently causes ureteral obstruction or reflux with hydronephrosis and renal infection. Many of these patients die of renal insufficiency rather than of cancer. A few will develop symptomatic hyperchloremic acidosis from absorption of the chloride ions in the urine. Hypokalemia may occur. The administration of potassium citrate will usually correct these electrolytic defects. The most popular method of urinary diversion today is anastomosis of the ureters to an isolated loop of ileum (or sigmoid) with one end of this loop brought to the skin to act as a conduit. Renal complications and electrolyte problems are minimized.

B. Radiation Therapy: In general, the more undifferentiated the tumor the more radiosensitive it is. It is therefore most useful in the grade III-IV, stage B_2 and C lesions. There is mounting evidence that radiotherapy in this type of neoplasm offers at least as good if not a better control rate than radical surgery without the mortality associated with the latter. The optimal dose is 6000 rads given over a period of 6 weeks or more. This is compatible with the maintenance of good vesical function. If, after irradiation, viable tumor is still demonstrable, cystectomy can still be considered. There has been recent enthusiasm for use of radiotherapy (4500 rads) followed by planned cystectomy 1-2 months later. It has been observed that 20-30% of these bladders are found to be free of tumor. This seems to reflect the significant value of modern radiation therapy.

C. Chemotherapy: Palliation of vesical neoplasms with 2 parenteral anticancer drugs has been reported (citral, 5-fluorouracil). Their effects are not dramatic. The instillation by catheter of 60 mg of triethylenethiophosphoramide (Thio-Tepa®) dissolved in 30-60 ml of normal saline has been suggested by Veenema in the treatment of superficial low-grade papillomas. Four to 6 weekly treatments should be given. This should be followed by instillations every month for 6-10 months. Success is judged by urinary cytology and cystoscopy. Similar therapy is indicated if new tumors appear following transurethral resection of a low-grade superficial neoplasm. This may change the nature of the mucosa; the appearance of new tumors may cease. Before each instillation, a white cell and platelet count should be obtained. Should the white count be less than 4000 or the platelets below 100,000 cu mm, treatment should be deferred until the hemogram improves.

D. Treatment of Complications: Infection can usually be controlled with antibiotics. It cannot be completely eradicated, however, as long as ulceration (either spontaneous or following electrosurgery) is present. Radiotherapy may control excessive bleeding. An infected hydronephrotic kidney, secondarily obstructed by the growth, may have to be removed.

Prevention

Employment in aniline dye factories should be restricted to 3 years, during which time periodic urinary Papanicolaou studies and cystoscopy are indicated. The clinical significance of endogenous carcinogenic agents has not been established. Schlegel has adduced evidence that the administration of ascorbic acid, 0.5 gm 3 times a day, may prevent the formation of vesical tumors through neutralization of urinary carcinogens. It seems worthwhile, therefore, to prescribe this drug in those in whom the diagnosis has been made.

Prognosis

The superficial, well-differentiated tumors may recur, or new papillomas may appear. Constant vigilance, with periodic cystoscopy, is therefore necessary for at least 3 years. New tumors may also be well controlled by transurethral means, but if they tend to recur they are apt to become progressively invasive and of higher grade. Cystectomy or radiation therapy must then be considered.

Prognosis with any vesical tumor varies, in general, with the stage (invasion) and grade (differentiation). The best results are obtained by transurethral resection of the grade I-II, stage O, A, B_1 tumors. Cystectomy cures about 15-25% of grade III-IV, stage B_2-C lesions with an accompanying mortality from the operation of 5-15%. Radiotherapy for the same serious neoplasms offers about 15-20% control at 5 years.

Barnes, R. W., & others: Control of bladder tumors by endoscopic surgery. J Urol **97**: 864-8, 1967.

Beck, A. D., Gaudin, H. J., & D. G. Bonham: Carcinoma of the urachus. Brit J Urol **42**: 555-62, 1970.

Boyland, E.: The Biochemistry of Bladder Cancer. Thomas, 1963.

Brinton, J.A., Ito, Y., & B.S. Olsen: Carcinosarcoma of the urinary bladder. Cancer 25:1183-6, 1970.

Caldwell, W.L., Bagshaw, M.A., & A.S. Kaplan: Efficacy of linear accelerator x-ray therapy in cancer of the bladder. J Urol 97:294-303, 1967.

Charron, J.W., & G. Gariepy: Neurofibromatosis of bladder: Case report and review of literature. Canad J Surg 13:303-6, 1970.

Connolly, J.G., & others: Use of the fractionated cystogram in the staging of bladder tumors. Canad J Surg 9:39-43, 1966.

Drew, J.E., & V.F. Marshall: The effects of topical thiotepa on the recurrence rate of superficial bladder cancers. J Urol 99:740-3, 1968.

Edland, R.W., Wear, J.B., Jr., & F.J. Ansfield: Advanced cancer of the urinary bladder. Am J Roentgenol 108:124-9, 1970.

Edsmyr, F., Moberger, F., & L. Wadström: Carcinoma of the bladder. Cystectomy after supervoltage therapy. Scandinav J Urol Nephrol 5:215-21, 1971.

Ellis, L.R., Udall, D.A., & C.V. Hodges: Further clinical experience with intestinal segments for urinary diversion. J Urol 105:354-7, 1971.

Falor, W.H.: Chromosomes in noninvasive papillary carcinoma of the bladder. JAMA 216:791-4, 1971.

Fein, R.L., & B.F. Horton: Vesical endometriosis: A case report and review of the literature. J Urol 95:45-50, 1966.

Goldstein, A.G.: Metastatic carcinoma to the bladder. J Urol 98:209-15, 1967.

Hendry, W.F., & J. Vinnicombe: Haemangioma of bladder in children and young adults. Brit J Urol 43:309-16, 1971.

Higgins, P.M., & G.C. Tresidder: Phaeochromocytoma of the urinary bladder. Brit MJ 3:274-7, 1966.

Jack, G.A.: Improved results of irradiation for carcinoma of the bladder. J Urol 102:330-2, 1969.

Jarman, W.D., & J.C. Kenealy: Polypoid rhabdomyosarcoma of the bladder in children. J Urol 103:227-31, 1970.

Jewett, H.J., King, L.R., & W.M. Shelley: A study of 365 cases of infiltrating bladder cancer: Relation of certain pathological characteristics to prognosis after extirpation. J Urol 92:668-78, 1964.

Kallet, H.A., & L. Lapco: Urine beta glucuronidase activity in urinary tract disease. J Urol 97:352-6, 1967.

Kaufman, J.J.: Treatment of carcinoma of the bladder with combined radiotherapy, chemotherapy, and surgery. Arch Surg 99:477-83, 1969.

Kerr, W.K., & others: The effect of cigarette smoking on bladder carcinogens in man. Canad MAJ 93:1-7, 1965.

Lacy, S.S., Whitley, J.E., & C.E. Cox: Vesical arteriography: An adjunct to staging of bladder tumors. Brit J Urol 42:50-5, 1970.

Lamb, D.: Correlation of chromosome counts with histological appearances and prognosis in transitional-cell carcinoma of bladder. Brit MJ 1:273-7, 1967.

Lang, E.K.: The roentgenographic assessment of bladder tumors. Surg Gynec Obst 23:717-24, 1969.

Laskowski, T.Z., Scott, R., Jr., & P.T. Hudgins: Combined therapy: Radiation and surgery in the treatment of bladder cancer. J Urol 99:733-9, 1968.

Leestma, J.E., & E.B. Price, Jr.: Paraganglioma of the urinary bladder. Cancer 28:1063-73, 1971.

Lerman, R.I., Hutter, R.V., & W.F. Whitmore, Jr.: Papilloma of the urinary bladder. Cancer 25:333-42, 1970.

Masina, F.: Segmental resection for tumours of the urinary bladder: Ten-year follow-up. Brit J Surg 52:279-83, 1965.

Melamed, M.R., Voutsa, N.G., & H. Grabstald: Natural history and clinical behavior of in situ carcinoma of the human urinary bladder. Cancer 17:1533-45, 1964.

Newman, D.M., & others: Squamous cell carcinoma of the bladder. J Urol 100:470-3, 1958.

Norehad, E.A., & others: Endometrosis of the bladder: case report. J Urol 96:901-5, 1966.

Park, C-H., & others: Reliability of positive exfoliative cytologic study of the urine in urinary tract malignancy. J Urol 102:91-2, 1969.

Poole-Wilson, D.S., & R.J. Barnard: Total cystectomy for bladder tumours. Brit J Urol 43:16-24, 1971.

Poole-Wilson, D.S.: Occupational tumours of the bladder. Proc Roy Soc Med 53:801-14, 1960.

Powel-Smith, C.J., & E.C. Reid: Preoperative irradiation and radical cystectomy in carcinoma of the bladder. Cancer 25:781-6, 1970.

Prout, G.R., Jr., Slack, N.H., & I.D.J. Bross: Preoperative irradiation as an adjuvant in the surgical management of invasive bladder carcinoma. J Urol 105:221-3, 1971.

Rubin, P.: Cancer of the urogenital tract: Bladder cancer. JAMA 206:2719-28, 1968.

Rubin, P., & others: Current concepts in Cancer-No. 22. The urogenital tract: Bladder cancer. JAMA 206:1761-76, 1968.

Santino, A.M., Shumaker, E.J., & J. Garces: Primary malignant lymphoma of the bladder. J Urol 103:310-3, 1970.

Schlegel, J.U., & others: The role of ascorbic acid in the prevention of bladder tumor formation. J Urol **103**:155-9, 1970.

Schulte, J.W.: Normal and pathologic cells in urine. Postgrad Med **33**:417-22, 1963.

Silber, I., Bowles, W.T., & J.J. Cordonnier: Palliative treatment of carcinoma of the bladder. Surg Gynec Obst **23**:586-8, 1969.

Smart, J.G.: Renal and ureteric tumours in association with bladder tumours. Brit J Urol **36**:380-90, 1964.

Sørensen, B.L., & others: Ultraviolet light cystoscopy in patients with bladder cancer. Scandinav J Urol Nephrol **3**:193-200, 1969.

Staszewski, J.: Smoking and cancer of the urinary bladder in males in Poland. Brit J Cancer **20**:32-5, 1966.

Thomas, D.G., Ward, A.M., & J.L. Williams: A study of 52 cases of adenocarcinoma of the bladder. Brit J Urol **43**:4-15, 1971.

Torres, H., & M.J. Bennett: Neurofibromatosis of the bladder: Case report and review of the literature. J Urol **96**:910-2, 1966.

Veenema, R.J., & others: Thiotepa bladder instillations: Therapy and prophylaxis for superficial bladder tumors. J Urol **101**: 711-5, 1969.

Wang, C.C., Scully, R.E., & W.F. Leadbetter: Primary malignant lymphoma of the urinary bladder. Cancer **24**:772-6, 1969.

Whitehead, E.D., & A.N. Tessler: Carcinoma of the urachus. Brit J Urol **43**:468-76, 1971.

Whitmore, W.F., Jr., & I.M. Bush: Ultraviolet cystoscopy in patients with bladder cancer. J Urol **95**:201-7, 1966.

Whitmore, W.F., Jr., & others: Preoperative irradiation with cystectomy in the management of bladder cancer. Am J Roentgenol **102**:570-6, 1968.

Whitmore, W.F., Jr., & V.F. Marshall: Radical total cystectomy for cancer of the bladder: 230 consecutive cases five years later. J Urol **87**:853-68, 1962.

Williams, D.I., & G. Schistad: Lower urinary tract tumours in children. Brit J Urol **36**: 51-65, 1964.

Yoshida, O., Brown, R.R., & G.T. Bryan: Relationship between tryptophan metabolism and heterotopic recurrences of human urinary bladder tumors. Cancer **25**:773-80, 1970.

TUMORS OF THE PROSTATE GLAND

The prostate is the urologic organ most often affected by benign or malignant neoplasm. Cancer of this organ is almost as common as malignancy of the lung or gastrointestinal tract.

The danger from adenomatous hypertrophy is not from the lesion per se but from the effects of obstruction: hydronephrosis and renal infection. The same is true, to a large extent, of prostatic cancer, although metastases may contribute to the death of the patient.

BENIGN PROSTATIC HYPERPLASIA (OR HYPERTROPHY)

There is some debate about the cause of the prostatic enlargement. One group believes that the obstructing tissue represents hyperplasia of the periurethral glands with compression of the true prostatic tissue peripherally to form the "surgical capsule." Thus, "prostatectomy" is not prostatectomy at all. The hyperplastic periurethral glandular tissue is removed; the prostate is not. Others believe that the prostatic lobes lying proximal to the verumontanum (the 2 lateral and subcervical lobes) undergo hyperplasia but in addition are invaded by the periurethral glands, thus giving the fibromuscular tissue its often striking glandular component. If this be true, then prostatectomy is accomplished.

Benign prostatic hyperplasia causes progressive obstruction to the flow of urine and, in the later stages, causes back pressure in the kidneys (hydronephrosis) and contributes to the establishment of infection in the urinary tract.

Etiology

Some enlargement begins to develop in most men by age 50. The majority have palpable evidence of hyperplasia by age 60. Not all have symptoms of obstruction, however, nor is the hyperplasia necessarily progressive.

The cause of this disease is not entirely clear, although its relationship to hormonal activity is borne out by much experimental and clinical evidence. Animal investigation reveals that prostatic obstruction is common in aging male dogs, but this does not develop if the animal has been previously castrated. Orchidectomy causes atrophy of the gland and therefore terminates the elaboration of prostatic fluid. Dogs with Sertoli cell (estrogen) tumors of the testis do not develop prostatic hyperplasia.

Previous castration also seems to prevent prostatic hypertrophy in men. However, administration of estrogens or even castration has little if any effect upon the gross size of the enlarged gland, although microscopically some atrophy of the epithelial structures may be noted. The administration of estrogens or androgens has little effect upon the amount of acid phosphatase elaborated by the gland.

Certainly androgens per se cannot be blamed for this hyperplasia, for the disease occurs at a time when the androgenic activity of the organism is decreasing. Therefore, an imbalance between androgens and estrogens may be the causative factor. It is not clear why hyperplasia of the prostate develops in some men and not in others and affects different individuals in varying degrees.

Pathogenesis (See chapter 10.)

The enlarged gland produces its harmful effects by obstructing the bladder neck and by upsetting the mechanisms which force open and funnel the vesical orifice.

A. Changes in the Bladder:

1. Early - As the degree of obstruction increases, the vesical detrusor undergoes compensatory hypertrophy in order to overcome the increasing urethral resistance. The muscle wall may become more than 2 cm thick. This power of compensation varies. One patient with a markedly obstructive gland may have few symptoms, whereas another may have great difficulty with a milder obstruction. There is therefore little relationship between the size of the gland and the severity of symptoms.

As compensatory hypertrophy develops, the following take place:

a. Trabeculation of the bladder wall - Taut, intertwined hypertrophic muscle bundles lift up the mucosa.

b. Hypertrophy of the trigone and interureteric ridge.

c. Diverticula - As the intravesical voiding pressure rises (as it must to overcome increased urethral resistance), the mucosal layer may be forced between the muscle fibers and finally balloon into the perivesical fat. It may then grow to large size. The diverticulum has no muscular wall and therefore cannot empty itself; the urine it contains easily becomes infected.

2. Late - In many men the power for further vesical compensation becomes exhausted when the muscle can no longer hypertrophy, and decompensation occurs. Urine is then retained in the bladder in increasing amounts, and symptoms may become severe. With chronic urinary retention, the hitherto thickened bladder wall may become markedly attenuated and atonic.

B. Changes in the Ureter and Kidney: With secondary hypertrophy of the trigonalureteral complex, there is increased downward traction on the intramural ureteral segments, thus increasing resistance to urine flow. This leads to progressive proximal dilatation and is the common cause of ureterohydronephrosis and its accompanying impaired renal function. Significant residual urine leading to chronic vesical distention may cause a vesicorenal reflux which is reflected in diminution in renal urinary secretion. In either case, vesical drainage by catheter leads to improvement in renal function.

In a few advanced cases of prostatic enlargement, the ureterovesical "valves" may give way. This not only hurts the kidney hydrodynamically but encourages the development and perpetuation of pyelonephritis.

C. Infection: Stagnation of urine leads to infection and its perpetuation. Cystitis may develop. If the organisms split urea, vesical stones may form. If the ureterovesical junction gives way, pyelonephritis develops. The renal lesion is the important complication of prostatic obstruction.

Pathology (See Fig 17-10.)

The prostate in the young adult may be compared to an apple; its true capsule is thin and intimately attached to the underlying secretory tissue. For this reason, intracapsular enucleation of the young man's prostate is impossible. The enlarged gland, on the other hand, is more like an orange. It has a thick "surgical" capsule (the peripherally compressed extraurethral prostate) which is poorly connected to the central obstructing tissue; this permits easy "shelling out" of the hyperplastic prostatic lobes, leaving the "surgical" capsule behind. It should be noted that the posterior prostatic lobe is left as part of this surgical capsule. Since it is in this lobe that carcinoma develops, intracapsular prostatectomy is not prophylactic against cancer developing later.

There are 3 lobes which commonly undergo hyperplasia: the 2 lateral lobes and the subcervical lobe. At times only the lateral lobes enlarge. Again, a fairly pure subcervical lobe hyperplasia is seen. In this instance the rectal examination may reveal a prostate of normal size, for this lobe cannot be felt. Very commonly, all 3 enlarge together. The gland becomes elongated and the lobes tend to herniate through the bladder neck; intravesical protrusion may be marked. Under these circumstances the true size of the gland, as judged by rectal palpation, will not be revealed.

On section the adenomatous pattern is usually obvious; multiple nodules are noted. The "surgical" capsule is composed of atrophic true extraurethral prostatic tissue which has been compressed and displaced to the periphery. It may be 2-5 mm in thickness. This capsule is poorly connected to the hyperplastic

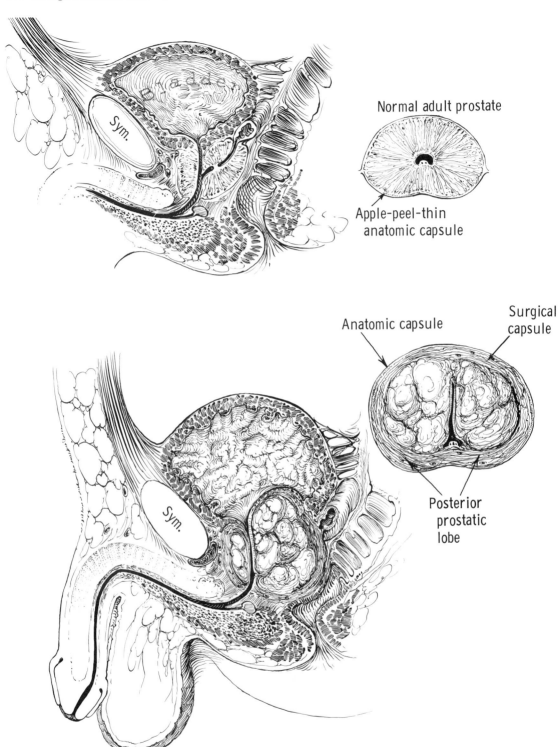

Fig 17-10. Pathogenesis of benign prostatic hyperplasia. Above: Normal bladder and prostate. Inset shows normal prostate (containing prostatic urethra) and thin fibrous anatomic capsule. **Below:** Enlarged prostate enclosed by relatively thick "surgical" capsule which is composed of the posterior prostatic lobe.

lobes, which therefore may be easily enucleated.

Microscopically, the hyperplasia affects glandular, muscular, and fibrous tissue in varying degrees. The epithelial cells are of the tall columnar type. They may pile up into a papillary pattern. There are no mitoses.

Clinical Findings

Benign prostatic enlargement seldom causes significant symptoms before age 50. The complaints are referable to the obstruction and may be increased by infection. Rectal examination may or may not reveal prostatic enlargement. Urinary infection may be present. The PSP may be depressed because of incomplete emptying of the bladder (residual urine); back pressure on the kidneys will cause true impairment of renal function. Cystoscopy will reveal hypertrophy of the prostate and secondary changes in the bladder wall.

A. Symptoms: (The physiologic explanation for the obstructive symptoms is discussed in chapter 10.) In the early stages, the patient may notice that if the bladder becomes too full there is a little hesitation in starting the stream and some loss of force and caliber of the stream. Later, the symptoms are more persistent and severe.

1. Bladder symptoms - Hesitancy in starting the stream may be marked. Considerable straining may be necessary. Because of the increased urethral resistance, decrease in caliber of the bladder neck, and derangement of the normal mechanisms which open the bladder neck, the stream is small and lacks force. This will be worse if the urge to urinate must be put off, for the smooth muscle of the bladder becomes overstretched and loses tone. Toward the end of urination the stream tends to diminish gradually and may end as a mere dribble. Frequency (both day and night) develops, depending on the degree of irritability of the bladder and the amount of residual urine; the greater this amount is, the smaller is the working capacity of the organ. If infection complicates the picture, all of the above symptoms are increased. The inflammatory edema of the prostate or bladder neck will increase the degree of obstruction and will cause more residual urine, thereby further increasing frequency. Hematuria is not uncommon. It may be due to rupture of dilated veins at the bladder neck which are apt to develop with straining. Acute urinary retention may develop suddenly in a patient who has had few premonitory symptoms. At other times it occurs after some months or years of increasing symptoms of prostatism. The patient then experiences great suprapubic pain and marked urgency; he is miserable until relieved by catheterization.

2. Renal symptoms - The hydronephrosis secondary to prostatic obstruction is usually painless unless it becomes infected. In a few men with vesicoureteral reflux, renal pain may be experienced during the act of voiding. In the advanced stage of the disease, symptoms of uremia may be noted: somnolence, vomiting, diarrhea, and loss of weight.

B. Signs: A visible mass low in the midline of the abdomen may be seen, felt, or percussed. In acute retention, it is quite tender. In chronic urinary retention, the bladder may be so flabby that only percussion will reveal it. On rectal examination the prostate may or may not be enlarged. One lobe may be larger than the other. The surface is usually smooth; it may be firm (fibromuscular) or unduly soft and boggy (adenomatous). Areas of induration should be sought (suggesting cancer).

It should be mentioned that the degree of obstruction is measured not by rectal examination but by the severity of the symptoms and the amount of residual urine.

Unless acute urinary infection is present or the patient is verging on complete urinary retention, the gland should be massaged. If pus is found in the secretion, conservative treatment may afford some relief from obstructive symptoms. Tenderness over a kidney may indicate renal infection. The maximum intravesical voiding pressure is significantly increased; voiding flow rate is reduced. Hypertension may be found. It may be caused by renal back pressure (ischemia).

C. Laboratory Findings: Urinalysis may reveal an otherwise completely silent complicating infection (pus, bacteria). Renal function as measured by PSP is a very important step in examination. It also indirectly estimates the presence or absence of residual urine (see p 52). If the PSP is 50% or more at 30 minutes after injection, and the urine volume is small, there can be no significant residual urine. If it is only 25%, either residual urine is present or renal function is depressed. The immediate passage of a catheter will quickly dispose of the question. If the PSP (including that found in the residual urine) is less than 30% in one-half hour, an estimation for nitrogen retention in the blood should be made.

D. X-Ray Findings: A plain film of the abdomen and excretory urograms may show complicating calculi. Often, ureterohydronephrosis is portrayed. This is usually caused by hypertrophy of the trigone which applies increased occlusive pull on the intravesical ureteral segments. Intravesical encroachment of the prostate and even ureteral reflux may be revealed on urethrography and cystography (Fig 17-11). The bladder may be raised well above the upper edge of the symphysis if the gland is significantly elongated.

E. Instrumental Examination: The amount of urine retained after voiding is a measure of the degree of decompensation of the bladder. This is ascertained by passing a catheter to the bladder immediately after voiding.

Cystoscopy or panendoscopy will show the degree of enlargement of the prostatic lobes and the secondary changes in the bladder wall (eg, trabeculation, diverticula, infection). It will also reveal complications such as vesical stone or incidental neoplasm.

Differential Diagnosis

The neurogenic bladder also causes difficulty with urination and a low maximum voiding flow rate. There is often a history of spinal cord or peripheral nerve injury. Neurologic examination may reveal definite abnormality (particularly perianal anesthesia), and the anal sphincter may be found to be atonic (relaxed). A cystometrogram is helpful. Cystoscopy may show little in the way of obstruction. A positive serologic test for syphilis of blood or spinal fluid may be suggestive. Herpes zoster involving the sacral spinal ganglia has caused urinary retention in a few patients.

Contracture of the vesical neck caused by chronic prostatitis (rare) mimics the symptoms of benign enlargement perfectly. A fibrous or nodular prostate is to be expected,

and its secretion will contain pus. Cystoscopy will settle the diagnosis.

Cancer of the prostate will be suggested by the finding of a hard gland. Besides the obstructive symptoms, lumbosacral backache with pain radiating down one or both legs suggests metastases to the bony pelvis or extension along the perineural lymphatics. If the disease is extensive, the serum acid phosphtase is increased. The levels of LDH and alkaline phosphatase in the urine are usually higher than normal. Osteoblastic metastases to the pelvic bones usually mean prostatic cancer. Biopsy is definitive.

Acute prostatitis will cause obstructive symptoms, but this disease is acute, is associated with marked febrile response, and often occurs in young individuals. Pyuria is always found. Rectal examination will reveal a prostate which is enlarged, but it is hot, exquisitely tender, and often fluctuant (abscess).

Urethral stricture also causes obstruction to urinary flow. A history of complicated gonorrhea (now rare) or perineal trauma should suggest the possibility. Urethral discharge, pyuria, and pus in the prostatic secretion usually accompany this abnormality. Urethral exploration with catheter or sound makes the diagnosis.

Sarcoma of the prostate is rare and affects younger men and boys. It is uniformly fatal. Symptoms are those of obstruction. A large, soft, or firm mass is felt in the prostatic area.

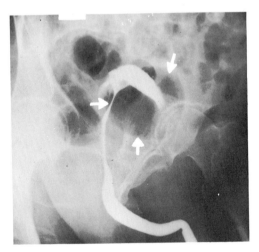 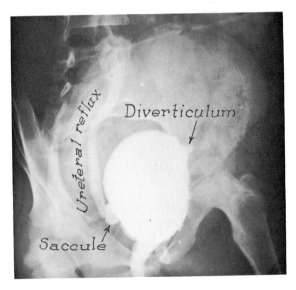

Fig 17-11. **Benign prostatic hypertrophy. Left:** Cystourethrogram. Thick radiopaque material seen in urethra and spreading over superior surface of greatly enlarged intravesical prostate. Arrows outline bladder filled with air. **Right:** Lateral voiding cystourethrogram showing diverticulum of the bladder ("Hutch" saccule; see Fig 11-4) and vesicoureteral reflux. Postoperative prostatectomy.

Vesical stone will be suggested by sudden interruption of the urinary stream accompanied by pain radiating down the penis. It will be revealed by radiography or cystoscopy.

Complications

Obstruction leads to infection. This may involve the bladder, kidneys, and the prostate itself. From the latter, epididymitis may develop. Stones may form in the bladder.

The obstruction may cause vesical diverticula. Hydronephrosis may occur from hypertrophy of the trigone or when a ureterovesical "valve" gives way.

Treatment

Since benign prostatic hyperplasia is not necessarily a progressive disease, conservative therapy should be used where applicable. The problem is to decide which patients can be treated in this manner and which require surgery. Criteria for operation vary, but the following seem feasible: (1) Impaired renal function due to the obstruction. (This indication is hardly debatable.) (2) A degree of symptoms which so upsets the patient that he requests relief. This will vary, since one man may be distressed at urinating 3 times during the night, whereas another may not be particularly inconvenienced by nocturia of 6 times.

A. Conservative Measures: Regular intercourse is the best means of combating prostatic congestion. If necessary, this may be replaced or augmented by 3 or 4 prostatic massages given at intervals of 14 days. At times improvement is striking.

Prostatitis should be treated with antimicrobials (effects will not be dramatic), prostatic massage (not oftener than once a week), and sitz baths.

If pyuria is present, antibiotics or sulfonamides may afford considerable relief. The choice of drug will depend upon the organism found. If there is a great deal of residual urine, drug therapy will probably not be successful.

To protect vesical tone, the patient should be conditioned to avoid excessive intake of fluids in a short period of time. Rapid distention of the bladder may cause the hypertrophic muscle to lose its tone and lead to sudden exacerbation of symptoms or even acute retention. For the same reason, the patient should void as soon as he feels the urge to do so, thus preventing the bladder from becoming overdistended.

The use of antiandrogen therapy (estrogens or orchidectomy) may have some beneficial effect upon benign prostatic hypertrophy, but the cost to the patient (impotence) is too high.

Men who are given testosterone for other reasons may notice improvement in their obstructive symptoms from increased vesical tone. Care should be taken that the patient does not have cancer of the gland, because androgen therapy will hasten its growth. The administration of cyproterone acetate has afforded some encouragement in the treatment of benign enlargement. Its use is still experimental.

Catheterization is mandatory for acute retention. If the patient is still unable to void spontaneously, and particularly if there have been few antecedent symptoms, a catheter should be left indwelling for 2-4 days. Thus, prostatic congestion is relieved, vesical tone is reestablished, and fairly normal voiding may return. If catheterization by any means is impossible, cystostomy must be performed. After a few days, the power of spontaneous urination may be restored. A permanent indwelling catheter (or cystostomy) may occasionally be indicated in the debilitated patient.

B. Surgery: There are 4 operations in vogue at present, but it is impossible to state the indications for each. The choice of operation is a personal matter for the surgeon.

Transurethral prostatectomy is most often used. In some hands only a small amount of tissue is removed; in others, this procedure is essentially a complete intracapsular removal. The latter method is to be preferred, since only this can compete with the results afforded by open surgery. The mortality is about 1-2%, and the urinary result is good in most instances. Potency is maintained, and hospitalization is relatively short.

Suprapubic transvesical prostatectomy is still the most popular open method of removal of the hypertrophied tissue. Its mortality is 2-4%. The urinary result is excellent, probably more consistently so than with the transurethral method. Potency is maintained.

Retropubic extravesical prostatectomy has a mortality rate of 2-4%. The urinary result is excellent. Potency is maintained.

Perineal prostatectomy involves little risk (2-3%), but impotence may occur, there is often some delay in regaining perfect urinary control, and on occasion some degree of stress incontinence persists. Rectourethral fistula has a definite incidence (1-5%), and is most distressing.

Cryosurgery: Some enthusiasm for this method of treatment is being evinced for the poor-risk patient. The instrument is passed down the urethra with the freezing unit placed in the prostatic urethra. Liquid nitrogen is circulated through the probe until the temperature in the prostatic capsule reaches 0-10°C. This leads to death and slough of the obstruct-

ing tissue. Blood loss is usually minimal.
The result in possibly 10% of patients is less
than optimal. Further evaluation of this method
is awaited.

Prognosis

Most patients can be given considerable
relief by conservative means. If on follow-up
their symptoms increase or renal function, as
measured by the PSP test, begins to diminish,
surgical intervention is indicated.

Allan, W.R., & G.J. Coorey: Retropubic
  prostatectomy. Brit J Urol 38:182-8,
  1966.
Baumrucker, G.O.: Transurethral resection:
  Accidents, hazards and pitfalls. J Urol 96:
  250-4, 1966.
Blandy, J.P.: Benign prostatic enlargement.
  Brit MJ 1:31-5, 1971.
Dowd, J.B., & others: Experiences with cryosurgery of the prostate in the poor-risk
  patient. S Clin North America 48:627-32,
  1968.
Finestone, A.J., & R.S. Rosenthal: Silent
  prostatism. Geriatrics 26:89-92, 1971.
Gernert, J.E., Bischoff, A.J., & E. Bors:
  Herpes zoster as a cause of urinary retention. Urol Internat 22:222-6, 1967.
Gill, W., & others: An experience with cryo-
  prostatectomy. Surg Gynec Obst 131:877-
  84, 1970.
Green, N.A.: Cryosurgery of the prostate
  gland in the unfit subject. Brit J Urol 42:
  10-20, 1970.
Holtgrewe, H.L., & W.L. Valk: Late results
  of transurethral prostatectomy. J Urol 92:
  51-5, 1964.
Hutch, J.A., & O.N. Rambo, Jr.: A study of
  the anatomy of the prostate, prostatic ure-
  thra and the urinary sphincter system. J
  Urol 104:443-52, 1970.
Lytton, B., Kupfer, D.J., & A.R. Traurig:
  The vesicorenal reflex. Invest Urol 4:
  521-30, 1967.
Mad, P., & others: Human prostatic hyperplasia. Arch Path 79:270-83, 1965.
Mostofi, F.K., & R.V. Thomson: Benign
  hyperplasia of the prostate gland. In:
  Urology, 3rd ed. Cambell, M.F., & J.H.
  Harrison (editors). Saunders, 1969.
Nadig, P.W., & W.L. Valk: Recovery from
  obstructive disease. J Urol 88:470-2, 1962.
Scott, F.B., & others: Uroflowmetry before
  and after prostatectomy. South MJ 60:
  948-52, 1967.
Scott, W.W., & J.C. Wade: Medical treatment
  of benign nodular prostatic hyperplasia
  with cyproterone acetate. J Urol 101:81-5,
  1969.
Semple, J.E.: Surgical capsule of the benign
  enlargement of the prostate. Brit MJ 1:
  1640-3, 1963.
Tanagho, E.A., & F.H. Meyers: Trigonal
  hypertrophy: A cause of ureteral obstruction. J Urol 93:678-83, 1965.
Walker, D., & others: Blood loss following
  cryosurgery of the prostate. J Urol 100:
  188-9, 1968.
Wildbolz, E.: Elective prostatectomy. Proc
  Roy Soc Med 51:1029-31, 1958.

CARCINOMA OF THE PROSTATE

Carcinoma of the prostate is rare before
age 60 and increases in frequency thereafter,
probably afflicting 25% of men in the eighth
decade. The disease is rare in Japanese and
Jews. Blacks are more commonly afflicted
than whites. There is a significant familial
incidence, which suggests a genetic component.
Multiple cancers are common in these patients.
It metastasizes primarily to the bones of the
pelvis and may damage the kidneys because of
the vesical obstruction which ensues.

Etiology

The true cause of prostatic carcinoma is
not known, but it is quite clear that its growth
is strikingly influenced by sex hormones. The
adult prostate is the major site of elaboration
of acid phosphatase. In advanced prostatic
cancer, particularly when it has metastasized
to bone, three-fourths of patients will have
markedly increased amounts of this enzyme
in the blood.

The administration of androgens usually
increases the rate of growth of this tumor and
increases the acid phosphatase level in the
serum. Estrogen therapy (or orchidectomy)
slows the growth of these tumors and maintains the amount of acid phosphatase in the
blood at a normal level. Determination of the
amount of acid phosphatase in the serum is
therefore an index of the extent of the tumor;
it also indicates the degree of success of antiandrogen therapy.

Pathogenesis and Pathology (See Fig 17-12.)

Cancer of the prostate is usually associated coincidentally with benign prostatic hyperplasia but does not develop from it. Most
malignancies originate in the posterior lobe
in the surgical capsule (compressed peripheral
prostatic tissue), although a few may be found
within the hyperplastic benign prostatic lobes.
These latter tumors are usually very small
("occult" or "academic" cancers) and apparently often completely removed by intracapsular enucleation of the enlarged gland.

The initial lesion is usually a firm area on
the postero-lateral surface. It gradually

spreads in the capsule (posterior lobe) and involves the hyperplastic tissue as well. The seminal vesicles then become involved. Later, the tumor may extend through the urethral mucosa or bladder wall; the external sphincter may be invaded. The rectal wall is singularly immune; only rarely does the tumor invade Denonvilliers' fascia.

The cancer spreads in the perineural lymphatics. The vesical, sacral, external iliac, and lumbar lymph nodes then become involved. The left supraclavicular node is occasionally affected. When the seminal vesicles are involved, 80% of patients will have invasion of the pelvic nodes.

Metastases also occur by way of the veins, particularly through the vertebrals. This mechanism accounts for the predilection of this tumor for the bones of the pelvis, heads of the femurs, and the lower lumbar spine. Other bones, including the skull, are occasionally involved. Visceral spread is also seen (eg, lungs, liver). Infiltration of the bone marrow is particularly common.

Grossly, cancers of the prostate are white or yellow. They may be quite hard, if fibrous; or merely firm, if more cellular. Multiple zones of cancer are not uncommon. Rarely, a tumor may be medullary and so soft as to simulate abscess.

On microscopic study, the tissue may be largely epithelial or may be scirrhous. The epithelial elements may assume a papillary pattern or may be anaplastic. Invasion of the stroma is usually obvious. Mitoses are common. Invasion of perineural sheaths is an outstanding feature but is not necessarily of prognostic importance.

After antiandrogen therapy, retrogressive changes may be marked. The gland becomes smaller and assumes a more normal consistency. This change may be marked within 3 months after therapy is instituted. Obstructive symptoms regress to some extent. Microscopically, the malignant cells have become smaller and stain more darkly. The cytoplasm becomes scanty. The number of these cells is markedly diminished. Similar changes occur in metastatic tumors.

A few transitional cell carcinomas arising from the epithelium of the ducts have been reported. Adenocarcinoma is rare; lymphomatous infiltration is occasionally seen.

Clinical Findings

A. Symptoms: The presenting symptoms in 95% of men with prostatic malignancy are from obstruction to the flow of urine, infection, or both. They are similar to those described in the discussion of benign prostatic enlargement.

1. Bladder symptoms - Hesitancy and straining to initiate the stream, loss of force and caliber of the stream, terminal dribbling, frequency with nocturia, symptoms of infection of the bladder, and urinary retention. Localized tumors unassociated with benign hyperplasia provoke no symptoms at all.

2. Symptoms due to metastases - One out of 20 patients have their first symptoms from metastases. Metastatic spread causes the following: pain in the lumbosacral region, which may radiate into the hips or down the legs; a mass in the right upper abdominal quadrant (ie, liver involvement), supraclavicular mass (ie, sentinel node metastasis), anemia and loss of weight, and hematuria late in the course of the disease when the bladder or urethra is invaded. Symptoms of renal insufficiency may be due to obstruction of the ureteral orifices by the primary tumor or by hypertrophy of the trigonal muscle; or to compression of the ureters by masses of iliac lymph nodes involved by metastatic cancer.

B. Signs: Rectal examination is the most important step in the diagnosis of cancer of the prostate. The early lesion is difficult to differentiate from certain benign conditions which cause areas of induration. A cancerous nodule is usually not raised above the surface of the gland. There is a sudden change in consistency between it and surrounding tissue (Fig 4-2). Diagnosis may not be possible without surgical biopsy.

The more advanced lesion is usually stony hard, and the gland is fixed. It may be nodular. The seminal vesicles may be indurated. Occlusion of the rectum by surrounding growth is very rare.

Other signs of prostatic cancer include an enlarged, nodular liver, pathologic fracture from metastasis (including sudden paraplegia from collapse of a vertebral body), and an enlarged, hard left supraclavicular node.

C. Laboratory Findings: Anemia may be extreme in the later stages, when bone marrow is replaced by tumor; hemorrhage and infection will also contribute to this. Urinalysis may or may not show infection. Red cells may be present.

In the early stages of obstruction, renal function is unimpaired. Later, if the ureters are occluded or if obstruction is so marked that renal back pressure develops, the PSP may be depressed because of renal impairment, residual urine, or both; serum creatinine or BUN may be increased.

Serum phosphatase determinations are important in the diagnosis of prostatic cancer. The normal serum acid phosphatase in men is

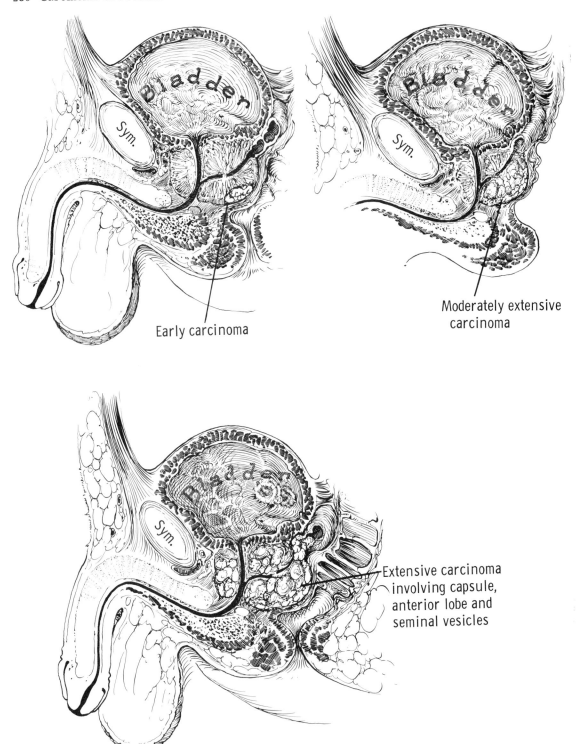

Early carcinoma

Moderately extensive carcinoma

Extensive carcinoma involving capsule, anterior lobe and seminal vesicles

Fig 17-12. Pathogenesis of carcinoma of prostate. Above left: Small, well-localized carcinoma in posterior aspect of prostate, easily felt on rectal examination. **Above right:** Extension of carcinoma into posterior half of prostate. **Below:** Advanced carcinoma of prostate; trabeculation of bladder wall.

1-5 King-Armstrong units (or 0.5-2 Bodansky or Gutman units). When the cancer extends outside the prostatic capsule and metastases are present, 75% of patients will have elevations to above 10 units. This is pathognomonic of advanced prostate carcinoma, whether metastases can be demonstrated or not. With antiandrogen therapy these abnormal levels tend to revert to normal.

The serum alkaline phosphatase (normally 5-13 King-Armstrong units, 2-4.5 Bodansky units, 3-10 Gutman units) will be elevated if there are bony metastases. This is a nonspecific reaction and merely reflects the amount of osteogenic activity in the body. After an initial further rise, it too tends to return to normal levels when hormonal treatment is instituted.

D. X-Ray Findings: A chest film may show evidence of metastases to the hilar nodes, lungs, or ribs. A plain film of the abdomen may reveal the typical osteoblastic metastases from prostatic tumor. The common sites include the pelvic bones, the lumbar spine, and the femoral heads. Excretory urograms may show hydronephrosis from bladder neck or ureteral obstruction (Fig 17-14).

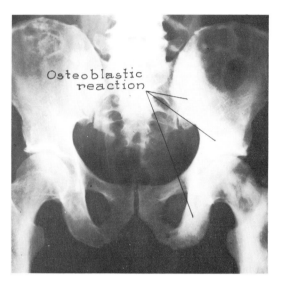

Fig 17-13. Metastases to bone from carcinoma of the prostate. Plain film of pelvis showing osteoblastic metastases to the lumbar vertebrae, ilium, ischium, and left femur.

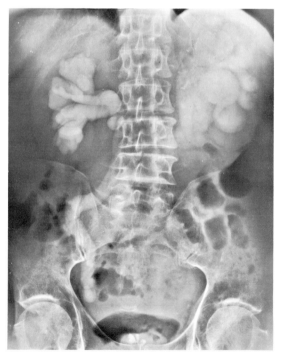 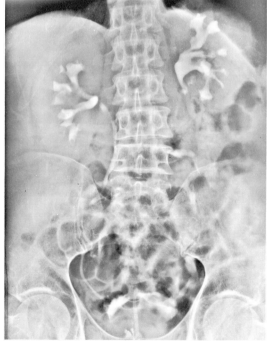

Fig 17-14. Cancer of prostate. Left: Excretory urogram at 75 minutes showing bilateral hydroureteronephrosis. **Right:** Fifteen minute urogram after 3 months of diethylstilbestrol. Significant reduction of obstruction.

E. An ^{85}Sr or ^{18}F scan (Fig 8-9) may reveal involvement of bones even though plain films seem normal.

F. Instrumental Examination: Passage of a catheter immediately after voiding will measure the amount of residual urine. Cystoscopy will usually show nonspecific vesical changes from obstruction (eg, trabeculation, diverticula, infection). Only very late will invasion of the base of the bladder be seen. Obstruction of the prostatic urethra will be evident. The gland may be found to be relatively fixed on movement of the instrument.

G. Cytology: Papanicolaou technics are of no value in the early cases. By the time malignant cells can be demonstrated in prostatic secretion, the diagnosis is usually quite evident clinically.

H. Biopsy: If the lesion is extensive, a positive diagnosis can be made on pathologic studies of tissue removed by transurethral resection. In early cases (limited to the capsule), this method fails. Needle biopsy through the perineum or transrectally is a useful procedure in order to establish the diagnosis in incurable cases before orchidectomy is done. Aspiration of marrow from the iliac crest may reveal malignant cells even in the absence of radiologic evidence of spread.

Differential Diagnosis

Benign prostatic hyperplasia can usually be differentiated by palpation of the prostate. Osteoblastic metastases in the pelvic bones as shown on x-ray or scan or an elevated serum acid phosphatase establishes the diagnosis of advanced cancer. At times only biopsy will clarify it.

Benign firm nodules may present difficulties in differential diagnosis. They may be caused by tuberculosis, chronic infection with fibrosis, granulomatous prostatitis, or calculi. The early cancerous nodule is usually not raised above the surface of the gland. The change in consistency from malignant to normal tissue is abrupt. Biopsy, however, is often necessary to make the diagnosis.

(1) Tuberculous nodules are often multiple. One or both seminal vesicles may be thickened. A nontender, thickened epididymis suggests tuberculosis. "Sterile" pyuria with the finding of tubercle bacilli establishes the diagnosis. Urograms may reveal the renal tuberculous lesion.

(2) The fibrous nodule associated with chronic prostatitis is usually raised above the surface of the gland. The induration gradually lessens as the finger approaches normal tissue. Pus is found in the prostatic secretion. Biopsy, however, may be necessary.

(3) Granulomatous prostatitis will cause development of a hard nodular prostate. A recent history of an acute prostatic infection can usually be elicited. Biopsy, however, may be needed for differentiation.

(4) Prostatic calculi often cause crepitation on palpation. An x-ray will usually reveal their presence just above or behind the symphysis. Occasionally a patient may have both calculi and cancer, however.

Paget's disease may present a mottled area of increased density of the pelvic bones on a radiogram which must be differentiated from metastatic prostatic cancer. Although Paget's disease may cause a slight increase in serum acid phosphatase, it is less than 10 King-Armstrong units. Higher levels mean prostatic cancer. X-rays of the skull and long bones will show the typical lesion of Paget's disease. Rectal examination should settle the diagnosis.

Prolonged intake of fluoride (in drinking water) has been reported to cause osteosclerosis that simulates the x-ray appearance of osseous metastases from carcinoma of the prostate.

Complications

Obstruction of the prostatic urethra may cause the formation of vesical diverticula or stones. Infection is common.

Renal damage may be due to functional obstruction of the ureterovesical junction secondary to trigonal hypertrophy, invasion of the intramural portion of the ureters by tumor, or compression of the ureters at the pelvic brim by iliac nodes containing metastatic tumor. Infection may further impair renal function.

Edema of the legs may occur from pressure of involved iliac nodes upon the great vessels.

Spontaneous fractures can develop at the site of bony metastases. Sudden spinal cord compression is not uncommon and may require immediate laminectomy.

Treatment

A. Curative (Radical) Measures: If, on palpating an indurated nodule in the prostate of a well-preserved man less than age 70, the clinician is unable to say that the patient does not have an early malignancy (and unless there is evidence of metastases to bone—by x-ray or scan—or elevation of the serum acid phosphatase), perineal exposure and immediate frozen section are indicated. If cancerous, the entire prostate, including its capsule, the seminal vesicles, and a portion of the bladder neck, can be removed through the same wound. The same radical procedure can be performed retropubically. Prostatovesiculectomy will cure about half of these favorable cases. Urinary control is usually normal after the operation, but impotence is to be expected. Some advise preliminary estrogen for 3-6 months before radical prostatectomy is performed, feeling that the overall control is thereby enhanced.

B. Palliative Measures:

1. Antiandrogen therapy - About 85% of prostatic cancers are androgen-dependent. These will show definite regression in size after a few weeks of antiandrogen therapy. The consistency of the gland tends to approach normal, the degree of urinary obstruction lessens, and bone pain disappears or decreases. The patient gains weight and strength, and anemia tends to correct itself. X-ray films often show healing of the metastatic lesions in bone. The price the patient must pay for this palliation includes impotence with loss of sexual desire, tender gynecomastia, and, at times, edema of the ankles. The edema can be controlled by restricted salt intake. Painful gynecomastia can usually be prevented by directing x-ray therapy to the region of the areola before estrogen treatment is begun.

There is no doubt that this mode of therapy affords much comfort to patients who formerly suffered greatly. It is also true that the life of these patients is slightly prolonged.

Although there is little doubt that antiandrogen therapy has a palliative effect on surgically incurable prostatic carcinoma, it has been shown that the administration of large doses of estrogen significantly increases the incidence of death from thromboembolic phenomena. Therefore, estrogens should be withheld until the patient develops symptoms or signs of metastases; when this happens, estrogens can be expected to cause regression of metastases in most patients.

Antiandrogen therapy includes orchidectomy and medical neutralization of testicular (and adrenal) androgens. The latter may be accomplished in the following ways:

a. Estrogen medication - Diethylstilbestrol, 1 mg/day, has proved effective and does not seem to be associated with secondary thromboembolic disorders. Other estrogens given in comparable dosage are equally efficient. A few advocate diethylstilbestrol, 5-100 mg/day for 3 months, and then 25 mg/day thereafter. Such large doses are of questionable value.

Therapy with massive doses of diethylstilbestrol diphosphate has been suggested for those patients with extensive disease or in those who are no longer being controlled by the usual dose of estrogen. The drug is given intravenously, undiluted. The following dosage schedule has been recommended: 500 mg 3 times a day for 10 days, 500 mg 2 times a day for 10 days, and then a similar dose daily for the next 10 days followed by 500 mg every week. Possibly half of patients will experience significant improvement.

b. Medical adrenalectomy - This can be accomplished by the administration of cortisone (or an equivalent drug), 50 mg/day in divided doses. Salt must be restricted (0.3 gm/day) and potassium added to the diet (3 gm/day). This should be tried when the effectiveness of estrogen therapy begins to wane.

c. Surgical adrenalectomy - This rather rigorous procedure offers so little more relief than is afforded by cortisone that it is probably not indicated. Hypophysectomy has few advocates, but ^{90}Yttrium or cryosurgical hypophysectomy has been shown to afford relief from severe diffuse bone pain in 75% of such patients.

2. Resection - If the degree of obstruction is severe or if antiandrogenic therapy fails to afford much relief, transurethral resection of the prostate will be necessary. Since cancer of the prostate invades the hyperplastic tissue, there is no longer any cleavage plane which will permit intracapsular enucleation, as is ordinarily practiced for benign hyperplasia (eg, suprapubic prostatectomy).

3. Cryosurgery - This technic has been used in the poor-risk patient instead of transurethral resection with some measure of successful relief of obstruction.

4. Testosterone and radioisotope therapy - If the tumor becomes androgen-independent and metastases are widespread, some regression may be obtained on the following regimen. Discontinue estrogens and steroids. Give testosterone, 100 mg/day for 17 days. Beginning on the sixth day of this course administer 1.8 mc of ^{32}P/day orally or IV for 7 days. The latter should be followed by therapy with iron, vitamin B complex, and liver extract to maintain an adequate hemogram. Dicalcium phosphate will contribute to reossification of healing bone. Estrogen therapy should then be resumed. Such a course of therapy can be repeated.

Tong reports dramatic results by giving parathyroid hormone followed by ^{32}P. The hormone seems to increase the degree of deposition of radioactive phosphorus in the bone.

5. Testosterone alone - When all else fails, the administration of testosterone alone can be tried. In most, it increases existing pain, but in a few cases relief may be afforded. The mechanism for this effect is not clear.

6. Injection of radioisotopes - The results of direct injection of radioactive isotopes (eg, gold) into the cancerous glands are equivocal.

7. Radiation therapy - There is increasing (and justified) enthusiasm for this mode of therapy in patients whose tumors do not lend themselves to radical surgery. The local lesion tends to decrease in size, and obstructive symptoms tend to regress. It has been

shown that x-ray therapy also acts favorably on metastases to lymph nodes as revealed on lymphangiograms. Whether such therapy can cure some of these tumors is still not known. The most favorable results are seen in the undifferentiated tumor group.

Prevention

At the present time, only 10% of men, when first seen by the urologist, have lesions that are amenable to cure by radical surgery. In order that this percentage may be significantly increased, careful palpation of the prostate in all men over 50 years of age is mandatory. Any suspicious induration requires immediate exploration.

Prognosis

Of the 10% of men with prostatic carcinoma whose illness is diagnosed early enough so that radical surgery would offer a reasonable hope of cure, at least half are over 70 years of age and may suffer from other infirmities of old age. For this reason they are not good subjects for radical procedures and most of them will live more comfortably and just as long with palliative treatment and will die of other causes. The curability rate of prostatic carcinoma is, therefore, about 2-4%. The prognosis in young men is the same as that of the older age groups.

Palliative treatment offers considerable temporary relief for most patients with advanced prostatic carcinoma. Death usually occurs within 3 years after the diagnosis has been made. A few patients will be controlled for 5 and even 10 years.

Alfthan, O., & L. R. Holsti: Prevention of gynecomastia by local roentgen irradiation in estrogen-treated prostatic carcinoma. Scandinav J Urol Nephrol 3:183-7, 1969.

Bailar, J. C., III, & D. P. Byar: Estrogen treatment for cancer of the prostate. Early results with 3 doses of diethylstilbestrol and placebo. Cancer 26:257-61, 1970.

Barnes, R. W., & others: Early prostatic cancer: Long-term results with conservative treatment. J Urol 102:88-9, 1969.

Bärring, N. E., Holmér, A., & B. I. Rudén: Interstitial irradiation of the pituitary gland with a ^{90}Sr-^{90}Y applicator having adjustable active length. Acta radiol (ther) 8:294-300, 1969.

Bennett, A. H., Dowd, J. B., & J. H. Harrison: Estrogen and survival data in carcinoma of the prostate. Surg Gynec Obst 130:505-8, 1970.

Bennett, J. E.: Treatment of carcinoma of the prostate by cobalt-beam therapy. Radiology 90:532-5, 1968.

Blackard, C. E., & others: Incidence of cardiovascular disease and death in patients receiving diethylstilbestrol for carcinoma of the prostate. Cancer 26:249-56, 1970.

Blackard, C. E., Soucheray, J. A., & D. F. Gleason: Prostatic needle biopsy with perineal extension of adenocarcinoma. J Urol 106:401-3, 1971.

Byar, D. P., & F. K. Mostofi: Cancer of the prostate in men less than 50 years old: An analysis of 51 cases. J Urol 102:726-33, 1969.

Chua, D. T.: Bone marrow biopsy in patients with carcinoma of the prostate. J Urol 102: 602-6, 1969.

Corriere, J. N., Jr., Cornog, J. L., & J. J. Murphy: Prognosis in patients with carcinoma of the prostate. Cancer 25:911-8, 1970.

Corwin, S. H., & others: Experiences with P-32 in advanced carcinoma of the prostate. J Urol 104:745-8, 1970.

Dees, J. E.: Radical perineal prostatectomy for carcinoma. J Urol 104:160-2, 1970.

Dow, J. A.: The technique of cryosurgery of the prostate. J Urol 105:286-90, 1971.

Dykhuizen, R. F., & others: The use of cobalt 60 teletherapy in the treatment of prostatic carcinoma. J Urol 100:333-8, 1968.

Fergusson, J. D., & W. F. Hendry: Pituitary irradiation in advanced carcinoma of the prostate: Analysis of 100 cases. Brit J Urol 43:514-9, 1971.

Gilbaugh, J. H., Jr., & G. J. Thompson: Fluoride osteosclerosis simulating carcinoma of the prostate with widespread bony metastases: A case report. J Urol 96:944-6, 1966.

Gilbertsen, V. A.: Cancer of the prostate gland. Results of early diagnosis and therapy undertaken for cure of the disease. JAMA 215:81-4, 1971.

Grout, D. C., & others: Radiation therapy in the treatment of carcinoma of the prostate. J Urol 105:411-4, 1971.

Jewett, H. J., & others: The palpable nodule of prostatic cancer. JAMA 203:403-6, 1968.

Jewett, H. J.: The case for radical perineal prostatectomy. J Urol 103:195-9, 1970.

Jorgens, J.: The radiographic characteristics of carcinoma of the prostate. S Clin North America 45:1427-40, 1965.

Kishev, S. V., Coughlin, J. D., & J. A. Dow: Late results following cryosurgery of the prostate (a clinical and panendoscopic study of 80 patients). J Urol 104:893-7, 1970.

Kopecky, A. A., Laskowski, T. Z., & R. Scott, Jr.: Radical retropubic prostatectomy in the treatment of prostatic carcinoma. J Urol 103:641-4, 1970.

Lynch, H. J., & others: Prostate carcinoma and multiple primary malignancies. Cancer 19:1891-7, 1966.

Mitch, W. E., Jr., & A. A. Serpick: Leukemic infiltration of the prostate: A reversible form of urinary obstruction. Cancer 26: 1361-5, 1970.

Morales, A., Connolly, J. G., & A. W. Bruce: Androgen therapy in advanced carcinoma of the prostate. Canad MAJ 105:71-2, 1971.

Morales, A.: The use of radioactive phosphorus to treat bone pain in metastatic carcinoma of the prostate. Canad MAJ 103:372-3, 1970.

Murphy, G. P., & others: Hypophysectomy and adrenalectomy for disseminated prostatic carcinoma. J Urol 105:817-25, 1971.

Olsen, B. S., & R. W. Carlisle: Adenocarcinoma of the prostate simulating primary rectal malignancy. Cancer 25:219-22, 1970.

Roy, R. R., & others: Eighteen fluorine total body scans in patients with carcinoma of the prostate. Brit J Urol 43:58-64, 1971.

Rubenstein, A. B., & M. E. Rubnitz: Transitional cell carcinoma of the prostate. Cancer 24:543-6, 1969.

Rubin, P.: Cancer of the urogenital tract: Prostatic cancer. Advanced and metastatic. JAMA 210:1072-81, 1969.

Rubin, P.: Cancer of the urogenital tract: Prostatic cancer. JAMA 209:1695-705, 1969.

Saglan, S., Wilson, C. B., & R. J. Seymour: Indications for hypophysectomy in diabetic retinopathy and cancer of the breast and prostate. California Med 113:1-6, Feb. 1970.

Schirmer, H. K. A., & W. W. Scott: Prostatic cancer and irradiation: Its possible mode of action and its clinical indication. South MJ 60:578-82, 1967.

Scott, R. J.: Needle biopsy in carcinoma of the prostate. JAMA 201:958-60, 1967.

Scott, W. W., & H. L. Boyd: Combined hormone control therapy and radical prostatectomy in the treatment of selected cases of advanced carcinoma of the prostate: A retrospective study based upon 25 years of experience. J Urol 101:86-92, 1969.

Silber, I., & M. H. McGavran: Adenocarcinoma of the prostate in men less than 56 years old: A study of 65 cases. J Urol 105:282-5, 1971.

The Veterans Administration Co-operative Urological Research Group: Treatment and survival of patients with cancer of the prostate. Surg Gynec Obst 124:1011-7, 1967.

Tong, E. C. K.: Parathormone and ^{32}P therapy in prostatic cancer with bone metastases. Radiology 98:343-51, 1971.

Welsh, J. F., & C. C. MacKinney: Experiences with aspiration biopsies of the bone marrow in the diagnosis and prognosis of carcinoma of the prostate gland. Am J Clin Path 41:509-12, 1964.

Wendel, R. G., & A. T. Evans: Complications of punch biopsy of the prostate gland. J Urol 97:122-6, 1967.

Wolf, H., Madsen, P. O., & H. Vermund: Prevention of estrogen-induced gynecomastia by external irradiation. J Urol 102: 607-9, 1969.

Woolf, C. M.: An investigation of the familial aspects of carcinoma of the prostate. Cancer 13:739-44, 1960.

Wynder, E. L., Mabuch, Y., & W. F. Whitmore, Jr.: Epidemiology of cancer of the prostate. Cancer 28:344-60, 1971.

SARCOMA OF THE PROSTATE

Sarcoma of the prostate is rare. It may arise from smooth or striated muscle or fibroplastic tissue. It is a disease of younger individuals, 50% occurring before the age of 5 years. Most sarcomas grow rapidly; all are highly malignant. They may extend into the base of the bladder and finally occlude the urethra. They may compress the rectum and cause obstipation. These tumors metastasize by way of the lymphatics to the pelvic and lumbar lymph nodes. Venous spread may occur, in which case the lungs, liver, and bone may become involved.

Clinical Findings

A. Symptoms: Symptoms are largely those of urinary obstruction. Rectal obstruction may cause increasing constipation and symptoms of bowel obstruction.

B. Signs: Since these tumors often grow to large size, they may be felt suprapubically. Rectal examination reveals a very large mass in the prostatic area. It may be firm, or may be soft enough to suggest abscess. Considerable residual urine is usually recovered upon catheterization.

C. X-Ray Findings: Cystograms or excretory urograms may show that the bladder has been lifted up by the tumor. A urethrogram will demonstrate the compression of the posterior urethra.

D. Instrumental Examination: Cystoscopy or panendoscopy will demonstrate the prostatic enlargement. Grape-like masses often fill the prostatic urethra and bladder neck.

Treatment and Prognosis

Sarcoma of the prostate is not radiosensitive, and attempts at treatment have so far been of little avail. Total prostatocystectomy has cured a very few. Postoperative radiotherapy has been advocated.

Lemmon, W. T., Jr., Holland, J. M., & A. S. Ketcham: Rhabodomyosarcoma of the prostate. Surgery **59**:736-44, 1966.
McPhail, J. L.: Rhabdomyosarcoma of the prostate. J Urol **87**:617-22, 1962.
Siegel, J.: Sarcoma of the prostate: A report of four cases and a review of current therapy. J Urol **89**:78-83, 1963.

TUMORS OF THE SEMINAL VESICLES

About 30 cases of primary carcinoma of the seminal vesicles have been reported in the literature; sarcoma is even rarer. The tumors cause symptoms suggesting obstruction from an enlarged prostate. Bloody ejaculation may be noted. Rectal examination will reveal a mass above the prostate and involving one vesicle. Radical extirpation of the lesion is indicated, but cure is rare.

Faruque, Hajdu, S. I.: Adenocarcinoma of the seminal vesicle. J Urol **99**:798-801, 1968.
Smith, B. A., Jr., Webb, E. A., & W. E. Price: Carcinoma of the seminal vesicle. J Urol **97**:743-50, 1967.

TUMORS OF THE URETHRA

BENIGN TUMORS

Benign tumors of the urethra are not common in men or women. They are usually papillary and may be found anywhere between the bladder neck and the external orifice. The most distal tumors may be visible; the others may make their presence known by bloody spotting. If the tumor is large enough, symptoms of urinary obstruction may develop. If the tumor arises in the prostatic urethra, bleeding may be noted in the last portion of the urine. If obstructive, infection is apt to be a complication. The diagnosis is made by biopsy. Transurethral electrocoagulation cures these lesions.

Malignant tumors of the urethra are not common; they occur more often in women than in men. Those arising from the most distal portion of the urethra are epidermoid carcinomas. Those originating more proximally are of the transitional cell type; though a few adenocarcinomas have been reported. Tumors involving the region of the external meatus metastasize to the superficial and deep subinguinal lymph nodes. The more proximal tumors spread to the vesical, sacral, hypogastric, and external iliac nodes (Figs 17-1 and 17-2).

If distal, either in men or women, these tumors may first present themselves as visible or palpable masses. Bloody discharge may be noted. Urinary obstruction may occur. The deeper tumors may be quite obstructive and are often complicated by infection. In men, they may be diagnosed and treated as urethral strictures. At times these tumors are complicated by periurethral abscesses which may lead to the formation of urinary fistulas.

The diagnosis is made by biopsy of the tumor, which is either palpated externally or seen directly by panendoscopy or on urethrograms (Fig 7-10).

Tumors of the distal urethra in women can often be cured by local excision. Similar tumors in men require amputation of the penis. Radical inguinal node dissection (which includes the superficial and deep subinguinal and the superficial inguinal nodes) is indicated if the nodes are involved.

Cancer of the perineal urethra may require radical penectomy with the formation of a perineal urethral orifice. If the bulb is involved, prostatocystectomy must be performed as well and the urinary stream diverted.

Although these tumors are relatively radioresistant, x-ray therapy may afford some palliation if groin dissection is contraindicated.

On the whole, these tumors are very malignant, and few cures are obtained in those patients whose lesions involve the proximal urethra.

Guinn, G. A., & A. G. Ayala: Male urethral cancer: Report of 15 cases including a primary melanoma. J Urol **103**:176-9, 1970.
Mandler, J. I., & T. L. Pool: Primary carcinoma of the male urethra. J Urol **96**:67-72, 1968.
Steyn, J., Hall, M., & N. J. Logie: Adenocarcinoma of the female urethra. Brit J Urol **39**:504-5, 1967.

Zeigerman, J. H., & S. F. Gordon: Cancer of the female urethra. A curable disease. Obst Gynec **36**:785-9, 1970.

TUMORS OF THE SPERMATIC CORD

About 300 cases of tumors of the spermatic cord have been reported. Most are benign and are composed of connective tissue elements. The malignant tumors tend to invade locally and to metastasize to the iliac and preaortic lymph nodes, liver, and lungs.

These tumors present palpable masses which may be associated with local pain. A blow to the area may bring the lesion to the attention of the patient. They must be differentiated from hernias, hydrocele of the cord, and spermatocele.

Benign tumors must be excised. Sarcomas require radical removal of the cord and the testicle. The external iliac and lumbar lymph nodes should also be treated with radiation therapy. Retroperitoneal node dissection should be given serious consideration.

Arlen, M., Grabstald, H., & W. F. Whitmore, Jr.: Malignant tumors of the spermatic cord. Cancer **23**:525-32, 1969.

Banowsky, L. H., & G. N. Shultz: Sarcoma of the spermatic cord and tunics: Review of the literature, case report and discussion of the role of retroperitoneal node dissection. J Urol **103**:628-31, 1970.

Dreyfus, W., & E. Goodsitt: Tumors of the spermatic cord. J Urol **84**:658-65, 1960.

Lundblad, R. R., Mellinger, G. T., & D. F. Gleason: Spermatic cord malignancies. J Urol **98**:393-6, 1967.

TUMORS OF THE TESTIS

With rare exception, all tumors of the testis are malignant. A few embryonal carcinomas and teratomas of the testis have been reported in childhood, but most occur between the ages of 20-35 years. Most of those seen after the age of 60 years are reticulum cell sarcomas, Sertoli cell tumors, or interstitial cell tumors. Only 25% arise from germ cells. They account for about 0.5% of all malignancies in men and 4% of all tumors affecting the genitourinary tract. Metastasis occurs relatively early. Some elaborate chorionic gonadotropins, and the prognosis in this type is exceedingly poor. Retroperitoneal germinomas without evidence of testicular involvement are occasionally seen.

Etiology

The cause of testicular tumors is not known. It may be significant, however, that they usually develop during the age of greatest sexual activity. Many authorities believe that the undescended testis, particularly in the pseudohermaphrodite, has a definite tendency to undergo carcinomatous change. Whether maldescent is the cause or whether some unknown factor causes both the lack of descent and tumor formation is not decided.

Pathogenesis and Pathology

A. Classification: Many classifications of tumor of the testis have been offered, most of them based upon morphology. Since about 10% of these tumors elaborate chorionic gonadotropin, a morphologic-endocrine grouping is feasible.

1. Teratoma - Most authorities agree that all of the teratomatous tumors of the testis, mixed or pure, arise from a totipotent cell which can develop in many directions. These cells have been likened to a twin of the host— a twin which develops in the host's own testis. Mixed tumors (teratomas) contain both mesenchymal and epithelial tissues. Fewer than 5% are benign; the rest are malignant. The malignant epithelial cells may overgrow the other elements and appear as the only cell in the tumor unless serial secretions are studied. However, one tumor frequently contains elements of 2 or even 3 of the common types.

a. Seminoma pattern (35%) - These tumors are made up of sheets of round epithelial cells with clear cytoplasm and large nuclei. Fibrous septa course through the tumor; these may be infiltrated with lymphocytes. Mitoses are common. Thirteen percent are chromatin positive (female).

b. Carcinoma pattern (33%) - This type tends to secrete chorionic gonadotropin and is often associated with hyperplasia of the interstitial cells. These tumors may therefore have arisen from primitive chorionic tissues. These embryonal epithelial cells may take on a papillary pattern. The cytoplasm is often granular. There is considerable variation in the size of the cells. Many mitoses are present. In some, syncytial cells are apparent; in others, the small Langhans' cells are seen. Typical chorio-epithelioma may be observed (2% of all testicular tumors). Embryonal carcinoma is the most common tumor in this group.

c. Teratoma pattern (28%) - These tumors contain numerous types of immature and mature mesenchymal and epithelial structures, including muscle, cartilage, nerve, and mucosa. One or more of these may predominate and present malignant change. These tumors probably represent malformed embryos. They ordinarily do not elaborate chorionic gonadotropin, and hyperplasia of Leydig's cells is not seen. An exception to this rule suggests that carcinoma or choriocarcinoma is present elsewhere. Positive chromatin patterns are found in 32% of this group.

2. Interstitial cell tumor - More than 50 cases have been reported; 90% are benign. Interstitial cell tumors secrete androgen and estrogen, which cause precocious sexual maturation in boys and gynecomastia in men.

3. Sertoli cell tumors - These rare, usually benign tumors are feminizing. Gynecomastia is a cardinal finding.

4. Lymphoma and reticulum cell sarcoma - These tumor types are occasionally observed. Leukemic infiltration has been reported.

B. Chorionic Gonadotropins: These substances may be found in the urine in abnormal amounts in about 5-10% of patients with testicular tumors. Usually such tumors have a carcinomatous pattern. If a positive hormone test is found in what seems to be a seminoma or teratoma, further sectioning will usually reveal tumor of the carcinoma type. Almost without exception the patient whose tumor secretes large amounts of hormone is dead within a year regardless of whether metastases are present or not and no matter what treatment is given. Clinically, these tumors must be considered chorioepitheliomas even though typical cells cannot be found in the testis. At autopsy, many of these patients will be found to have the hemorrhagic metastases typical of choriocarcinoma.

C. Metastases: Except for choriocarcinoma, the major route for metastases is lymphatic. The lumbar and mediastinal nodes are most commonly involved. The left supraclavicular node is at times affected. The lesion will spread to the superficial inguinal and subinguinal nodes only if the scrotum becomes invaded (and this is unusual) or if previous orchidopexy or hernioplasty has been performed. In 20% of cases with lymph node metastases, the abdominal (lumbar) lymph nodes on the side opposite the primary tumor will contain metastatic cancer.

Masses of lumbar lymph nodes may displace the ureters or kidneys. Ureteral occlusion occasionally is observed. Bowel may also be displaced.

Metastases are commonly found in the lungs and liver; other organs are involved less frequently. Probably 30-40% of the patients have metastases when they are first seen.

Clinical Findings

A painless lump in the testis must be regarded as tumor until proved otherwise. The common sites of metastases are the preaortic lymph nodes and the lungs. Gynecomastia suggests the presence of a functioning tumor and is a bad prognostic sign. About 10% of tumors produce this symptom. If carcinoma of the testis cannot be unequivocally ruled out, orchidectomy must be done immediately.

A. Symptoms: The most common presenting symptom is enlargement of the testis. It may be discovered quite by accident, or attention may be drawn to it because of mild discomfort caused by its weight. On rare occasion it can be quite painful if bleeding occurs into its own substance.

If the tumor is elaborating large amounts of chorionic gonadotropins, gynecomastia may be seen. This change is also seen with Sertoli and Leydig cell tumors, both of which cause secretion of estrogen.

Symptoms from metastases include a supraclavicular or abdominal mass (lymph nodes), abdominal pain from bowel or ureteral obstruction, cough from metastases to the lung, and nonspecific symptoms of loss of weight and anorexia.

In the rare instance of a Leydig cell tumor, a preadolescent boy may undergo precocious development of sexual organs and secondary sexual characteristics. The adult experiences no accentuation of sex characteristics; in fact, he is apt to become impotent. The boy with Sertoli cell tumor may develop a female escutcheon and gynecomastia.

B. Signs: The testis is usually definitely enlarged and diffusely involved. The tumor is ordinarily smooth and in general maintains its ovoid shape. It is firm and gives the sensation of abnormal weight. It does not transilluminate. Of the greatest importance is the fact that pressure on the organ fails to cause the typical sickening testicular discomfort. The epididymis can be distinguished from the testis in the early stages, but later it is lost in the mass. A very early tumor may present as a firm, nontender nodule embedded in the testis.

The spermatic cord is usually normal on palpation. It is rare for the scrotum to be involved except in the last stage of the disease. Hydrocele develops secondary to tumor in about 10% of cases. In such instances in young men, if adequate palpation of the testis cannot be done, the hydrocele must be aspirated.

Metastases without an evident primary source occurring in a young cryptorchid should suggest the possibility of tumor of that testis. A hard mass in the left supraclavicular area in a young man should be regarded as testicular malignancy until proved otherwise, since tumor of the testis is the most common malignancy in that age group. Gynecomastia should suggest the presence of a functioning testicular neoplasm. Metastases should be sought along the aorta; masses of involved lymph nodes are often palpable.

In the later stages, evidence of weight loss and even cachexia may be seen.

C. Laboratory Findings: The patient may be anemic if metastases are widespread. Urinalysis is of no help in diagnosis. Renal function is usually normal even though unilateral ureteral occlusion develops. An estimate of the level of urinary chorionic gonadotropins should be done. Its presence means testicular tumor of the carcinoma type or chorio-epithelioma, and is a grave prognostic sign. A negative test has no diagnostic significance.

The 17-ketosteroids are elevated with Leydig cell tumor. Urinary estrogens may be increased with both Leydig cell and Sertoli cell neoplasms.

A serologic test for syphilis is indicated in every case, for gumma can simulate tumor.

D. X-Ray Findings: A chest film may show evidence of metastases. Excretory urograms are indicated in all cases of testicular tumor; masses of carcinomatous lumbar nodes may displace the ureter or kidney (Fig 17-15) and may cause ureteral stenosis. Retrograde ureterograms (Fig 17-15) or venacavagrams (Fig 7-16) may more clearly delineate an extra-ureteral mass. Lymphangiography is proving to be an excellent method for demonstrating lymph node metastases (Fig 17-15), although a number of false-positives and a few false-negatives have been observed.

Differential Diagnosis

A. Painless Scrotal Swellings: Hydrocele may be quite tense and even firm if the tunica vaginalis is thickened. It will transilluminate. Hydrocele, it must be remembered, develops secondary to some testicular malignancies. In case of doubt, aspirate the hydroceles of young men to afford adequate palpation of the testis.

A spermatocele is a free cystic mass lying above and behind the testis.

Tuberculosis of the epididymis may present itself as an enlargement, but palpation should reveal that the testis is separate from the mass. If the testis has become secondarily involved, differentiation may be more difficult.

The diagnosis of tuberculosis will be enhanced by finding beading of the vas, induration of the prostate or seminal vesicles, and pus and tubercle bacilli in the urine.

Gumma is a very rare nontender testicular lesion which causes enlargement. A history of syphilis and a positive serologic test should suggest this diagnosis.

About 75 instances of epidermoid cyst of the testis have been reported. The correct diagnosis is made by the pathologist. Occasionally other tumors may metastasize to the testes. The primary sites are the prostate, the kidneys, and the gastrointestinal tract.

B. Painful Scrotal Swellings: It is rare for testicular tumors to be exquisitely painful, but moderate discomfort is present in 40% of patients. Nonspecific epididymitis, if acute, is exceedingly painful. If seen early it is obvious that only the epididymis is involved. After some hours, the entire testis becomes swollen. Pyuria and symptoms of lower tract infection are usually present. Chronic epididymitis should not be confusing, for the induration will involve the epididymis only.

Mumps orchitis is usually much more painful than tumor and is quite tender. Parotitis is almost always evident, and fever may be quite high.

Torsion of the spermatic cord is a disease of childhood, at which age tumor is unusual. Torsion is suggested if the epididymis can be felt anterior to the testis. Also, elevation of the testis onto the pubis increases the torsion and therefore the pain.

Complications

Complications arise from the metastases. Rarely a ureter may become occluded by extrinsic pressure from involved lymph nodes.

Treatment

A. Orchidectomy: If after careful examination a testicular tumor cannot be ruled out, the testicle should be removed. Orchidectomy is performed through an inguinal incision. This permits high ligation of the cord at the internal ring. Furthermore, the blood supply of the testis should be divided before the tumor itself is handled, thus decreasing the risk of vascular dissemination. At this time, the peritoneum should be opened so that the lumbar and iliac chain of lymph nodes can be palpated.

B. Bilateral Radical Resection: Radical resection of the retroperitoneal (iliac and lumbar) lymph nodes is indicated for almost all testicular tumors except the seminoma, which is highly radiosensitive. It appears to be of little value in cases of chorionepithelioma,

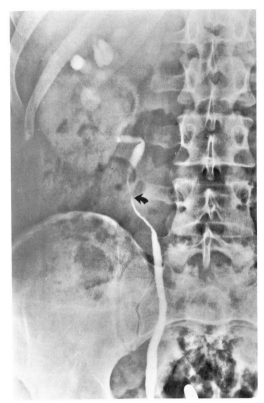

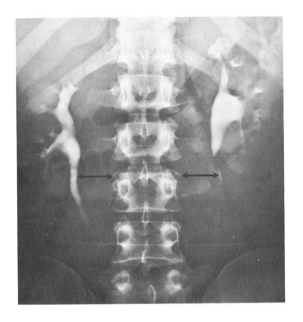

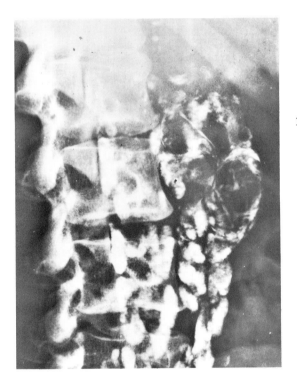

Fig 17-15. **Carcinoma of the testis. Above left:** Excretory urogram showing lateral displacement of both upper ureters by metastases to lumbar lymph nodes. **Above right:** Retrograde bulb ureterogram showing hydronephrosis and ureteral deviation at L4 secondary to metastases in right lumbar lymph nodes. (See Fig 7-16 for venacavagram on same patient.) **Left:** Lymphangiogram demonstrating enlarged lumbar lymph nodes involved by metastatic tumor.

but, on theoretical grounds, it might be worth trying. The presence of massive metastases in these nodes is considered a contraindication to resection. Preoperative lymphangiography allows radiograms to be taken on the operating table to be sure that all nodes have been removed.

Lobectomy has been successfully employed in a few patients with isolated pulmonary metastases.

C. X-Ray Therapy: Radiation therapy is given in all cases of testicular neoplasm, whether metastases have been discovered or not. It is the treatment of choice for seminoma. For the other tumors, radiotherapy is given following lymphadenectomy. A few clinicians advise radiation both before and after node dissection. There seems to be increasing interest in routine therapy to the mediastinum and left supraclavicular area as well.

D. Chemotherapy: It has been shown that the employment of 3 cancericidal drugs is effective in palliation of metastatic chorionic tumor. These comprise an alkylating agent (eg, chlorambucil), an antimetabolite (eg, methotrexate), and the antitumor antibiotic dactinomycin. Given in combination as a first course, they are repeated at intervals. Mithramycin is also reported to be effective in the treatment of embryonal carcinoma, teratocarcinoma, and choriocarcinoma.

This method of treatment is apt to cause subsidence of lumbar lymph node involvement and pulmonary metastases. In most cases the urinary chorionic gonadotropin titer falls sharply to normal; this demonstrates the effect of chemotherapy upon trophoblastic tissue.

Toxic effects include nausea and vomiting, stomatitis, diarrhea, leukopenia, thrombocytopenia, skin eruptions, and loss of hair. Serious toxic symptoms necessitate withholding the drug until the side effects have cleared.

Prognosis

The presence of demonstrable metastases implies a poor prognosis, except in seminomas.

The type of tumor is of great prognostic significance. Seminomas are the least malignant, particularly if they contain lymphoid stroma microscopically. Ten percent of patients are dead 5 years after operation. Teratomas are more often fatal; 55% are dead 5 years after operation. Fifty-five percent of those with tumors of the carcinoma pattern are dead in 5 years. Almost all patients with chorio-epithelioma are dead within 2 years of diagnosis.

Hyperplasia of interstitial cells is a bad prognostic sign. The majority of these patients also have increased levels of urinary gonadotropins. The finding of chorionic gonadotropin in the urine is a serious sign. Most of these patients die within 2 years.

Abell, M. R., Fayos, J. V., & I. Lampe: Retroperitoneal germinomas (seminomas) without evidence of testicular involvement. Cancer 18:273-90, 1965.

Abell, M. R., & F. Holtz: Testicular and paratesticular neoplasms in patients 60 years of age and older. Cancer 21:852-70, 1968.

Ansfield, F. J., & others: Triple drug therapy in testicular tumors. Cancer 24:442-6, 1969.

Asif, S., & O. T. Uehling: Microscopic tumor foci in testes. J Urol 99:776-9, 1968.

Busch, F. M., Sayegh, E. S., & O. W. Chenault, Jr.: Some uses of lymphangiography in the management of testicular tumors. J Urol 93:490-5, 1965.

Castro, J. R., & M. Gonzalez: Results in treatment of pure seminoma of the testis. Am J Roentgenol 111:355-9, 1971.

Chiappa, S., & others: Combined testicular and foot lymphangiography in testicular carcinomas. Surg Gynec Obst 123:10-4, 1966.

Collins, D. H., & R. C. B. Pugh: The pathology of testicular tumors. Brit J Urol 36:1-111, 1964, Supplement.

Dykhuizen, R. F., & others: The use of cobalt 60 telecurietherapy or x-ray therapy with and without lymphadenectomy in the treatment of testis germinal tumors: A 20-year comparative study. J Urol 100: 321-8, 1968.

Earle, J. D., Bagshaw, M. A., & H. S. Kaplan: Linear accelerator supervoltage radiation therapy: testicular tumor. Radiology 91: 1008-12, 1968.

Haggar, R. A., MacMillan, A. B., & D. G. Thompson: Leukemic infiltration of testes. Canad J Surg 12:197-201, 1969.

Hanash, K. A., Carney, J. A., & P. P. Kelalis: Metastatic tumors to testicles: Routes of metastases. J Urol 102:465-8, 1969.

Hobson, B. M.: Male chorionic gonadotropin excretion. Acta endocrinol 49:337-48, 1965.

Hopkins, G. B.: Interstitial cell tumor of the testes: Case report and review of the literature. J Urol 103:449-51, 1970.

Jacobs, E. M.: Combination chemotherapy of metastatic testicular germinal cell tumors and soft part sarcomas. Cancer 25:324-32, 1970.

Johnson, D. E., Kuhn, C. R., & G. A. Guin: Testicular tumors in children. J Urol 104: 940-3, 1970.

Johnson, D. E., & others: Cryptorchism and testicular tumorigenesis. Surgery 63:919-22, 1968.

Kennedy, B. J.: Mithramycin therapy in advanced testicular neoplasms. Cancer 26: 755-66, 1970.

Kiely, J. M., & others: Lymphoma of the testes. Cancer **26**:847-52, 1970.

Marin-Padilla, M.: Histopathology of the embryonal carcinoma of the testis. Arch Path **85**:614-22, 1968.

McCullough, D. L., Carlton, C. E., & H. M. Seybold: Testicular tumors in infants and children: Report of 5 cases and evaluation of different modes of therapy. J Urol **105**: 140-8, 1971.

Mendelson, D., & A. A. Serpick: Combination chemotherapy of testicular tumors. J Urol **103**:619-23, 1970.

Price, E. B., Jr.: Epidermoid cysts of the testis: A clinical and pathologic analysis of 69 cases from the testicular tumor registry. J Urol **102**:708-13, 1969.

Price, E. B., Jr., & F. K. Mostofi: Epidermoid cysts of the testis in children: A report of four cases. J Pediat **77**:676-9, 1970.

Rigby, C. C.: Chromosome studies in ten testicular tumours. Brit J Cancer **22**:480-5, 1968.

Rolnick, D., & D. Presman: Acute pain as presenting symptom of testicular tumor. J Urol **88**:529-32, 1962.

Rosvoll, R. V., & J. R. Woodard: Malignant sertoli cell tumor of the testis. Cancer **22**: 8-13, 1968.

Rubin, P., & others: Cancer of the urogenital tract: Testicular tumors. JAMA **213**:89-106, 1970.

Shiffman, M. A.: Androblastoma (Sertoli cell tumor): Case report. J Urol **98**:493-6, 1967.

Silva-Inzunza, E., & W. E. Coutts: Sex of testicular tumors. Brit J Urol **31**:333-5, 1959.

Skinner, D. G., Leadbetter, W. F., & E. W. Wilkins, Jr.: The surgical management of testis tumors metastatic to the lung: A report of 10 cases with subsequent resection of from one to seven pulmonary metastases. J Urol **105**:275-82, 1971.

Skinner, D. G., & W. F. Leadbetter: The surgical management of testis tumors. J Urol **106**:84-93, 1971.

Smithers, D., Wallace, E. N. K., & D. M. Wallace: Radiotherapy for patients with tumours of the testicle. Brit J Urol **43**: 83-92, 1971.

Tamoney, H. J., Jr., & A. Noriega: Malignant interstitial cell tumor of the testis. Cancer **24**:547-51, 1969.

Walsh, P. C., & others: Retroperitoneal lymphadenectomy for testicular tumors. JAMA **217**:309-12, 1971.

Young, P. G., & others: Embryonal adenocarcinoma in the prepubertal testis. A clinicopathologic study of 18 cases. Cancer **26**: 1065-75, 1970.

TUMORS OF THE EPIDIDYMIS

Tumors of the epididymis are quite rare, but most are benign (adenomatoid tumors). They may arise from epithelial or connective tissue structures. The malignant group spreads by lymphatics (same as testis) and veins and offers a poor prognosis. Tumors metastasizing to the epididymis are rare.

These tumors often present as painless enlargements, although mild discomfort may be felt. Hydrocele may be the only change present; this, of course, is also true of tumors of the testis. Aspiration of hydroceles is imperative if the testicle cannot be properly palpated.

These lesions must be differentiated from tuberculous or nonspecific epididymitis; this may prove impossible without surgical exploration.

Treatment consists of epididymectomy if one can be sure the lesion is benign. Orchidectomy must be undertaken for cancer or sarcoma. X-ray therapy to regional lymph nodes is also indicated.

Broth, G., Bullock, W. K., & J. Morrow: Epididymal tumors: 1. Report of 15 new cases including review of literature. 2. Histochemical study of the so-called adenomatoid tumor. J Urol **100**:530-6, 1968.

Fisher, E. R., & H. Klieger: Epididymal carcinoma (malignant adenomatoid tumor, mesonephric, mesodermal carcinoma of epididymis). J Urol **95**:568-72, 1966.

Wachtel, T. L., & D. J. Mehan: Metastatic tumors of the epididymis. J Urol **103**:624-7, 1970.

Williams, G., & R. Banerjee: Paratesticular tumours. Brit J Urol **41**:332-9, 1969.

TUMORS OF THE PENIS

Almost all of the tumors of the penis are of epithelial origin and almost always involve the prepuce or glans. They are similar in all respects to tumors of the skin elsewhere on the body.

Etiology

There seems to be no doubt that the most common cause of cancer of the penis is chronic inflammation from infection of the foreskin and glans. In China, Africa, and Southeast

Asia, 10-15% of all tumors are of the penis. On the other hand, the incidence is less than 5% where circumcision is the rule.

Pathogenesis and Pathology

Certain precancerous lesions can be recognized. Leukoplakia may rarely involve the penis. It consists of a white scaly lesion which causes some thickening of the skin. Microscopically, hyperplasia of the squamous cell layer is evident. There is no invasion of the subcutaneous tissue. Considerable small round cell infiltration is seen.

Erythroplasia of Queyrat is strictly a lesion of the penis. Its surface is ordinarily red and indurated and may ulcerate. On microscopic examination, considerable overdevelopment of the rete pegs is noted, yet their basement membranes remain intact. Mitoses are present, but the cells are fairly uniform in size. Some increase in vascularity is noticeable. It may respond to fluorouracil applied locally.

Bowen's disease, or carcinoma in situ, may be found on any skin surface. A raised indurated red plaque may be noted; its center may be ulcerated. Microscopic study reveals anaplasia of epithelial elements with considerable hyperplasia of the squamous cell layers and mitotic activity. The basement membrane, however, remains intact.

Epidermoid carcinoma of the penis is rarely found in a man who has been circumcised during infancy. The growth arises on the glans or the inner surface of the foreskin. It may first appear as a raised, red, firm plaque or as an ulcer. As it grows it may be proliferative or ulcerative. It is usually painless, although severe secondary infection may cause discomfort. Because of the tumor and the edema from infection, retraction of the prepuce may be impossible.

The microscopic picture in epidermoid carcinoma is the same as that of epidermoid cancer anywhere on the skin or mucous surfaces. Hyperkeratosis is prominent. Hyperplasia of the rete is marked, and mitoses are frequent. Invasion of the connective tissue is obvious. Metastases occur through lymph channels which drain to the superficial and deep subinguinal and superficial inguinal nodes; the iliac nodes may also become involved. Enlarged lymph nodes are commonly found in these patients; some are inflammatory and others contain metastatic tumor cells. Widespread metastases by way of veins are not common.

Among the rare growths reported are leiomyosarcoma, melanoma, Kaposi's sarcoma, and vascular tumors.

Clinical Findings

Neoplasms of the penis are usually epithelial and malignant. They involve the foreskin or glans and may be papillary or infiltrating. Metastases to the subinguinal and inguinal lymph nodes are common and have a poor prognosis.

A. Symptoms: The patient may notice an enlarging warty growth or a spreading ulcer on the glans or foreskin. These lesions are usually painless unless secondary infection is marked. Tumors of the shaft are rare.

If the foreskin cannot be retracted, the patient may complain of local pain from infection; a foul, often bloody discharge emanating from the preputial pouch; and a firm lump in the region of the glans.

Masses in the inguinal region may be noted. They can be quite painful and tender if inflammatory, although this finding does not rule out the presence of metastases. In the late stages the metastatic nodes may be quite large, may ulcerate, and can cause hemorrhage which may be difficult to control.

B. Signs: A papillary or ulcerating tumor may be seen. The latter type may be quite destructive. If tumor is suspected and the foreskin cannot be retracted, a dorsal slit of the prepuce should be done.

Enlarged lymph nodes may be found both above and below the inguinal ligament. These can be due to metastases, infection, or both. In the advanced stage, these masses may be quite large. They may ulcerate through the skin.

C. Laboratory Findings: Anemia may be evident in the later stages of the disease. Leukocytosis may be secondary to local infection. The urine bathing an unretractable foreskin will show pus, bacteria, and often red cells. Biopsy is necessary in all patients suspected of having tumors. This can usually be done under local anesthesia. A slit in the dorsal surface of the foreskin may be necessary to properly visualize the lesion.

D. X-Ray Findings: A lymphangiogram may show metastases to the iliac lymph nodes (Fig 7-15).

Differential Diagnosis

Syphilitic chancre may simulate a small ulcerating epithelioma. Dark field examination should reveal Treponema pallidum. In case of doubt, biopsy is indicated.

Chancroid can at times cause some confusion in diagnosis. It is ordinarily a rapidly spreading ulcerative lesion which is quite painful. Complement fixation tests or the finding of Hemophilus ducreyi on smears from the lesion is diagnostic.

Condylomata acuminata are soft warty growths usually of venereal origin and probably caused by a virus. They are usually not invasive. If any doubt exists, biopsy should be done.

Complications

The common complications of tumors of the penis are infection of the tumor and inguinal adenitis, metastatic involvement, and, rarely, invasion of the urethra with urinary obstruction.

Treatment

Before treatment is instituted, a biopsy must be obtained and a positive diagnosis of cancer established.

A. The Local Lesion: Small lesions without evidence of metastases can be destroyed by local excision or by x-ray or radium therapy. More extensive lesions may require partial amputation, though evidence is mounting that irradiation offers a comparable cure rate (50%). Amputation should be done at a level 2 cm proximal to the tumor. Local recurrence after amputation is rare.

B. The Inguinal and Subinguinal Lymph Nodes:
1. Surgical therapy - If the primary lesion is small and no adenopathy is demonstrable, radical resection of the inguinal areas is not indicated. These wounds are often slow to heal, and considerable lymphedema of the area develops.

If a few metastatic nodes are present, as judged by examination or biopsy, bilateral radical inguinal node dissection must be done because of the cross-connections between the 2 sides. It must be remembered that the adenitis may be entirely on an inflammatory basis.

In the presence of advanced metastases, either local or general, excision of these nodes is valueless.
2. X-ray therapy - Metastases in lymph nodes are radioresistant. X-ray treatment can be used, however, to palliate large growths or to stop bleeding from ulceration of the tumor.

Prevention

The evidence seems to be quite clear that circumcision in infancy will almost certainly prevent carcinoma of the penis in later life.

Prognosis

The prognosis is good in small epitheliomas. Sexual intercourse may be completely satisfactory even though half of the penis has been amputated. When a few metastases are present in the resected inguinal nodes, the outlook is fair. Extensive metastatic involvement, however, offers a very poor outlook.

Alexander, L. L., & others: Radium management of tumors of penis. New York J Med **71**:1946-50, 1971.

Das Gupta, T. K.: Radical groin dissection. Surg Gynec Obst **129**:1275-80, 1969.

Dehner, L. P., & B. H. Smith: Soft tissue tumors of the penis. Cancer **25**:1431-47, 1970.

Fronstin, M. H., & J. B. Hutcheson: Malignant melanoma of the penis: A report of two cases. Brit J Urol **41**:324-6, 1969.

Hanash, K. A., & others: Carcinoma of the penis. J Urol **104**:291-7, 1970.

Hayes, C. W., Clark, R. M., & V. A. Politano: Kaposi's sarcoma of the penis. J Urol **105**:525-7, 1971.

Hueser, J. N., & R. P. Pugh: Erythroplasia of Queyrat treated with topical 5-fluorouracil. J Urol **102**:595-7, 1969.

Lewis, R. J., & B. J. Bendl: Erythroplasia of Queyrat. Report of a patient successfully treated with topical 5-fluorouracil. Canad MAJ **104**:148-9, 1971.

McAninch, J. W., & C. A. Moore: Precancerous penile lesions in young men. J Urol **104**:287-90, 1970.

Paymaster, J. C., & P. Gangadharin: Cancer of the penis in India. J Urol **97**:110-3, 1967.

Pratt, R. M., & R. T. A. Ross: Leiomyosarcoma of the penis. Brit J Surg **56**:870-2, 1969.

Vaeth, J. M., Green, J. P., & R. O. Lowy: Radiation therapy of carcinoma of the penis. Am J Roentgenol **108**:130-5, 1970.

TUMORS OF THE SCROTUM

Tumors of the scrotal skin are rare. Most of them arise from occupational exposure to various carcinogens, including soot, tars, creosote, and petroleum products. While a few benign tumors of the skin or subcutaneous tissues occur, most are epitheliomas. They metastasize by lymphatic channels to the superficial inguinal and subinguinal nodes.

The diagnosis should be considered in any lesion of the scrotal skin in a man who gives a history of prolonged exposure to carcinogens. Biopsy is necessary if any doubt exists. Treatment consists of wide excision of the primary tumor. If a few inguinal metastases are noted, bilateral inguinal node dissection is indicated.

El-Domeiri, A. A., & M. A. Paglia: Carcinoma of the scrotum, radical excision and repair using ox fascia: Case report. J Urol **106**:575-7, 1971.

Kickham, C. J. E., & M. Dufresne: An assessment of carcinoma of the scrotum. J Urol **98**:108-10, 1967.

Tucci, P., & G. Haralambides: Carcinoma of the scrotum: Review of literature and presentation of 2 cases. J Urol **89**:585-90, 1963.

•   •   •

General References

Arduino, L. J.: Chemotherapy in urologic cancer. S Clin North America **45**:1351-64, 1965.

Hiatt, H. H.: Cancer chemotherapy—present status and prospects. New England J Med **276**:157-66, 1967.

Rubin, P.: Current concepts in genitourinary oncology: A multidisciplinary approach. J Urol **106**:315-38, 1971.

18...

Oliguria

Richards P. Lyon, MD *

When the urine output is so low that the end products of metabolism cannot be effectively excreted, the patient is said to be in a state of oliguria. It is not possible to define oliguria in terms of so many milliliters of urine excreted. A patient who can concentrate urine to a specific gravity of 1.040 does not become oliguric until his daily urine volume falls below 500 ml; the patient who can concentrate only to a specific gravity of 1.006 is oliguric when his daily urine volume falls below 1000 ml.

The causes of oliguria may be classified as follows: (1) organic renal lesions, eg, acute tubular necrosis (lower nephron syndrome), acute glomerulonephritis, and terminal chronic renal disease†; (2) severe fluid and electrolyte imbalance, eg, dilution or hypotonicity, hypertonic dehydration; and (3) urinary tract obstruction. This classification has clinical value since the diagnostic approach and the treatment of each is specific. For example, although groups (1) and (2) have in common a small urine volume and rising nitrogen levels, restriction of potassium and fluid is essential in the acute organic group whereas the administration of potassium and fluid may be lifesaving in the physiologic imbalance group.

ACUTE TUBULAR NECROSIS
(Lower Nephron Nephrosis; Acute Reversible Renal Failure)

The most common causes of acute tubular necrosis are shock, exposure to nephrotoxic chemicals (eg, carbon tetrachloride), intravascular hemolysis (eg, due to transfusion reactions or following transurethral resection), severe crushing injuries with myohemoglobinuria, and prolonged and severe fluid and electrolyte imbalances.‡ The majority of lesions are due to a combination of causes. Damage to the renal tubules is more prone to occur among elderly persons.

Acute tubular necrosis was at one time commonly termed "lower nephron nephrosis" because Lucké and others first observed the lesion in the distal tubule only. Subsequent studies have demonstrated that the proximal tubule and the glomerulus are often involved. The essential lesion is cellular necrosis which does not begin to heal for 6-10 days or longer. Repair is ultimately complete upon gross clinical examination, but more sensitive tests of renal function indicate that some residual damage is always present. In rare instances the basement membrane of the tubules sloughs away, in which case cellular replacement cannot take place; the lesion is irreversible. Anuria is a common finding in these cases, and implies a much less favorable prognosis.

Clinical Findings

A. Symptoms and Signs: The clinical picture is not distinctive. The patient with carbon tetrachloride poisoning may have no complaint other than progressive edema, whereas a patient who has undergone abdominal surgery or one with severe hemorrhage resulting from a ruptured aortic aneurysm will present with all of the signs that follow surgical procedures in the abdomen. When acute tubular necrosis is suspected, the physician should survey renal function by means of the usual tests and observe body water changes (reflected by changes in body weight). A daily urine output of less than 400 ml in spite of adequate intake is the presenting complaint. Acute tubular necrosis must always be suspected following clinical shock.

Body weight: In the presence of shock or following transurethral resection (but in the absence of cardiac failure), an early postopera-

---

*Associate Clinical Professor of Urology, University of California School of Medicine, San Francisco, California.
†Only acute tubular necrosis will be discussed here.
‡An increasing number of instances of the hemolytic-uremic syndrome are being reported in the literature.

tive increase in body weight suggests the oliguria of acute tubular necrosis.

B. Laboratory Findings: The diagnosis may be established by simple laboratory tests.
1. Specific gravity of urine - The urine specific gravity is near 1.010 within 48 hours of the onset of shock or poisoning. This test may mislead the physician during the first 48 hours because the urine specific gravity may be as high as 1.026 during this interval. It is not known whether elevation of specific gravity in the first 48 hours is due to transudative material in the urine or whether it reflects the specific gravity of the urine already present in the bladder before renal shutdown occurred.
2. PSP excretion - 0 to trace per hour, regardless of urine volume.
3. Urine chloride concentration* - Fixed between 30-40 mEq/L in the classic case where the urine contains no blood. A urine chloride measurement between 40-100 mEq/L is compatible with a partial tubular lesion. These concentrations tend to remain fixed throughout the oliguric period. A urine chloride of less than 20 mEq/L or more than 100 mEq/L rules out acute tubular necrosis. Urine sodium tends to remain fixed between 30-60 mEq/L. Urine potassium tends to be 25 mEq/L.
4. Serum electrolytes - Sodium and chloride concentrations may be low, normal, or high, depending on salt and water intake. Serum potassium concentration is rarely elevated during the first 72 hours except in the patient with severe crush injuries. Serum CO_2 will reflect the degree of acidosis, although this may not be significant in terms of need for correction.
5. Tests of retention - Serum creatinine and urea nitrogen tend to rise together at a 1:10 ratio. In rare instances, the serum creatinine may rise precipitously (possibly due to end products of muscle trauma) out of proportion to urea nitrogen. If the cause of the oliguria is obstruction, urea nitrogen tends to rise faster than serum creatinine. If oliguria results from intra- or extraperitoneal urinary extravasation, the rise in urea nitrogen is precipitous while serum creatinine stays close to normal.
6. Urine/plasma creatine ratio < 10:1.
7. Urine urea concentration - A value of 1.1 gm% or more in a random urine specimen seems to guarantee that acute tubular necrosis has not occurred.
8. Renograms - The radioisotope renogram can be diagnostic in differentiating the oliguria of obstruction from that of acute tubular necrosis. The tubular phase of concentration of radioactive material remains elevated, as is shown by comparing curve D with curve B in Fig 8-8.
9. Mannitol - The mannitol diuresis test has been suggested as a means of differentiating the oliguria of acute tubular necrosis from that caused by physiologic imbalance. If the above criteria in differential diagnosis of oliguria are followed, the mannitol test could be useful only when urine specific gravity is 1.010, PSP excretion is 0 to a trace, and urine chloride is fixed in the range of 40-100 mEq/L. If, after correction of the fluid-ion imbalance, diuresis does not occur, the mannitol test might be used to satisfy the physician's concern that the diagnosis was still being missed. If a diuresis is achieved in this manner, the fluid-ion imbalance posing the problem would still have to be discovered.
10. If the mannitol diuresis test is inconclusive, 2 other powerful diuretic agents may be tried—ethacrynic acid (Edecrin®), 150-200 mg, or furosemide (Lasix®), 160 mg, as single doses IV.

Treatment

A. During the Phase of Oliguria:
1. Fluid intake and body weight - Attention to total body water is of primary importance. The patient who is taking no food by mouth produces 300-500 ml/day of water in the process of metabolism. This is termed water of oxidation or metabolic water. This water contains no electrolytes and is therefore analogous to an infusion or a drink of salt-free water. To prevent overhydration (and therefore dilution) this amount of water must be excreted by the body each day. Therefore, to maintain a normal water-electrolyte relationship, the patient must be allowed to lose 1 lb/day. A chart should be made and a declining "weight line" should be plotted beginning on the day of onset of oliguria. Parenteral water should be ordered only if body weight falls below this weight line. Because invisible cutaneous and respiratory losses are 800 ml/day, about 300 ml/day of parenteral water will maintain this balance. If too much water has been given before the diagnosis is made, water must be completely withheld until the desired weight is reached no matter how many days that requires.

Overhydration to the point of pulmonary edema ("drowning") rarely occurs during the first several days of oliguria if the patient is carefully watched. However, cardiac failure not uncommonly occurs between the 8th and

---

*Urine chloride is measured with Scribner's Bedside Chloride Set, which permits accurate determination of the chloride concentration in any body fluid (eg, serum, urine, gastrointestinal fluid) in less than 60 seconds. (See p 54.)

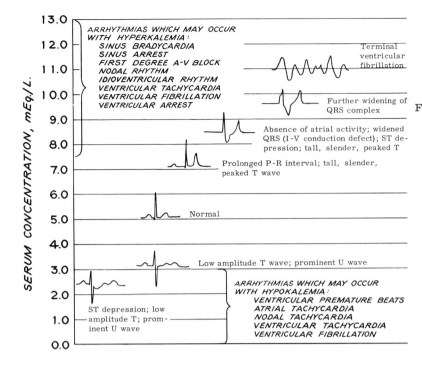

ARRHYTHMIAS WHICH MAY OCCUR
WITH HYPERKALEMIA:
   SINUS BRADYCARDIA
   SINUS ARREST
   FIRST DEGREE A-V BLOCK
   NODAL RHYTHM
   IDIOVENTRICULAR RHYTHM
   VENTRICULAR TACHYCARDIA
   VENTRICULAR FIBRILLATION
   VENTRICULAR ARREST

Terminal ventricular fibrillation

Further widening of QRS complex

Absence of atrial activity; widened QRS (I-V conduction defect); ST depression; tall, slender, peaked T

Prolonged P-R interval; tall, slender, peaked T wave

Normal

Low amplitude T wave; prominent U wave

ARRHYTHMIAS WHICH MAY OCCUR
WITH HYPOKALEMIA:
   VENTRICULAR PREMATURE BEATS
   ATRIAL TACHYCARDIA
   NODAL TACHYCARDIA
   VENTRICULAR TACHYCARDIA
   VENTRICULAR FIBRILLATION

ST depression; low amplitude T; prominent U wave

SERUM CONCENTRATION, mEq./L.

Fig 18-1. Correlation of the ECG with serum potassium levels. Provided there is no parallel change in sodium and calcium. (Reproduced, with permission, from Krupp, M.A., & M.J. Chatton: Current Diagnosis & Treatment. Lange, 1972.)

12th days unless a regimen of relative dehydration is rigidly enforced. The danger of slight overhydration during this interval is greater than the danger of slight dehydration.

2. Extracellular electrolytes - Serum sodium, chloride, CO_2, and pH should be determined every 48 hours if possible, and serum potassium must be determined every 24 hours. A base-line electrocardiogram should be taken immediately and should be repeated every 2 or 3 days or whenever serum potassium elevations occur. (Note: Dangerous hyperkalemia is most to be feared in the young patient with crush injury. It is rare in the elderly patient if close attention is given to body weight and water restriction.) Salt or sodium should be added to parenteral solutions only if the serum sodium falls below 126 mEq/L. Sodium in the form of sodium lactate or sodium bicarbonate is indicated primarily where clinical acidosis is noted. Serum nitrogen or creatinine levels may be determined, but they have no practical value in treatment.

3. Osmotic diuresis - The usefulness of mannitol in therapy is open to question. If obstruction of the tubule by such a material as acid hematin is considered a possibility, osmotic diuresis by mannitol (or 50% dextrose) should be effective through its osmotic diuretic action.

4. Nutrition - 100 gm of dextrose daily (supplying 400 Calories) is accepted as the amount necessary to minimize protein catabolism. The concentration of dextrose in the parenteral solution must be adjusted so as not to require an excessive water intake. (Note: An increased rate of serum potassium elevation as a consequence of insufficient caloric intake has not been observed.)

B. Phase of Recovery: If close attention is paid to body weight and the patient loses 1 lb/day, intensive diuresis is rare. During the recovery phase, urine volume rapidly increases to 1500 ml/day at a specific gravity of 1.010, and removal of metabolic wastes again increases. At this point, urine chloride concentration will shift either up or down, depending upon serum chloride excess or lack. Tubular reabsorption of salt is still impaired at this time, and 2 gm (35 mEq) of sodium chloride over normal intake should be allowed for every liter of urine to compensate the loss. The increasing urine volume will remove potassium (15 mEq/L or more of urine) from the extracellular space rapidly, and hypokalemia may suddenly occur if oral or parenteral potassium is not supplied. In the usual case, oral intake is adequate and potassium supplements are sufficient. The body weight line will level out as the kidneys regain control of water and electrolyte balance and as oral intake supplies body needs. Attempts to force fluids at this time increase the danger of cardiac failure just when the patient is recovering. If urine volume falls off in the phase of diuresis, cardiac failure should be suspected rather than a reactivation of the renal tubular lesion.

Complications

Rapidly advancing acidosis is a rare complication which leads to fatiguing hyperventilation, movement of potassium from the cells with consequent hyperpotassemia, and other serious physiologic disturbances which are not fully understood. The most easily available emergency aid is parenteral sodium—preferably administered as NaHCO₃—which minimizes acidosis and thus favors the motion of potassium back into the cell. Insulin with 50% dextrose may be helpful if given aggressively by venous cannula. However, the rapidity with which peritoneal dialysis can be instituted makes it the most decisive treatment. Moderate serum potassium elevations may be controlled and further elevations prevented by oral administration of exchange resins, used in combination with sorbitol to promote evacuation.

In the rare instance where serious edema with overhydration has occurred, peritoneal dialysis with 7.5% dextrose solution may be life-saving.

Prevention With Mannitol

The osmotic diuresis produced by mannitol is apparently effective in preventing acute tubular necrosis, particularly where poisons such as hemoglobin and myohemoglobin are presented to the kidney for filtration and excretion. Presumably, the osmotic ability of mannitol prevents the usual absorption of H_2O from the filtrate and enables the drug to literally wash out the tubule. In this way, stasis of toxic materials is prevented.

Mannitol is most effective when used at the time of insult (as in intravascular hemolysis during cardiac bypass and as shock is controlled after injury or during surgery). An initial dose of 25 gm of mannitol as a 20-50% solution may be followed by a 5% solution allowing a maximum 24-hour intake of 100 gm of mannitol. Because salt tends to be lost at the rate of 4-6 gm/L of urine during mannitol diuresis, the drug should be administered in 0.45% saline. Where diuresis is in excess of the intake of the 5% mannitol solution, 0.45% saline is required by itself to compensate for the urine increment. If diuresis does not occur with the primary dose, mannitol should be promptly discontinued.

Ajik, M.: Prevention of acute renal failure. Am J Surg 108:384-91, 1964.

Briggs, J. D., & others: Renal function after acute tubular necrosis. Brit MJ 2:513-6, 1967.

Figueroa, J. E.: Acute renal failure: Its unusual causes and manifestations. M Clin North America 51:995-1002, 1967.

Flanagan, W. J., Henderson, L. W., & J. P. Merrill: The clinical application and technique of peritoneal dialysis. GP 28:98-109, Nov. 1963.

Freeman, R. B., & others: Renal tubular necrosis due to nephrotoxicity of organic mercurial diuretics. Ann Int Med 57:34-43, 1962.

Gianantonio, C. A., & others: The hemolytic-uremic syndrome. J Pediat 72:757-65, 1968.

Hammond, D., & others: Hemolytic-uremic syndrome. Am J Dis Child 114:440-9, 1967.

Handa, S. P., & M. Z. Lazor: Acute tubular necrosis. A review of 44 necropsied cases. Am J M Sc 251:29-36, 1966.

Hedger, R. W.: The conservative management of acute oliguric renal function. M Clin North America 55:121-35, 1971.

Huffer, J. C., & R. P. Lyon: The conservative management of acute renal failure by a controlled dehydration regimen. J Urol 85:459-61, 1961.

Lunding, M., Steiness, L., & J. H. Thaysen: Acute renal failure due to tubular necrosis. Acta med scandinav 176:103-19, 1964.

Lyon, R. P.: Measurement of urine chloride as a test of renal function. J Urol 85:884-8, 1961.

Lyon, R. P.: Nonobstructive oliguria—differential diagnosis. California Med 99:83-9, 1963.

Maher, J. F., O'Connell, J. M. B., & G. E. Schreiner: Traumatic acute renal failure. Postgrad Med 39:70-80, 1966.

Merrill, J. P.: Acute renal failure. JAMA 211:289-91, 1970.

Mueller, C. B.: The mechanism of acute renal failure after injury and transfusion reaction and its prevention by solute diuresis. S Clin North America 45:499-508, 1965.

Myler, R. K., Lee, J. C., & J. Hopper, Jr.: Renal tubular necrosis caused by mushroom poisoning. Arch Int Med 114:196-204, 1964.

Nielsen, V. K., & J. Larsen: Acute renal failure due to carbon tetrachloride poisoning. Acta med scandinav 178:363-74, 1965.

Powers, S. R., Jr., & others: Prevention of postoperative acute renal failure with mannitol in 100 cases. Surgery 55:15-22, 1964.

Reidenberg, M. M., & others: Acute renal failure due to nephrotoxins. Am J M Sc 247:25-9, 1964.

Stahl, W. M.: Effect of mannitol on the kidneys. New England J Med 272:381-6, 1965.

Stremple, J. F., Ellison, E. H., & L. C. Carey: Osmolar diuresis: success and/or failure.

A collective review. Surgery 6:924-37, 1966.

Trinkle, J.K., & W.S. Kiser: Acute renal failure: Diagnosis of etiology by radioisotope renography. J Urol **91**:199-202, 1964.

Vertel, R.M., & J.P. Knochel: Nonoliguric acute renal failure. JAMA **200**:598-602, 1967.

Weeks, R.S.: The crush syndrome. Surg Gynec Obst **127**:369-75, 1968.

Wennberg, J.E., & others: Renal toxicity of oral cholecystographic media. JAMA **186**: 461-7, 1963.

PHYSIOLOGIC IMBALANCES CAUSING OLIGURIA

Three-fourths of oliguria cases are due to physiologic imbalances involving the body fluids, electrolytes, and blood volume rather than to acute tubular necrosis or ureteral obstruction. Functional renal failure, in contrast to the organic lesion, requires prompt therapy with solutions that are usually withheld from a patient with acute tubular necrosis. The most common imbalances are (1) hypotonic dehydration or overhydration (dilutional syndrome), (2) acute normotonic dehydration, (3) hypertonic dehydration, and (4) circulatory failure.

Pathologic Physiology

Reasonably good kidney function is essential if fluid and electrolyte balance is to be maintained by the patient himself. The kidney excretes or retains various substances, including salt, potassium, water, and the end products of metabolism, thus maintaining a normal body water and electrolyte balance (or normotonicity) by means of the selective excretion of electrolytes with respect to water.

The second most important function of the kidney is the maintenance of normal body pH; the kidney accomplishes this by selectively excreting acid and base.

Unimpaired renal blood flow is necessary if these activities are to be carried out in the normal way. Any fluid or electrolyte imbalance affects all tissue cells; when the renal tubular cell is so affected, its ability to compensate losses (eg, from the gastrointestinal tract) becomes limited. Thus, decreased tubular function, when superimposed upon an existing water and electrolyte imbalance, compounds the clinical problem. The return of adequate renal function is necessary if normal fluid and electrolyte balance is to be maintained by the patient himself. The correction of tonicity (serum sodium concentration) is most important in returning renal tubular function to normal.

Diagnosis and Treatment

There are no characteristic clinical patterns for any particular fluid or electrolyte imbalance. Varying degrees of lethargy, weakness, ileus, and many other nonspecific symptoms are common to all. The physician must rely on a careful history of the route and volume of loss, must observe weight changes closely, and must use the appropriate tests and measurements in order to establish a diagnosis and prescribe treatment.

A. Dilution Syndrome (Hypotonic Overhydration or Dehydration): This is the most common fluid and electrolyte imbalance of iatrogenic etiology and often leads to severe oliguria. It is due to the overzealous use of salt-free solutions in the immediate postoperative period, when the action of the antidiuretic hormone leads to water retention. It is even more apt to develop if during the preoperative period the patient did not eat, lost electrolytes by vomiting, and was able to retain only water and thus came to surgery already in a mildly hypotonic state. The diagnosis is established by serum sodium and chloride levels 10 mEq/L or more below normal, a PSP excretion of 5% or more per hour, and a history suggestive of salt deficit. Despite the low serum sodium and chloride levels, urine salt concentrations may be as high as 100 mEq/L, which indicates that further salt is being lost by the kidney.

In the presence of overhydration, treatment requires at the least aggressive water restriction. Where a rapid recovery is important, as with the elderly patient immobilized in bed by the fluid-ion problem, 3-5% salt solution given slowly intravenously, over a period of 24-48 hours, will provide an early diuresis. In the presence of dehydration (as measured by body weight), normal saline solution (0.9%) is indicated. The number of mEq of NaCl to make such a correction is determined by assuming that body water is 50% of body weight and that the administered salt will diffuse into this volume. Thus, the desired rise in serum sodium concentration, multiplied by the number of liters of estimated body water, provides the correction requirement.

B. Simple Dehydration: A diagnosis of simple dehydration can be made if weight loss is out of proportion to the severity of the illness (greater than 0.5-1 lb/day), the serum sodium and chloride concentrations are reasonably normal, and the urine specific gravity is 1.022 or higher. A normal serum creatinine or nitrogen level in the presence of oliguria is rare, but establishes the fact that kidney function is normal. If dehydration is severe and prolonged, the concentrating power of the kidney may have begun to fail and a specific gravity in the range of 1.010 suggests renal tubular damage. PSP excretion of 5% or more in 1 hour rules out acute tubular necrosis. The presence of anemia and a long history of chills and fever, nausea, weight loss, or pyuria suggest chronic renal failure. A urine chloride of less than 5 or more than 150 mEq/ L speaks against a chronic renal lesion.

Treatment consists of administering hypotonic solutions such as 0.45% sodium chloride, with added potassium as urine volume increases. When rehydration is complete, the patient's weight will return to normal less starvation losses (0.5 lb/day).

C. Diminished Renal Blood Flow: Preclinical shock, cardiac failure, and a relative hypotension in a normally hypertensive patient are the most common disorders in this group. Shock, preclinical shock, and heart failure present no diagnostic difficulties. Oliguria may occur in the patient whose established systolic blood pressure is 200 mm Hg who, because of the administration of antipressor agents or serious primary disease, sustains a drop in systolic blood pressure to the usual normal range of 120 mm Hg.

Treatment is directed at the restoration of blood pressure, primarily by blood volume replacement and on occasion with vasoconstrictors. Attempts to promote diuresis by the addition of fluids and salt are to be condemned, except in cases where salt and water deficits are present. Digitalization of the patient with cardiac failure will lead to improved renal blood flow and diuresis.

Bell, H., Hayes, W.L., & J. Vosburgh: Hyperkalemic paralysis due to adrenal insufficiency. Arch Int Med 115:418-20, 1965.

Berlyne, G.M., & others: Treatment of hyperkalemia with a calcium-resin. Lancet 1:169-72, 1966.

Berman, L.B.: The hypokalemic syndromes. GP 29:105-9, June 1964.

Bruck, E., Abul, G., & T. Aceto, Jr.: Therapy of infants with hypertonic dehydration due to diarrhea. Am J Dis Child 115:281-301, 1968.

Bruck, E., Abul, G., & T. Aceto, Jr.: Pathogenesis and pathophysiology of hypertonic dehydration with diarrhea. Am J Dis Child 115:122-44, 1968.

Burns, R.O., & others: Peritoneal dialysis. New England J Med 267:1060-6, 1962.

Carpenter, C.C.J., & others: Clinical evaluation of fluid requirements in Asiatic cholera. Lancet 1:726-7, 1965.

Cohn, H.E., & J.P. Capelli: The diagnosis and management of oliguria in the postoperative period. S Clin North America 47:1187-1206, 1967.

Doolin, R.D., & others: Evaluation of intermittent peritoneal lavage. Am J Med 26:831-44, 1959.

Flinn, R.B., Merrill, J.P., & W.R. Welzant: Treatment of the oliguric patient with a new sodium-exchange resin and sorbitol. New England J Med 264:111-5, 1961.

Forland, M., & T.N. Pullman: Electrolyte complications of drug therapy. M Clin North America 47:113-29, 1963.

Forland, M., & T.N. Pullman: Aspects of cardiac disease: M Clin North America 50:255-69, 1966.

Gerst, P.H., Porter, M.R., & R.A. Fishman: Symptomatic magnesium deficiency in surgical patients. Ann Surg 159:402-6, 1964.

Kassirer, J.P., & others: The critical role of chloride in the correction of hypokalemic alkalosis in man. Am J Med 38:172-89, 1965.

Kleeman, C.R., & M.P. Fichman: The clinical physiology of water metabolism. New England J Med 277:1300-7, 1967.

Klein, D.E., Wright, H.K., & L. Persky: Electrolyte and osmolality changes attending electroresection. Arch Surg 90:871-5, 1965.

Leaf, A.: The clinical and physiologic significance of the serum sodium concentration. New England J Med 267:25-30, 77-83, 1962.

Leaf, A., & R.F. Santos: Physiologic mechanisms in potassium deficiency. New England J Med 264:335-41, 1961.

Levinsky, N.G.: Management of emergencies. VI. Hyperkalemia. New England J Med 274:1076-7, 1966.

Lyon, R.P.: Measurement of urine chloride as a test of renal function. J Urol 85:884-8, 1961.

Moore, F.D.: Regulation of the serum sodium concentration. Origin and treatment of tonicity disorders in surgery. Am J Surg 103:302-7, 1962.

Moyer, C.A., Margraf, H.W., & W.W. Monafo, Jr.: Burn shock and extravascular sodium deficiency—treatment with Ringer's solution with lactate. Arch Surg 90:799-811, 1965.

Pullen, H., Doig, A., & A.T. Lambie: Intensive intravenous potassium replacement therapy. Lancet 2:809-11, 1967.

Schwartz, W.B., & A.S. Relman: Effects of electrolyte disorders on renal structure and function. New England J Med 276:383-9, 452-8, 1967.

Symposium on fluid and electrolyte problems. P Clin North America 11:789-1103, 1964.

Teree, T.M., & others: Stool losses and acidosis in diarrheal disease of infancy. Pediatrics 36:704-13, 1965.

Winters, R.W.: Terminology of acid-base disorders. Ann Int Med 63:873-84, 1965.

Winters, R.W.: Studies of acid-base disturbances. Pediatrics 39:700-12, 1967.

Zimmerman, B.: Pituitary and adrenal function in relation to surgery. S Clin North America 45:299-315, 1965.

BILATERAL URETERAL OBSTRUCTION*

The causes of bilateral ureteral stenosis are (1) occlusion by masses of metastatic (or lymphomatous) iliac or lumbar lymph nodes (eg, cancer of the cervix or prostate); (2) retroperitoneal fasciitis; (3) bilateral ureteral calculi (or ureteral calculus blocking an only kidney); and (4) trauma to or ligation of the ureters in conjunction with gynecologic surgery or abdominoperineal resection of the rectum. Ligation of only one ureter will not cause oliguria if the other kidney is normal.

Complete anuria (not oliguria) is rare with acute tubular necrosis, fluid and electrolyte aberrations, and in association with diminished renal blood flow. Immediate anuria following surgery in the lower abdomen means bilateral ureteral injury until proved otherwise.

Clinical Findings

A. Symptoms and Signs: If obstruction is due to surgical injury, the patient suffers undue and prolonged ileus. If renal pain is present, renal tenderness may be elicited. If excess fluids have been given, edema may be noted. Signs of ileus are evident (eg, a quiet, distended abdomen, vomiting). A few days after surgical ureteral injury, urine may begin to leak through the wound or the vagina.

B. Laboratory Findings: The hematocrit may be low, particularly if edema is present. The urine specific gravity is often of no value, although it tends to be below 1.010 regardless of the state of hydration. If any urine is being secreted, some PSP will be recovered. The urine chloride concentration will depend upon water and salt relationships. Blood nitrogen may be elevated out of proportion to creatinine. The excretory urogram with "delayed" films taken up to 24 hours will often demonstrate an increasing density of the kidney (nephrogram effect) typical of obstruction and adequate renal function.

C. Instrumental Examination: Cystoscopy should be done and ureteral catheterization attempted. If the catheters are arrested in the lower ureters, radiopaque fluid can be introduced and x-rays taken. In this way the diagnosis of bilateral injury can be established.

Differential Diagnosis

If the patient has just undergone pelvic surgery and if there is no evidence of diminished renal blood flow (eg, cardiac failure, hemorrhage) or fluid-ion imbalance, bilateral ureteral obstruction should be suspected. A radioisotope renogram should clearly differentiate between acute renal failure and bilateral ureteral ligation (Fig 8-8).

Complications, Treatment, and Prognosis

For injuries to the ureter, see p 234.

• • •

---

*See also Injuries to the Ureter, p 234, Acquired Diseases of the Ureter, p 361, and associated references.

19...

The Neurogenic Bladder

Normal vesical action depends upon an intact nerve supply. If either the sensory or motor nerves are interrupted, bladder function will be impaired. The type of abnormality is determined by the site and degree of the injury.

Spinal cord trauma secondary to vertebral fracture is the most common cause of neurogenic bladder dysfunction. Certain diseases (eg, tabes dorsalis, diabetes mellitus, multiple sclerosis) and cord tumors or herniated intervertebral disks also may cause abnormalities in micturition. Certain congenital anomalies (myelomeningocele, spina bifida, absence of the sacrum) are also associated with neurogenic vesical dysfunction. Cordotomy to relieve intractable pain may affect perception of the need for voiding; abdominoperineal resection of the rectum disturbs the innervation of the bladder and may be followed by at least temporary difficulty with urination.

NORMAL VESICAL FUNCTION

ANATOMY

Detrusor Muscle

The bladder wall is composed of a mesh of muscle fibers running in every direction except when they approach the internal orifice, where they are rearranged to form 3 definite layers: internal longitudinal, middle circular, and external longitudinal. The outer layer extends down the whole length of the female urethra and to the distal end of the prostate but is circularly and spirally oriented; thus, it functions as the major involuntary sphincter. The middle circular detrusor muscle layer ends at the internal orifice of the bladder; it is best developed anteriorly. The internal component remains longitudinal and reaches the distal end of the urethra in the female and the end of the prostate in the male. These

converging fibers cause a thickening that forms the so-called vesical neck, but anatomically there is no true sphincter at this point.

External Sphincters

There are 2 voluntary external sphincter mechanisms formed of striated muscle. The major one, which lies between the fascial layers of the urogenital diaphragm, is maximally condensed around the middle third of the female urethra (external to the external layer of urethral musculature) while in the male these fibers surround the distal portion of the prostate and the membranous urethra. The striated muscles of the pelvic floor (eg, levator ani) further contribute to sphincteric function.

Diaphragm and Abdominal Muscles

These play only secondary roles in micturition. Their contraction may further increase intravesical pressure in the female.

Nerve Supply

The sacral portion of the spinal cord, which contains the center controlling micturition (S2-4), is housed within the vertebral bodies T12 to L1. Fractures in the region of the 12th thoracic and first lumbar vertebrae or below lead to flaccid neurogenic bladder because they destroy the voiding reflex center or the pelvic nerves (or both). Injuries above this level cause a spastic type of neurogenic bladder due to damage of the upper motor neurons.

A. Motor Nerves: (Fig 19-1.)

1. To the detrusor - These nerves are part of the parasympathetic nervous system. They arise from S2-4 and reach the bladder wall through the pelvic nerves. The trigonal portion of the bladder, because of its different embryologic origin, is innervated by motor fibers from the thoracolumbar outflow (T11 to L2) of the sympathetic nervous system. In dogs, intravenously administered epinephrine causes contraction of the trigone, the function of which is twofold. First, its tone pulls downward upon the ureterovesical junction, thus combating reflux; second, its contracture at

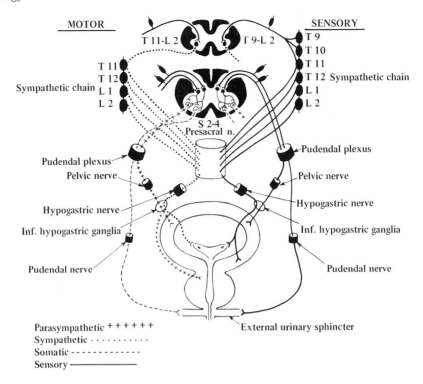

MOTOR   SENSORY

T 11-L 2   T 9-L 2   T 9
                               T 10
T 11   T 11
T 12   T 12 Sympathetic chain
Sympathetic chain L 1   L 1
                   L 2   L 2
                    S 2-4
                 Presacral n.

Pudendal plexus   Pudendal plexus
Pelvic nerve   Pelvic nerve

Hypogastric nerve   Hypogastric nerve

Inf. hypogastric ganglia   Inf. hypogastric ganglia

Pudendal nerve   Pudendal nerve

Parasympathetic + + + + + +
Sympathetic · · · · · · · · · ·   External urinary sphincter
Somatic - - - - - - - - - - - -
Sensory ─────────

Fig 19-1. Segmental and peripheral innervation of the urinary bladder. (Reproduced, with permission, from E. Bors: J Nerv Ment Dis **116**:572-8, 1952.)

the time of voiding helps open the bladder neck. Interruption of the sympathetic pathways may denervate the genital ducts and cause loss of the power of ejaculation.

2. To the external sphincter - The motor nerve supply to the external sphincter and perineal muscles is somatic (voluntary) and reaches those structures through the pudendal nerves. They also arise from S2-4. The motor fibers descend in the pyramidal tracts.

B. Sensory Nerves: Sensation from the urethra and bladder is returned to the central nervous system by fibers which travel with both the parasympathetic and somatic (S2-4) and the sympathetic motor nerves (T9 to L2). The parasympathetic nerves carry the sensory stretch perceptors. The sensory fibers ascend in the lateral spinothalamic tracts and fasciculus gracilis.

C. Voiding (Spinal) Reflex: The afferent and efferent fibers of the sacral portion of the cord (S2-4) form a simple spinal reflex which controls vesical function. Its activity is under the voluntary control of the cerebral cortex through the mediation of suprasegmental connections.

PHYSIOLOGY

Neurophysiology

Urinary control is largely centered in the simple reflex reaction between the bladder and the sacral cord. The normal bladder is able to distend gradually to normal capacity (400 ml) without appreciable increase in intravesical pressure. At this point, sensations of fullness are transmitted to the sacral cord where, if voluntary (cerebral) control is lacking (as in infants), discharges through the motor side of the reflex arc cause powerful, sustained detrusor contraction and spontaneous involuntary urination. As myelinization and training of the young child progress, cerebral inhibitory functions suppress the sacral reflex and the individual voids at his convenience.

Vesical Physiology

The normal act of urination is initiated by voluntary suppression of cerebral inhibition. Relaxation of the muscles of the pelvic floor and the striated external sphincter occur first. This operates to drop the vesical base, thereby further contributing to minimizing urethral resistance. The muscle fibers of the bladder wall begin to contract; intravesical pressure begins to rise. Because the vesical longitudinal muscles insert into the urethra, their contraction along with the trigone tends to pull the internal vesical sphincter open, forming a funnel. The increased hydrostatic pressure (30-40 cm of water) exerted by the detrusor is directed down the urethra. Reciprocally, the urethral counterpressure drops and voiding ensues. The detrusor maintains its contraction until complete emptying has occurred.

When the bladder is empty, the detrusor muscle relaxes and the bladder neck is allowed to close; urethral and perineal muscle tone then returns to normal. Should the person choose to interrupt the urinary stream, the external sphincter is contracted voluntarily. Detrusor muscle spasm then relaxes by reciprocal reflex action and the bladder neck closes.

CYSTOMETRIC STUDY

Cystometry has contributed much to our understanding of normal vesical function and is of value in diagnosing the types of nervous system lesions which cause neurogenic vesical dysfunction. A normal cystometrogram is shown in Fig 19-2. A cystometer is shown at left.

The normal bladder can usually perceive the first injection of fluid through a catheter. The desire to void is felt initially when 100-200 ml of fluid have been instilled. As fluid is introduced, intravesical pressure remains fairly constant at 8-15 cm of water. There are no sharp rises of pressure (uninhibited contractions) until 350-450 ml of fluid have been introduced, at which point a definite sensation of fullness (capacity) and distress is noted and the pressure increases sharply to 40-100 cm

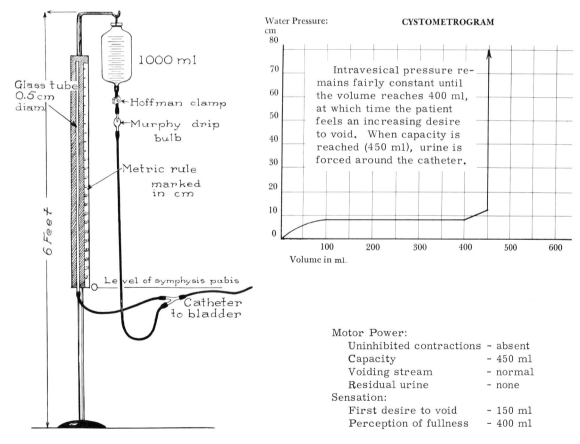

Fig 19-2. Cystometry. Left: A simple water manometer (see p 111 for technic of cystometry). Right: Normal cystometrogram. As fluid is slowly introduced into the bladder, the detrusor gradually relaxes to accept increasing amounts of fluid without change in intravesical pressure. At a volume of 400 ml the patient felt an urge to void. Shortly thereafter, an involuntary contraction of the detrusor occurred which was reflected in a sharp increase in intravesical pressure.

water. This results in involuntary voiding around the catheter. If the catheter is withdrawn, the patient voids with a forceful, continuous stream. If bladder function is normal, there is no residual urine. Should the patient voluntarily strain to void, the resulting intravesical pressure recorded by the manometer will be a summation of true intravesical pressure and intra-abdominal pressure. The patient, therefore, should be cautioned against straining.

More sophisticated methods have been developed to study intravesical pressure and urethral resistance during the resting phase and while voiding, but these methods are not generally available for clinical use. Measurement of intravesical pressure and urethral resistance afford more information of a dynamic nature. Urinary continence requires that urethral pressure exceed intravesical pressure. In the normal person, during voiding, intravesical pressure rises to 30-40 cm of water, exceeding urethral resistance which drops reciprocally. If urethral resistance is high (eg, benign prostate hyperplasia, spasm of the striated periurethral muscles), voiding will require an abnormally high intravesical pressure. Should urethral resistance be low, even normal intravesical pressure or increased intra-abdominal pressure may be associated with incontinence.

ABNORMAL VESICAL FUNCTION

The following descriptions assume that the upper and lower motor neuron lesions are complete, but it must be realized that many incomplete lesions occur.

The bladder and the lower extremities respond similarly to injury or disease since their innervation arises from essentially the same segments of the spinal cord. Thus, an upper motor neuron (suprasegmental) lesion causes spasticity in both; lower motor neuron (segmental or infrasegmental) lesions cause flaccidity. Any lesion that damages the sacral cord on either side of the arc (sensory or motor) causes flaccidity.

There are, then, 2 main types of neurogenic bladder: spastic and flaccid. Each may be complete or incomplete. Mixed lesions are not uncommon.

SPASTIC (REFLEX OR AUTOMATIC) NEUROGENIC BLADDER
(Caused by Upper Motor Neuron Lesion)

This type of bladder disorder is caused by any lesion of the cord above the voiding reflex arc. Trauma is the most common cause, but the disorder may also be produced by tumor or multiple sclerosis. The lesion usually affects both the suprasegmental motor and sensory fibers (Fig 19-6). The sacral reflex arc remains intact, but the loss of conscious sensation and cerebral motor control lead to severe aberrations of function. This is potentially the most serious type of injury because the cord below the lesion is hyperirritable rather than ''dead'' and affects the bladder most adversely. For this reason the incidence of renal damage is relatively high in this group. Injury to the pyramidal tracts deprives the bladder of cortical inhibition; uninhibited contractions then occur with filling, and vesical capacity is diminished. Voiding is interrupted, involuntary, and incomplete. Hypertrophy of the detrusor develops, often leading to vesicoureteral reflux. Trigonal hypertrophy may cause functional obstruction of the ureterovesical junctions. Dilatation of the internal sphincter occurs. The external sphincter and perineal muscles become spastic (upper motor neuron lesion) and obstructive. This causes increased resistance to the flow of urine and results in an impaired stream and residual urine. The sensory lesion deprives the patient of the perception of vesical fullness if the lesion is complete.

In summary, the spastic neurogenic bladder is typified by (1) reduced capacity, (2) involuntary detrusor contractions, (3) high intravesical voiding pressure, (4) marked hypertrophy of the bladder wall (trabeculation), and (5) spasm of the striated urinary sphincters. The diagram in Fig 19-6 illustrates these findings.

UNINHIBITED NEUROGENIC BLADDER
(Mild Spastic Neurogenic Bladder)

The uninhibited neurogenic bladder, a mild form of the spastic neurogenic bladder, may develop following a cerebral vascular accident or arteriosclerotic degeneration in the spinal cord. It may also occur as the first sign of multiple sclerosis. The lesion is centered either in the inhibitory centers of the cortex or in the pyramidal tracts (upper motor neuron). Minor lesions due to myelomeningocele or spina bifida may occasionally affect the supra-segmental motor fibers, in which case the cortical inhibition to the vesical stretch reflex is lost and voiding may become precipitate and involuntary. Because all other mechanisms, including the sacral reflex arc, are normal, the sensation of fullness is retained, the stream is free, and there is no residual urine. Capacity is, however, diminished. The cystometrogram and the site of the lesion are diagrammed in Fig 19-7.

FLACCID (ATONIC, NONREFLEX, OR AUTONOMOUS) NEUROGENIC BLADDER
(Caused by Lower Motor Neuron Lesion)

The most common cause of flaccid neurogenic bladder is trauma, although tumors, herniated intervertebral disks, tabes dorsalis, poliomyelitis, and certain congenital defects, including meningomyelocele, can affect the

same centers. Vesical dysfunction arises when there is injury to the center of micturition in the cord (S2-4), cauda equina, or sacral roots or nerves (Fig 19-8), thereby interrupting the sacral reflex arc. Loss of the perception of fullness permits overstretching of the detrusor and atony of the muscle, and this further contributes to weak and inefficient detrusor contraction. Thus, capacity is increased and the amount of residual urine is often large. Mild to moderate trabeculation (hypertrophy) of the bladder wall develops, accompanied by dilatation of the vesical outlet. External sphincter and perineal muscle tone is usually diminished, as is typical of striated muscle when a lower motor neuron lesion is present. Voluntary urination does not occur, but fairly efficient emptying can be accomplished by increased intra-abdominal and suprapubic (manual) pressure. The vesical (motor) paralysis which occurs occasionally in poliomyelitis usually clears quickly and spontaneously.

Myelomeningocele and spina bifida are associated with mild to severe vesical dysfunc-

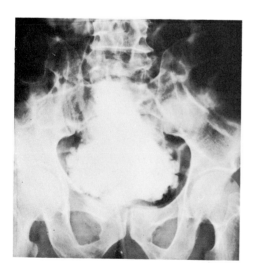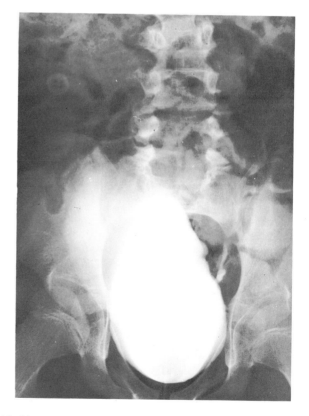

Fig 19-3. The spastic and flaccid neurogenic bladders as seen on cystography. Left: Spastic neurogenic bladder showing "Christmas tree" or "pine tree" effect. Heavy trabeculation, cellules, and small diverticula. Right: Flaccid neurogenic bladder showing oval-shaped bladder of large capacity in a boy eight years old. The bladder, characteristically, is tipped to one side. Note severe spina bifida (myelomeningocele) and left ureteral reflux.

tion, usually of the flaccid type, because the lesion affects the cauda equina and at times the sacral portion of the cord. Incontinence is the major symptom because of atony of the pelvic floor (external sphincter). Occasionally, in conjunction with somatic (external sphincter) flaccidity, there may be visceral (bladder) spasticity as well; this is a difficult combination to treat.

In summary, flaccid neurogenic bladder is typified by (1) large capacity, (2) no involuntary detrusor contractions, (3) low intravesical pressure, and (4) mild (but at times even marked) trabeculation (hypertrophy) of the bladder wall. These findings are shown in Fig 19-8.

RECOVERY OF VESICAL FUNCTION AFTER SPINAL CORD INJURY

Initial Phase

A. Spinal Shock: Immediately following a severe injury to the spinal cord or cauda equina, no matter at what level, there is complete anesthesia and flaccid paralysis below the level of the lesion. The bladder, innervated as it is from the lowest part of the spinal cord, is similarly affected. Perception of fullness and detrusor contraction are absent. The bladder gradually fills until overflow incontinence occurs.

The cystometrogram (Fig 19-4) shows a very large bladder capacity, no involuntary detrusor contractions, and low intravesical pressure.

B. Recovery From Spinal Shock: Spinal shock may last for a period of a few weeks to 6 months or more. The early clues to the return of reflex activity include movement of a toe, spontaneous spasm in a leg, return of sensation in some area, and spontaneous voiding around the indwelling catheter.

Cystometric studies (Fig 19-5) may then demonstrate a large bladder capacity (but smaller than during the shock period), a few weak involuntary contractions of the detrusor, and the beginning of return of intravesical pressure (tone).

If the injury involves the cord above the sacral area, anal sphincter tone and the bulbocavernosus reflex may return.

The "ice water test" should be tried periodically. Ninety ml of saline solution at 3° C (38° F) should be introduced forcefully into the bladder through a straight catheter. If the catheter is immediately ejected, the reaction is "positive." Should this not occur, the catheter should be removed quickly; if the fluid is ejected within 1 minute this is also considered a "positive" test. "Negative" responses occur during the stage of spinal shock, but this reaction is one of the first to return with recovery if the sacral reflex arc is intact (upper motor neuron lesion). This test is therefore of value in differentiating an upper from a lower motor neuron lesion early in the recovery phase.

Final Phase

When spinal shock is over, the resulting condition of the bladder depends upon the level and extent of the lesion in the spinal cord.

A. Upper Motor Neuron (Suprasegmental) Lesion: Toward the end of the stage of spinal shock, more obvious evidence of reflex activity is observed: movement of an extremity; vigorous spasm of an extremity, often accompanied by voiding around the catheter; progressive return of sensation in one or more areas; and hyperactive peripheral reflex activity and muscle tone. On removal of the catheter, spontaneous though inefficient urination occurs.

Cystometry (Fig 19-6) will show the changes typical of a spastic neurogenic bladder: bladder capacity below normal (100-300 ml); forceful, involuntary detrusor contractions; and increased intravesical pressure.

B. Lower Motor Neuron (Segmental or Infrasegmental) Lesion: When spinal shock has cleared, the following may occur: progressive return of sensation in some areas, hypoactive reflexes, and flaccid muscle tone. It is difficult to know when a patient is coming out of a spinal shock, for this phase of recovery presents a similar picture. On removal of the catheter, spontaneous urination does not occur. As capacity is reached, overflow dribbling develops. The bladder can be partially emptied by manual pressure over the bladder.

The usual reactions seen with the flaccid neurogenic bladder are shown on cystometric study (Fig 19-8): bladder capacity above normal (600-1000 ml), absence of uninhibited detrusor contractions, and decreased intravesical pressure.

CYSTOMETROGRAM

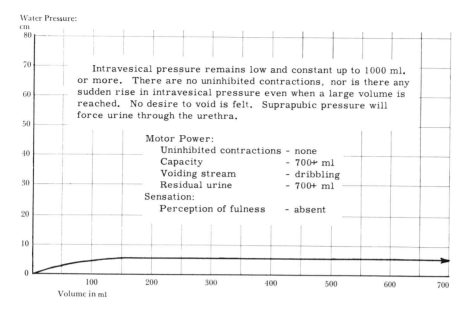

Intravesical pressure remains low and constant up to 1000 ml. or more. There are no uninhibited contractions, nor is there any sudden rise in intravesical pressure even when a large volume is reached. No desire to void is felt. Suprapubic pressure will force urine through the urethra.

Motor Power:
    Uninhibited contractions - none
    Capacity   - 700+ ml
    Voiding stream   - dribbling
    Residual urine   - 700+ ml
Sensation:
    Perception of fulness - absent

Fig 19-4. Stage of spinal shock. Cystometrogram showing flaccidity and lack of response of the bladder during the first few weeks after injury.

CYSTOMETROGRAM

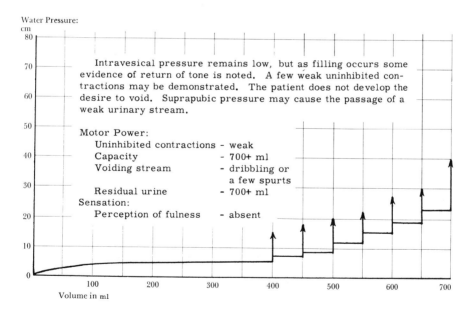

Intravesical pressure remains low, but as filling occurs some evidence of return of tone is noted. A few weak uninhibited contractions may be demonstrated. The patient does not develop the desire to void. Suprapubic pressure may cause the passage of a weak urinary stream.

Motor Power:
    Uninhibited contractions - weak
    Capacity   - 700+ ml
    Voiding stream   - dribbling or
                     a few spurts
    Residual urine   - 700+ ml
Sensation:
    Perception of fulness - absent

Fig 19-5. Stage of recovery of vesical function after severe injury to the spinal cord or cauda equina. Cystometrogram demonstrating the activity of the bladder during the early stages of recovery from spinal shock.

SPECIFIC TYPES OF
NEUROGENIC BLADDERS

The diagnosis of neurogenic bladder depends upon a complete history and physical (including neurologic) examination and the application of such specialized urologic tests as cystoscopy, cystography, excretory urography, and cystometry, including determination of residual urine. These tests may have to be repeated several times as recovery progresses.

COMPLETE SPASTIC (REFLEX, AUTOMATIC) NEUROGENIC BLADDER

This type of cord bladder is the result of a partial or complete transection of the cord above the sacral level (above the lumbar spine) following recovery from spinal shock. The common causes are trauma, tumor, and multiple sclerosis. Cerebral control is lacking; the bladder functions in conjunction with its sacral reflex arc. The principal findings are diminished bladder capacity, increased intravesical pressure, spasm of the external urinary sphincters, and involuntary contractions of the vesical muscle.

Clinical Findings

A. Symptoms: The severity of symptoms depends on the site and extent of the lesion. Urinary symptoms include involuntary urination, often frequent and scanty, which may occur with involuntary spasm of the extremities. True sensation of fullness is lacking, although vague lower abdominal sensations due to stretching of the overlying peritoneum may be felt. The major nonurologic symptoms are spastic paralysis and subjective sensory changes.

B. Signs: Complete neurologic examination will establish the site of the lesion. The anal sphincter tone is normal or increased; the bulbocavernosus reflex is intact or hyperactive (upper motor neuron lesion). Palpation and percussion usually do not reveal a distended bladder, since the bladder automatically discharges a portion of its contents when the urine volume reaches 150-300 ml. Stimulation of the skin of the abdomen, thigh, or genitals may initiate voiding. Such stimulation may cause involuntary contraction of the extremities.

If the lesion is in the upper thoracic or cervical cord, distention of the bladder (plugged catheter, cystometry, cystoscopy) may excite hyperactive autonomic reflexes, which include severe hypertension, bradycardia, and pilomotor and sudomotor responses above the neurologic level. Headache may be severe; the hypertension may cause a cerebrovascular accident. Patients reacting in this manner should have an indwelling catheter open at all times. Should instrumentation be necessary, spinal anesthesia or the administration of a ganglionic or postganglionic blocking agent will protect the patient from this reaction.

C. Laboratory Findings: Anemia may be found if infection of the urinary tract has been prolonged and poorly controlled. If secondary renal damage is severe and uremia has developed, anemia is to be expected. The urine is infected. Red cells may be found if calculi have developed. Renal function may be normal or impaired, depending on the efficacy of treatment and the absence of renal complications (hydronephrosis, pyelonephritis, calculosis).

D. X-Ray Findings: Excretory urograms and retrograde cystograms are essential since renal complications (eg, calculi, hydronephrosis) are common. Urinary stones may be seen. A trabeculated bladder of small capacity is typical of this type of neurogenic bladder. Ureteral reflux may be noted on the cystograms (Figs 11-5 and 19-3), which will almost certainly show a dilated bladder neck. If the cause of the neurogenic abnormality is undetermined, a plain film may reveal fracture or disease (eg, metastases) of the spine above the lumbar area.

E. Instrumental Examination: Cystoscopy and panendoscopy usually show moderate to severe trabeculation of the bladder wall, vesical diverticula, and changes compatible with infection. Stones may be visualized. The bladder is often hyperirritable to instrumentation.

The site of the lesion and the type of cystometrogram are diagrammed in Fig 19-6. As fluid is introduced into the bladder, strong, uninhibited contractions are noted until a contraction of such strength develops that involuntary urination occurs around the catheter. Capacity is diminished to 100-300 ml, and significant amounts of residual urine are found (50-150 ml). Although a true sense of fullness is lacking, various auras may be experienced (eg, sweating, vague low abdominal pain, intense spasm of the legs) when capacity is reached.

The "ice water test" is positive.

UNINHIBITED NEUROGENIC BLADDER
(Mild Spastic Neurogenic Bladder)

Incomplete lesions of the cortex or the pyramidal (motor) tracts may weaken or abolish cerebral restraint. The patient may have frequency and nocturia, and may suffer episodes of incontinence due to uncontrollable urgency. Brain tumors, multiple sclerosis, arteriosclerotic changes within the cord, and, at times, cerebrovascular accidents may be etiologic factors, but the cause is not always known. This type of reaction is often found in those suffering from anxiety (see chapter 31). The symptoms and clinical findings in adults are similar to those seen in normal infants.

Clinical Findings

A. Symptoms: Frequency, nocturia, and urgency are the principal symptoms and are similar to those of cystitis. If symptoms are due to organic neurologic disorders (eg, cerebral vascular accident, brain tumor), characteristic symptoms of these lesions may be found.

B. Signs: General and neurologic examinations are normal unless primary central nervous system disease is present, in which case hyperreflexia and abnormal peripheral reflexes may be elicited (eg, multiple sclerosis).

C. X-Ray Findings: Some patients with multiple sclerosis may develop vesicoureteral reflux or ureterovesical obstruction. Urethrograms and cystograms are usually normal, but reflux may be seen.

D. Instrumental Examination: Cystoscopy and panendoscopy are normal, although some vesical irritability and diminished capacity may be demonstrated.

The sites of the possible lesions and the type of cystometrogram are diagrammed in Fig 19-7. As the bladder is filled, strong, uninhibited contractions are noted; long before "normal" capacity is reached, involuntary urination occurs around the catheter. Perception of sensation is normal, and there is no residual urine.

FLACCID (ATONIC, NONREFLEX, OR AUTONOMOUS) NEUROGENIC BLADDER

Injury to the sacral portion of the cord or to the motor or sensory roots of the cauda equina impairs the reflex arcs of the bladder. The common causes of this type of vesical re-action are trauma, tumors, tabes dorsalis, and congenital anomalies (eg, meningomyelocele). It may be seen following surgery in which the pelvic nerves are inadvertently injured (eg, abdominoperineal resection of the rectum). The bladder is also flaccid during the stage of spinal shock (Fig 19-4). This type of neurogenic bladder is characterized by large vesical capacity, low intravesical pressure, and the absence of involuntary detrusor contractions.

Clinical Findings

A. Symptoms: The patient complains of muscular paralysis and loss of peripheral sensation. The main urinary symptom is overflow incontinence. Suprapubic pressure may be required to initiate urination. Perception of fullness is absent.

B. Signs: Neurologic examination reveals evidence of a lower motor neuron lesion: absent or hypoactive peripheral reflexes, flaccid paralysis, absence of the bulbocavernosus reflex, and loss of anal sphincter tone. Sensation is diminished or absent. If perianal anesthesia alone is present, only one arm of the sacral reflex arc is damaged.

An overdistended bladder may be discovered on palpation or percussion. Pressure over the organ will cause passage of a stream of urine.

C. Laboratory Findings: Anemia may be noted, due either to chronic pyelonephritis or to uremia secondary to advanced renal damage (eg, infection hydronephrosis, calculi). Pus cells and bacteria are found in the urine. Because of the amount of residual urine in the bladder, the PSP test must be performed with a catheter in place. Nitrogen retention may be associated with severe renal complications.

D. X-Ray Findings: A plain film of the abdomen may reveal a fracture of the lumbar spine or extensive spina bifida. Calcific shadows compatible with urinary stone may be visualized. Excretory urograms and retrograde cystograms should be performed routinely, since complications are common. These include vesical and renal calculi and hydroureteronephrosis. However, the latter change is usually less marked than that seen with the spastic neurogenic bladder because the incidence of ureteral reflux and functional ureterovesical obstruction is lower. The bladder will appear large on the urogram.

E. Instrumental Examination: Cystoscopy and panendoscopy, when performed some weeks after the injury, reveal mild to moderate trabeculation (hypertrophy) of the detrusor.

Motor Power:
    Uninhibited contractions - present
    Capacity   - 260 ml
    Voiding stream   - weak to strong but
                             involuntary and
                             interrupted
    Residual urine   - 125 ml
Sensation:
    Perception of fulness   - absent

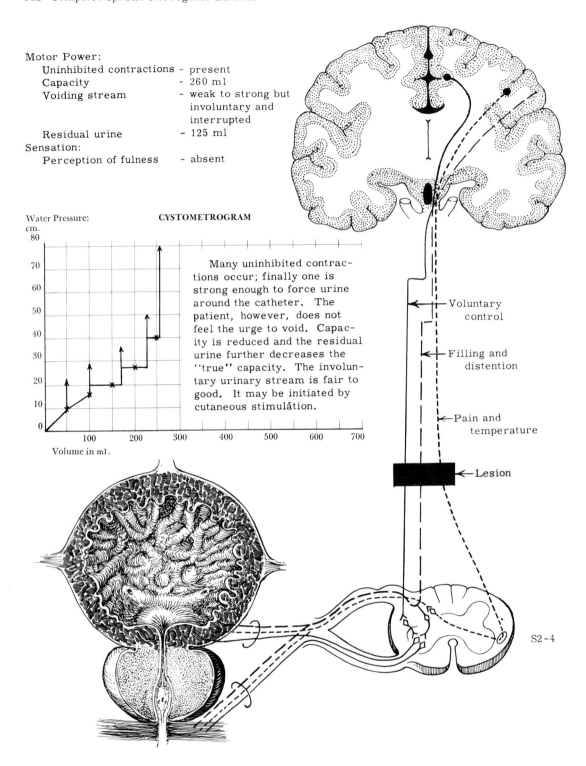

Water Pressure:
cm.

CYSTOMETROGRAM

Many uninhibited contrac-
tions occur; finally one is
strong enough to force urine
around the catheter. The
patient, however, does not
feel the urge to void. Capacity is reduced and the residual
urine further decreases the
"true" capacity. The involuntary urinary stream is fair to
good. It may be initiated by
cutaneous stimulation.

Volume in ml.

Voluntary control

Filling and distention

Pain and temperature

Lesion

S2-4

Fig 19-6. Complete spastic neurogenic bladder. Caused by a more or less complete transection
of the spinal cord above S2. Cystometric study of a typical case shows function after recovery
from spinal shock. (Modified after Nesbit, Lapides, and Baum: Fundamentals of Urology.
Edwards, 1953.)

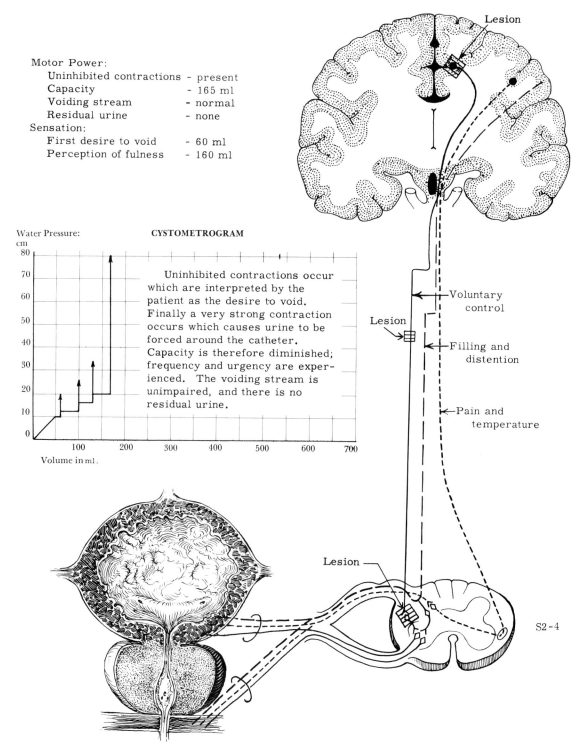

Motor Power:
    Uninhibited contractions - present
    Capacity   - 165 ml
    Voiding stream   - normal
    Residual urine   - none
Sensation:
    First desire to void   - 60 ml
    Perception of fulness   - 160 ml

CYSTOMETROGRAM

Water Pressure:
cm

Uninhibited contractions occur which are interpreted by the patient as the desire to void. Finally a very strong contraction occurs which causes urine to be forced around the catheter. Capacity is therefore diminished; frequency and urgency are experienced. The voiding stream is unimpaired, and there is no residual urine.

Volume in ml.

Lesion

Voluntary control

Lesion

Filling and distention

Pain and temperature

Lesion

S2-4

Fig 19-7. Uninhibited neurogenic bladder. Caused by a lesion of the inhibitory centers of the cortex or pyramidal tracts. Cystometric study of a typical case. (Modified after Nesbit, Lapides, and Baum: Fundamentals of Urology. Edwards, 1953.)

Motor Power:
    Uninhibited contractions - absent
    Capacity   - 700+ ml
    Voiding stream   - weak; improved
                               by suprapubic
                               pressure

    Residual urine   - 150 ml
Sensation:
    Perception of fulness   - absent

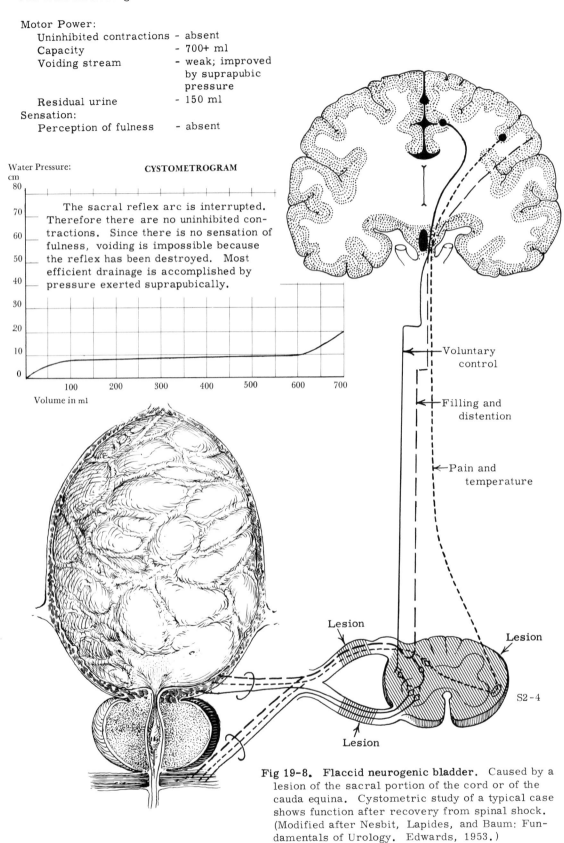

CYSTOMETROGRAM

The sacral reflex arc is interrupted. Therefore there are no uninhibited contractions. Since there is no sensation of fulness, voiding is impossible because the reflex has been destroyed. Most efficient drainage is accomplished by pressure exerted suprapubically.

Water Pressure: cm

Volume in ml

Voluntary control

Filling and distention

Pain and temperature

Lesion

Lesion

Lesion

S2-4

Fig 19-8. **Flaccid neurogenic bladder.** Caused by a lesion of the sacral portion of the cord or of the cauda equina. Cystometric study of a typical case shows function after recovery from spinal shock. (Modified after Nesbit, Lapides, and Baum: Fundamentals of Urology. Edwards, 1953.)

Vesical capacity is increased. Inflammatory changes may be present. The bladder neck is usually dilated. Stones may be visualized. The patient may experience little discomfort with instrumentation because of loss of local sensation.

Cystography will show a bladder of increased capacity (Fig 19-3). Reflux of the radiopaque fluid to the kidneys may be demonstrated.

Urethrography may reveal some laxness of the external urinary sphincter (lower motor neuron lesion). The bladder neck is usually wide open.

Cystometric examination and the site of the lesion are diagrammed in Fig 19-8). Vesical capacity is increased, the intravesical pressure is decreased, and there are no uninhibited contractions. Even after abdominal pressure is used to expel the bladder contents, as much as 250 ml of urine may be retained.

Lapides has described a simple test which is diagnostic of a lower motor neuron lesion. The intravesical pressure is noted after the instillation of 100 ml of water. Urecholine, 2.5 mg, is injected subcutaneously. A cystometric reading is made 10, 20, and 30 minutes later. If the rise is more than 15 cm of water, a lower motor neuron lesion is present.

DIFFERENTIAL DIAGNOSIS OF NEUROGENIC BLADDERS

The diagnosis of most cases of neurogenic bladder is obvious. Sacral nerve damage is evident, as judged by the bulbocavernosus reflex, anal sphincter tone, and perianal sensation. Too often the diagnosis of neurogenic bladder is made on very tenuous grounds.

Cystitis

Inflammations of the bladder, both non-specific and tuberculous also cause frequency of urination and urgency, even to the point of incontinence. Pyuria and bacteriuria are found, although it must be remembered that the neurogenic bladder is usually secondarily infected because of the presence of residual urine (or a retention catheter).

The cystometrogram of the inflamed bladder is similar to that obtained with uninhibited neurogenic bladder (Fig 19-7), but this reaction and the symptoms disappear after appropriate treatment. Should definitive antibiotic therapy not relieve symptoms, a primary neurologic lesion should be sought.

Chronic Urethritis

Symptoms of frequency, nocturia, and burning on urination may be due to chronic inflammation of the urethra. The urine is not infected. Panendoscopy will often reveal urethral stenosis and signs of urethral inflammation. Neurologic and cystometric studies are normal.

Vesical Irritation Due to Psychic Disturbance

The patient gives a long history of periodic bouts of urinary frequency, usually occurring only in the morning. Comparable nocturia is absent. The symptoms are precipitated by anxiety. The urine is normal.

Cystometric studies reveal a hyperirritable bladder of diminished capacity. The pressure curve is similar to that seen with the uninhibited neurogenic bladder (Fig 19-7). If the patient's anxiety can be allayed the intravesical pressure and vesical capacity may return to normal.

Interstitial Cystitis

The patient with submucous fibrosis is almost always a woman over 40 years of age. She complains of great frequency, nocturia, urgency, and suprapubic pain when the bladder reaches its markedly limited capacity (60-100 ml). The urinalysis is usually normal, and there is no residual urine. Cystometry usually shows a hypertonic detrusor reaction with some uninhibited contractions. The voiding pressure is usually quite high, and voiding is involuntary. Cystoscopy shows typical scarring; the mucosa is apt to split and bleed with vesical distention.

Cystocele

Relaxation of the pelvic floor following childbirth may cause some frequency, nocturia, and stress incontinence. Since residual urine is often found, infection may be demonstrated on urinalysis.

Pelvic examination usually reveals relaxation of the anterior vaginal wall and descent of the urethra and bladder when the patient strains to urinate. Cystoscopy will reveal similar findings.

Infravesical Obstruction

Congenital urethral valves or strictures and benign or malignant enlargements of the prostate usually cause impairment of the urinary stream. Hypertrophy (trabeculation) of the detrusor occurs, and residual urine accumulates. During this compensatory stage, bladder neck obstruction may resemble the spastic neurogenic bladder.

If decompensation occurs, the vesical wall becomes attenuated and atonic; and capacity may be markedly increased. Overflow incontinence may develop. The cystometrogram may simulate that of the flaccid neurogenic bladder (Fig 19-8).

If the difficulty is nonneurogenic, the anal sphincter tone is normal and the bulbocavernosus reflex is intact. Peripheral sensation, motor power, and reflexes are normal. Cystoscopy and panendoscopy will reveal the local lesion causing the obstruction. Even though appropriately treated, prolonged catheter drainage of the decompensated bladder may be necessary before the vesical tone returns to normal.

COMPLICATIONS
OF NEUROGENIC BLADDER

The principal complications of neurogenic bladder are infection, hydronephrosis, and calculus formation. The primary factors which contribute to these complications are the presence of residual urine, ureteral reflux of urine, and confinement to bed. Sexual problems are common (see below).

Infection
In neurovesical disease, the bladder loses the power to empty itself. Under these circumstances, infection is almost inevitable. With acute trauma to the spinal cord, the bladder is temporarily paralyzed and a retention catheter is therefore necessary. The introduction of an indwelling catheter always causes cystitis no matter what mechanical or medical measures are taken to prevent infection. The key to whether the kidneys will become involved is the ureterovesical junction.

If the ureterovesical valves become incompetent, reflux of infected urine from the bladder reaches the kidneys. This may be caused by elevation of intravesical pressure from irrigations or expression of urine by the Credé maneuver, in which case these procedures must be discontinued.

If a large catheter is placed in the male bladder, periurethral abscess may ensue. This may rupture to the outside, producing a urinary fistula. If spontaneous drainage does not occur, urethral diverticulum may develop. Epididymitis secondary to prostatocystitis is not uncommon. The testis may become secondarily involved.

Hydronephrosis
The incidence of vesicoureteral reflux, particularly in the patient with a spastic neurogenic bladder, is significant. The etiologic factor appears to be the trabeculation which

develops in association with this bladder condition. Secondary ureterohydronephrosis is the rule. Hypertrophy of the trigone is associated with vesical trabeculation. This causes an abnormal pull upon the ureterovesical junction which may lead to functional obstruction and therefore proximal dilatation.

Calculus
A number of factors may contribute to stone formation in the bladder or kidneys. Bed rest and inactivity cause demineralization of the skeleton and therefore hypercalciuria. Recumbency also contributes to urinary stasis.

If the infection is due to urea-splitting bacteria, the urine remains alkaline, in which medium calcium is less soluble.

In order to "build up" the injured patient, the physician may mistakenly encourage the drinking of milk (thereby increasing the calcium intake and urinary output) and prescribe vitamin preparations including vitamin D. The latter only increases the efficiency of the bowel to absorb calcium into the blood stream; increased urinary calcium excretion then occurs.

Renal Amyloidosis
Secondary amyloidosis of the kidneys is a common cause of death in patients with neurogenic bladder. Its incidence is highest in those patients who have had decubitus ulcers or urethral infection.

Sexual Problems
Men who have suffered traumatic cord or cauda equina lesions experience varying degrees of sexual trouble. Those with upper motor lesions fare well; 95% will have psychic or reflex erections. In patients with complete lower motor neuron lesions, impotence occurs in 80%, but if the lesion is incomplete the incidence is 25%. The patient with an upper motor neuron defect has little chance of experiencing ejaculation or orgasm, although the patient with an incomplete lesion has a better prognosis.

TREATMENT OF NEUROGENIC BLADDER

The treatment of any form of neurogenic bladder is aimed at maintaining a relatively good functional capacity, controlling incontinence, and preserving renal function. Functional capacity is measured by the difference between true capacity and the amount of urine retained after voiding. The desirable interval between voidings should be at least 2 and preferably 3 hours.

Urinary continence should not be sought at the expense of vesical capacity or renal function. Few paralytics are so confident of their control that they appear in public without some type of collecting apparatus (Fig 19-10).

Treatment of Stage of Spinal Shock

Following severe injury to the spinal cord, the bladder is temporarily paralyzed. During the next few months it undergoes gradual improvement. If the sacral cord or cauda equina is damaged, the end result is a flaccid bladder. If the injury is higher, the bladder becomes spastic in type.

During spinal shock, when the bladder is paralyzed, some type of vesical drainage must be instituted immediately and then maintained.

It has become increasingly clear that the presence of a permanent indwelling catheter always leads to persistent bacteriuria. Intermittent catheterization prevents this complication in a high percentage of cases, but it requires intensive nursing care. If this is not possible, an indwelling catheter must be used.

Either a No. 16 F balloon (Foley) or a No. 8 or 10 F Gibbon (polythene) catheter can be used. The latter, because of its small size, may decrease the incidence of urethral complications (eg, periurethral abscess, urethral diverticulum). The Foley catheter in the male should be taped to the abdomen so that sharp angulation does not occur at the penoscrotal junction. It should be changed every week. The Gibbon catheter usually need only be changed once a month.

Some advocate the use of cystostomy rather than a urethral catheter, thus circumventing the often serious urethral and genital tract complications. Should these develop in association with urethral catheter drainage, cystostomy should be seriously considered; it will allow removal of the offending catheter.

Vesical hygiene contributes to the control of infection, lowers the incidence of vesical calculi, and possibly maintains optimum vesical capacity when a urethral catheter is used. A simple apparatus for closed irrigation and drainage is shown in Fig 19-9. Any sterile solution may be used. A 10% solution of hemiacridin (Renacidin®) tends to prevent the precipitation of calcium salts in the lumen of the catheter. The capacity of the bladder should be determined by periodic cystometric observations and no more than this amount of fluid allowed to enter the bladder. It is then drained off. The bladder should be irrigated 3 times a day. If done faithfully, this is a much simpler procedure than tidal drainage and is probably just as efficient in maintaining vesical capacity. The Gibbon catheter is not irrigated.

Cystograms should be taken periodically. If they reveal ureteral reflux, forceful irrigation is contraindicated.

In order to control infection a fluid intake of at least 3000 ml/day must be maintained (200 ml of fluid every hour when awake). This reduces stasis and decreases the concentration of calcium in the urine. Renal and ureteral drainage are enhanced by raising the head of the bed, moving the patient frequently, and, above all, ambulating the patient in a wheel chair as early as possible. These measures lessen the incidence of acute pyelonephritis and renal and vesical calculosis. Sulfonamides or antibiotics should be vigorously administered if febrile reactions occur. Little is gained by prolonged prophylactic medication, for sterilization of the urine is impossible when a catheter is in place.

Prevention of calculosis requires a low-calcium diet (eliminate dairy products) containing no vitamin D. As mentioned above, early ambulation in a wheel chair reduces the incidence of calculosis. If hypercalciuria is demonstrated by periodic Sulkowitch tests, other prophylactic measures should be considered (see chapter 15).

TREATMENT OF SPECIFIC TYPES OF NEUROGENIC BLADDER

Once the specific type of neurogenic bladder is established (including the post-traumatic group after emergence from spinal shock), the following steps should be taken to attain optimum function.

Spastic Neurogenic Bladder

A. Patient With Large Bladder Capacity: To successfully train the spastic neurogenic bladder, the patient must be able to wait 2-3 hours between involuntary voidings. He should not leak during this period, and he must be able to initiate voiding by manual stimulation or squeezing of the abdomen, genitalia, or thighs. This can be done by the patient unless he is quadriplegic.

B. Patient With Markedly Diminished Functional Vesical Capacity: If the functional capacity is only 50-100 ml, involuntary voidings may occur as often as every 15-30 minutes; and satisfactory bladder training cannot be attained (see cystometrogram in Fig 19-9). The alternatives are:

1. Permanent retention catheter, cutaneous vesicostomy, cutaneous ureterostomy, uretero-ileocutaneous anastomosis, or cystostomy, particularly if ureteral reflux can be demonstrated on cystograms.

2. Urinal or other collecting apparatus constantly in place.

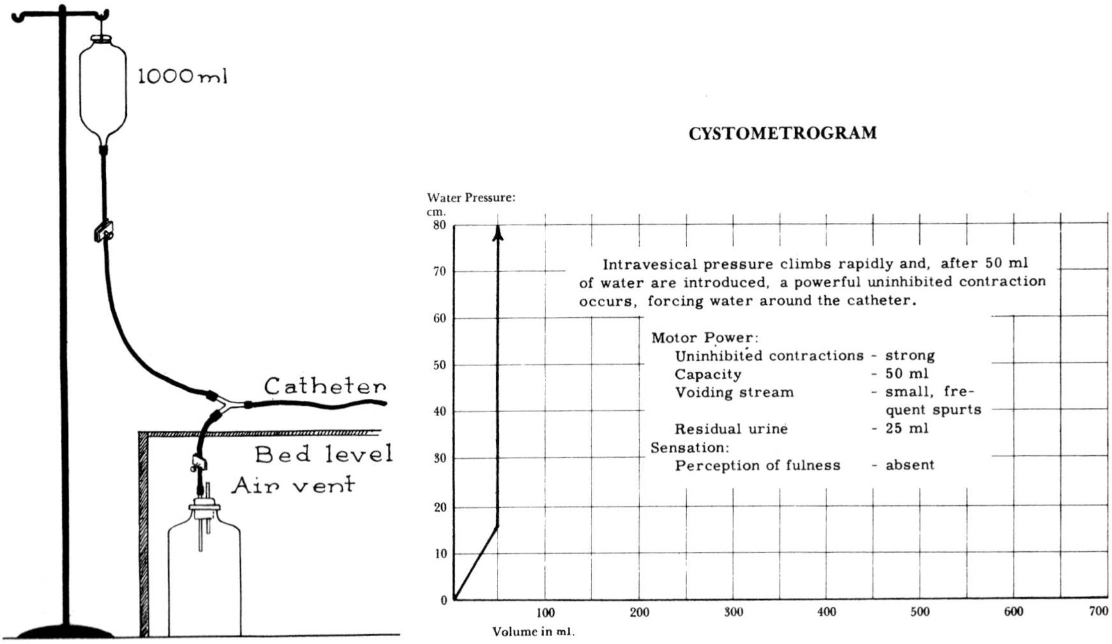

CYSTOMETROGRAM

Water Pressure: cm.

Intravesical pressure climbs rapidly and, after 50 ml of water are introduced, a powerful uninhibited contraction occurs, forcing water around the catheter.

Motor Power:
　Uninhibited contractions - strong
　Capacity - 50 ml
　Voiding stream - small, frequent spurts
　Residual urine - 25 ml
Sensation:
　Perception of fulness - absent

Volume in ml.

1000 ml

Catheter

Bed level

Air vent

Fig 19-9. Left: Closed system for vesical irrigation and vesical drainage. **Right:** Cystometrogram typical of severely spastic bladder.

3. If low functional capacity is due to the retention of a large volume of urine, transurethral resection of the bladder neck may be undertaken. If this fails to improve emptying power satisfactorily, the pudendal nerves (somatic supply to the perineal and external urinary sphincter muscles) should be blocked with procaine in order to decrease urethral resistance. If this proves effective, pudendal neurectomy can be done. Transurethral destruction of the external sphincter may be necessary.

4. If the true capacity is very low, and particularly if the patient suffers involuntary spasm of the extremities when he voids, his spastic bladder (and extremities) should be made flaccid.

If, despite catheter drainage, progressive ureterohydronephrosis develops, the conversion of an upper motor to a lower motor neuron lesion may cause regression of the upper tract changes. This can be accomplished by 1 of the following technics:

a. Subarachnoid injection of absolute alcohol - This should be preceded by spinal anesthesia. If voiding can be accomplished manually under spinal anesthesia, then the alcohol injection should be done. It acts by destroying the conus and the cauda equina.

b. Anterior and posterior rhizotomy from T12 to and including S5 also converts the lesion to a lower neuron type.

c. Sacral neurotomy of S2-4 has a similar effect upon the bladder but is not complete enough to eradicate annoying spasms of the extremities.

These procedures may have to be combined with resection of the bladder neck if stenosis of that structure is found.

5. Progressive upper tract deterioration may require urinary diversion.

C. Parasympatholytic Drugs: The quaternary ammonium amines methantheline bromide (Banthine®), 50-100 mg 3-4 times daily orally, and propantheline bromide (Pro-Banthine®), 15-30 mg 3-4 times daily orally, reduce vesical tone and thereby increase vesical capacity. Because of the prolonged nature of the disease, these agents have proved of little practical value except in patients with mildly spastic bladders (uninhibited neurogenic bladder).

Flaccid Neurogenic Bladder

If the neurologic lesion is complete, volitional voiding cannot be accomplished without manual suprapubic pressure augmented, if possible, by abdominal and diaphragmatic contraction. If the lesion is incomplete, spontaneous voiding may occur but the size and force of the stream is impaired and residual urine remains in the bladder. Proper care of the flaccid bladder requires:

A. Bladder Training and Care: Voiding every 2 hours by the clock protects the bladder from overdistention, which the patient is unable to perceive, and preserves maximum tone. Catheter drainage must be used for the patient who has ureteral reflux on cystography.

B. Surgery: Transurethral resection of the bladder neck for hypertrophy or spasm, which causes the retention of a large volume of residual urine. At times this operation may fail to reduce the amount of residual urine to a point where a proper interval between voidings is afforded, in which case transurethral resection of the external sphincter may be considered. This will require the use of a collection device.

C. Parasympathomimetic Drugs: The stable derivatives of acetylcholine are at times of value in initiating and increasing the efficiency of the contraction of the detrusor. They may therefore be helpful in the symptomatic treatment of the milder types of flaccid neurogenic bladder. Their usefulness may be gauged during cystometric study. When the bladder has been filled to a volume of 400 ml, the minimal recommended dose should be given subcutaneously. If intravesical pressure rises appreciably within a few minutes, the drug can be expected to be helpful clinically.

Bethanechol chloride (Urecholine®) is the drug of choice. It is given either orally, 10-50 mg every 4-6 hours (the latter dose is usually necessary), or subcutaneously, 5-10 mg every 4-6 hours. Methacholine chloride (Mecholyl®) is given orally, 0.2-0.4 gm every 4-6 hours, or subcutaneously, 10-20 mg every 4-6 hours.

D. Implanted Electrodes: An attempt is being made to implant electrodes into the bladder wall with an external stimulator mechanism in order to cause efficient detrusor action. When perfected, this technic may prove to be an important step in the treatment of the flaccid bladder.

Neurogenic Bladder Associated With Spina Bifida

Following the repair of meningocele or myelomeningocele, the cauda equina and sacral cord are apt to be involved by scar tissue. These patients usually have neurogenic vesical dysfunction which may be of the atonic or spastic type but is often of the mixed type (spastic bladder—upper motor neuron lesion; atony of the pelvic floor—lower motor neuron lesion).

The goals of therapy are to control incontinence and to preserve renal function.

A. Conservative Treatment:

1. Mild symptoms - If there is occasional dribbling or some residual urine associated with lack of desire to void, have the patient void every 2 hours when awake. Manual suprapubic pressure will enhance the efficiency of emptying. An external condom catheter (Fig 19-10) will protect the male who still suffers small losses. A similar complaint in a female will require an indwelling catheter.

2. More severe symptoms - If true urinary incontinence associated with residual urine and ureteral reflux is found, the following steps should be taken.

a. Mostly atonic bladder - If reflux is demonstrated, "triple voiding" should be prescribed as follows: The patient is instructed to void with strain; walk around for a few minutes, void again; and walk and void a third time. In most instances the entire urinary tract will be completely emptied by this maneuver.

If incontinence is marked, an indwelling catheter may be necessary. The same treatment is indicated if reflux has led to significant impairment of renal function.

b. Mostly spastic bladder - The problem with patients in this category is more serious because the bladder is hypertonic and has a small capacity but the external sphincter is atonic. Almost constant dribbling may result.

A female will require an indwelling catheter; the condom catheter may suffice for the male. If reflux is demonstrated the male will require a catheter also in order to protect the kidneys from high intravesical pressure.

B. Surgical Treatment: If significant residual urine is found and is associated with considerable dribbling, transurethral resection of the bladder neck will reduce the residual urine and will cure 30% of cases. A few may notice increased incontinence, however.

If the bladder is of the spastic type with diminished capacity, sacral nerve block, internal pudendal neurectomy, or selective neurectomy (S3) may improve capacity and stop ureteral reflux.

If the refluxing patient suffers recurrent fever (pyelonephritis) despite the presence of an indwelling catheter, vesicoureteroplasty may be indicated. If incontinence cannot be controlled, urinary diversion must be considered. The Bricker operation (uretero-ileal cutaneous conduit) is the method of choice.

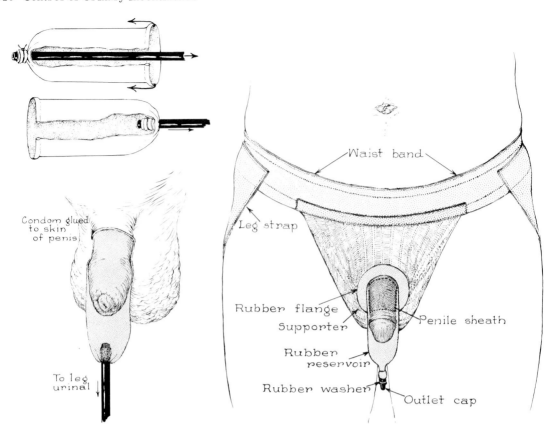

Condom glued
to skin
of penis

To leg
urinal

Waist band

Leg strap

Rubber flange

Supporter

Rubber
reservoir

Rubber washer

Penile sheath

Outlet cap

Fig 19-10. **Left:** Condom catheter. **Right:** McGuire urinal.

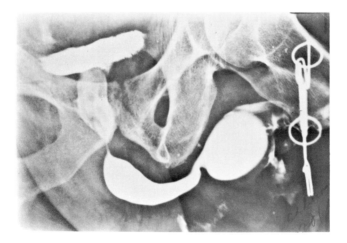

Fig 19-11. **Urethral diverticulum.** Atonic neurogenic bladder after transurethral resection. Diverticulum is a complication of prolonged use of a Cunningham clamp.

THE CONTROL OF
URINARY INCONTINENCE

In the Hospital

Urinary incontinence is a distressing aspect of neurovesical dysfunction, particularly if the patient achieves a bladder which otherwise functions adequately. This difficulty is minimized in men under hospital conditions, for with close supervision and the ever-present urinal, the urine can usually be properly collected. Women have a greater problem because of the need for placement of the bedpan, and bedwetting may be frequent. Even an indwelling catheter does not guarantee dryness for the incontinent woman, since leakage around the catheter often occurs. No simple satisfactory solution to this problem has yet been reached. Urinary diversion may be necessary.

After Discharge

When the time comes for discharge from the hospital almost all men, even though they have achieved "excellent" bladder control, must wear a "condom catheter" (Fig 19-10). This consists of a condom with a catheter at the distal end for drainage of any urine unexpectedly lost. The catheter drains into a leg urinal. The condom may be secured to the penis by elastoplast, cellulose tape, or cement.

A McGuire urinal (Fig 19-10) consists of a heavy condom incorporated into an athletic supporter. If there is considerable leakage of urine the dependent end can be drained through a tube into a leg urinal.

Urethral compression by means of a Cuningham clamp is preferred by some patients. It may, however, lead to the development of a urethral diverticulum (Fig 19-11).

TREATMENT OF COMPLICATIONS

The most common and significant complications can be discovered by cystography, cystometry, cystoscopy, and excretory urography repeated at least once a year.

Hydronephrosis

Ureteral reflux, as shown by cystography, is an indication for an indwelling catheter. Over a period of months, the ureterovesical junction may again become competent. If, despite prolonged drainage, reflux persists, vesicoureteroplasty may be indicated. Progressive hydroureteronephrosis, found on urography, may require nephrostomy or urinary diversion as a lifesaving measure.

Pyelonephritis

Bouts of renal infection must be treated by antimicrobials. If the pyelonephritis is associated with ureteral reflux, constant vesical drainage must be instituted. Urinary diversion should be considered.

Epididymitis

In acute epididymitis secondary to prostatitis initiated by the urethral catheter, prophylactic vasoligation is indicated during a quiescent period. Should this not suffice, removal of the urethral catheter and placement of a suprapubic tube will be necessary.

Calculi

A. Vesical: Vesical calculi, diagnosed by x-ray or cystoscopy, can usually be washed out through an instrument or crushed and removed transurethrally. If they are large, suprapubic removal will be required.

B. Ureteral: These can usually be diagnosed by excretory urograms; if no radiopaque fluid is excreted, cystoscopy and the passage of a ureteral catheter may be necessary. Most ureteral stones can be removed cystoscopically. Surgical intervention may be indicated.

C. Renal: The diagnosis of renal calculi is made by radiography. If the calculus is obstructive, it must be removed; if not, conservative treatment is the rule, for the recurrence rate is high because of the presence of urea-splitting organisms in the kidney.

If stones form despite the prophylactic steps listed on p 317, an even more rigorous regimen should be instituted.

PROGNOSIS

The greatest threat to the patient with a neurogenic bladder is progressive renal damage (pyelonephritis, calculosis, and hydronephrosis). Some degree of hydronephrosis is found in 25% of these patients; a few will die because of it unless appropriate treatment is instituted.

The quadriplegic patient presents a serious problem. If his bladder is spastic, he cannot initiate voiding by self-stimulation; if his bladder has been made flaccid, he is unable to exert suprapubic pressure. An indwelling catheter may be the best solution. Most paraplegics can eventually achieve comfortable bladder function, although many must continue to wear some type of collecting apparatus.

· · ·

General References

Abramson, A. S., Roussan, M. S., & G. D'Oronzio: Method for evaluating function of the neurogenic bladder. JAMA **195**:554-8, 1966.

Bors, E., & A. E. Comarr: Neurological Urology. Physiology of Micturition, Its Neurological Disorders and Sequelae. University Park Press, 1971.

Bors, E., & R. W. Porter: Neurosurgical considerations in bladder dysfunction. Urol Internat **25**:114-33, 1970.

Bucy, J. G.: Patterns of urological disease in patients with myelomeningocele. J Urol **106**:541-7, 1971.

Chapman, W. H., & others: A prospective study of the urinary tract from birth in patients with meningomyelocele. J Urol **102**:363-6, 1969.

Comarr, A. E.: Sexual function among patients with spinal cord injury. Urol Internat **25**:134-68, 1970.

Comarr, A. E.: Traumatic cord bladder: management and complications. S Clin North America **45**:1509-22, 1965.

Cooper, D. G. W.: Detrusor action in children with myelomeningocele. Arch Dis Child **43**:427-32, 1968.

Culp, D. A., Bekhrad, A., & R. H. Flocks: Urological management of the meningomyelocele patient. JAMA **213**:753-8, 1970.

Currie, R. J., & others: External sphincterotomy in paraplegics: Technique and results. J Urol **103**:64-8, 1970.

Dalton, J. J., Jr., Hackler, R. H., & R. C. Bunts: Amyloidosis in the paraplegic: Incidence and significance. J Urol **93**:553-5, 1965.

Eckstein, H. B.: Urinary control in children with myelomeningocele. Brit J Urol **40**:191-5, 1968.

Emmett, J. L., & J. G. Love: Vesical dysfunction caused by protruded lumbar disk. J Urol **105**:86-91, 1971.

Ericsson, N. O., & others: Micturition urethrocystography in children with myelomeningocele. Acta radiol (diag) **11**:321-36, 1971.

Ferguson, D. E., & R. W. Geist: Pre-school urinary tract diversion for children with neurogenic bladder from myelomeningocele. J Urol **105**:131-6, 1971.

Gottlieb, R. J., & J. Cuttner: Vincristine-induced bladder atony. Cancer **28**:674-5, 1971.

Guttman, L., & H. Frankel: The value of intermittent catheterization in the early management of traumatic paraplegia and tetraplegia. Paraplegia **4**:63-83, 1966.

Hald, T., & others: Clinical experience with a radio-linked bladder stimulator. J Urol **97**:73-8, 1967.

Halverstadt, D. B.: Electrical stimulation of the human bladder: 3 years later. J Urol **106**:673-7, 1971.

Hodgkinson, C. P., & J. E. Morgan: Basic pressures of voiding in the adult female. Am J Obst Gynec **103**:755-70, 1969.

Kahan, M., Goldberg, P. D., & E. E. Mandel: Neurogenic vesical dysfunction and diabetes mellitus. New York J Med **70**:2448-55, 1970.

Koontz, W. W., Jr., & G. R. Prout, Jr.: Agenesis of the sacrum and the neurogenic bladder. JAMA **203**:481-6, 1968.

Kuru, M.: Nervous control of micturition. Physiol Rev **45**:425-94, 1965.

Lapides, J., Friend, C. R., & P. Ajemian: Denervation supersensitivity as a test for neurogenic bladder. Surg Gynec Obst **114**:241-4, 1962.

Lapides, J.: Urecholine regimen for rehabilitating the atonic bladder. J Urol **91**:658-9, 1964.

Manfredi, R. A., & J. F. Leal: Selective sacral rhizotomy for the spastic bladder syndrome in patients with spinal cord injuries. J Urol **100**:17-20, 1968.

Marchetti, L. J., & P. Gonick: A comparison of renal function in spinal cord injury patients with and without reflux. J Urol **104**:365-7, 1970.

McCoy, R. M., & R. K. Rhamy: Ileal conduits in children. J Urol **103**:491-5, 1970.

Miller, H., Simpson, C. A., & W. K. Yeates: Bladder dysfunction in multiple sclerosis. Brit MJ **1**:1265-9, 1965.

Morales, P.: Neurogenic bladder in traumatic paraplegia. New York J Med **68**:2031-7, 1968.

Nieder, R. M., O'Higgins, J. W., & J. A. Aldrete: Autonomic hyperreflexia in urologic surgery. JAMA **213**:867-9, 1970.

Peha, L. J., Comarr, A. E., & E. Bors: Cinecystourethrography in patients with spinal cord injuries. Am J Roentgenol **104**:375-9, 1968.

Ray, B., & G. J. Wise: Urinary retention associated with herpes zoster. J Urol **104**:422-5, 1970.

Ross, J. C., Biggon, N. O. K., & M. Damanski: Bladder dysfunction in non-traumatic paraplegia. Lancet **1**:779-82, 1964.

Ross, J.C., & R.M. Jameson: Vesical dysfunction due to prolapsed disc. Brit MJ **3**:752-4, 1971.

Stark, G.: Pudendal neurectomy in management of neurogenic bladder in myelomeningocele. Arch Dis Childhood **44**:698-704, 1969.

Stenberg, C.C., Burnette, H.W., & R.C. Bunts: Electrical stimulation of human neurogenic bladders: Experience with 4 patients. J Urol **97**:79-84, 1967.

Sussit, J.G., & others: Implantable electrical stimulator: Review of the literature and report of a successful case. Canad MAJ **95**:1128-31, 1966.

Symposium. The neurogenic bladder. Acta neurol scandinav, Suppl. 20, 1966.

Tanagho, E.A., Meyers, F.H., & D.R. Smith: The trigone: Anatomical and physiological considerations. 1. In relation to the ureterovesical junction. J Urol **100**:623-32, 1968.

Tanagho, E.A., & E.R. Miller: Initiation of voiding. Brit J Urol **42**:175-83, 1970.

Woodburne, R.T.: Anatomy of the bladder and bladder outlet. J Urol **100**:474-87, 1968.

20...

Disorders of the Perirenal Area

Disorders of the perirenal area include those of the adrenal gland as well as retroperitoneal extrarenal cysts and tumors. Diseases of this area are of interest to the urologist because their definitive radiologic diagnosis and localization is best accomplished through urologic modes of examination and because the urologist is most familiar with the area from the standpoint of surgical approach.

DISEASES OF THE ADRENAL CORTEX

Hyperplasia and almost all tumors of the adrenal cortex present clinical symptoms and signs whose characteristics depend upon the types of adrenal hormones that are elaborated in excess. The clinical entities in question are therefore medical or endocrinologic rather than urologic in type. They include congenital adrenal hyperplasia, Addison's disease, cyst, Cushing's syndrome (tumor or hyperplasia), adrenogenital syndrome (tumor or hyperplasia), and aldosteronism. For details concerning the etiology, pathogenesis, pathology, clinical findings (including laboratory tests), and treatment of these syndromes, the reader is referred to the appropriate sources.

Cysts of the adrenal gland usually cause no symptoms; endocrine function is absent. Adrenal cysts are usually discovered on abdominal palpation or incidentally on a plain film of the abdomen. Calcifications in the wall of the cyst are often seen.

Spontaneous hemorrhage into the adrenals is occasionally observed in infants and in association with severe sepsis (eg, meningitis). Signs of hemorrhage or findings compatible with adrenal insufficiency are usually noted. Later, the adrenals may undergo calcification.

Bennett, A. H., Harrison, J. H., & G. W. Thorn: Neoplasms of the adrenal gland. J Urol **106**:607-14, 1971.

Biglieri, E. G., & others: Diagnosis of an aldosterone-producing adenoma in primary aldosteronism. JAMA **201**:510-4, 1967.

Cerny, J. C., & others: The preoperative diagnosis of adrenal cysts. J Urol **104**:787-9, 1970.

Colapinto, R. F., & B. L. Steed: Arteriography of adrenal tumors. Radiology **100**:343-50, 1971.

Conn, J. W.: Preoperative diagnosis of primary aldosteronism. Arch Int Med **123**:113-23, 1969.

Cope, C. L.: The adrenal cortex in internal medicine. Brit MJ **2**:847-53, 914-21, 1966.

Eisenstein, A. B.: Addison's disease: Etiology and relationship to other endocrine disorders. M Clin North America **52**:327-38, 1968.

Fishman, L. M., & others: Incidence of primary aldosteronism in "essential" hypertension. JAMA **205**:497-502, 1968.

Gabrilove, J. L., & others: Feminizing adrenocortical tumors in the male. Medicine **44**:37-79, 1965.

George, J. M., & others: The syndrome of primary aldosteronism. Am J Med **48**:343-56, 1970.

Hartman, G. W., Witten, D. M., & R. E. Weeks: The role of nephrotomography in the diagnosis of adrenal tumors. Radiology **86**:1030-4, 1966.

Hendren, W. H., & J. D. Crawford: Adrenogenital syndrome: The anatomy of the anomaly and its repair. Some new concepts. J Pediat Surg **4**:49-58, 1969.

Herrera, M. G., Cahill, G. F., Jr., & G. W. Thorn: Cushing's syndrome: Diagnosis and treatment. Am J Surg **107**:144-52, 1964.

Hutter, A. M., & D. E. Kayhoe: Adrenal cortical carcinoma. Clinical features of 138 patients. Am J Med **41**:572-80, 1966.

Hutter, A. M., & D. E. Kayhoe: Adrenal cortical carcinoma. Results of treatment with o, p'DDD in 138 patients. Am J Med **41**:581-92, 1966.

Kenny, F. M., & others: Virilizing tumors of the adrenal cortex. Am J Dis Child **115**:445-58, 1968.

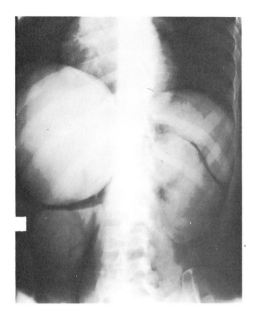

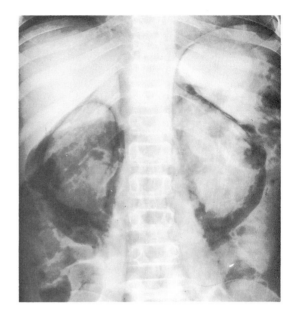

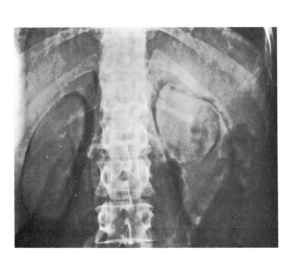

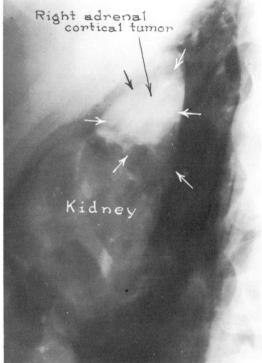

Fig 20-1. The adrenal gland and retroperitoneal insufflation. Above left: Pneumogram showing large androgenic tumor of right adrenal. Upper pole of kidney saucerized by pressure; kidney displaced downward. Spleen seen above left kidney. **Above right:** Pneumogram delineating small right adrenal cortical tumor. **Below left:** Presacral oxygen showing large pheochromocytoma overlying upper half of left kidney. Upper renal pole has been displaced laterally. **Below right:** Pneumogram showing a large right adrenal tumor.

Lawson, D. W., & others: Massive retroperitoneal adrenal hemorrhage. Surg Gynec Obst 129:989-94, 1969.

Lewis, V. G., Ehrhardt, A. A., & J. Money: Genital operations in girls with the adrenogenital syndrome. Subsequent psychologic development. Obst Gynec 36:11-5, 1970.

Marks, L. J.: Carcinoma of the lung and Cushing's syndrome. Geriatrics 19:881-6, 1964.

McAlister, W. H., & P. R. Koehler: Diseases of the adrenal. Radiol Clin North America 5:205-20, 1967.

Mikaelsson, C. G.: Retrograde phlebography of both adrenal veins. Acta radiol (diagn) 6:348-54, 1967.

O'Neal, L. W.: Correlation between clinical pattern and pathological findings in Cushing's syndrome. M Clin North America 52:313-26, 1968.

Sober, I., & M. Hirsch: Unilateral massive adrenal hemorrhage in newborn infant. J Urol 93:430-4, 1965.

Tank, E. S., & others: Surgery of the adrenal glands in infancy and childhood. J Urol 106: 280-6, 1971.

Tucci, J. R., & others: Rapid dexamethasone suppression test for Cushing's syndrome. JAMA 199:379-82, 1967.

Van De Walter, J. M., & E. W. Fonkalsrud: Adrenal cysts in infancy. Surgery 60: 1267-70, 1966.

Visser, H. K. A.: The adrenal cortex in childhood. Arch Dis Child 41:2-16, 1966.

DISEASES OF THE ADRENAL MEDULLA

PHEOCHROMOCYTOMA

With few exceptions, pheochromocytomas are benign tumors. About 40% of them secrete epinephrine, which stimulates metabolic functions and increases cardiac output. The remainder elaborate norepinephrine, which is a powerful vasoconstrictor; this type of pheochromocytoma is most apt to cause sustained hypertension. Many tumors excrete mixtures of the 2 hormones. In the adult, about 85% of these tumors arise in the adrenal gland. Other sites of origin are the sympathetic chain, the organs of Zuckerkandl, the thorax, and the bladder wall. One instance of involvement of the ovary has been reported. Norepinephrine-secreting tumors are apt to be extra-adrenal. In children, about 30% are extra-adrenal and a similar percentage are multiple. Familial series have been reported.

Clinical Findings

A. Symptoms: The patient with periodic attacks of hypertension may complain of paroxysms of severe headache, palpitations, sweating, nausea and vomiting, and visual disturbances. Tumors that stimulate metabolic functions may also cause nervousness, and loss of weight in spite of increased appetite. Patients with sustained hypertension usually have symptoms compatible with essential hypertension.

B. Signs: Hypertension is the rule, either sustained or in attacks. Postural tachycardia or hypotension may be noted. Cardiac enlargement is usual. In a few cases the tumor may be large enough to be palpated.

C. Laboratory Findings: The cold pressor response is negative. The BMR is elevated but the PBI is normal. Glycosuria or hyperglycemia may be noted.

If pheochromocytoma is suspected, but the patient is normotensive, histamine phosphate, 0.02 mg IV, should be given. Immediate significant hypertension constitutes a positive test. Glucagon has also been suggested as a provocative test for the normotensive patient. Give 0.5 mg crystalline glucagon in 1 ml of diluent intravenously. Should this fail to cause a hypertensive response, give 1 mg of the drug. Tyramine has also been used in this group of patients. The dose is 1 gm IV. If the blood pressure rises 20 points or more, the test is positive. These substances are thought to be safer than histamine. Should the pressure rise to dangerous levels, give phentolamine (Regitine®), 5 mg IV, promptly.

If the patient is hypertensive, phentolamine, 5 mg IV, is given. If the blood pressure drops 25 mm Hg or more, the test is considered positive.

Urinary VMA levels are increased with pheochrome tumors, but the most reliable test is direct assay of epinephrine and norepinephrine in urine or blood. In the patient with paroxysmal hypertension, these tests must be done during or just following an attack.

Localization of the tumor may be accomplished by catheterization of the vena cava. Venous samples are collected at various levels and subjected to quantitative estimation of epinephrine and norepinephrine.

D. X-Ray Findings: Excretory urograms may show the tumor itself and, in addition, downward displacement of the kidney with the upper pole pushed laterally. Retroperitoneal gas insufflation (Fig 20-1) is a useful method of outlining an adrenal tumor. Since these tumors are quite vascular, angiography may be diagnostic (Fig 20-2).

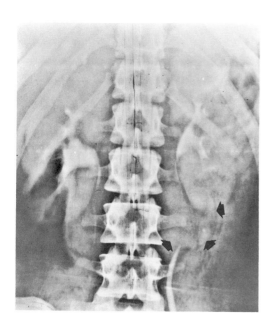 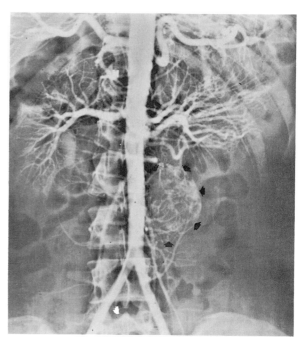

Fig 20-2. Extraadrenal pheochromocytoma. Left: Excretory urogram showing normal kidneys but a soft tissue mass just below and medial to left kidney. **Right:** Angiogram, same patient. Vascular mass below left renal arteries. **Surgical diagnosis:** Pheochromocytoma.

Differential Diagnosis

Thyrotoxicosis may be mimicked by epinephrine-producing tumors. In the latter the PBI is normal; in the former, provocative tests are negative and urinary VMA levels are normal.

Diabetes may cause confusion since some patients with pheochromocytomas have glycosuria and hyperglycemia. The finding of sustained or periodic hypertension, positive provocative tests, and normal urinary VMA levels are the basis for differentiation.

Essential hypertension and pheochromocytoma with sustained hypertension are often clinically indistinguishable; the definitive tests outlined above will establish the presence of a tumor.

Pheochromocytoma may be misdiagnosed as psychoneurosis if the leading symptoms are nervousness, irritability, headache, and weight loss. The finding of hypertension, particularly during an attack, and the application of diagnostic tests will clarify the diagnosis.

Complications

Hypertensive crises with sudden blindness or cerebrovascular accidents may be precipitated by emotional stress or palpation of the tumor or may occur during anesthetic induction or surgical excision of the tumor.

Treatment

Although the use of oral phenoxybenzamine (Dibenzyline®) to exert a blocking effect upon catecholamines has been suggested for chronic medical therapy, most authorities believe that surgical excision of the tumor (or tumors) is required. These patients have diminished blood volume, and shock may occur at the time of surgery. This deficiency can be overcome before surgery by giving oral phentolamine (50-100 mg every 2-4 hours until the hematocrit falls) or by suitable transfusions. If normal blood volume is restored, it is unusual to have any major difficulty at the time of surgery. The patient can be titrated with IV phentolamine during surgery if hypertensive episodes occur; with IV cortisone if hypotension develops.

Persistence of hypertension after excision of a tumor suggests the presence of another pheochromocytoma. Catecholamines should again be assayed.

Prognosis

If the tumor is removed before irreversible cardiovascular damage has developed, the outlook is good. The surgical mortality rate is less than 5%.

Albores-Saavedra, J., & others: Pheochromocytoma of the urinary bladder. Cancer 23: 1110-8, 1969.

Allen, S. D., Karafin, L., & A. R. Kendall: Non-visualization of the kidney due to a ureteral pheochromocytoma. J Urol 105: 571-4, 1971.

Brown, W. G., & others: Vanilmandelic acid screening test for pheochromocytoma and neuroblastoma. Am J Clin Path 46:599-602, 1966.

Carey, L. C., & E. H. Ellison: Adrenelectomy: technique, errors and pitfalls. S Clin North America 46:1283-92, 1966.

Downs, A. R., & C. B. Schoemperlen: Intrathoracic pheochromocytoma. Canad J Surg 9:180, 1966.

Engelman, K., & A. Sjoerdsma: Chronic medical therapy for pheochromocytoma. Ann Int Med 61:229-41, 1964.

Engelman, K., & others: Further evaluation of the tyramine test for pheochromocytoma. New England J Med 278:705-9, 1968.

Freis, J. G., & J. A. Chamberlin: Extra-adrenal pheochromocytoma: Literature review and report of a cervical pheochromocytoma. Surgery 63:268-79, 1968.

Harrison, T. S., & others: Localization of pheochromocytomata by caval catneterization. Arch Surg 95:339-43, 1967.

Lanner, L. O., & M. Rosencrantz: Arteriographic appearances of phaeochromocytomas. Acta radiol (diag) 10:35-48, 1970.

Lawrence, A. M.: Glucagon provocation test for pheochromocytoma. Ann Int Med 66: 1091-6, 1967.

Rosenberg, J. C., & R. L. Varco: Physiologic and pharmacologic considerations in the management of pheochromocytoma. S Clin North America 47:1453-60, 1967.

Rossi, P., & W. F. Panke: Arteriography in pheochromocytoma. JAMA 205:547-53, 1968.

Spergel, G., & others: A modified phentolamine test for the diagnosis of pheochromocytoma. JAMA 211:266-9, 1970.

Thomas, J. E., Rooke, E. D., & W. F. Kvale: The neurologist's experience with pheochromocytoma. JAMA 197:755-8, 1966.

Weber, A. L., Janover, M. L., & N. T. Griscom: Radiologic and clinical evaluation of pheochromocytoma in children: Report of 6 cases. Radiology 88:117-23, 1967.

NEUROBLASTOMA

Neuroblastomas may arise in the adrenal gland, but just as many are found in the retroperitoneal area (ganglioneuroblastoma) and mediastinum. The retroperitoneal and adrenal tumors have the poorest prognosis. The majority are seen before the age of 3 years; a few present as late as the sixth decade. Most patients have lymphocytes which are cytotoxic to neuroblastoma cells in tissue culture. Most members of the patient's family show the same lymphocytic reaction. It has been observed that the more lymphocytes found in the patient's peripheral blood or in the tumor, the better the prognosis. Abnormalities of muscle and heart and hemihypertrophy have been observed in association with neuroblastoma.

Metastases occur through both the blood stream and lymphatics. Common sites include the skull and long bones, regional lymph nodes, the liver, and the lungs. Local invasion is common.

Clinical Findings

A. Symptoms: Most commonly an abdominal mass is noted by parents, the physician, or the patient himself. Symptoms relating to metastases are fever, malaise, bone pain, and failure to gain weight.

B. Signs: A flank mass is usually palpable, even visible. The tumor is usually nodular and fixed, since it tends to be locally invasive. Evidence of metastases may be noted: ocular proptosis from metastases to the skull, enlarged nodular liver, or a mass in bone.

C. Laboratory Findings: Anemia is common; 70% of patients have metastases when first seen. Urinalysis and renal function are normal. Because neuroblastomas elaborate various catecholamines, urinary VMA is elevated in most cases. Bone marrow aspiration may reveal tumor cells.

D. X-Ray Findings: Excretory urography usually reveals a large area of grayness in one of the upper abdominal quadrants. At least 50% of these tumors contain calcific deposits. The ipsilateral kidney, which usually functions normally, is displaced by the suprarenal mass (Fig 20-3).

An inferior venacavagram may show evidence of occlusion from invasion by the tumor. Such a finding indicates the need for preliminary radiotherapy before surgical excision is attempted.

A bone survey should be done. Metastases to the skull and long bones are common; those to the long bones are apt to be symmetrical.

Differential Diagnosis

Nephroblastoma (Wilms's tumor) is also a disease of childhood. Intravenous urograms show the distortion characteristic of an intrin-

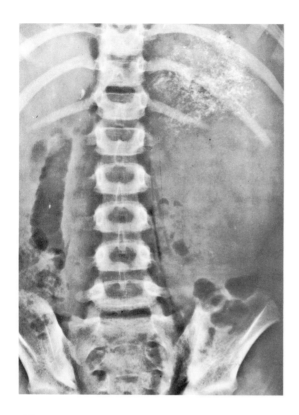

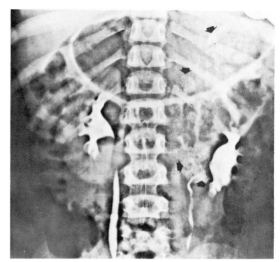

Fig 20-3. Neuroblastoma of adrenal gland. Left: Plain film, child age 7 years, showing large mass occupying left flank. Punctate calcification in upper portion which is typical of neuroblastoma. **Right:** Excretory urogram, child age 4 years, revealing lateral and downward displacement and rotation of left kidney by suprarenal mass. No calyceal deformity; calcific areas in mass compatible with neuroblastoma.

sic renal tumor; no such distortion is shown in neuroblastoma. Urinary VMA levels are normal with Wilms's tumor and elevated in neuroblastoma. Urinary LDH may be increased with Wilms's tumor but is normal with neuroblastoma.

Hydronephrosis may also present as a mass in the flank but is not ordinarily hard and nodular; evidence of urinary infection is common. Hydronephrosis is often bilateral, in which case the PSP excretion is depressed. Excretory or retrograde urograms will reveal the dilated pelvis and calyces and the site of obstruction.

Treatment

Surgical excision of the tumor is required, with preoperative radiotherapy if necessary. In all cases, postoperative irradiation should be given. There is increasing evidence that chemotherapy, given periodically for a 2 year period, is helpful particularly if the patient is under 1 year of age. Useful drugs include cytophosphamide (Cytoxan®) and vincristine (Oncovin®).

Chemotherapy or radiation therapy may be used for metastatic disease.

Although vitamin B_{12} has been suggested as an adjunct in therapy, it appears to be of no value.

Prognosis

Retroperitoneal and adrenal neuroblastomas have a poor prognosis because of late diagnosis. Collins' "period of risk" operates just as it does with Wilms's tumor in judging cure.

Bill, A. H.: Immune aspects of neuroblastoma. Current information. Am J Surg **122**:142-6, 1971.

Gitlow, S. E., & others: Diagnosis of neuroblastoma by qualitative and quantitative determination of catecholamine metabolites in urine. Cancer **25**:1377-83, 1970.

Langman, M. J. S.: Treatment of neuroblastoma with vitamin B_{12}. Arch Dis Childhood **45**:385-7, 1970.

McDonald, P., & H. A. Hiller: Angiography in abdominal tumors in childhood with particular reference to neuroblastoma and Wilms's tumor. Clin Radiol 19:1-18, 1968.

Miller, R.W., Fraumeni, J.F., Jr., & J.A. Hill: Neuroblastoma: Epidemiologic approach to its origin. Am J Dis Child 115: 253-61, 1968.

Rice, M.S.: Neuroblastoma in childhood: A review of 69 cases. Australian Paediat J 2:1-15, 1966.

Schneider, K.M., Becker, J.M., & I.H. Krasna: Neonatal neuroblastoma. Pediatrics 36:359-66, 1965.

Sy, W., & J.H. Edmondson: The developmental defects associated with neuroblastoma—etiologic implications. Cancer 22: 234-8, 1968.

Symposium. Cancer of the urogenital tract. Neuroblastoma. JAMA 205:153-66, 1968.

RETROPERITONEAL EXTRARENAL TUMORS

Although these tumors and cysts are rare, they must be considered in the differential diagnosis of renal and suprarenal masses since they present as masses in the flank. Most of these neoplasms arise from mesothelial tissues of the retroperitoneum and are therefore of connective tissue origin. They may be comprised of a single type of cell (eg, lipoma, fibroma), but more commonly are mixed tumors (eg, chondrolipomyxoma). Many are malignant (eg, lipomyxorhabdomyosarcoma). Others, for the most part, arise from the mesonephros and its duct, and the gonads. The cystic tumors are benign; the solid growths may be benign or malignant. Even if benign, however, they tend to grow to large size and to surround and displace adjacent organs.

The most common finding is the discovery of a mass in the flank. Gastrointestinal symptoms caused by displacement or invasion of intraperitoneal organs may also be noted. Edema of the legs may occur if the vena cava is occluded. A plain film of the abdomen may show a large soft tissue mass in the upper abdomen. The kidney may be displaced, yet its calyceal system is not distorted; this is a cardinal sign of retroperitoneal extrarenal tumor (Fig 20-3). Hydronephrosis may develop from ureteral compression. Gastrointestinal studies may reveal displacement of the stomach or colon. Renal tumors or cysts cause distortion of the pelvis and calyces. Extrarenal tumors ordinarily do not.

Adrenal tumors are rarely large enough to be palpable. The x-ray findings are the same in both, but most adrenal tumors are associated with symptoms and signs of hyperfunction.

An enlarged spleen may present as a mass in the left upper abdomen and at times can displace the kidney. Hematologic changes may accompany splenomegaly; findings elsewhere consistent with lymphoma may be helpful.

The main complication is displacement or invasion of adjacent organs (eg, spleen, stomach, liver, ureter, kidney, vena cava, and aorta).

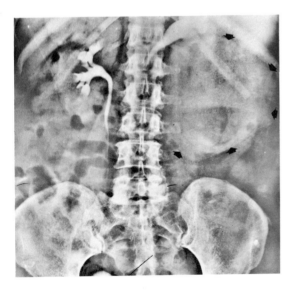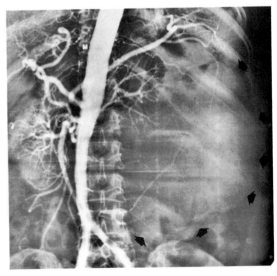

Fig 20-4. Retroperitoneal lipoma. Left: Excretory urogram showing large soft tissue mass in left upper quadrant displacing kidney superomedially. Right kidney is normal. **Right:** Renal angiogram, same patient, revealing large, relatively avascular mass in left abdomen. Left renal vasculature displaced medially and superiorly.

Surgical removal of the cyst or tumor is the only method of cure. The solid tumors are difficult to remove in toto because of their penchant for invading and surrounding vital structures. These tumors are radioresistant.

The prognosis after the excision of cysts is good. The recurrence rate after removal of the solid tumors is high even though the neoplasm is benign.

Adlerman, E. J., & others: Primary retroperitoneal leiomyosarcoma. New York J Med **63**:1709-14, 1963.

Armstrong, J. R., & I. Cohn, Jr.: Primary malignant retroperitoneal tumors. Am J Surg **100**:937-43, 1965.

Braasch, J. W., & A. B. Mon: Primary retroperitoneal tumors. S Clin North America **47**:663-78, 1967.

Dassel, P. M.: Primary retroperitoneal tumors. Am J Roentgenol **78**:333-42, 1957.

•   •   •

21...
Disorders of the Kidneys

CONGENITAL ANOMALIES OF THE KIDNEYS

Congenital anomalies occur more frequently in the kidney than in any other organ. Some cause no difficulty, but many (eg, hypoplasia, polycystic kidneys) cause impairment of renal function. It has been noted that the child with a gross deformity of an external ear associated with ipsilateral maldevelopment of the facial bones is apt to have a congenital abnormality of the kidney (eg, ectopy, hypoplasia) on the same side as the visible deformity. Lateral displacement of the nipples has been observed in association with bilateral renal hypoplasia.

Fleisher, D. S.: Lateral displacement of the
    nipples, a sign of bilateral renal hypoplasia.
    J Pediat **69**:806-9, 1966.
Taylor, W. C.: Deformity of ears and kidneys.
    Canad MAJ **93**:107-10, 1965.

AGENESIS

One kidney may be absent. This is probably due to the fact that the ureteral bud (from the wolffian duct) fails to develop or, if it does develop, does not reach the metanephros (adult kidney). Without a drainage system, the metanephric mass undergoes atrophy. The ureter is usually absent on the side of the unformed kidney, although a blind duct may be found. (See chapter 2.)

Renal agenesis causes no symptoms; it is usually found by accident on urography. It is not an easy diagnosis to establish even though the ureteral ridge is absent and no orifice is visualized, for the kidney could be present but be drained by a ureter whose opening is ectopic (into the urethra, seminal vesicle, or vagina).

Hynes, D. M., & E. M. Watkin: Renal agenesis.
    Am J Roentgenol **110**:772-7, 1970.

Rizza, J. M., & S. E. Downing: Bilateral renal
    agenesis in two female siblings. Am J Dis
    Child **121**:60-3, 1971.

HYPOPLASIA

Hypoplasia implies a small kidney. The total renal mass may be divided in an unequal manner, in which case one kidney is small and the other kidney correspondingly larger than normal. Some of these congenitally small kidneys prove, on pathologic examination, to be dysplastic.

Differentiation from acquired atrophy is difficult. Atrophic pyelonephritis usually reveals typical distortion of the calyces. Vesicoureteral reflux in the infant may cause a dwarfed kidney even in the absence of infection. Stenosis of the renal artery leads to shrinkage of the kidney.

Goldman, R. L., & N. B. Friedman: Epididymal tubules in the dysplastic kidney.
    J Urol **99**:148-53, 1968.
Kanasawa, M., & others: Dwarfed kidneys in
    children. Am J Dis Child **109**:130-40, 1965.

SUPERNUMERARY KIDNEYS

The presence of a third kidney is very rare; the presence of 4 separate kidneys in one individual has only been reported once. This anomaly must not be confused with duplication (or triplication) of the pelvis in one kidney, which is not uncommon.

DYSPLASIA

Renal dysplasia presents protean manifestations. Multicystic kidney of the newborn is almost always unilateral, nonhereditary, and characterized by an irregularly lobulated mass of cysts; the ureter is usually absent or atretic. It may develop because of faulty union of the nephron and the collecting system. At most, only a few embryonic glomeruli and tubules are observed. The only finding is the discovery of an irregular mass in the flank. Nothing is shown on urography. Cystoscopy usually fails to reveal the ipsilateral ureteral orifice. In order to rule out tumor, surgical exploration is indicated.

Dysplasia of the renal parenchyma is also seen in association with ureteral obstruction or reflux. It is relatively common as a segmental renal lesion involving the upper pole of a duplicated kidney whose ureter is obstructed by a congenital ureterocele. It may also be found in urinary tracts severely obstructed by posterior urethral valves; in this instance, the lesion may be bilateral.

Microscopically, the renal parenchyma is "disorganized." Tubular and glomerular cysts may be noted; these elements are fetal in type. Islands of metaplastic cartilage are often seen. The common denominator seems to be fetal obstruction.

Bernstein, J.: The morphogenesis of renal parenchymal maldevelopment (renal dysplasia). P Clin North America **18**:395-407, 1971.

Greene, L. F., Feinzaig, W., & D. C. Dahlin: Multicystic dysplasia of the kidney: With special reference to the contralateral kidney. J Urol **105**:482-7, 1971.

Risdon, R. A.: Renal dysplasia. Part I. A clinicopathological study of 76 cases. Part II. A necropsy study of 41 cases. J Clin Path **24**:57-71, 1971.

POLYCYSTIC KIDNEYS

Polycystic kidney disease is an almost always bilateral (95% of cases) hereditary disease. The kidneys are usually much larger than normal, and are studded with cysts of various sizes. Impairment of renal function is the rule. In severe cases, symptoms occur during infancy; otherwise, symptoms do not appear until after the age of 40 years. Cystic disease of the lung, liver, spleen, and pancreas may also be noted.

Etiology and Pathogenesis

The evidence suggests that the cysts develop because of defects in the development of the collecting and uriniferous tubules and in the mechanism of their joining. Blind secre-

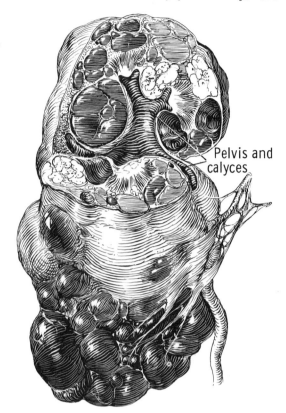

Pelvis and calyces

Fig 21-1. Polycystic kidney. Multiple cysts deep in the parenchyma and on the surface. Note distortion of the calyces by the cysts.

tory tubules which are connected to functioning glomeruli become cystic. As these cysts enlarge, they compress adjacent parenchyma, destroy it by ischemia, and occlude normal tubules. The result is progressive functional impairment. It would appear that medullary sponge kidney is part of this spectrum but in a milder form.

Pathology

Grossly, the kidneys are usually much enlarged. Their surfaces are studded with cysts of various sizes (Fig 21-1). On section the cysts are found to be scattered throughout the parenchyma. The fluid in the cyst is usually amber-colored but may be hemorrhagic.

Microscopically, the lining of the cysts consists of a single layer of cells. The renal parenchyma may show peritubular fibrosis and evidence of secondary infection. There appears to be a reduction in the number of glomeruli, some of which may be hyalinized. Renal arteriolar thickening is a prominent finding in the adult.

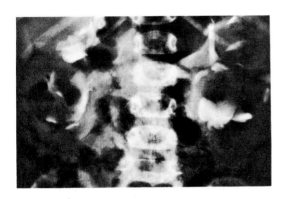
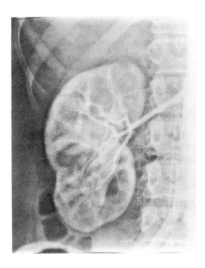
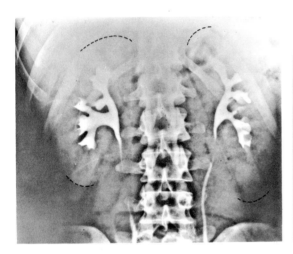
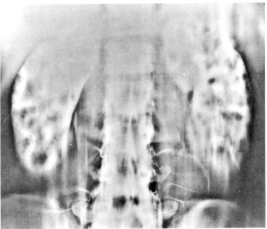

Fig 21-2. Polycystic kidneys. Above left: Excretory urogram in a child showing elongation, broadening, and bending of the calyces around cysts. Good renal function. **Above right:** Angiogram of right kidney showing "negative" shadows of cysts. **Below left:** Excretory urogram without gross abnormality. However, the right kidney is 16.5 cm long, and the left kidney 18.5 cm long, which suggests the possibility of polycystic disease. All calyces are broad; a few are distorted. **Below right:** Angiogram with tomography on same patient. Multiple cysts are seen as "negative" shadows. This is an example of the mild form of the disease. Good renal function; normotension.

Clinical Findings

A. Symptoms: Pain over one or both kidneys may occur because of the drag on the vascular pedicles by the heavy kidneys or from hemorrhage into a cyst. Gross total hematuria is not uncommon and may be severe; the cause for this is not clear. Colic may be present if blood clots are passed. The patient may notice an abdominal mass.

Infection (chills, fever, renal pain) commonly complicates polycystic disease. Symptoms of vesical irritability may be the first complaint. When renal insufficiency ensues, headache, nausea and vomiting, weakness, and loss of weight occur.

B. Signs: One or both kidneys are usually palpable. They may feel nodular. If infected, they may be tender. Hypertension is found in 60-70% of these patients. Evidence of cardiac enlargement is then noted.

Fever may be present if pyelonephritis exists or if cysts have become infected. In the stage of uremia, anemia and loss of weight may be evident. Ophthalmoscopic examination may show changes typical of moderate or severe hypertension.

C. Laboratory Findings: Anemia may be noted, either caused by chronic loss of blood or, more commonly, by the hematopoietic depression which accompanies uremia. Proteinuria and microscopic (if not gross) hematuria are the rule. Pus cells and bacteria are commonly found.

Progressive loss of concentrating power occurs. The PSP and clearance tests will show varying degrees of renal impairment. About a third of patients with polycystic kidney disease are uremic when first seen.

D. X-Ray Findings: Both renal shadows are usually enlarged on a plain film of the abdomen, even as much as 5 times normal size. Kidneys more than 16 cm in length are suspect.

Excretory urograms are helpful if, as is true in most cases, the PSP excretion is better than 30% in 1 hour, in which event excretion of the medium may be sufficient to delineate the calyceal system and thus establish the diagnosis. On these or on retrograde urography the renal masses are usually enlarged, and the calyceal pattern is quite bizarre (spider deformity). The calyces are broadened and flattened, enlarged, and often curved, as they tend to hug the periphery of adjacent cysts (Fig 21-2). Often the changes are only slight or may even be absent on one side, leading to the erroneous diagnosis of tumor of the other kidney.

If cysts are infected, perinephritis may obscure the renal and even the psoas shadows.

Angiography will reveal bending of small vessels around the cysts and the "negative" shadows (nonvascular) of the cysts (Fig 21-2).

Photoscan (see chapter 8) will reveal multiple "cold" avascular spots in large renal shadows.

E. Instrumental Examination: Cystoscopy may show evidence of cystitis, in which case the urine will contain abnormal elements. Bleeding from a ureteral orifice may be noted.

After catheterization of the ureters, the collected pelvic urine may be found to contain pus and bacteria microscopically and by culture. The PSP test will usually reveal bilateral impairment of kidney function.

Differential Diagnosis

Bilateral hydronephrosis (on the basis of congenital or acquired ureteral obstruction) may present bilateral flank masses and signs of impairment of renal function, but urography will show changes quite different from those of the polycystic kidney.

Bilateral renal tumor is rare but may mimic polycystic kidney disease perfectly on

urography. Differentiation of a unilateral tumor may be quite difficult if one of the polycystic kidneys shows little or no distortion on urography. However, tumors are usually localized to one portion of the kidney, whereas cysts are quite diffusely distributed. The total renal function should be normal with unilateral tumor but is usually depressed in the patient with polycystic kidney disease. Renal angiography may be needed, at times, to differentiate between the 2 conditions (Fig 21-2).

In Lindau's disease (angiomatous cerebellar cyst, angiomatosis of the retina, tumors or cysts of the pancreas), multiple bilateral cysts or adenocarcinomas of both kidneys may develop. Urograms or nephrotomograms may suggest polycystic kidney disease. The presence of other stigmas should make the diagnosis. Angiography should be definitive.

Tuberous sclerosis (convulsive seizures, mental retardation, and adenoma sebaceum) is typified by hamartomatous tumors often involving the skin, brain, retinas, bones, liver, heart, and kidneys. The renal lesions are usually multiple and bilateral and microscopically are angiomyolipomas. If seen in the stage of uremia, the urograms are apt to suggest polycystic disease; the presence of other stigmas and angiography should make the differentiation.

Simple cyst (see below) is usually unilateral and single; total renal function should be normal. Urograms will show a single lesion (Fig 21-3), whereas polycystic kidney disease is bilateral and the filling defects are multiple.

Complications

Pyelonephritis, for reasons which are not clear, is a common complication of polycystic kidney disease. It may be asymptomatic; pus cells in the urine may be few or absent. Stained smears or quantitative cultures make the diagnosis.

Infection of cysts will be associated with pain and tenderness over the kidney and a febrile response. The differential diagnosis between infection of cysts and pyelonephritis may be difficult.

In rare instances gross hematuria may be so brisk and persistent as to endanger life.

Treatment

Except for unusual complications, the treatment is conservative and supportive.

A. General Measures: Place the patient on a low-protein diet (0.5-0.75 gm/kg/day of protein) and force fluids to 3000 ml or more per day. Physical activity may be permitted within reason, but strenuous overexercise is contraindicated. When the patient is in the state of absolute renal insufficiency, treat as

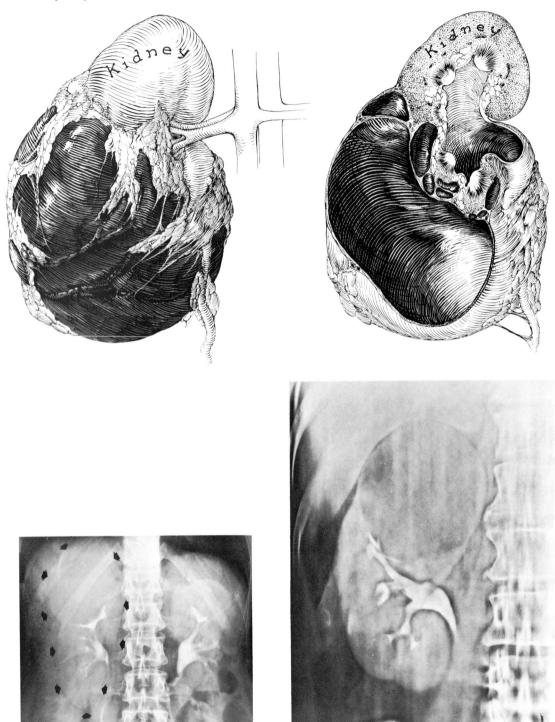

Fig 21-3. Simple cyst. **Above left:** Large cyst displacing lower pole laterally. **Above right:** Section of kidney showing one large and a few small cysts. **Below left:** Excretory urogram showing soft tissue mass in upper pole of right kidney. Elongation and distortion of upper calyces by cyst. **Below right:** Angionephrotomogram showing large cyst in upper renal pole distorting upper calyces and dislocating kidney laterally.

for uremia from any cause. Hemodialysis
may be indicated.

B. Surgery: There is no evidence that excision or decompression of cysts improves
renal function. Should a large cyst be found
to be compressing the upper ureter, causing
obstruction and further embarrassing renal
function, it should be resected. When the degree of renal insufficiency becomes life-
threatening, renal transplantation should be
considered.

C. Treatment of Complications: Pyelonephritis must be rigorously treated to prevent
further renal damage. Infection of cysts requires surgical drainage. If bleeding from one
kidney is so severe as to threaten exsanguination, nephrectomy must be considered as a
lifesaving measure.

Concomitant diseases (eg, tumor, obstructing stone) may require definitive surgical treatment.

Prognosis

If the disease is so severe as to present
symptoms in infancy or childhood, the prognosis is very poor. The larger group, presenting clinical signs and symptoms after the age
of 35-40 years, has a somewhat more favorable prognosis. Although there is wide variation, these patients usually do not live longer
than 5 or 10 years after the diagnosis is made.

Anderson, D., & R. L. Tannen: Tuberous
sclerosis and chronic renal failure. Potential confusion with polycystic kidney disease. Am J Med 47:163-8, 1969.
Bernstein, J.: Heritable cystic disorders of
the kidney: The mythology of polycystic
disease. P Clin North America 18:435-44,
1971.
Gwinn, J. L., & B. H. Landing: Cystic diseases of the kidneys in infants and children.
Radiol Clin North America 6:191-204, 1968.
Halpern, M., Dalrymple, G., & J. Young:
The nephrogram in polycystic disease: An
important radiographic sign. J Urol 103:
21-3, 1970.
Hurwitz, R. A., & J. Weigel: Polycystic kidneys: A diagnostic study with continuous
drip infusion pyelography, nephrotomography, and renal scans. J Urol 94:639-46,
1965.
Ivemark, B. I., Lagergren, C., & N. Lindvall:
Roentgenologic diagnosis of polycystic kidney and medullary sponge kidney. Acta
radiol (diag) 10:225-35, 1970.
Lazarus, J. M., & others: Hemodialysis and
transplantation in adults with polycystic
renal disease. JAMA 217:1821-4, 1971.
Lieberman, E., & others: Infantile polycystic
disease of the kidneys and liver. Medicine
50:277-318, 1971.
Milam, J. H., Magee, J. H., & R. C. Bunts:
Evaluation of surgical decompression of
polycystic kidneys by differential renal
clearances. J Urol 90:144-9, 1963.
Osathanondh, V., & E. L. Potter: Pathogenesis of polycystic kidneys. Arch Path 77:
459-512, 1964.
Rho, Yong-Myun: Von Hippel-Lindau's disease.
Canad MAJ 101:135-42, 1969.
Wenzl, J. E., Lagos, J. C., & D. D. Albers:
Tuberous sclerosis presenting as polycystic
kidneys and seizures in an infant. J Pediat
77:673-6, 1970.

SIMPLE (SOLITARY) CYST

Simple cyst of the kidney is usually unilateral and single but may be multiple and
multilocular and, more rarely, bilateral. It
differs from polycystic kidneys both clinically
and pathologically.

Etiology and Pathogenesis

Whether simple cyst is congenital or acquired is not clear. Its origin may be similar
to that of polycystic kidneys, ie, the difference
may be merely one of degree. On the other
hand, simple cysts have been produced in animals by causing tubular obstruction and local
ischemia, which suggests that the lesion can
be acquired.

As a simple cyst grows it compresses and
thereby destroys renal parenchyma, but rarely
is a significant amount of renal tissue destroyed
unless numerous cysts are present. A solitary
cyst may be placed in such a position as to
compress the ureter, causing progressive
hydronephrosis. Infection may then complicate the picture.

Pathology

Simple cysts usually involve the lower pole
of the kidney. They average about 10 cm in
diameter when producing symptoms, but a few
are large enough to fill the entire flank. They
usually contain a clear amber fluid. Their
walls are quite thin, and the cysts are "blue-
domed" in appearance. Calcification of the
sac is occasionally seen. About 15% contain
hemorrhagic fluid, and of these about one-half
have papillary cancers on their walls.

Simple cysts are usually superficial but
may be deeply situated, in which case destruction of renal parenchyma is more extensive.
When situated deep in the kidney, the cyst wall
is adjacent to the epithelial lining of the pelvis

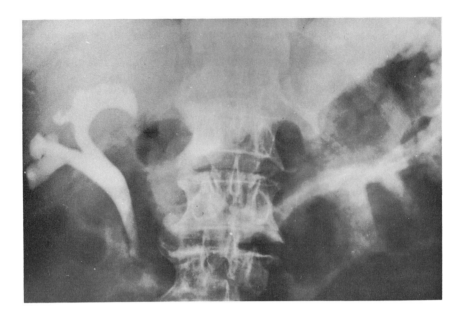

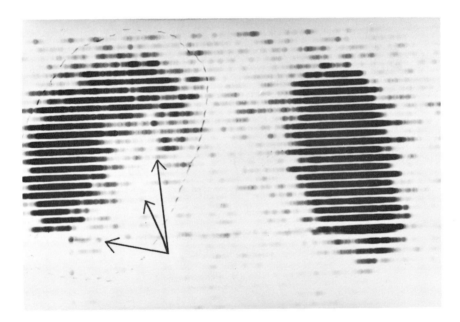

Fig 21-4. Mass in right kidney. Above: Retrograde urogram showing gross distortion of upper calyx and displacement of lower pole laterally. **Below:** Rectilinear scan, same patient, revealing "cold" spot in medial and lower parts of right kidney (left scan normal). **Surgical diagnosis:** Renal cyst.

or calyces, from which it may be separated only with great difficulty. Cysts do not communicate with the renal pelvis (Fig 21-3). Microscopic examination of the cyst wall shows heavy fibrosis and hyalinization; areas of calcification may be seen. The adjacent renal tissue is compressed and fibrosed.

Clinical Findings

A. Symptoms: Pain in the flank or back, usually intermittent and dull, is not uncommon. Should bleeding suddenly distend the cyst wall, pain may come on abruptly and be severe. Gastrointestinal symptoms are frequently noted and may suggest peptic ulcer or gallbladder disease. The patient may discover a mass in the abdomen, although cysts of this size are unusual. Should the cyst become infected the patient usually complains of pain in the flank, malaise, and fever.

B. Signs: Physical examination is usually normal, although occasionally a mass in the region of the kidney may be palpated. Tenderness in the flank may be noted if the cyst becomes infected.

C. Laboratory Findings: Urinalysis is usually normal. Microscopic hematuria is rare. Renal function tests are normal unless the cysts are multiple and bilateral (rare). Even in the face of extensive destruction of one kidney, compensatory hypertrophy of the other kidney will maintain normal total function.

D. X-Ray Findings: An expansion of a portion of the kidney shadow or a mass superimposed upon it can usually be seen on a plain film of the abdomen (Fig 7-2, top left). The axis of the kidney may be abnormal because of rotation due to the weight or position of the cyst. Streaks of calcium can sometimes be seen in the border of the mass.

Excretory urograms (Figs 21-3 and 21-4) will accentuate the cyst because the secretory tissue will become more dense whereas the cyst will not. The urogram will show changes compatible with a space-occupying lesion. One or more calyces or the pelvis will sometimes be bent around the cyst and will be broadened and flattened, even obliterated. Oblique and lateral films may be helpful. If a mass occupies the lower pole of the kidney, as is usually the case, the upper part of the ureter may be displaced toward the spine. The kidney itself may be rotated.

Nephrotomography (Fig 21-3) will usually establish the diagnosis of cyst by revealing lack of opacification of the lesion. Retrograde urograms may be necessary if excretory urograms are not diagnostic.

These cysts tend to be relatively superficial and well rounded. In rare instances a cyst may be so superficial that it fails to encroach upon the calyceal system.

Angiography (Fig 21-5) may demonstrate a cyst quite clearly since the functioning renal parenchyma will be strikingly outlined by the dense contrast medium, whereas the cyst will not be opacified at all. However, lack of opacification may be seen in relatively avascular or necrotic tumors and cysts with papillary tumors on their walls.

A rectilinear scan (Fig 21-4) will clearly delineate the mass but it does not differentiate cyst from tumor. The technetium scan, made with the camera, will reveal that the mass is,

indeed, avascular (see chapter 8).

If all indications point to a simple cyst and if the patient's condition precludes surgical exploration, a renal cystogram can be made (Fig 21-5). If the aspirated fluid is clear, the cyst wall smooth, and cytologic study of the fluid negative, the presence of a benign cyst can be assumed.

Differential Diagnosis

Carcinoma of the kidney also consumes space but tends to lie more deeply in the organ and therefore causes more distortion of the calyces. Hematuria is common with tumor, rare with cyst. If a solid tumor overlies the psoas muscle, the edge of the muscle is obliterated on the plain film; it can be seen through a cyst, however. Evidence of metastases (ie, loss of weight and strength, palpable supraclavicular nodes, chest film showing metastatic nodules), erythrocytosis, hypercalcemia, and increased sedimentation rate suggest cancer. It must be remembered, however, that the walls of a simple cyst may undergo cancerous degeneration. If the renal vein is occluded by cancer the excretory urogram may be visualized only faintly or not at all. Angiography (Fig 17-3) or nephrotomography (Fig 17-4) may reveal the "pooling" of the medium in the highly vascularized tumor, whereas the density of a cyst is not affected. It is wise to assume that all space-occupying lesions of the kidneys are cancers. If metastases are not demonstrable, surgical exploration is indicated.

Polycystic kidney disease is almost always bilateral, as shown by urography (Fig 21-2). Diffuse calyceal and pelvic distortion is the rule. Simple cyst is usually solitary and unilateral. Polycystic kidney disease is usually accompanied by impaired renal function and hypertension. Simple cyst is not.

Renal carbuncle is a rare disease. A history of skin infection a few weeks before the onset of fever and local pain may be obtained. Urograms may show changes similar to cyst or tumor, but the renal outline as well as the edge of the psoas muscle may be obscured because of perinephritis. The kidney may be fixed, as demonstrated by comparing the position of the kidney in the supine and upright positions. Angiography will demonstrate an avascular lesion (Fig 12-6). Surgery is indicated in either case.

Hydronephrosis may present the same symptoms and signs as simple cyst, but the urograms are quite different. Cyst causes calyceal distortion; with hydronephrosis, dilatation of the calyces and pelvis due to an obvious ureteral obstruction is present. Acute or subacute hydronephrosis usually produces more local pain because of increased intra-

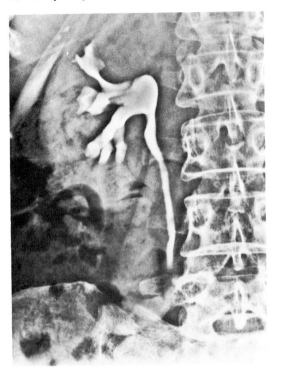

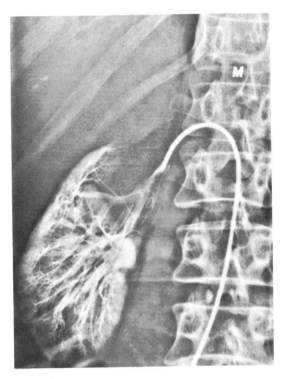

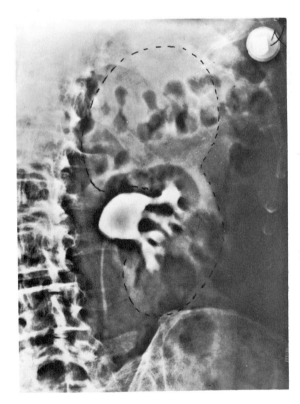

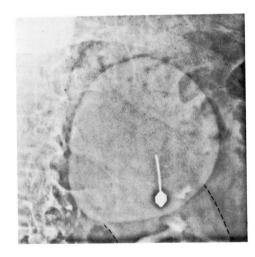

Fig 21-5. **Diagnosis of simple renal cyst.**
Above left: Excretory urogram showing lateral and inferior displacement and distortion of upper calyx, right kidney. **Differential diagnosis:** Cyst versus tumor. **Upper right:** Same patient. Selective femoral angiogram showing a completely avascular mass typical of cyst. **Below left:** Excretory urogram showing lateral displacement of upper pole, left kidney, by suprarenal mass. **Below right:** Same patient. Renal cystogram showing smooth-walled cyst. Cytology was negative. (Courtesy of Frank Hinman, Jr., MD.)

pelvic pressure and is more apt to be complicated by infection.

Extrarenal tumor (eg, adrenal, mixed retroperitoneal sarcoma) may displace a kidney, but rarely does it invade it and distort its calyces.

If an echinococcus cyst of the kidney does not communicate with the pelvis it may be difficult to differentiate from solitary cyst, for no scolices or hooklets will be present in the urine. Often the wall of a hydatid cyst reveals calcification on x-ray examination (Fig 13-3). A skin sensitivity test (Casoni) for hydatid disease may prove helpful.

Complications (Rare)

Spontaneous infection in a simple cyst is rare, but when it occurs it is difficult to differentiate from carbuncle.

Hemorrhage into the cyst sometimes occurs. If sudden, it causes severe pain. The bleeding may come from a complicating carcinoma arising on the wall of the cyst.

Hydronephrosis may develop if a cyst of the lower pole impinges upon the ureter. This in itself may cause pain from back pressure of urine in the pelvis. This obstruction may lead to renal infection.

Treatment

A. Specific Measures: Surgical exploration is indicated even though the diagnosis seems established for it is surprising how commonly cyst and renal tumor are confused. Furthermore, 3-5% of cysts have cancer on their walls, so all cysts must be assumed to be malignant until proved benign. Fortunately, they are not so dangerous as the parenchymal carcinoma.

It is rare for the kidney to be significantly damaged by a simple cyst. Therefore, only that portion of the sac external to the kidney need be excised. If, however, the kidney is severely damaged (and if its mate is normal), nephrectomy may be indicated.

B. Treatment of Complications: If the cyst should become infected, intensive antibiotic therapy should be instituted. If this proves unsuccessful, surgical excision of the extrarenal portion of the cyst and drainage will prove curative.

If, on exploration, the cyst appears to contain blood (and the other kidney is normal), immediate nephrectomy should be strongly considered without preliminary incision into the cyst, for this finding makes the presence of neoplasm likely. Drainage of the contents of a cancerous cyst, either by incision or needle, invites growth of carcinoma in the wound.

If hydronephrosis is present, excision of the cyst will relieve the ureteral obstruction.

Pyelonephritis in the involved kidney should suggest urinary stasis secondary to impaired ureteral drainage. Removal of the cyst and consequent relief of urinary back pressure will make antimicrobial therapy more effective.

Prognosis

Without complications the prognosis is excellent if the cyst is excised. If untreated, progressive damage to the kidney may occur.

Deliveliotis, A., & C. Kavadis: Parapelvic cysts of the kidney: Report of seven cases. Brit J Urol **41**:386-93, 1969.

Deliveliotis, A., Zorzos, S., & M. Varkarakis: Suppuration of solitary cyst of the kidney. Brit J Urol **39**:472-8, 1967.

Evans, A.T., & J.P. Coughlin: Urinary obstruction due to renal cysts. J Urol **103**: 277-80, 1970.

Genert, J.E., Stein, J., & A.J. Bischoff: Solitary renal cysts: Experience with 100 cases. J Urol **100**:251-3, 1968.

Khorsand, D.: Carcinoma within solitary cysts. J Urol **93**:440-4, 1965.

Kropp, K.A., & others: Morbidity and mortality of renal exploration for cyst. Surg Gynec Obst **125**:803-6, 1967.

Weitzner, S.: Clear cell carcinoma of the free wall of a simple renal cyst. J Urol **106**: 515-7, 1971.

Williams, G., Blandy, J.P., & G.C. Tresidder: Communicating cysts and diverticula of the renal pelvis. Brit J Urol **41**:161-70, 1969.

RENAL FUSION

About one out of 1000 individuals has some type of renal fusion, the most common being the horseshoe kidney. The fused renal mass almost always contains 2 excretory systems and therefore 2 ureters. The renal tissue may be divided equally between the 2 flanks, or the entire mass may be on one side. Even in the latter case the 2 ureters open at their proper places in the bladder.

Etiology and Pathogenesis

It appears that this fusion of the 2 metanephroi occurs early in embryologic life when the kidneys lie low in the pelvis. For this reason, they seldom ascend to the high position which normal kidneys assume. They may even remain in the true pelvis. Under these circumstances such a kidney may derive its blood supply from many vessels in the area (eg, aorta, iliacs).

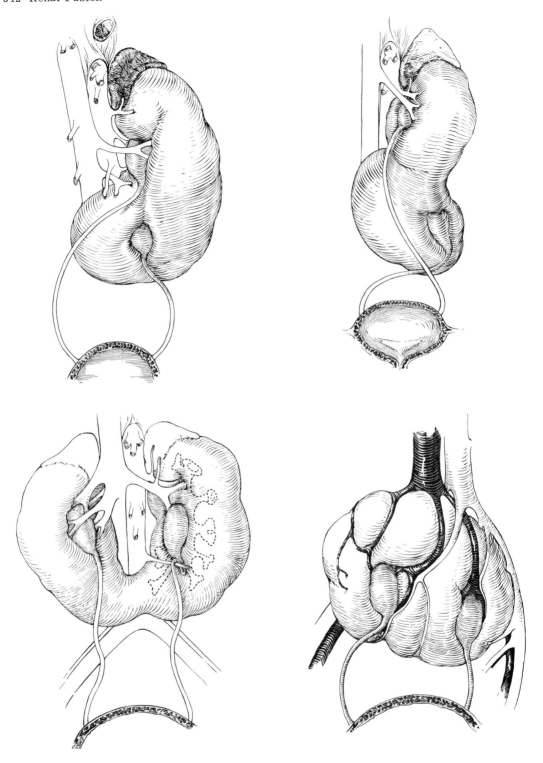

Fig 21-6. Renal fusion. Above left: Crossed renal ectopy with fusion. The renal mass lies in the left flank. The right ureter must cross over the midline. **Above right:** Example of "sigmoid" kidney. **Below left:** Horseshoe kidney. Pelves are anterior. Note aberrant artery obstructing left ureter; low position of renal mass. **Below right:** Pelvic "cake" kidney. Pelves are placed anteriorly. Note aberrant blood supply.

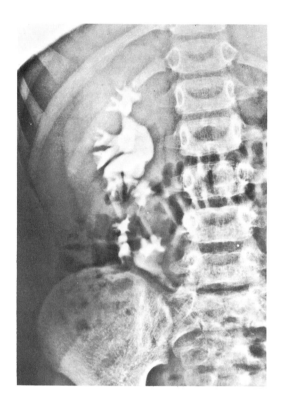

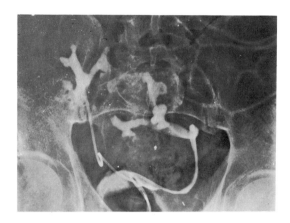

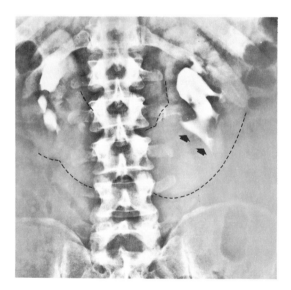

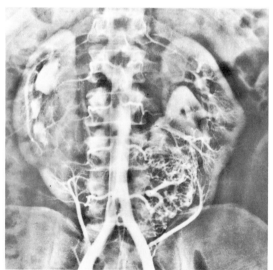

Fig 21-7. Renal fusion. Above left: Excretory urogram showing fused renal masses on the right side. Both kidneys are normal. Crossed renal ectopy. **Above right:** Retrograde urogram showing pelvic "cake" kidney. **Below left:** Excretory urogram showing horseshoe kidney with expansion of left side of isthmus and compression of lower left calyceal system. **Lower right:** Angiogram on same patient. Hypervascular mass in left side of isthmus typical of adenocarcinoma.

Pathology

Because the renal masses fuse early, normal rotation cannot occur; therefore, each pelvis lies on the anterior surface of its organ. Thus the ureter must ride over the isthmus of a horseshoe kidney or traverse the anterior surface of the fused kidney. Some degree of ureteral compression may arise from this or from obstruction by one or more aberrant blood vessels. The incidence of hydronephrosis and therefore infection is significant.

In horseshoe kidney the isthmus usually joins the lower poles of each kidney; each renal mass lies lower than normal. The axes of these masses are vertical, whereas the axes of normal kidneys are oblique to the spine since they lie along the edges of the psoas muscles.

On rare occasion the 2 nephric masses are fused into one mass ("cake kidney") containing 2 pelves and 2 ureters. The mass may lie in the midline (usually in the pelvis) or in one flank, in which case one ureter crosses the midline to open into the bladder at the proper point (crossed renal ectopy with fusion).

Clinical Findings

A. Symptoms: Most patients with fused kidneys have no symptoms. Some, however, develop ureteral obstruction. Gastrointestinal symptoms (reno-digestive reflex) mimicking peptic ulcer, cholelithiasis, or appendicitis may be noted. Infection is apt to occur if ureteral obstruction and hydronephrosis develop.

B. Signs: Physical examination is usually negative unless the abnormally placed renal mass can be felt. With horseshoe kidney it may be possible to palpate a mass over the lower lumbar spine (the isthmus). In the case of crossed ectopy, a mass may be felt in the flank.

C. Laboratory Findings: Urinalysis is normal unless there is infection. Renal function is normal unless disease coexists in each of the fused renal masses.

D. X-Ray Findings: In the case of horseshoe kidney the axes of the 2 kidneys, if visible on a plain film, are parallel to the spine. At times the isthmus can be identified. The plain film may also reveal a large soft tissue mass in one flank yet not show a renal shadow on the other side ("cake kidney"). (Fig 21-7.)

Excretory urograms establish the diagnosis if the renal parenchyma has maintained good function. The increased density of the kidney tissue may make its position or configuration more distinct. Urograms will also visualize the pelves and ureters.

1. With horseshoe kidney, the renal pelves usually lie on the anterior surfaces of their respective kidney masses, whereas the normal kidney has its pelvis lying mesial to it. The most valuable clue to the diagnosis of horseshoe kidney is the presence of calyces in the region of the lower pole which point medially and overlie the psoas muscles or even reach the vertebrae (Figs 21-6, 21-7).

2. Crossed renal ectopy with fusion shows 2 pelves and 2 ureters leading from it. One ureter must cross the midline in order to empty into the bladder at the proper point (Figs 21-6, 21-7).

3. A cake or lump kidney may lie in the pelvis (fused pelvis kidney), but again its ureters and pelves will be shown (Figs 21-6, 21-7).

Tomograms will clearly outline the renal mass but are seldom necessary.

With pelvic fused kidney or one lying in the flank, the plain film taken with ureteral catheters in place will give the first hint of the diagnosis. Retrograde urograms will show the position of the pelves and demonstrate changes compatible with infection or obstruction (Fig 21-8). Renal scanning will delineate the renal mass and its contour (see chapter 8).

Differential Diagnosis

Separate kidneys which fail to undergo the normal rotation may be confused with horseshoe kidney. They lie along the edges of the psoas muscles, whereas the poles of a horseshoe kidney lie parallel to the spine and their lower poles are placed on the psoas muscles. The calyces in the region of the isthmus of a horseshoe kidney point medially and lie close to the spine.

The diagnosis of cake or lump kidney may be missed on excretory urograms if one of its ureters is markedly obstructed so that a portion of the kidney and its pelvis and ureter fail to visualize. Catheterization of the ureters and retrograde urograms will demonstrate both excretory tracts in the renal mass.

Complications

Fused kidneys are prone to ureteral obstruction because of a high incidence of aberrant renal vessels and the necessity for one or both ureters to arch around or over the renal tissue. Hydronephrosis and infection therefore are common.

A large cake kidney occupying the concavity of the sacrum may cause dystocia.

Treatment

No treatment is necessary unless there is obstruction or infection. Drainage of a horseshoe kidney may be improved by dividing its isthmus. If one pole of a horseshoe is badly damaged it may require resection.

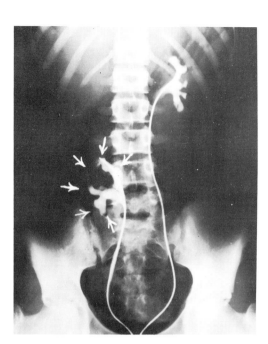 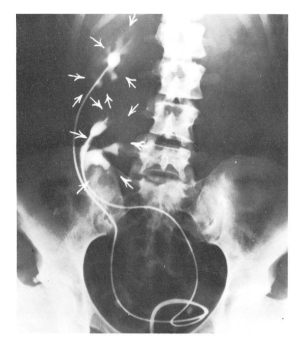

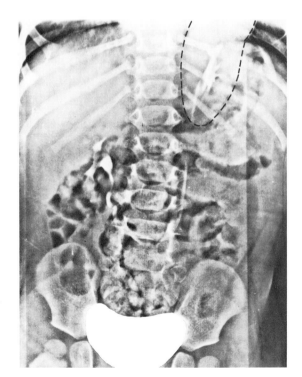

Fig 21-8. Renal ectopy. **Above left:** Retrograde urogram showing simple congenital ectopy.
Above right: Retrograde urogram showing crossed renal ectopy. In this film the differentiation
between fusion and nonfusion cannot be made. **Below:** Left kidney, ectopic in the chest.

Prognosis

In most cases, the outlook is excellent. Should ureteral obstruction and infection occur, renal drainage must be improved by surgical means so that antimicrobial therapy will be effective.

Blackard, C. E., & G. T. Mellinger: Cancer in a horseshoe kidney. Arch Surg **97**:616-27, 1968.

Dretler, S. P., Olsson, C., & R. C. Pfister: The anatomic, radiologic and clinical characteristics of the pelvic kidney: An analysis of 86 cases. J Urol **105**:623-7, 1971.

Dworin, J. W.: Crossed ectopia of a solitary kidney. J Urol **102**:289-90, 1969.

Grégoir, W.: Conservative surgery in horseshoe-kidney. Urol Internat **16**:129-38, 1963.

ECTOPIC KIDNEY

Congenital ectopic kidney usually excites no symptoms unless complications such as ureteral obstruction or infection develop.

Simple Ectopy

Simple congenital ectopy is a low kidney on the proper side which failed to ascend normally. It may lie over the pelvic brim or in the pelvis. (Rarely, it may be found in the chest.) It takes its blood supply from adjacent vessels, and its ureter is short. It is prone to ureteral obstruction and infection, which may lead to pain or fever. At times such a kidney may be palpable, leading to an erroneous presumptive diagnosis (eg, cancer of the bowel, appendiceal abscess).

Excretory or retrograde urograms (Fig 21-8) will reveal the true position. Hydronephrosis, if present, will be evident. There is no redundancy of the ureter, as is the case with nephroptosis or acquired ectopy (eg, displacement by large suprarenal tumor).

Obstruction and infection may complicate simple ectopy and should be treated by appropriate means.

Crossed Ectopy Without Fusion

In crossed ectopy without fusion the kidney lies on the opposite side of the body but is not attached to its normally placed mate. Unless 2 distinct renal shadows can be seen it may be difficult to differentiate this condition radiologically from crossed ectopy with fusion (Fig 21-6).

Arduino, L. J.: Crossed renal ectopia without fusion. J Urol **93**:125-6, 1965.

Burke, E. C., Wenzl, J. E., & D. C. Utz: The intrathoracic kidney. Am J Dis Child **113**:487-90, 1967.

Ward, J. N., Nathanson, B., & J. W. Draper: The pelvic kidney. J Urol **94**:36-9, 1965.

ABNORMAL ROTATION

Normally, when the kidney ascends to the lumbar region the pelvis lies on its anterior surface. Later, the pelvis comes to lie mesially. Such rotation may fail to occur, although this seldom leads to renal disease. Urography demonstrates the abnormal position.

MEDULLARY SPONGE KIDNEY
(Cystic Dilatation of the Renal Collecting Tubules)

Medullary sponge kidney is a congenital defect characterized by widening of the distal collecting tubules. It is usually bilateral, affecting all of the papillae, but it may be unilateral. At times, only one papilla is involved. Cystic dilatation of the tubules is often present also. Infection and calculi are occasionally seen as a result of urinary stasis in the tubules. Potter believes that medullary sponge kidney is related to polycystic renal disease. Its occasional association with hemihypertrophy of the body has been noted.

The only symptoms are those arising from infection and stone formation. The diagnosis is made on the basis of excretory urograms (Fig 21-9). The pelvis and calyces are normal, but dilated (streaked) tubules are seen just lateral to them; many of the dilated tubules contain round masses of radiopaque material (the cystic dilatation). If stones are present, a plain film will reveal small round calculi in the pyramidal regions just beyond the calyces. Retrograde urograms often do not reveal the lesion unless the mouths of the collecting ducts are widely dilated.

The differential diagnosis includes tuberculosis, healed papillary necrosis, and nephrocalcinosis. Tuberculosis is usually unilateral, and urography shows ulceration of calyces; tubercle bacilli are found on bacteriologic study. Papillary necrosis may be complicated by calcification in the healed stage, but may be distinguished by its typical calyceal deformity, the presence of infection, and, usually, impaired renal function (Fig 12-4). The tubular and parenchymal calcification seen in nephrocalcinosis is more diffuse than that seen with sponge kidney (Fig 15-12); the symp-

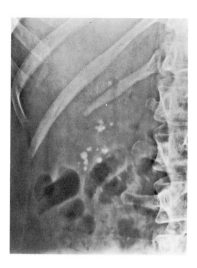 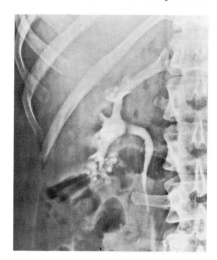

Fig 21-9. Medullary sponge kidneys. Left: Plain film of right kidney showing multiple small stones in its midportion. **Right:** Excretory urogram showing relationship of calculi to calyces. Typically, the calyces are large; the stones are located in the dilated collecting tubules.

toms and signs of primary hyperparathyroidism or renal tubular acidosis may be found.

There is no treatment for medullary sponge kidney. Therapy is directed toward the complications (eg, pyelonephritis and renal calculi). Only a small percentage of people with sponge kidney develop complications. The over-all prognosis is good. A few may pass small stones occasionally.

Goldman, S. H., & others: Hereditary occurrence of cystic disease of the renal medulla. New England J Med **274**:984-92, 1966.

Harrison, A. R., & J. P. Williams: Medullary sponge kidney and congenital hemihypertrophy. Brit J Urol **43**:552-61, 1971.

MacDougall, J. A., & W. G. Prout: Medullary sponge kidney. Brit J Surg **55**:130-3, 1968.

Potter, E. L., & V. Osathanondh: Medullary sponge kidney. Two cases in young infants. J Pediat **62**:901-7, 1963.

Pyrah, L. N.: Medullary sponge kidney. J Urol **95**:274-83, 1966.

ABNORMALITIES OF RENAL VESSELS

As a rule, each kidney receives one renal artery from the aorta and has one vein passing to the vena cava. Aberrant veins and especially arteries are common. Three or 4 renal arteries may be depicted on angiography. An aberrant artery passing to the lower pole of the kidney may compress and thereby obstruct the ureter, causing hydronephrosis. On urography

it is impossible to differentiate between an obstructing vessel and an intrinsic ureteral stenosis. The final diagnosis is made at the operating table.

ACQUIRED LESIONS OF THE KIDNEYS

RENO-ALIMENTARY FISTULA

Over 100 instances of reno-alimentary fistula have been reported. They usually involve the stomach, duodenum, or adjacent colon, although fistula formation with the esophagus, small bowel, appendix, and rectum has been reported.

The underlying cause is usually a pyonephrotic kidney which becomes adherent to a portion of the alimentary tract and then ruptures spontaneously, thus creating a fistula (Fig 21-10). The patient is therefore apt to suffer symptoms and signs of acute pyelonephritis. Urography may show radiopaque material escaping into the gastrointestinal tract. Gastrointestinal series may also reveal the connection with the kidney. The treatment is nephrectomy with closure of the opening into the gut.

Arthur, G. W., & D. G. Morris: Reno-alimentary fistulae. Brit J Surg **53**:396-402, 1966.

Baird, J. M., & H. M. Spence: Ingested foreign bodies migrating to the kidney from the

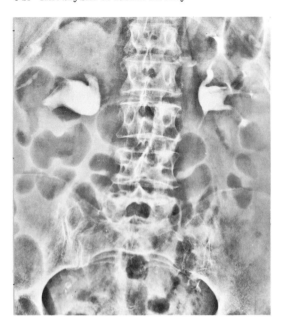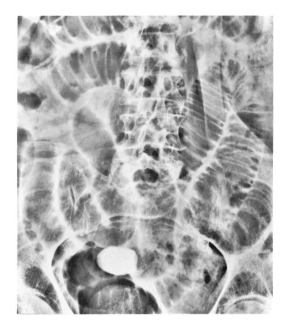

Fig 21-10. Nephroduodenal fistula and small bowel obstruction from renal staghorn calculus.
Left: Excretory urogram showing nonfunction of right kidney; staghorn stone. **Right:** Patient presented with symptoms and signs of bowel obstruction 4 years later. KUB showing dilated loops of small bowel down to a point just proximal to ileocecal valve. Obstruction due to stone which was extruded into duodenum. (Courtesy of C. D. King, MD.)

gastrointestinal tract. J Urol **99**:675-80, 1968.

Brown, R. B.: Spontaneous nephrocolic fistula. Brit J Urol **38**:488-91, 1966.

Ehrenfeld, W. K., & others: Cutaneous nephrogastric fistula: case report. J Urol **97**: 33-5, 1967.

Schwartz, D. T., & others: Pyeloduodenal fistula due to tuberculosis. J Urol **104**:373-5, 1970.

Shukri, A. M.: Reno-alimentary fistulae. Brit J Surg **55**:551-4, 1968.

Wise, H. M., Jr., & T. Shimada: Pyeloduodenal fistula: a case report. J Urol **97**: 987-9, 1967.

Yue, K. P., & H. W. Johnson: Foreign body in the kidney: Transintestinal migration. J Urol **98**:172-4, 1967.

ANEURYSM OF THE RENAL ARTERY

Aneurysm of the renal artery is rare. It usually results from degenerative arterial disease which weakens the wall of the artery so that intravascular pressure may balloon it out. It is most commonly caused by arteriosclero-sis or periarteritis nodosa, but it may develop secondary to trauma or syphilis. Congenital aneurysm has been reported.

Aneurysmal dilatation has no deleterious effect upon the kidney unless the mass compresses the renal artery, in which case some renal ischemia and therefore atrophy is to be expected. A true aneurysm may rupture, thus producing a false aneurysm. The extravasated blood occupying the retroperitoneal space finally becomes encapsulated by a fibrous covering as organization occurs. An aneurysm may involve a small artery within the renal parenchyma. It may rupture into the renal pelvis or a calyx.

Most aneurysms cause no symptoms unless they rupture, in which case there may be severe flank pain and even shock. If an aneurysm ruptures into the renal pelvis, marked hematuria occurs. The common cause of death is severe hemorrhage from rupture of the aneurysm. Hypertension is not usually present. A bruit should be sought over the costovertebral angle or over the renal artery anteriorly. If spontaneous or traumatic rupture has occurred, a mass may be palpated in the flank.

A plain film of the abdomen may show a ring-like calcification (Fig 21-11), either

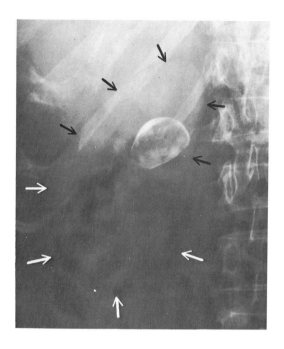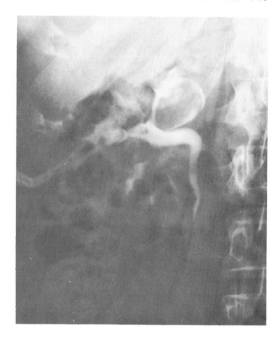

Fig 21-11. Intrarenal aneurysm of renal artery. Left: Plain film showing calcified structure over right renal shadow. **Right:** Excretory urogram which relates calcific mass to pelvis and upper calyx. (Courtesy of C. D. King, MD.)

intra- or extrarenal. Urograms may be normal, or reveal renal atrophy. Some impairment of renal function may be noted if compression or partial obstruction of the renal artery has developed. Aortography will delineate the aneurysm. The renal scan may show changes compatible with a renovascular lesion.

The differential diagnosis of rupture of an aneurysm and injury to the kidney is difficult unless a history or evidence of trauma is obtained. A hydronephrotic kidney may present a mass, but urography will clarify the issue.

Since the incidence of spontaneous rupture of noncalcified and large calcified aneurysms is significant, the presence of such a lesion is an indication for surgical intervention. The repair of extrarenal aneurysms may be considered, but complications (eg, thrombosis) are not uncommon. If an intrarenal aneurysm is situated in one pole, heminephrectomy may be feasible. If, however, it is in the center of the organ, nephrectomy will be required. Those few patients found to have hypertension may become normotensive following definitive surgery.

Cerny, J. C., Chang, Cheng-Yang, & W. J. Fry: Renal artery aneurisms. Arch Surg **96**:653-62, 1968.

Glass, P. M., & A. C. Uson: Aneurisms of the renal artery: A study of 20 cases. J Urol **98**:285-92, 1967.

Hogbin, B. M., & C. G. Scorer: Spontaneous rupture of an aneurism of the renal artery with survival. Brit J Urol **41**:218-21, 1969.

McClure, P. H., & J. L. Westcott: Periarteritis nodosa with perirenal hemorrhage: A case report with angiographic findings. J Urol **102**:126-9, 1969.

Poutasse, E. F.: Renal artery aneurisms: Their natural history and surgery. J Urol **95**:297-306, 1966.

Smith, J. N., & F. Hinman, Jr.: Intrarenal arterial aneurisms. J Urol **97**:990-6, 1967.

RENAL INFARCTS

Renal infarcts are caused by arterial occlusion. The major causes are subacute bacterial endocarditis, atrial or ventricular thrombi, arteriosclerosis, polyarteritis nodosa, and trauma. A thrombotic process in the abdominal aorta may gradually extend upward to occlude the renal artery.

If smaller arteries or arterioles become obstructed, the tissue receiving blood from such a vessel will first become swollen and then undergo necrosis and fibrosis. Multiple infarcts are the rule. Should the main renal artery become occluded, the entire kidney will react in kind. The kidney may therefore become functionless and atrophic as it undergoes necrosis and fibrosis.

Partial renal infarct is usually a silent disease. Sudden and complete infarction may cause renal pain and at times gross or microscopic hematuria. Tenderness over the flank may then be elicited. The kidney is not significantly enlarged by arterial occlusion. Serum glutamic oxaloacetic transaminase will be elevated for 1 or 2 days after the incident.

Excretory urograms may fail to visualize a portion of the kidney with partial infarction; with complete infarction, none of the radiopaque fluid is excreted. In this instance, retrograde urography will reveal no obstruction and, in fact, ureteropyelograms will be normal, but no urine will drain from the ureteral catheter; there is no function. Even though complete loss of measurable function has occurred, renal circulation may be restored spontaneously in some instances.

Renal angiography makes the definitive diagnosis. A rectilinear scan may reveal no tubular function in a kidney of normal size. Lack of tracer activity may be noted in one pole if a segmental artery becomes occluded. A dynamic technetium scan will reveal no perfusion of the affected renal vasculature.

During the acute phase, infarction may mimic ureteral stone. With stone the excretory urogram may also show lack of renal function, but even so there is usually enough of the medium in the tubules so that a "nephrogram" is obtained (Fig 15-8). This will not occur with complete infarction. Evidence of a cardiac or vascular lesion is helpful in arriving at a proper diagnosis.

The complications are related to those arising from the primary cardiovascular disease. In a few cases, hypertension may develop a few days or weeks after the infarction. It may later subside.

If the diagnosis of thrombosis or embolism of the renal artery is made promptly, embolectomy should be considered. If not, anticoagulants must be used as a means of preventing further thrombotic accidents; such treatment has a good chance of contributing to the return of some renal function. Should permanent hypertension ensue in a patient with partial occlusion of the renal artery, renal endarterectomy or nephrectomy may cure the hypertension.

Fergus, J. N., Jones, N. F., & M. L. Thomas: Kidney function after arterial embolism. Brit MJ **4**:587-90, 1969.

Goldsmith, E. I., & others: Embolectomy of the renal artery. J Urol **99**:366-70, 1968.

Grablowsky, O. M., & others: Renal artery thrombosis following blunt trauma: Report of four cases. Surgery **67**:895-900, 1970.

Lang, E. K., Mertz, J. H. O., & M. Nourse: Renal arteriography in the assessment of renal infarction. J Urol **99**:506-12, 1968.

Parker, J. M., & J. D. Lord: Renal artery embolism: A case report with return of complete function of the involved kidney following anticoagulant therapy. J Urol **106**: 339-41, 1971.

Peterson, N. E., & D. F. McDonald: Renal embolization. J Urol **100**:140-5, 1968.

Ranniger, K., Abrams, E., & T. A. Borden: Pseudotumor resulting from a fresh renal infarct. Radiology **92**:343-4, 1969.

THROMBOSIS OF THE RENAL VEIN

Thrombosis of the renal vein is rare in the adult. It may develop secondary to various inflammatory lesions, including intrarenal or perirenal suppuration, or from ascending thrombosis of the vena cava associated with phlebothrombosis, or disseminated malignant disease. Thrombosis of the renal vein may occur as a complication of ileocolitis of infancy. The thrombosis may extend from the vena cava into the peripheral venules or may originate in the peripheral veins and propagate to the main renal vein. The severe passive congestion which develops causes the kidney to swell and to become engorged. Degeneration of the nephrons ensues. Pain in the flank is usually experienced, and symptoms and signs of sepsis are occasionally seen. Hematuria may be noted. A large tender mass is often felt in the flank. The blood count may reveal changes compatible with sepsis. Thrombocytopenia may be noted. The urine contains albumin, red cells, and frequently pus cells and bacteria. Urograms show poor or absent secretion of the radiopaque material in a large kidney. Stretching and thinning of the calyceal infundibula may be noted. Clots in the pelvis may cause filling defects. Later the kidney may undergo atrophy. The typical picture of the nephrotic syndrome develops in many of these patients.

Renal angiography reveals stretching and bowing of small arterioles. In the nephrographic phase, the pyramids may become quite dense. Venacavagraphy or, preferably, selective renal venography will demonstrate the thrombus in the renal vein (Fig 21-12) and, at times, in the vena cava.

The symptoms and signs may suggest acute renal infection or obstruction from a ureteral calculus. Acute pyelonephritis will cause the greatest difficulty in differential diagnosis, since the complaints and physical findings in the 2 diseases are similar. Excretory urography will prove helpful, for simple pyelonephritis will not appreciably depress renal function and there are no significant changes in the calyceal pattern. The presence of a stone in the ureter should be obvious; some degree of dilatation of the ureter and pelvis should then also be expected.

If the diagnosis of unilateral infected renal venous thrombosis can be established, immediate nephrectomy should be considered. Although this disease is a rare complication of thrombophlebitis of the iliac veins or vena cava, modern treatment of the latter by early vein ligation or the use of anticoagulants may be expected to prevent propagation of the thrombosis. A few cases of successful thrombectomy have been reported. This appears to lead to some improvement in renal function. If nephrotic syndrome develops, appropriate treatment is indicated.

Prognosis is poor if bilateral renal vein thrombosis occurs. The outlook in the unilateral type is good if the primary cause can be controlled.

Alexander, F., & W. A. B. Campbell: Congenital nephrotic syndrome and renal vein thrombosis in infancy. J Clin Path 24:27-40, 1971.

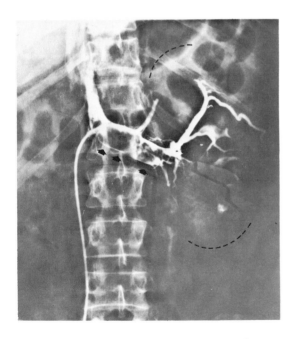

Fig 21-12. Thrombosis of renal vein. Selective left renal venogram showing almost complete occlusion of vein. Veins to lower pole failed to fill. Note large size of kidney.

Belman, A. B., & others: Nonoperative treatment of unilateral renal vein thrombosis in the newborn. JAMA 211:1165-8, 1970.

Cohn, L. H., & others: The treatment of bilateral renal vein thrombosis and nephrotic syndrome. Surgery 64:387-96, 1968.

Fein, R. L., Chait, A., & A. Leviton: Renal vein thrombectomy for the treatment of renal vein thrombosis associated with the nephrotic syndrome. J Urol 99:1-12, 1968.

Mauer, S. M., & others: Bilateral renal vein thrombosis in infancy: Report of a survivor following surgical intervention. J Pediat 78:509-12, 1971.

Rosenmann, E., Pollak, V. E., & C. L. Pirani: Renal vein thrombosis in the adult: a clinical and pathologic study based on renal biopsies. Medicine 47:269-335, 1968.

Taylor, L.: Renal vein thrombosis in malignant disease. Arch Int Med 111:449-51, 1963.

Wegner, G. P., & others: Renal vein thrombosis. A roentgenographic diagnosis. JAMA 209:1661-7, 1969.

ARTERIOVENOUS FISTULA

Arteriovenous fistula may be congenital or acquired. A number of these fistulas have been reported following renal needle biopsy and as a complication of ligation of the renal pedicle in nephrectomy. A few have been recognized in association with adenocarcinoma of one kidney.

A thrill can often be palpated and a murmur heard both anteriorly and posteriorly. In cases with a wide communication, the systolic blood pressure is elevated and a widened pulse pressure is noted. Renal angiography establishes the diagnosis. Surgical repair is indicated, but nephrectomy is often necessary. Those that develop secondary to renal biopsy tend to seal spontaneously.

DeWeerd, J. H.: Arteriovenous fistula in hypernephroma. J Urol 93:666-8, 1965.

Ekelund, L., & T. Lindholm: Arteriovenous fistulae following percutaneous renal biopsy. Acta radiol (diag) 11:38-48, 1971.

Gold, D., Latts, E. M., & H. M. Wexler: Congenital arteriovenous fistulae of kidney. Arch Int Med 115:208-13, 1965.

Goldstein, A. G., Delaurentis, D. A., & A. J. Schwartz: Post-nephrectomy arteriovenous fistula. J Urol 98:44-7, 1967.

Riba, L. W., & M. P. Simon: Intrarenal arteriovenous fistula treated with partial nephrectomy. J Urol 98:293-5, 1967.

Tunner, W. S. , & others: Repair of an intrarenal arteriovenous fistula with preservation of the kidney. J Urol **103**:286-9, 1970.

Tynes, W. V. , & others: Surgical treatment of
renal arteriovenous fistulas: Report of 5
cases. J Urol **103**:692-8, 1970.

RENAL CORTICAL NECROSIS

Acute necrosis of the renal cortex is, with
few exceptions, a complication of severe hemorrhage often occurring secondary to premature
separation of the placenta occurring in the third
trimester of pregnancy. The entire cortex of
each kidney commonly exhibits coagulation necrosis. The cause is thought to be spasm of
the glomerular afferent arteries and disseminated intravascular coagulation. Microscopically, the glomeruli and proximal convoluted
tubules are necrotic. The medulla is intact.
After a few weeks peripheral cortical calcification is noted. It may be seen on lamino-
grams.

The onset is usually characterized by
sudden severe abdominal pain secondary to
severe uterine hemorrhage. Oliguria develops
promptly and leads to progressive uremia.
(For a discussion of the differential diagnosis
and treatment of oliguria, see p 296.)

Blood loss must be promptly replaced.
Hyperkalemia may require dialysis. The use
of ganglionic blocking agents, eg, trimethaphan
(Arfonad®), may relieve the cortical ischemia.

The prognosis depends upon the degree of
renal damage. In many cases the renal lesion
is irreversible. In most patients who recover,
some degree of permanent renal damage is
evident.

Carter, B. : Premature separation of the normally implanted placenta. Six deaths due
to gross bilateral cortical necrosis of the
kidneys. Obst Gynec **29**:30-3, 1967.

Cramer, G. G. , & J. R. Fuglestad: Cortical
calcification in renal cortical necrosis.
Am J Roentgenol **95**:344-8, 1965.

Effersøe, P. , Raaschou, F. , & A. C. Thomsen:
Bilateral renal cortical necrosis. Am J
Med **33**:455-8, 1962.

Leonidas, J. C. , Berdon, W. E. , & D. Gribetz:
Bilateral renal cortical necrosis in the new-
born infant: Roentgenographic diagnosis.
J Pediat **79**:623-7, 1971.

Tessler, A. N. , & R. S. Hotchkiss: Renal cortical necrosis. J Urol **85**:471-5, 1961.

• • •

22...

Disorders of the Ureters

CONGENITAL ANOMALIES OF THE URETER

Congenital ureteral anomalies are common. Since most of them cause obstruction to or stasis of urine, hydronephrosis with secondary renal infection is a common sequel.

INCOMPLETE URETER

The ureter may be entirely absent or may extend from the bladder only part way to the renal area. Either the ureteral bud fails to develop from the urogenital segment during embryologic development, or it is arrested in its development before it reaches the kidney. Absence of the kidney or multicystic renal disease is to be expected.

DUPLICATION OF THE URETER

Complete or incomplete duplication of the ureter is one of the most common congenital ureteral anomalies. Familial inheritance has been noted. The incomplete (**Y**) type (Fig 22-1) is more common than 2 complete ureters on one side (Figs 22-1, 22-3). The condition may be bilateral. Duplication presupposes 2 renal pelves in the renal mass. Most cases occur in females. An instance of 5 ureters on one side has been reported.

These abnormalities usually cause no difficulty; in the **Y** type, however, obstruction at the point where the 2 ureters join may be observed. One segment may become dilated because of retrograde flow (reflux) from one ureter into the other.

In complete duplication, the ureter from the upper pole opens at a point closest to the bladder neck. It follows that the ureter to the major lower pole has a relatively short intravesical ureteral segment. Thus, vesicoureteral reflux to the lower portion of the kidney

may be seen (Fig 11-4). Most ureteroceles in children involve the ureter which drains the upper portion of the duplicated kidney. The ureter to the upper renal pole may open ectopically into the vulva, urethra, or seminal vesicle (Fig 22-3). Such ureters are always obstructed to some degree (Figs 22-1, 22-8).

Duplication of the ureter is clinically significant only when obstruction or reflux is present, in which case dilatation and tortuosity of the ureter and hydronephrosis are found (Fig 22-1).

The symptoms and signs are those of persistent or recurrent infection. Urologic investigation (urograms) will reveal the congenital abnormality. If complete hydronephrotic atrophy of one renal pole has occurred, excretory urograms may show only one normal pelvis and ureter (Fig 22-4). The clue to duplication will be the observation that the visualized pelvis and calyces fail to drain a relatively large area of the renal shadow. The visualized ureter may be displaced by its dilated obstructed mate.

If the anomaly causes obstruction or reflux, surgical repair should be attempted if at all practicable. It may be necessary to resect the hydronephrotic pole of the kidney. Nephrectomy may be indicated if renal damage is severe.

Amar, A. D.: Lateral ureteral displacement: Sign of non-visualized duplication. J Urol **105**:638-41, 1971.

Amar, A. D., & K. Chabra: Reflux in duplicated ureters: Treatment in children. J Pediat Surg **5**:419-30, 1970.

Diaz-Ball, F. L., & others: Pyeloureterostomy and ureteroureterostomy: Alternative procedures to partial nephrectomy for duplication of the ureter with only one pathological segment. J Urol **102**:621-6, 1969.

Lundin, E., & W. Riggs: Upper urinary tract duplication associated with ectopic ureterocele in childhood and infancy. Acta radiol (diag) **7**:13-24, 1968.

Parker, R. M., Pohl, D. R., & J. R. Robison: Ureteral triplication with ectopia. J Urol **103**:727-31, 1970.

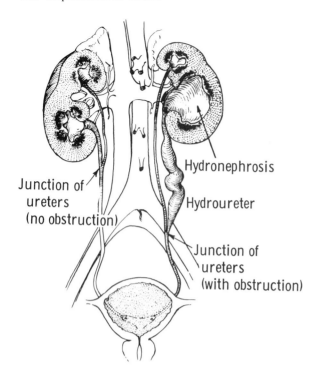

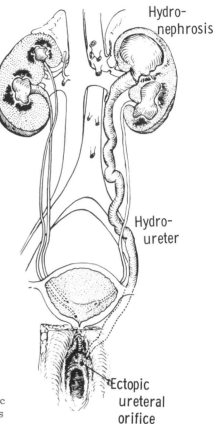

Fig 22-1. Duplication of ureters. Left: Incomplete Y type with hydroureteronephrosis on left. Right: Complete duplication with obstruction to one ureter with ectopic orifice on left. The ureter with the ectopic opening always drains the upper pole of the kidney.

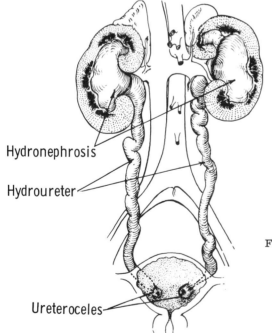

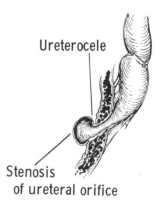

Fig 22-2. Ureterocele. Left: Obstructing ureteroceles (adult type) with hydroureteronephrosis. Above: Sagittal section through ureterocele and ureter to show pathologic changes. Resection of this ureterocele will be followed by vesicoureteral reflux.

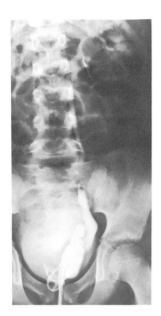
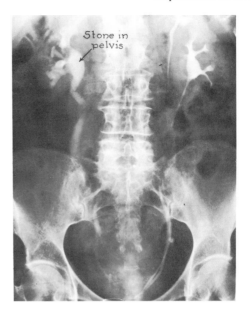

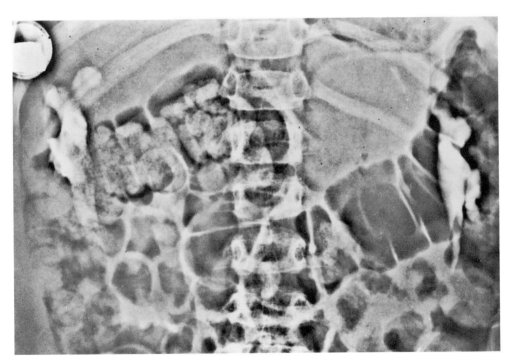

Fig 22-3. **Duplication of ureters.** **Above left:** Ureteral catheters passed through opening in region of verumontanum. Injection of radiopaque fluid reveals duplicated ureter to upper renal pole joining seminal vesicle (ectopic ureteral ostium). Second ureter not shown. **Above right:** Excretory urogram showing complete duplication of left ureters and renal pelves, which are otherwise normal. Staghorn calculus in right kidney; dilatation of upper ureter suggests possibility of presence of stone in lower portion of right ureter. **Below:** Excretory urogram showing marked displacement of visualized renal masses by giant functionless hydronephroses of upper renal segments. Ureters to upper poles opened into prostatic urethra.

Peterson, C., Jr., & M. L. Silbiger: Five ureters: A case report. J Urol **100**:160-2, 1968.

Whitaker, J., & D. M. Danks: A study of the inheritance of duplication of the kidneys and ureters. J Urol **95**:176-8, 1966.

URETEROCELE

A ureterocele is a ballooning of the submucosal ureter into the bladder, secondary probably to congenital stenosis of the epithelial lining at the vesical end of the ureter; thus the urine cannot easily escape into the bladder. The pressure produced by ureteral peristalsis pushes the periureteral vesical mucosa into the bladder, causing a cystic protrusion. This urine-filled cyst is covered by vesical mucosa on the outside and lined by ureteral mucosa internally (Fig 22-2). Its complications, basically caused by the obstruction, are hydroureter, hydronephrosis, and upper tract infection. Stones may develop in the cyst. If large enough, ureterocele may cause bladder neck obstruction (ectopic ureterocele) and may even prolapse through the female urethra.

Ureterocele is most commonly encountered in little girls and usually involves the ureter which drains the upper pole of a duplicated kidney (Figs 11-4 and 22-4). Ureteroceles in adults tend to be bilateral, and are smaller and less obstructive than those seen in children.

The history and physical signs are compatible with ureteral obstruction or urinary tract infection. A history of an obstructed urinary stream, even incontinence, may be elicited if the ureterocele impinges on the bladder neck. Pyuria and bacteriuria may be present. Total renal function is normal unless both kidneys are affected. Excretory urograms may show cystic dilatation of the lower end of the ureter (Fig 22-4, left) or a round space-occupying lesion in a cystogram. Some changes from back pressure above this point are to be expected (eg, hydroureter, hydronephrosis, changes due to infection). A cystogram may reveal reflux into the lower renal pole.

Catheterization of the pinpoint ureteral opening may be impossible, but it is helpful in establishing the presence of infection in the

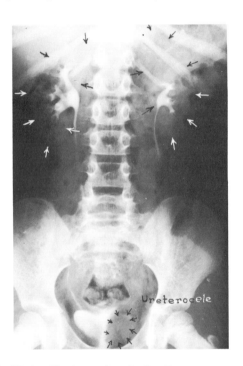
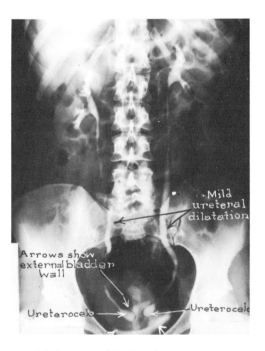

Fig 22-4. Ureterocele. Left: Excretory urogram in a girl 8 years old, showing a space-occupying lesion on the left side of the bladder caused by ureterocele. Absence of calyceal system in the upper portion of the left kidney implies duplication of the ureters and pelves and nonfunction (advanced hydronephrosis) of the upper pole; its dilated ureter drains into the obstructing ureterocele and displaces the visualized ureter laterally just below the kidney. **Right:** Excretory urogram in an adult female, showing "cobra head" deformity of the distal ends of both ureters; bilateral ureteroceles causing minimal obstruction; pressure on bladder from uterus. No treatment is indicated.

kidney. If poor renal function has precluded adequate secretion of opaque material given intravenously, retrograde urography should be attempted.

The small, mildly obstructive ureterocele can usually be destroyed transurethrally. In children it may be necessary to open the bladder suprapubically so that the cyst can be resected. This may be followed, however, by vesicoureteral reflux because the obstruction has caused wide dilatation of the ureteral hiatus, thus shortening the intravesical ureter (Fig 11-4). At times, the obstructing ureterocele may so dilate the intramural ureter that reflux up the noninvolved ureter may occur. Excision of the cystic structure combined with simultaneous vesicoureteroplasty should, therefore, probably be done. Removal of this obstruction will usually cause the pathologic changes of the ureter and kidney to regress. Secondary infection can then more readily be controlled or cured. Reimplantation of both ureters as one unit should be done. If the affected portion of a duplicated kidney is destroyed, heminephrectomy and complete ureterectomy are indicated.

Berdon, W. E., & others: Ectopic ureterocele. Radiol Clin North America 6:205-14, 1968.
Clark, C. W., & G. W. Leadbetter, Jr.: General treatment, mistreatment and compli-cations of ureteroceles. J Urol 106:518-20, 1971.
Johnston, J. H., & L. M. Johnson: Experiences with ectopic ureteroceles. Brit J Urol 41: 61-70, 1969.
Leadbetter, G. W.: Ectopic ureterocele as a cause of urinary incontinence. J Urol 103: 223-6, 1970.
Royle, M. C., & W. E. Goodwin: The management of ureteroceles. J Urol 106:42-7, 1971.
Stephens, F. D.: Caecoureterocele and concepts on the embryology and aetiology of ureteroceles. Aust New Zeal J Surg 40: 239-48, 1971.
Williams, D. I., & M. Royle: Ectopic ureter in the male child. Brit J Urol 41:421-7, 1969.

POSTCAVAL URETER

The rare postcaval or retrocaval ureter is one which (from above downward) passes medially and behind the vena cava, turns forward along the great vein's left wall, and then passes laterally on the anterior surface of the vena cava and resumes its normal course to the bladder. It actually "hooks" around the cava.

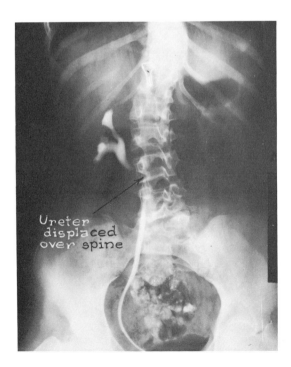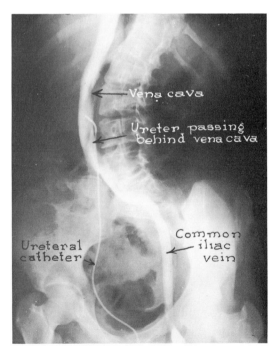

Fig 22-5. Postcaval ureter. Left: Retrograde ureteropyelogram showing upper ureter displaced onto the vertebral bodies, suggesting postcaval ureter. Note the congenital deformity of the spine. **Right:** Femoral venacavagram (right oblique view) showing ureter in retrocaval position.

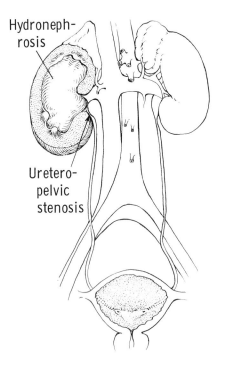

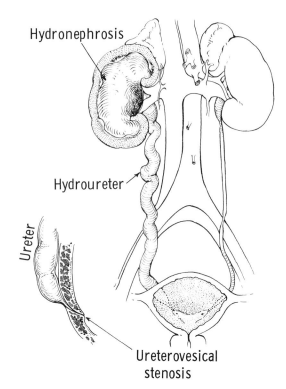

Fig 22-6. Congenital ureteral obstruction. Left: Right ureteropelvic stenosis with hydronephrosis. **Right:** Ureterovesical obstruction with hydroureteronephrosis. The common causes are (1) reflux, (2) hypertrophy of the ureterotrigonal complex secondary to distal obstruction, and (3) hypertrophy of the circular musculature of the juxtavesical ureter (Tanagho).

This anomalous position is due to an abnormal development of the vena cava.

The significance of postcaval ureter lies in the ureteral obstruction which is usually caused by the cava. This leads to hydronephrosis and, at times, infection. A catheter passed up such a ureter will take a course, in its midportion, overlying the spine. A ureterogram will show this defect graphically. A simultaneous femoral venogram will relate the vena cava to the ureter (Fig 22-5).

Division of the ureter where it courses around the cava, with end-to-end anastomosis in the normal position, relieves the obstruction. It has also been recommended that the vena cava be divided, the ureter replaced in its normal position, and the vena cava then repaired. Nephrectomy may be necessary if secondary renal damage is advanced.

Hyams, B. B., Schneiderman, C., & A. B. Mayman: Retrocaval ureter. Canad MAJ **98**:45-9, 1968.

Shown, T. E., & C. A. Moore: Retrocaval ureter: 4 cases. J Urol **105**:497-501, 1971.

STRICTURE OF THE URETER

Evidence of obstruction at the ureteropelvic or ureterovesical junction has heretofore been interpreted as stricture. It is now clear that most cases of the latter type really represent changes secondary to ureterovesical reflux (Fig 22-6). Some ureteropelvic obstructions also develop as a complication of reflux. A similar picture develops secondary to hypertrophy of the trigone which arises in association with distal obstruction. Creevy has observed what he calls achalasia of the lower ureteral segment which produces a functional obstruction. Tanagho & others find that this obstruction is caused by congenital hypertrophy of the circular smooth musculature of the juxtavesical ureter.

Symptoms are often absent, for many of these strictures are so mild that sudden renal capsular distention does not take place even though the kidney is completely destroyed by hydronephrotic atrophy. Some patients, however, may have costovertebral angle pain from the obstruction; others may complain only of reflex gastrointestinal complaints; and some have both. Ureteral stricture not uncommonly simulates appendicitis. Symptoms of infection may be elicited. It should be remembered, however, that chronic pyelonephritis may cause no symptoms.

Physical examination may reveal nothing unless the hydronephrotic kidney is large and tense and can be felt or percussed. Tenderness may be present with complicating renal infection. Urinalysis may provide evidence of urinary infection. Renal function will be normal unless there is bilateral renal disease.

A plain film of the abdomen may reveal an enlarged renal shadow. Excretory urograms will demonstrate dilatation of the excretory tract above the site of constant narrowing (Fig 22-7); one must not be confused by "pseudo-strictures," which represent normal systolic ureteral contraction. Advanced renal damage may cause lack of excretion of the radiopaque medium. A voiding cystourethrogram may reveal ureterovesical reflux.

Retrograde passage of a ureteral catheter may be arrested by a severe stricture. It may, however, pass through the site of obstruction, only to be stopped by the acute ureteral angulations proximal to the stricture. On the other hand, an area of functional obstruction may accept a large catheter easily although stasis persists. Retrograde ureteropyelograms will furnish a graphic picture of the obstruction and the changes secondary to it.

Little significance should be attached to the ease of passage of various sizes of catheters in the diagnosis of stricture. Unjustified diagnoses of stricture have also been made by passing a catheter with a fusiform bulge at its tip up the ureter. On withdrawal, a "hang" or sudden resistance to withdrawal is sometimes mistaken for evidence of stricture. It should be pointed out that it is the nature of the ureter to go into spasm even on being touched lightly during surgery. The diagnosis of true stricture is made on urographic study, preferably by the "nontraumatic" intravenous type. The point of narrowing should show in every film, and dilatation above this point should be noted.

Repair of the stricture is usually indicated if the kidney retains some degree of function. Severe renal damage is treated by nephrectomy. Should the changes be secondary to vesicoureteral reflux or hypertrophy of the juxtavesical ureter, repair of this junction may be indicated.

Allen, T. D.: Congenital ureteral strictures. J Urol **104**:196-204, 1970.

Tanagho, E. A., Smith, D. R., & T. H. Guthrie: Pathophysiology of functional ureteral obstruction. J Urol **104**:73-88, 1970.

ECTOPIC URETERAL ORIFICE

In rare instances the ureter opens at a point other than the lateral horn of the interureteric ridge. If it drains distal to the external sphincter, a constant dripping (incontinence) of urine is noted. Ectopy results from an abnormality of embryologic development (see chapter 2). The wolffian duct arises from the cloaca and acts as the drainage tube for the pronephros (primitive kidney) and the mesonephros. From this duct, at a point near the cloaca (which divides to form the rectum and lower urinary tract), the ureteral bud develops, then extends to and joins the metanephros. This junction forms the permanent kidney. As development progresses, the ureteral opening in the wolffian duct gradually moves caudally until the wolffian and ureteral ducts have separate openings in the urethrovesical area. Normally in the male the wolffian ducts form the vasa deferentia and seminal vesicles. Their cranial ends drain the spermatogenic tubules of the testes. In the female, the superior portion atrophies and the caudal portion becomes Gartner's duct.

If abnormalities of development occur, the ureter may enter the urinary tract at a position below the normal point. In the male, its orifice may be found in the posterior urethra; in the female, just outside the bladder neck.

Should the ureteral orifice not disengage itself from the proximal end of the wolffian duct (Fig 22-3), it is obvious that in the male the ureter will drain into the seminal tract (eg, seminal vesicle, vas deferens). In the female it will drain into the remnants of Gartner's duct. In this instance urine will empty into the vagina, cervix, uterus, or the vaginal vestibule. The latter is the most common site (Figs 22-1, 22-8). Most ectopic orifices are seen in the female.

Most ureters with ectopic openings are one of a pair to a single kidney, and the ectopic ureter almost always drains the rudimentary upper renal pole. Since ureters which open in abnormal positions are usually obstructed at their terminations, hydroureter and hydronephrosis develop. Secondary infection is common. Those ureters opening in the proximal urethra usually reveal vesicoureteral reflux on cystography.

In the male, since all ectopic orifices are proximal to the external sphincter, no incontinence ensues. In the female, vaginal or vestibular ureters are devoid of sphincteric control, and a constant drainage of urine occurs in spite of normal voiding.

Symptoms therefore depend upon the site of the opening. If proximal to the sphincter, there may be flank pain, fever, and vesical

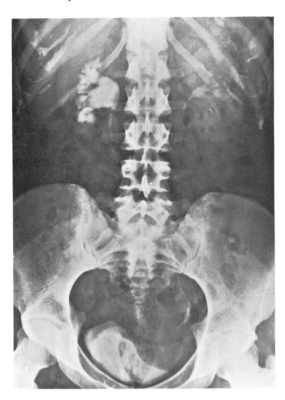
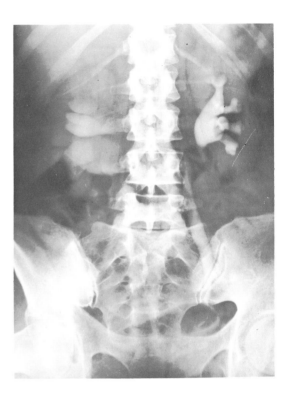

Fig 22-7. Ureteral obstruction. Left: Right ureteropelvic stenosis with mild hydronephrosis due to aberrant blood vessel. Pressure defect of left side of bladder from uterus. **Right:** Excretory urogram taken 2 weeks after Wertheim operation showing bilateral ureteral obstruction and advanced hydronephrosis on right.

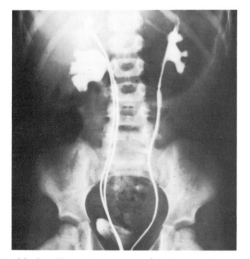
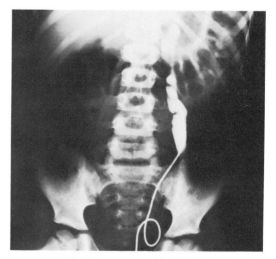

Fig 22-8. Ectopic ureter. (Girl, age 6, complained of partial urinary incontinence.) **Left:** Cystoscopy revealed 2 ureteral orifices on right, one on left; these were catheterized and urograms made. **Right:** Same patient. Ectopic ureteral orifice near urethral meatus catheterized. Retrograde urogram demonstrates second left hydronephrotic renal pelvis. Resection of upper pole and ureter cured incontinence.

irritability. If the opening is without sphincteric control, "incontinence" is the complaint. Symptoms of renal infection and pain may also be experienced. In the female, careful inspection of the vestibule or anterior vaginal wall may reveal an orifice from which urine or purulent material may drain. Renal tenderness or enlargement may be present. Epididymitis is a common complication when the ureter drains into the seminal vesicle.

The urine may be infected. Excretory urograms will usually show duplication of the renal pelves with hydronephrosis of the upper pole whose ureter may be markedly dilated and tortuous. Distally it may be traced beyond the trigonal area. If renal destruction is severe, no opaque medium may be excreted. Absence of calyces in the upper portion of the renal shadow and lateral displacement of the upper portion of the visualized ureter will suggest the diagnosis.

Cystoscopy may reveal the orifice in the urethra. If catheterization can be performed (it may be possible if a vaginal or vestibular orifice is identified), urine can be obtained for study and urograms made (Fig 22-8).

It may be feasible to resect the lowermost portion of the ureter and to implant the distal end of the ureter into the bladder. However, resection of the superior renal pole and its ureter is usually indicated because of the degree of parenchymal damage.

Johnston, J. H., & T. J. Davenport: The single ectopic ureter. Brit J Urol **41**:428-33, 1969.

Orquiza, C. S., & others: Ectopic opening of the ureter into the seminal vesicle: Report of case. J Urol **104**:532-5, 1970.

Wiggishoff, C. C., & J. H. Kiefer: Ureteral ectopia: Diagnostic difficulties. J Urol **96**: 671-3, 1966.

Williams, D. I.: The ureter, the urologist and the paediatrician. Proc Roy Soc Med **63**: 595-602, 1970.

ACQUIRED DISEASES OF THE URETER

ACQUIRED URETERAL STRICTURE

Most ureteral strictures are congenital, but some are acquired. The most common causes of acquired stenosis are the following:

(1) Injury to the ureters during extensive pelvic surgery or from intensive radiotherapy (Fig 22-7).

(2) Renal or ureteral injury secondary to external trauma with perirenal and periureteral hematoma which leaves periureteral scar tissue following absorption.

(3) Compression of the ureters by lymph nodes involved by cancer (metastases, lymphomas) (Fig 17-15).

(4) Contracture due to infection, and ischemia caused by prolonged impaction of a ureteral stone.

(5) Prolonged pressure upon the ureter by aberrant blood vessels.

(6) Pyeloureteritis - Tuberculosis or bilharzial infections may cause fibrosis of the ureter, which may lead in turn to contracture (Fig 13-2).

(7) Retroperitoneal fibrosis.

(8) Aneurysm of the aorta or following aortofemoral bypass grafts.

(9) Ureteropelvic or ureterovesical obstruction secondary to vesicoureteral reflux (see chapter 11).

(10) Occlusion of the ureterovesical junction by cancer of the bladder or prostate (Fig 17-14).

(11) Obstruction of the ureterovesical junction caused by hypertrophy of the trigone secondary to benign prostatic hyperplasia or posterior urethral valves.

(12) Compression of the lower ureters secondary to severe constipation in women and children.

(13) Endometriosis involving the ureter.

(14) Compression of the ureter by the right ovarian vein (rare).

The effects upon the kidney and the clinical findings, complications, and treatment of acquired ureteral stricture are the same as those described under congenital stricture and urinary obstruction and stasis.

Abercrombie, G. F., & W. F. Hendry: Ureteric obstruction due to peri-aneurysmal fibrosis. Brit J Urol **43**:170-3, 1971.

Alkema, H. D., & R. K. Ratliff: Successful treatment of post-radiation ureteral stricture by simple linear incision. J Urol **97**: 251-3, 1967.

Bates, J. S., & C. T. Beecham: Retroperitoneal endometriosis with ureteral obstruction. Obst Gynec **34**:242-8, 1969.

Brooks, R. T., Jr., Fraser, W. E., & W. E. Lucas: Endometriosis involving the urinary tract: A report of 2 cases with ureteral obstruction. J Urol **102**:185-7, 1969.

Derrick, F. C., & others: Incidence of right ovarian vein syndrome in pregnant females. Obst Gynec **35**:37-8, 1970.

Dykhuizen, R. F., & J. A. Roberts: The ovarian vein syndrome. Surg Gynec Obst **130**:443-52, 1970.

Graham, J. B., & R. S. Abad: Ureteral obstruction due to radiation. Am J Obst Gynec **99**:409-12, 1967.

Green, T. H., Jr., & others: Urologic complications of radical Wertheim hysterectomy: Incidence, etiology, management, and prevention. Obst Gynec **20**:293-312, 1962.

Mallouh, C., & C.M. Pellman: Scrotal herniation of the ureter. J Urol **106**:38-41, 1971.

Wagenknecht, L.V., & P.O. Madsen: Bilateral ureteral obstruction secondary to aortic aneurism. J Urol **103**:732-6, 1970.

Waggoner, C.M., & J.S. Spratt, Jr.: Prognostic significance of radiographic ureteropathy before and after irradiation therapy for carcinoma of the cervix uteri. Am J Obst Gynec **105**:1197-1200, 1969.

RETROPERITONEAL FASCIITIS
(Chronic Retroperitoneal Fibroplasia, Idiopathic Retroperitoneal Fibrosis)

One or both ureters may be compressed by a chronic inflammatory process of unknown etiology which involves the retroperitoneal tissues over the lower lumbar vertebrae. Patients treated for migraine with methysergide (Sansert®) may also develop retroperitoneal fibrosis. Sclerosing Hodgkin's disease and other malignancies have occasionally been found to cause this reaction.

The symptoms, which are nonspecific, include renal pain, low back pain, and the syndrome of uremia. The only pathognomonic sign is the presence of a palpable firm mass over the sacral promontory.

Infection of the urinary tract is not usually present. Renal function tests are normal unless both ureters are obstructed; anemia may be found during the stage of uremia.

The diagnosis can be made if excretory urograms reveal medial deviation of the ureters involved in the fibrous plaque in the lumbar area (Fig 22-9). Secondary to obstruction, there is dilatation of the ureters and renal pelves proximal to that point. When uremia has supervened, retrograde urograms may be needed to delineate the excretory tracts.

If radiographic changes are moderate and the patient is not uremic, corticosteroid therapy should be instituted; rather dramatic response in a matter of a few weeks has been reported. Begin with 30-60 mg of prednisone per day. If serial urograms show lessening hydronephrosis, the dosage can be gradually decreased to a maintenance dose of 5-15 mg/day. If the degree of obstruction is severe, the ureters should be freed from the fibrous plaque and either transplanted intraperitoneally or displaced lateral to the psoas muscles so that they do not again become involved. Since there is a tendency for the disease to progress, prophylactic corticosteroid therapy should be instituted.

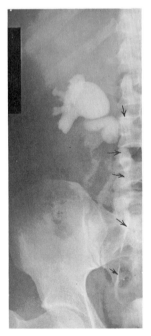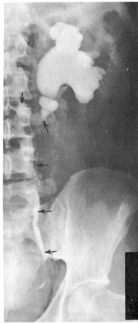

Fig 22-9. Retroperitoneal fasciitis. Right and left kidneys of same patient as shown by excretory urography. Note medial deviation of the upper portions of the ureters (see arrows) with marked obstruction. (Courtesy of J.A. Hutch, MD.)

If the patient has been on methysergide, withdrawal of the drug is often followed by spontaneous regression of the obstruction.

Bianchine, J. R., & A. P. Friedman: Metabolism of methysergide and retroperitoneal fibrosis.   Arch Int Med **126**:252-4, 1970.

Cerny, J. C., & T. Scott: Non-idiopathic retroperitoneal fibrosis.   J Urol **105**:49-55, 1971.

Kerr, W. S., Jr., & others: Idiopathic retroperitoneal fibrosis: Clinical experiences with 15 cases, 1956-1967.   J Urol **99**:575-84, 1968.

Mitchinson, M. J., Withycombe, J. F. R., & R. A. Jones: The response of idiopathic retroperitoneal fibrosis to corticosteroids.   Brit J Urol **43**:444-9, 1971.

Morandi, L. P., & P. J. Grob: Retroperitoneal fibrosis: Response to corticosteroid therapy.   Arch Int Med **128**:295-8, 1971.

Nitz, G. L., & others: Retroperitoneal malignancy masquerading as benign retroperitoneal fibrosis.   J Urol **103**:46-9, 1970.

Packham, D. A., & J. G. Yates-Bell: The symptomatology and diagnosis of retroperitoneal fibrosis.   Brit J Urol **40**:207-22, 1968.

Ross, J. C., & H. J. Goldsmith: The combined surgical and medical treatment of retroperitoneal fibrosis.   Brit J Surg **58**:422-7, 1971.

Wright, F. W., & R. C. Sanders: Is retroperitoneal fibrosis a self-limiting disease?   Brit J Surg **44**:511-4, 1971.

23...

Disorders of the Bladder, Prostate, and Seminal Vesicles

CONGENITAL ANOMALIES OF THE BLADDER*

EXSTROPHY

Exstrophy of the bladder is a complete ventral defect of the urogenital sinus and the overlying skeletal system (see chapter 2). Other congenital anomalies are frequently associated with it. The lower central abdomen is occupied by the inner surface of the posterior wall of the bladder, whose mucosal edges are fused with the skin. Urine spurts onto the abdominal wall from the ureteral orifices.

The rami of the pubic bones are widely separated. The pelvic ring thus lacks rigidity, the femurs are rotated externally, and the child "waddles like a duck." Since the rectus muscles insert on the rami, they are widely separated from each other inferiorly. A hernia, made up of the exstrophic bladder and surrounding skin, is therefore present. Epispadias almost always accompanies it.

Renal infection is common, and hydronephrosis caused by ureterovesical obstruction is often found on urography. These films also reveal the separation of the pubic bones.

The possibility of complete definitive repair of the defect is being explored. The defective organs have been successfully reconstructed in a few girls who have then gained complete urinary control, but these are the exceptions. The results are even poorer in the male. The main problem is establishing normally functioning sphincteric mechanisms. Vesicoureteral reflux is a common complication of reconstructive procedures. Carcinomatous degeneration of such a bladder is not uncommon.

Treatment usually consists, therefore, of early urinary diversion (ureteroileal cutaneous conduit) followed later by resection of the blad-

---

*Congenital vesicorectal fistulas are discussed with urethrorectal fistulas.

der and repair of the hernia of the lower abdominal wall. Reconstruction of the epispadiac penis must also be performed.

Treatment is, unfortunately, less than ideal. The male is infertile. Without urinary diversion, death from renal failure usually occurs by 20 years of age.

Engel, R. M., & H. A. Wilkinson: Bladder exstrophy. J Urol **104**:699-704, 1970.

Marshall, V. F., & E. C. Muecke: Functional closure of typical exstrophy of the bladder. J Urol **104**:205-12, 1970.

Muecke, E. C., & V. F. Marshall: Subsymphyseal epispadias in the female patient. J Urol 99:622-8, 1968.

O'Kane, H. O. J., & J. McI. Megaw: Carcinoma in the exstrophic bladder. Brit J Surg 55: 631-5, 1968.

Smith, M. J. V., & J. K. Lattimer: The management of bladder exstrophy. Surg Gynec Obst 123:1015-8, 1966.

Stagner, R. V., & C. V. Hodges. Experiences with exstrophy of the bladder. J Urol 89: 53-6, 1963.

Williams, D. I., & J. Savage: Reconstruction of the exstrophied bladder. Brit J Surg 53: 168-73, 1966.

PERSISTENT URACHUS

Embryologically, the allantois connects the urogenital sinus with the umbilicus. Normally the allantois is obliterated and is represented by a fibrous cord (urachus) extending from the dome of the bladder to the navel (see chapter 2).

Incomplete obliteration sometimes occurs. If obliteration is complete except at the superior end, a draining umbilical sinus may be noted. If it becomes infected, the drainage will be purulent. If the inferior end remains open it will communicate with the bladder, but this does not usually produce symptoms. Rarely, the entire tract remains patent, in

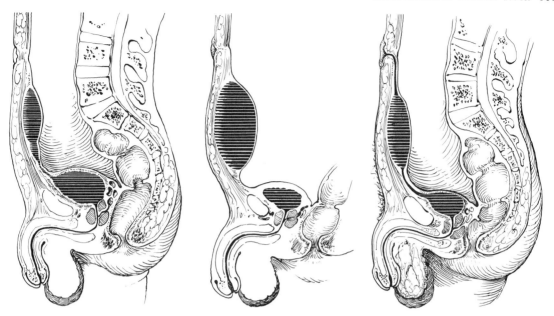

Fig 23-1. Types of Persistent Urachus. Left: Communicating urachus continuous with the bladder. This is a "pseudodiverticulum," and usually causes no symptoms. **Center:** Urachal cyst; usually causes no symptoms or signs unless it becomes large or infected. **Right:** Patent urachus. There is constant drainage of urine from the umbilicus.

which case urine drains constantly from the umbilicus. This is apt to become obvious within a few days of birth. If only the ends of the urachus seal off, a cyst of that body may form and may become quite large, presenting a low midline mass (Fig 23-1). Should the cyst become infected, signs of general and local sepsis will develop.

Adenocarcinoma may occur in a urachal cyst, particularly at its vesical extremity, and will tend to invade the tissues beneath the anterior abdominal wall. It may be seen cystoscopically. Stones may develop in a cyst of the urachus. These can be identified on a plain x-ray film.

Treatment consists of excision of the urachus, which lies on the peritoneal surface. If adenocarcinoma is present, radical resection is required.

Blichert-Toft, M., & O.V. Nielsen: Diseases of the urachus simulating intra-abdominal disorders. Am J Surg **122**:123-8, 1971.

Constantian, H.M., & E.L. Amaral: Urachal cyst: Case report. J Urol **106**:429-31, 1971.

Nadjmi, B., & others: Carcinoma of the urachus: Report of two cases and review of the literature. J Urol **100**:738-43, 1968.

Ney, C., & R.M. Friedenberg: Radiographic findings in anomalies of the urachus. J Urol **99**:288-91, 1968.

CONTRACTURE OF THE BLADDER NECK

There is considerable debate about the incidence of congenital narrowing of the bladder neck. Some feel that its presence is a common cause of vesicoureteral reflux, vesical diverticula, a bladder of large capacity, and the syndrome of irritable bladder associated with enuresis. A few observers consider this contracture a rare phenomenon and believe that the diagnosis is purely presumptive. The diagnosis is based upon endoscopic observation, which is an unreliable method. Voiding cystourethrography has been used to depict such narrowing, but interpretation of the films varies from urologist to urologist and radiologist to radiologist.

Recently, Nunn studied the intravesical and urethral pressures during voiding in cases with the signs mentioned above. He found no evidence of bladder neck obstruction. The 2 recorded pressures were essentially equal. It appears that the bladder neck would have to be extremely stenotic to truly obstruct urine flow. It is becoming increasingly clearer that, in the little girl, the obstructive lesion is spasm of the periurethral striated muscle which develops secondary to distal urethral stenosis (see chapter 25).

Empirical treatment is often employed, consisting of suprapubic bladder neck revision or transurethral resection. Making the bladder neck incompetent in the male child may later cause retrograde ejaculation and, therefore, infertility. Revision of the bladder neck in the female may cause urinary incontinence. This diagnosis must therefore be made with caution.

Grieve, J.: Bladder neck stenosis in children is it important? Brit J Urol **39**:13-6, 1967.

Harrow, B.R., Sloane, J.A., & W.S. Witus: A critical examination of bladder neck obstruction in children. J Urol **98**:613-7, 1967.

Kaplan, G.W., & L.R. King: An evaluation of Y-V vesicourethroplasty in children. Surg Gynec Obst **130**:1059-66, 1970.

Leadbetter, G.W., Jr.: Urinary tract infection and obstruction in children. Clin Pediat **5**:377-84, 1966.

Moir, J.C.: Vesicovaginal fistulae caused by wedge-resection of the bladder neck. Brit J Surg **53**:102-4, 1966.

Murphy, J.J., Schoenberg, H.W., & T.A. Tristan: The prevention of chronic pyelonephritis. Brit J Urol **37**:58-62, 1965.

Nunn, I.N.: Bladder neck obstruction in children. J Urol **93**:693-9, 1965.

Ochsner, M.G., Burns, E., & H.H. Henry, Jr.: Incidence of retrograde ejaculation following bladder neck revision in the child. J Urol **104**:596-7, 1970.

Shopfner, C.E.: Roentgenologic evaluation of bladder neck obstruction. Am J Roentgenol **100**:162-76, 1967.

Smith, D.R.: Critique on the concept of vesical neck obstruction in children. JAMA **207**:1686-92, 1969.

ACQUIRED DISEASES OF THE BLADDER

INTERSTITIAL CYSTITIS
(Hunner's Ulcer, Submucous Fibrosis)

Interstitial cystitis is primarily a disease of middle-aged women. It is characterized by fibrosis of the vesical wall, with consequent loss of bladder capacity. Frequency is the principal symptom.

Pathogenesis and Pathology

Infection does not appear to be the cause of fibrosis of the bladder wall, for the urine is usually normal. It has been postulated that the fibrosis is due to obstruction of the vesical lymphatics secondary to pelvic surgery or infection, but many of these patients fail to give such a history. It may be secondary to thrombophlebitis complicating acute infections of the bladder or pelvic organs, or may be the result of prolonged intrinsic arteriolar spasm secondary to psychogenic impulses.

Recently, evidence has been adduced which suggests that interstitial cystitis is an autoimmune collagen disease. Oravisto and his associates studied 54 women afflicted with this disease. Antinuclear antibodies were found in 85%. A significant number had allergy of the reagin type or hypersensitivity to drugs. Such an etiology would account for the favorable responses to corticosteroids.

The primary change is fibrosis in the deeper layers of the bladder. The capacity of the organ is decreased, sometimes markedly. The mucosa is thinned, especially where mobility is greatest as the bladder fills and empties (ie, over the dome), and small ulcers or cracks in the mucous membrane may be seen in this area. In the most severe cases, the normal mechanism of the ureterovesical junctions is destroyed, leading to vesicoureteral reflux. Hydroureteronephrosis and pyelonephritis may then ensue.

Microscopically, the mucosa may be thinned or even denuded. The capillaries of the tunica propria are often engorged, and signs of inflammation are apparent. The muscle is replaced by varying amounts of fibrous tissue, which is often quite avascular. The lymphatics may be engorged.

Clinical Findings

Interstitial cystitis should be considered when a middle-aged woman with clear urine complains of severe frequency and nocturia and suprapubic pain on vesical distention.

A. **Symptoms:** There is a long history of slowly progressive frequency and nocturia, both of which may be severe. The history does not suggest infection (burning on urination, cloudy urine). Suprapubic pain is usually marked when the bladder is full. Pain may also be experienced in the urethra or perineum. It is relieved on voiding. Gross hematuria is occasionally noted, usually when urination has had to be postponed (ie, following vesical overdistention). The patient is tense and anxious. Whether this is secondary to the prolonged and severe symptoms or is the primary cause of the vesical changes is not clear (see chapter 31).

B. **Signs:** Physical examination is usually normal. Some tenderness in the suprapubic area may be noted. There may be some tenderness in the region of the bladder when palpated through the vagina.

C. Laboratory Findings: If the patient has had no previous treatment (eg, instrumentation), the urine is almost always free of infection. Microscopic hematuria may be noted. Renal function (as measured by the PSP test) is normal except in the occasional patient in whom vesical fibrosis has led to vesicoureteral reflux or obstruction.

D. X-Ray Findings: Excretory urograms are usually normal unless reflux has occurred, in which case hydronephrosis is found. The accompanying cystogram will reveal a bladder of small capacity; reflux into a dilated upper tract may be noted on cystography.

E. Instrumental Examination: Cystoscopy is diagnostic. As the bladder fills, increasing suprapubic pain is experienced. The vesical capacity may be as low as 60 ml. In a patient not previously treated (by fulguration or hydraulic overdistention), the bladder lining may look fairly normal. But if distention is continued in spite of increasing pain, punctate hemorrhagic areas may appear over the most distensible portion of the wall. With further distention, an arcuate split in the mucosa will occur and bleeding from it may be profuse.

Differential Diagnosis

Tuberculosis of the bladder may cause true ulceration but is most apt to involve the region of the ureteral orifice which drains the tuberculous kidney. Typical tubercles may be identified, pyuria is present, and tubercle bacilli can usually be found. Furthermore, urograms will often show the typical lesion of renal tuberculosis.

Nonspecific vesical infection seldom causes ulceration. Pus and bacteria will be found in the urine. Antimicrobial treatment will be effective.

Complications

Gradual ureteral stenosis or reflux and its sequelae (e.g., hydronephrosis) may develop.

Treatment

A. Specific Measures: There appears to be no definitive treatment for interstitial cystitis. The therapy usually employed frequently affords partial relief but may be completely ineffective.

Hydraulic overdistention, with or without anesthesia, in some cases gradually improves the bladder capacity. Vesical lavage with increasing strengths of silver nitrate (1:5000-1:100) may have the same effect. Superficial (transcystoscopic) electrocoagulation of the split mucosa is commonly practiced and may afford temporary relief of pain.

Corticotropin causes an increase in vesical capacity in many patients and affords complete or partial relief from pain. The effective dose is in the range of 25 mg IM 4 times daily for 1 month.

Cortisone acetate, 100 mg, or prednisone (Meticorten®), 10-20 mg/day, in divided doses orally for 21 days, followed by decreasing amounts for an additional 21 days, has also been found effective. Transcystoscopic injection of the lesions with prednisone has its proponents.

Antihistamines (eg, pyribenzamine, 50 mg 4 times a day) may also afford some relief. Heparin sodium (long-acting), 20,000 units/day IV, also blocks the action of histamine, and its use in the treatment of Hunner's ulcer is encouraging.

Bilateral section of the third sacral nerve may increase bladder capacity significantly and relieve the pain associated with vesical distention.

If corticosteroids fail to afford any relief, subtotal cystectomy and enlargement of the bladder by adding a patch of colon (colocystoplasty) should be considered.

B. General Measures: General or vesical sedatives may be prescribed but seldom afford relief. If urinary infection is found (usually following instrumentation), it should be treated by appropriate antibiotics. If senile urethritis is discovered diethylstilbestrol vaginal suppositories may prove helpful.

C. Treatment of Complications: If progressive hydronephrosis develops secondary to ureteral stenosis, little will be gained by ureteral dilatations. Diversion of the urinary stream (eg, uretero-ileal cutaneous anastomosis) may therefore be necessary.

Prognosis

Only a minority of patients are apparently cured or have their symptoms controlled by the treatment outlined above. Most are not relieved, and remain bladder invalids.

Geist, R.W., & S.J. Antolak, Jr.: Interstitial cystitis in children. J Urol 104:922-5, 1970.

Hanash, K.A., & T.L. Pool: Interstitial cystitis in men. J Urol 102:427-8, 1969.

Oravisto, K.J., Alfthan, O.S., & E.J. Jokinen: Interstitial cystitis: Clinical and immunological findings. Scandinav J Urol Nephrol 4:37-42, 1970.

Silk, M.R.: Bladder antibodies in interstitial cystitis. J Urol 103:307-9, 1970.

Simmons, J.L.: Interstitial cystitis: an explanation for the beneficial effect of an antihistamine. J Urol 85:149-55, 1961.

Weaver, R.G., Dougherty, T.F., & C.A. Natoli: Recent concepts of interstitial cystitis. J Urol **89**:377-83, 1963.

EXTERNAL VESICAL HERNIATION

The bladder of a young girl may protrude through a patulous urethra and present itself externally. Treatment requires gentle pressure upon the mass, with the patient in the Trendelenburg position. After reduction, a small urethral catheter should be left in the bladder for a few days. If herniation recurs, the bladder and urethra should be sutured to the linea alba.

INTERNAL VESICAL HERNIATION

One side of the bladder may become involved in an inguinal hernia (in men) or a femoral hernia (in women) (Fig 23-2). Such a mass may recede on urination. It is most often found as a previously unsuspected complication during the surgical correction of a hernia.

Soloway, H.M., Portney, F., & A. Kaplan: Hernia of the bladder. J Urol **84**:539-43, 1960.

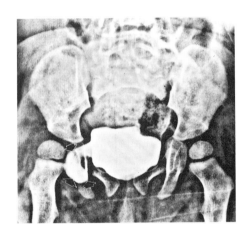

Fig 23-2. **Internal vesical hernia; lateral cystograms in stress incontinence. Left:** Female, 6 months old. Cystogram of excretory urogram showing tongue of bladder in right femoral hernia (see arrows). **Below left:** Stress incontinence. Upright lateral cystogram showing sagging of the bladder below a line extending from the sacrococcygeal joint to the inferior edge of the pubic bone. **Below right:** Upright voiding film showing abnormal descent of bladder with complete loss of the posterior urethrovesical angle. (Courtesy of Dr. J.A. Hutch.)

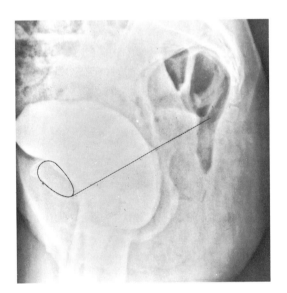

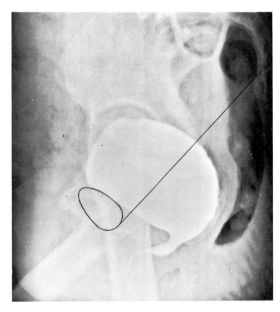

URINARY STRESS INCONTINENCE

Stress incontinence, the loss of urine with physical strain (eg, coughing, sneezing), is a common complaint of older women. Although it usually occurs as an aftermath of childbirth, it has been observed in girls and nulliparous women also.

Normal urethral resistance is about 125 cm of water; this is the sum of the smooth muscle urethral sphincter (50 cm of water) and the striated midurethral sphincter (75 cm of water). Normally, with strain or cough, intraperitoneal pressure rises sharply but the resistance in the mid urethra rises also, thus maintaining the relatively high urethra-to-detrusor pressure ratio. In patients with stress incontinence, the basic lesion is loss of normal midurethral resistance caused by weakening and attenuation of the striated muscle sphincter and tissues that afford support to the bladder neck and proximal urethra (this includes the whole pelvic floor). In addition, the area of the posterior urethra and bladder neck has fallen out of the true pelvis so that the strain which suddenly increases intravesical pressure is associated with decreased resistance in the proximal and mid urethra thereby leading to incontinence. These mechanical defects are revealed by a standing-straining cystourethrogram utilizing a beaded chain.

Lapides is convinced that the basic pathologic defect in stress incontinence is shortening of the urethra to less than 3 cm as measured in the upright position. This theory, however, has not been generally accepted, and many exceptions to this explanation have been cited. The definitive method of study requires the actual measurement of intravesical and intraurethral pressures under conditions of physical stress (eg, cough, strain).

Clinical Findings

The patient complains of loss of urine only with straining in the upright position. Some degree of urethrocele is usually noted. Of some diagnostic value is the demonstration that support to the bladder neck will cause the patient to be continent with cough or strain. This test must be performed with the patient standing. The region of the bladder neck is lifted well up under the symphysis pubis with 2 fingers or 2 clamps. (If clamps are used infiltration with a local anesthetic is required.) False position tests, however, are sometimes elicited.

An important test in establishing the diagnosis of true stress incontinence is the standing-straining lateral urethrocystogram with a beaded chain in the urethra and bladder. The normal urethral axis in relation to the per-pendicular is 30°; the posterior urethrovesical angle is about 90°. In less severe degrees of incontinence, the normal urethral axis is maintained but the normal urethrovesical angle is lost. In the more severe types there is widening of the angle of the urethral axis as well as complete obliteration of the urethrovesical angle. A similar finding can be recorded by taking lateral cystographic views in both horizontal and upright positions and with and without voiding. Normally, the base of the bladder is well supported and remains "flat." The vesical base should be above a line drawn from the bottom of the symphysis pubis to the sacrococcygeal joint (Fig 23-2). The base sags downward in the patient with stress incontinence and the vesical floor tends to take on a "funnel" shape which is the same as the contour of normal voiding.

Differential Diagnosis

Careful history taking will differentiate between stress and urgency incontinence. The latter implies the presence of a local inflammatory disease. The following diseases must be differentiated from the lesion causing stress incontinence if good surgical results are to be obtained: ectopic ureteral orifice, neurogenic bladder, senile urethritis, urethral diverticulum, and local lesions of the urethra and bladder (eg, cystitis, urethritis). The history, physical examination, urinalysis, and PSP test as well as cystoscopy, excretory urography, and cystometry should make the differentiation. None of these diseases exhibit the changes on cystourethrography described above.

Treatment

If hypoestrogenism of the vagina and urethra is discovered, give estrogens locally or by mouth. Kegel exercises may afford considerable improvement or even cure. Tanagho has shown that it is largely deficiency of the striated external sphincter that causes stress incontinence. Such exercises may improve tone of the muscles of the pelvic floor. The patient should be instructed to rhythmically contract and relax the anal sphincter (which can be sensed by the patient) 30 times a session 3 times a day for months. If these measures fail, either a vaginal repair with particular attention to support of the bladder neck or a urethrovesical suspension (Marshall-Marchetti) operation will usually be successful. In the type showing more severe derangement of urethrovesical relationships, urethrovesical suspension is the procedure of choice. It may be combined with vaginal repair if local conditions warrant. For the few failures, a sling of rectus fascia should be brought under the bladder neck in order to afford maximum support.

Prognosis

If the proper diagnosis has been made, the cure rate approaches 85%. Unfortunately, after a year or so, stress incontinence recurs in a few cases.

Bates, C.P., & others: Synchronous cine/ pressure/flow/cysto-urethrography with special reference to stress and urge incontinence. Brit J Urol 42:714-22, 1970.

Benson, R.C.: Retropubic vesicourethropexy - success or failure? Obst Gynec 35:665-70, 1970.

Cochrane, K.W.: Applied anatomy and surgical treatment of stress incontinence. New Zealand MJ 72:117-22, 1970.

Low, J.A.: Management of severe anatomic deficiencies of urethral sphincter function by a combined procedure with a fascial sling. Am J Obst Gynec 105:149-55, 1969.

Marshall, V.F., & R.M. Segaul: Experience with suprapubic vesicourethral suspension after previous failures to correct stress incontinence in women. J Urol 100:647-8, 1968.

Noll, L.E., & J.A. Hutch: The SCIPP line - an aid in interpreting the voiding lateral cystourethrogram. Obst Gynec 33:680-9, 1969.

Sanders, S., & W. Mathisen: Stress incontinence. A follow-up study of retropubic suspension. Urol Internat 22:324-31, 1967.

Shute, W.B.: Vaginal support and stress incontinence. Am J Obst Gynec 91:824-36, 1965.

Steinhausen, T.B., & others: Chain urethrocystography before and after urethrovesical suspension for stress incontinence. Obst Gynec 35:405-15, 1970.

Uhle, C.A.W., Kohler, F.P., & C.R. Mackinney: Urinary stress incontinence in the female patient. J Urol 99:613-6, 1968.

URINARY INCONTINENCE

Complete urinary incontinence can occur following any type of prostatectomy, though it is relatively rare. Some intrinsic damage to the smooth muscle periurethral sphincter is implied. The patient may be able to hold his urine as long as the external urinary sphincter is held tight, but this can only be maintained for minutes. Numerous operations for cure of total incontinence have been devised. Berry has employed a plastic device which is placed in the perineum so that it compresses the urethra. The success rate is less than 30% and pain from the prosthesis is a problem.

Hinman and co-workers have placed a segment of rib in the perineum in such manner that it compresses the perineal urethra. About 33% receive some benefit.

Tanagho has designed a procedure based upon sound anatomic principles that has enjoyed significant success in restoring urinary continency. A strip of the heavy layer of the middle circular layer of the detrusor muscle, anteriorly, is formed into a tube, thus affording sphincteric action. This is anastomosed to the bladder neck or prostatic urethra. Preliminary results are encouraging.

Berry, J.L., & C.P. Dahlen: Evaluation of a procedure for correction of urinary incontinence in men. J Urol 105:105-6, 1971.

Engel, R.M., & J.C. Wade: Experience with the Berry prosthesis. J Urol 102:78-80, 1969.

Hinman, F.J., Schmaelzle, J.F., & A.S. Cass: Autogenous perineal bone graft for post-prostatectomy incontinence. II. Technique and results of prosthetic fixation of urogenital diaphragm in men. J Urol 104:888-92, 1970.

Mathisen, W.: A new operation for urinary incontinence. Surg Gynec Obst 130:606-8, 1970.

Raney, A.M.: Re-evaluation of post-prostatectomy urinary incontinence with the Berry procedure. J Urol 102:81-3, 1969.

Symmonds, R.E.: Loss of the urethral floor with total urinary incontinence. A technique for urethral reconstruction. Am J Obst Gynec 103:665-76, 1969.

Tanagho, E.A., & others: Mechanism of urinary continence. II. Technique for surgical correction of incontinence. J Urol 101:305-13, 1969.

Tanagho, E.A., & D.R. Smith: Clinical evaluation of a technique for correction of complete urinary incontinence. J Urol 107:402-11, 1972.

Wendel, R.M., & L.R. King: The treatment of total urinary incontinence. J Pediat Surg 5:543-9, 1970.

FOREIGN BODIES INTRODUCED INTO THE BLADDER AND URETHRA

Numerous objects have been found in the urethra and bladder of both men and women. Some of them find their way into the urethra in the course of inquisitive self-exploration. Others are introduced (in the male) as contraceptive devices in the hope that plugging the urethra will block the drainage of the ejaculate.

The presence of a foreign body causes cystitis. Hematuria is not uncommon. Embarrassment may cause the victim to delay medical consultation. A plain x-ray of the bladder area will disclose metal objects. Nonopaque objects sometimes become coated with calcium. Cystoscopy will visualize them all.

Cystoscopic or suprapubic removal of the foreign body is indicated. If not removed, the foreign body will lead to infection of the bladder. If the infecting organisms are urea-splitting, the alkaline urine (causing increased insolubility of calcium salts) contributes to rapid formation of stone upon the foreign object.

Jameson, R.M.: Foreign bodies and damage to the female urethra and bladder. Brit J Urol 39:506-8, 1967.
Thomas, W.J.C.: Unusual presentation of retained urethral foreign bodies with review of other cases. Brit J Surg 51:921-2, 1964.

VESICAL MANIFESTATIONS OF ALLERGY

So many mucous membranes are affected by allergens that the possibility of allergic manifestations involving the bladder must be considered. Hypersensitivity is occasionally suggested in cases of recurrent symptoms of acute "cystitis" in the absence of urinary infection or other demonstrable abnormality. During the attack, general erythema of the vesical mucosa may be seen and some edema of the ureteral orifices noted.

A careful history may reveal that these attacks follow the ingestion of a certain food not ordinarily eaten (eg, fresh lobster). Sensitivity to spermicidal creams is occasionally observed. If vesical allergy is suspected, it may be aborted by the subcutaneous injection of 0.5-1 ml of 1:1000 epinephrine. Control may also be afforded by the use of one of the antihistamines. Skin testing has not generally proved helpful.

Pastinszky, I.: The allergic diseases of the male genitourinary tract with special reference to allergic urethritis and cystitis. Urol Internat 9:288-305, 1960.
Powell, N.B., Boggs, P.B., & J.P. McGovern: Allergy of lower urinary tract. Ann Allerg 28:252-5, 1970.
Unger, D.L., Kubik, F., & L. Unger: Urinary tract allergy. JAMA 170:1308-9, 1959.

DIVERTICULUM

Most vesical diverticula are acquired and are secondary to either obstruction distal to the vesical neck or the upper motor neuron type of neurogenic bladder. Increased intravesical pressure causes vesical mucosa to insinuate itself between hypertrophied muscle bundles so that a mucosal extravesical sac develops. Often, this sac lies just superior to the ureter and causes vesicoureteral reflux (see chapter 11). The diverticulum is devoid of muscle and therefore has no expulsive power; residual urine is the rule, and infection is perpetuated. At the time of prostatectomy, diverticulotomy should be considered.

Goldman, H.J.: A rapid safe technique for removal of a large vesical diverticulum. J Urol 106:379-81, 1971.
Schiff, M.J., & B. Lytton: Congenital diverticulum of the bladder. J Urol 104:111-5, 1970.

VESICAL FISTULAS

Vesical fistulas are common. The bladder may communicate with the skin, intestinal tract, or gynecologic organs. The primary disease is usually not urologic. The causes are as follows: (1) Primary intestinal disease. Cancer of the rectosigmoid, tuberculosis of the cecum, diverticulitis of the rectosigmoid, appendiceal abscess, and regional enteritis. (2) Primary gynecologic disease. Pelvic inflammatory disease and cancer of the cervix or uterus. (3) Physical, surgical, or obstetric trauma.

Malignant tumors of the small or large bowel, uterus, or cervix may invade and perforate the bladder. Inflammations of adjacent organs may also erode through the vesical wall. Severe injuries involving the bladder may lead to perivesical abscess formation, and these abscesses may rupture through the skin of the perineum or abdomen. The bladder may be inadvertently injured during gynecologic or intestinal surgery; cystotomy for stone or prostatectomy may lead to a persistent cutaneous fistula.

Clinical Findings
A. Vesicointestinal Fistula: Symptoms arising from a vesicointestinal fistula include vesical irritability, the passage of feces and gas through the urethra, and usually a change in bowel habits (eg, obstipation, abdominal distention, diarrhea) caused by the primary

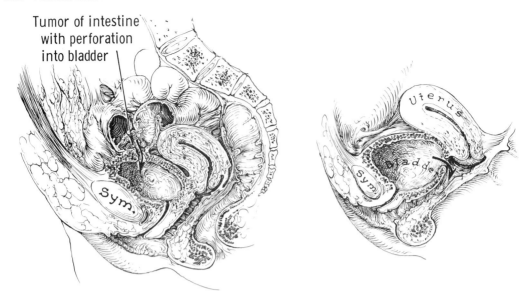

Tumor of intestine
with perforation
into bladder

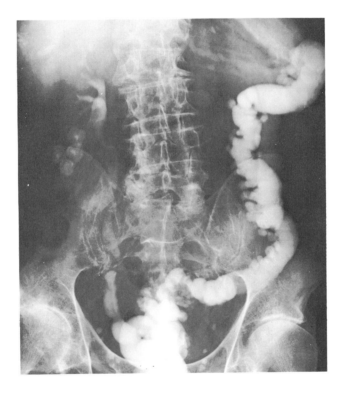

Fig 23-3. Vesical fistulas. Above left: Primary carcinoma of the sigmoid with perforation through bladder wall. **Above right:** Injury to base of bladder following delivery by forceps. **Below:** Cystogram showing radiopaque fluid entering sigmoid containing multiple diverticula; right urethral reflux, gallbladder calculi.

intestinal disease. Signs of bowel obstruction may be elicited; abdominal tenderness may be found if the cause is inflammatory. The urine is always infected.

A barium enema, upper gastrointestinal series, or sigmoidoscopic examination may demonstrate the communication. Following a barium enema, centrifuged urine should be placed on an x-ray cassette and an exposure made. The presence of radiopaque barium will establish the diagnosis of vesicocolonic fistula. Cystograms may reveal reflux of the opaque material into the bowel (Fig 23-3). Cystoscopic examination will show a severe localized inflammatory reaction from which bowel contents may exude. Catheterization of the fistulous tract may be feasible; the instillation of radiopaque fluid will establish the diagnosis.

B. Vesicovaginal Fistula: This relatively common fistula is secondary to obstetric, surgical, or radiation injury or to invasive cancer of the cervix. The constant leakage of urine is most distressing to the patient. Pelvic examination usually reveals the fistulous opening, which can also be visualized with the cystoscope. It may be possible to pass a ureteral catheter through the fistula into the vagina. Vaginography often successfully shows ureterovaginal, vesicovaginal, and rectovaginal fistulas. A 30 ml Foley catheter is inserted into the vagina and the balloon is distended. A radiopaque solution is then instilled and appropriate x-rays taken. Biopsy of the edges of the fistula may show carcinoma.

C. Vesicoadnexal Fistula: This rare fistula can be diagnosed by vaginal examination and by seeing the fistulous opening through the cystoscope.

Differential Diagnosis

It is necessary to differentiate ureterovaginal from vesicovaginal fistula. Instill methylene blue solution into the bladder and insert 3 cotton pledgets into the vagina; then have the patient ambulate. If the proximal cotton ball is wet but colorless, the lesion is ureterovaginal. If the deep cotton pledget contains blue fluid, the diagnosis is vesicovaginal fistula. If only the distal cotton is blue, the patient probably has urinary incontinence.

Treatment

A. Vesicointestinal Fistula: Treatment consists of proximal colostomy (if the lesion is in the rectosigmoid). When the inflammatory reaction has subsided, resection of the involved bowel may be done with closure of the opening in the bladder. Later the colostomy can be closed. Small bowel or appendiceal

vesical fistulas require bowel or appendiceal resection and closure of the vesical defect.

B. Vesicovaginal Fistula: Those fistulas secondary to surgical or obstetric injury respond readily to surgical repair. Fistulas which develop following radiation therapy for cancer of the cervix are much more difficult to close because of the avascularity of the tissues. Surgical closure of fistulas which arise from direct invasion of the bladder by cervical carcinoma is impossible; diversion of the urinary stream above the level of the bladder (eg, ureterosigmoidostomy) is therefore necessary.

C. Vesicoadnexal Fistula: These fistulas are cured by removal of the involved gynecologic organs with closure of the opening in the bladder.

Aldrete, J. S., & W. H. Re Mine: Vesicocolic fistula - a complication of colonic cancer. Arch Surg 94:627-34, 1967.

Boronow, R. C.: Management of radiation-induced vaginal fistulas. Am J Obst Gynec **110**:1-7, 1971.

Cushing, R. M., Tovell, H. M., & L. M. Liegner: Major urologic complications following radium and x-ray therapy for carcinoma of the cervix. Am J Obst Gynec **101**:750-5, 1968.

Falk, H. C., & M. L. Tancer: Urethrovesicovaginal fistula. Obst Gynec **33**:422-31, 1969.

Gross, M., & B. Peng: Appendico-vesical fistula. J Urol **102**:697-8, 1969.

Henderson, M. A., & W. P. Small: Vesicocolic fistula complicating diverticular disease. Brit J Urol **41**:314-9, 1969.

Hutch, J. A., & L. E. Noll: Prevention of vesicovaginal fistulas. Obst Gynec **35**:924-7, 1970.

Moir, J. C.: Vesicovaginal fistula: Thoughts on the treatment of 350 cases. Proc Roy Soc Med **59**:1019-22, 1966.

Russell, C. S.: The vesical fistula high in the vagina. Proc Roy Soc Med **59**:1022-4, 1966.

Su, C. T.: A flap technique for repair of vesicovaginal fistula. J Urol **102**:56-9, 1969.

Wolfson, J. S.: Vaginography for demonstration of ureterovaginal, vesicovaginal and rectovaginal fistulas, with case reports. Radiology **83**:438-41, 1964.

PERIVESICAL LIPOMATOSIS

The syndrome of perivesical lipomatosis has only been recognized in the past few years. The cause is not known. The disorder seems to affect principally black males in the 20-40 year age group. There are no pathognomonic symptoms. There may be some dysuria or mild urinary obstructive symptoms. Examination may demonstrate a distended bladder. Excretory urograms and cystography may show dilatation of both upper tracts and an upward displacement and lateral compression of the bladder. In the perivesical area, x-ray reveals areas of radiolucency compatible with fatty tissue. Angiography shows no evidence of neoplastic vessels.

On surgical exploration, lipomatous tissue surrounding the bladder at the lower ureteral zones is found. Wide excision of this tissue is indicated, but the results in terms of relief of ureteral obstruction have been equivocal.

Lucey, D.T., & M.J.V. Smith: Pelvic lipomatosis. J Urol **105**:341-5, 1971.

Mahlin, M.S., & B.W. Dovitz: Perivesical lipomatosis. J Urol **100**:720-2, 1968.

Morettin, L.B., & M. Wilson: Pelvic lipomatosis. Am J Roentgenol **113**:181-4, 1971.

RADIATION CYSTITIS

Many women receiving radiation treatment for carcinoma of the cervix develop some degree of vesical irritability. These symptoms may develop months after cessation of treatment. The urine may or may not be sterile. Vesical capacity is usually appreciably reduced. Cystoscopy will reveal a pale mucous membrane with multiple areas of telangiectatic blood vessels. Vesical ulceration may be noted, and vesicovaginal fistulas may develop. If symptoms are severe and prolonged, diversion of the urine from the bladder may be necessary.

Mallik, M.K.B.: Study of radiation necrosis of the urinary bladder following treatment of carcinoma of the cervix. Am J Obst Gynec **83**:393-400, 1962.

CONGENITAL ANOMALIES OF THE PROSTATE AND SEMINAL VESICLES

Congenital anomalies of the prostate are rare. Cysts of the prostate and the seminal vesicles have been reported. Enlargements of the prostatic utricle are often found in association with penoscrotal or perineal hypospadias. They are usually small, lying in the midline posterior to the prostate and emptying through the verumontanum. These cysts represent embryologic remnants of the distal end of the müllerian ducts (see chapter 2). Rarely they become large enough to be easily palpable rectally or even abdominally. Through local pressure, they may cause symptoms of obstruction of the bladder neck.

Heetderks, D.R., Jr., & L.C. Delambre: Cyst of the seminal vesicle. J Urol **93**: 725-8, 1965.

Rieser, C., & T.L. Griffin: Cysts of the prostate. J Urol **91**:282-6, 1964.

Syme, G.: Müllerian duct cyst. Australian New Zealand J Surg **35**:56-60, 1965.

BLOODY EJACULATION

The most common cause of bloody ejaculation is hypertrophy of the mucosa of the seminal vesicles. It usually responds to the administration of diethylstilbestrol, 5 mg/day for one week. Rare causes include prostatic ductal carcinoma and tumors of the seminal vesicles. It has also been postulated that there may be an anomalous venous communication with the seminal vesicles.

Ross, J.C.: Haemospermia. Practitioner **203**:59-62, 1969.

•   •   •

24...

Disorders of the Penis and Male Urethra

CONGENITAL ANOMALIES OF THE PENIS AND MALE URETHRA

Congenital absence of the penis is exceedingly rare. A few cases of duplication have been reported, occasionally with 2 complete urethral channels. Megalopenis (hyperplasia) may be seen in boys suffering from interstitial cell tumor or hyperplasia or tumor of the adrenal cortex. Micropenis (hypoplasia) is often seen in male intersexes who have other feminizing traits (eg, hypospadias).

Tripanthi, V.N.P., & V.S. Dick: Complete duplication of the urethra. J Urol 101:866-9, 1969.

STENOSIS OF THE EXTERNAL URINARY MEATUS

Stenosis of the external meatus is common and should be sought in all newborn males. It may be congenital or can be acquired after circumcision from trauma to the meatus by rough diapers. If it is severe, dilatation of the entire urinary tract, up to and including the renal pelvis (hydronephrosis), may develop, and death from uremia may occur. The usual symptom is bloody spotting and crusting of the meatus, which is caused by infection and ulceration just within the orifice. Meatotomy is indicated, following which the parents must dilate the urethra once every day for 2 weeks and at lengthening intervals for 2 more weeks. The small end of an oral thermometer is an excellent and available instrument for this purpose.

URETHRAL STRICTURE

Congenital urethral stricture occasionally occurs in male infants. The 2 most common sites are in the region of the corona (fossa navicularis) and in the membranous urethra. Severe strictures cause back pressure (from obstruction), which is followed by dilatation of the urethra, hypertrophy of the vesical musculature, and functional ureterovesical obstruction or reflux, both leading to hydronephrosis. Symptoms may be those of obstruction (eg, urinary stream of small caliber, hyperdistended bladder) or secondary infection (eg, fever, dysuria).

Excretory urograms may show the changes caused by obstruction (vesical trabeculation, hydronephrosis). The post-voiding film may reveal residual urine. A urethrogram (Figs 7-10 and 24-1) will delineate the degree and length of the stricture.

Every child with the symptoms mentioned above should be examined cystoscopically. The passage of the instrument will be arrested by the stricture. Urethral dilatations with sounds or filiforms and followers will keep the stricture open, but the prognosis depends upon the degree of damage suffered by the upper urinary tract. Surgical repair of the stricture is usually necessary. Congenital diaphragmatic strictures respond to overdilatation or internal urethrotomy.

Cobb, B.G., Wolf, J.A., Jr., & J.S. Ansell: Congenital stricture of the proximal urethral bulb. J Urol 99:629-31, 1968.
Leadbetter, G.W., Jr.: The etiology, symptoms, and treatment of urethral strictures in male children. Pediatrics 31:80-6, 1963.

POSTERIOR OR PROSTATIC URETHRAL VALVES

Posterior (prostatic) urethral valves or diaphragms are folds of mucous membrane on the floor of the prostatic urethra (Fig 24-1). They are one of the most common causes of congenital urethral obstruction in boys. Since they are obstructive, they cause dilatation of the prostatic urethra, hypertrophy of the de-

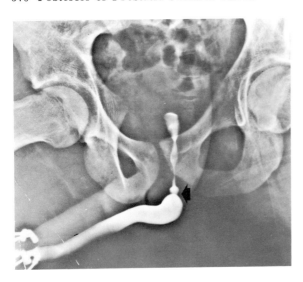 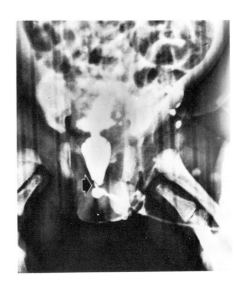

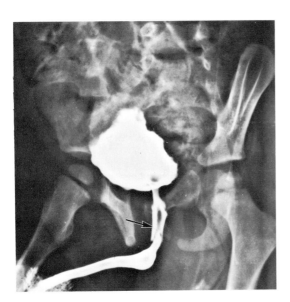 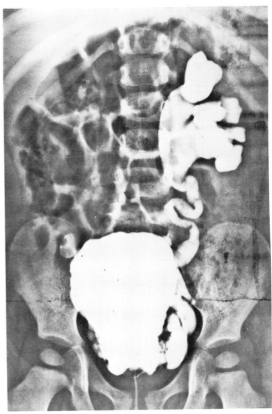

Fig 24-1. **Above left:** Retrograde urethrogram showing congenital diaphragmatic stricture. **Above right:** Posterior urethral valves revealed on voiding cystourethrography. Arrow points to area of severe stenosis at distal end of prostatic urethra. **Below left:** Posterior urethral valves. Patient would not void with cystography. Retrograde urethrogram showing valves (see arrow). **Below right:** Cystogram, same patient. Free vesicoureteral reflux and vesical trabeculation with diverticula.

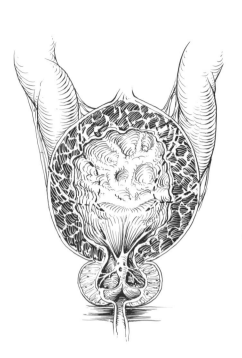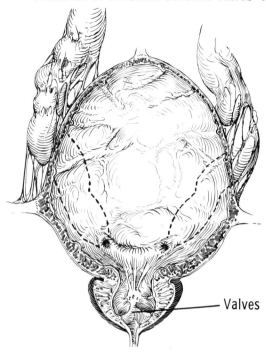

— Valves

Fig 24-2. Posterior urethral valves. Left: Dilatation of the prostatic urethra, hypertrophy of vesical wall and trigone in stage of compensation; bilateral hydroureters secondary to trigonal hypertrophy. **Right:** Attenuation of bladder musculature in stage of decompensation; advanced ureteral dilatation and tortuosity, usually secondary to vesicoureteral reflux.

trusor (trabeculation), vesical diverticula, and hypertrophy of the trigonal muscles. The latter development tends to cause a functional obstruction of the intravesical ureter; hydro-ureteronephrosis is therefore the rule. In the advanced stage, vesicoureteral reflux may occur, but less than half of these boys exhibit reflux. Infection under these circumstances is almost inevitable, but it is apt to occur late because of the normally sterile proximal urethra. A few cases of intraperitoneal rupture of the kidney and bladder with urinary ascites have been reported in such newborns.

Clinical Findings

A. Symptoms: Difficulty in initiating urination and a weak urinary stream are the principal symptoms. A distended bladder may be noted by the parents. Infection causes frequency, enuresis, and burning on urination. High fever suggests renal infection, but infection can be present without febrile response or vesical symptoms.

In the later stages, after renal insufficiency has developed, the child may suffer from anorexia, loss of weight, and anemia.

B. Signs: A distended bladder may be seen, felt, or percussed. More commonly,

however, a hard mass is felt deep in the pelvis. This represents the severely hypertrophied bladder. A poor urinary stream may be observed. Often, however, examination may reveal nothing more than evidence of chronic illness.

C. Laboratory Findings: Anemia due to chronic infection or uremia may be noted. The urine is often infected. Impairment of renal function may be discovered by noting loss of concentrating power of the kidneys or elevation of the BUN.

A diaper PSP test should be performed on all infants suspected of having urinary tract obstruction. Excretion of less than 30% of the dye in 3 hours requires explanation. Little dye will be recovered when valves are present because of the combination of impaired renal function and transport of urine.

D. X-Ray Findings: Excretory urograms may demonstrate hydroureters and hydronephroses as well as irregularity in the outline of the bladder (trabeculation) or diverticula. The post-voiding film will reveal considerable retention of urine. Voiding cystourethrograms may reveal wide dilatation of the prostatic urethra and the negative shadows representing

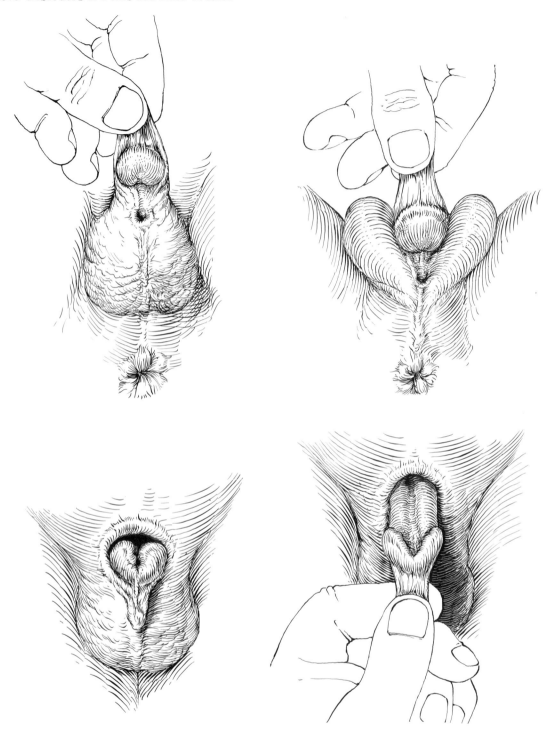

Fig 24-3. Hypospadias and epispadias. Above left: Hypospadias, penoscrotal type. Redundant dorsal foreskin which is deficient ventrally; ventral chordee. **Above right:** Hypospadias, mid-scrotal type. Chordee more marked. Penis often small. **Below left:** Epispadias. Redundant ventral foreskin which is absent dorsally; severe dorsal chordee. **Below right:** Traction on foreskin reveals dorsal defect.

the valves (Fig 24-1). This procedure is the definitive diagnostic step. The cystograms may demonstrate reflux of the radiopaque material into the ureters and kidneys. The urograms which result usually preclude the need for ureteral catheterization and retrograde urograms. If the child cannot be induced to void, retrograde urethrography may show the valves (Fig 24-1).

E. Instrumental Examination: A catheter can usually be passed without difficulty, thereby ruling out stricture. These valves are only obstructive from within outward. Cystoscopy and panendoscopy show trabeculation of the bladder wall, occasionally diverticula, and hypertrophy of the trigone. The mucosal diaphragms may be visualized on the floor of the prostatic urethra, although they may be torn during instrumentation and therefore may be missed.

Treatment

Treatment consists of destruction of the valves. The simplest method is to pass very large sounds (up to 30 F) through a perineal urethrotomy. Transurethral resection has its advocates, but 10-15% may be left incontinent. If ureteral reflux is demonstrated, prolonged suprapubic or catheter urinary drainage may cause ureterovesical valvular competence to return and reduce upper tract dilatation and stasis. Repair of the ureterovesical junctions, however, may be required. If severe secondary ureteral kinks have developed which have themselves become obstructive, nephrostomy or loop ureterostomy drainage may be necessary to maintain or improve renal function. Repair of such ureters may be accomplished later.

Complicating urosepsis should be treated by whatever drug is indicated by culture and sensitivity tests. In many cases infection cannot be eradicated even after definitive surgical repair; suppressive therapy should then be applied.

Prognosis

The prognosis depends upon the degree of destruction of the upper urinary tract. Diagnosis is too often not made until renal damage has become severe. Some of these children continue to lose function from incurable renal infection even after the obstruction has been relieved.

Early diagnosis requires that a competent nurse in the newborn nursery—or the pediatrician—make it a point to observe the size and force of the urinary stream in all male infants before they leave the hospital.

Hendren, W. H.: Posterior urethral valves in boys: A broad clinical spectrum. J Urol 106:298-307, 1971.

Leonidas, J. C., Leiter, E., & D. Gribetz: Congenital urinary tract obstruction presenting with ascites at birth: Roentgenographic diagnosis. Radiology 96:111-2, 1970.

Marsden, R. T. H.: Posterior urethral valves in adults. Brit J Urol 41:586-91, 1969.

Nesbit, R. M., & M. M. Labardini: Urethral valves in the male child. J Urol 96:218-28, 1966.

Robertson, W. B., & J. A. Hayes: Congenital diaphragmatic obstruction of the male posterior urethra. Brit J Urol 41:592-8, 1969.

Waldbaum, R. S., & V. F. Marshall: Posterior urethral valves: Evaluation and surgical management. J Urol 103:801-9, 1970.

URETHRORECTAL AND VESICORECTAL FISTULAS

Urethrorectal and, more rarely, vesicorectal fistulas are sometimes seen. They are almost always associated with imperforate anus occurring when the urorectal fold which divides the rectum from the urogenital sinus fails to develop completely. This permits a communication between the rectum and the urethra (in the region of the verumontanum) or bladder. (See chapter 2.)

An infant with such a fistula passes fecal material and gas through the urethra. The anus may develop normally (open externally), in which case urine may be passed through the rectum.

Cystoscopy and panendoscopy usually visualize the fistulous opening. Barium given by mouth will reach the blind rectal pouch, and appropriate radiograms will measure the distance between the end of the rectum and the perineum. The imperforate anus must be opened immediately and the fistula closed, or, if the rectum lies quite high, temporary sigmoid colostomy must be performed. Definitive surgery, with repair of the urethral fistula, can be undertaken later.

Culp, O. S., & H. W. Calhoun: A variety of rectourethral fistulas: Experiences with 20 cases. J Urol 91:560-71, 1964.

HYPOSPADIAS

Hypospadias in the male is evidence of feminization. The hypospadiac penis presents

ventral curvature (chordee) distal to the urethral meatus. The meatus opens on the ventral
side of the penis proximal to the tip of the
glans penis; it may present as far back as the
perineum. When the orifice is in the scrotal
or perineal area, the scrotum is bifid, thereby
assuming the appearance of labia majora. The
foreskin is deficient on the ventrum (Fig 24-3).
In extreme degrees of hypospadias, the penis
may be unusually small, simulating a hypertrophied clitoris (see p 404).

The penoscrotal and perineal types (Fig
24-3) are usually associated with enlargement
of the prostatic utricle, which represents a
remnant of the fused ends of the müllerian
ducts. At times a rudimentary or even complete vaginal tract and uterus are present (see
p 406). For this reason, chromatin (genetic)
sex should be established by a buccal smear.
The incidence of cryptorchism is high. There
is no deficiency of the sphincters, so incontinence does not occur.

Adequate surgical correction demands,
above all, straightening of the shaft so that
normal intercourse is possible. This must be
followed by formation of a urethra which extends to or near the tip of the glans so that semen can be deposited deep in the vagina. For
psychologic reasons, it is best that this cor-
rective surgery be completed before school age.

Aarskog, D.: Clinical and cytogenetic studies
  in hypospadias. Acta paediat scandinav,
  Suppl 203, 1970.
Allen, T.D., & H.M. Spence: The surgical
  treatment of coronal hypospadias and re-
  lated problems. J Urol 100:504-8, 1968.
Broadbent, T.R., & R.M. Woolf: Hypospadias:
  One-stage repair. Brit J Plast Surg 18:406-
  12, 1965.
Cronin, T.D., Guthrie, T., & D. Herr: Ex-
  periences in the surgical correction of
  hypospadias. Am J Surg 110:818-25, 1965.
Culp, O.S.: Struggles and triumphs with hypo-
  spadias and associated anomalies: Review
  of 400 cases. J Urol 96:339-51, 1966.
Fuqua, F.: Renaissance of urethroplasty:
  The Belt technique of hypospadias repair.
  J Urol 106:782-5, 1971.
Hodgson, N.B.: A one-stage hypospadias re-
  pair. J Urol 104:281-3, 1970.
Horton, C.E., & C.J. Devine, Jr.: One-stage
  repair for hypospadias cripples. Plast
  Reconstr Surg 45:425-30, 1970.
Persky, L., Kiehn, C.L., & J.D. Des Prez:
  A one-stage hypospadias repair. J Urol
  88:259-61, 1962.
Smith, D.R.: Repair of hypospadias in the
  preschool child: A report of 150 cases.
  J Urol 97:723-30, 1967.

EPISPADIAS

Epispadias is considerably less common
than hypospadias, but it is more disabling. It
is quite rare in females. The urethra opens
on the dorsum of the penis at some point proximal to the glans. The most common site is at
the abdominopenile junction. Dorsal curvature
(chordee) is also present (Fig 24-3). More
serious, however, is the fact that this dorsal
defect usually extends proximally, so that a
defect of the urinary sphincters is present.
This causes urinary incontinence. The pubic
bones are separated as seen with exstrophy of
the bladder. It should be noted that epispadias
is but a relatively mild degree of exstrophy.

Treatment requires correction of urinary
incontinence and of the inability to copulate.
Operations upon the urinary sphincters have
not been too successful. Plastic repair of the
penis requires reduction of the chordee followed by urethroplasty, which advances the
urinary orifice to the distal end of the shaft.
If urinary continence cannot be gained, some
type of urinary diversion may have to be provided (eg, uretero-ileal conduit).

Burkholder, G.V., & D.I. Williams: Epispadias and incontinence: Surgical treatment of 27 children. J Urol 94:674-9, 1965.
Dey, D.L., & D. Cohen: The surgery of female epispadias. Surgery 69:542-5, 1971.
Michalowski, E., & W. Modelski: The surgical treatment of epispadias. Surg Gynec
  Obst 117:465-8, 1963.
Spence, H.M., & others: Panel discussion:
  Anomalies of external genitalia in infancy
  and childhood. J Urol 93:1-23, 1965.

ACQUIRED DISEASES OF THE PENIS AND MALE URETHRA

PRIAPISM

Priapism is a rather rare affliction. It
consists of a prolonged erection, unassociated
with sexual stimulation, which is usually painful. The blood in the cavernous spaces becomes sludge-like rather than clotted. It may
last for many days. About 25% of the cases
are associated with leukemia, metastatic carcinoma, or sickle cell disease, but as a rule
the mechanism is not clear. Priapism is
occasionally seen following injuries to the
spinal cord.

If spontaneous subsidence of priapism does not occur within a few hours, the following regimen should be instituted: Ice water enemas should first be ordered; temporary (even permanent) subsidence of the erection may occur. Evacuation of the sludged blood of the corpora by needle and syringe should next be tried. The corpora should then be thoroughly irrigated with an anticoagulant followed by bandage compression. Controlled hypotension with trimethaphan (Arfonad®) should be instituted; a systemic anticoagulant should be used. Unless the erection subsides promptly, either spontaneously or in response to treatment, the septa of the corpora cavernosa undergo fibrosis. This results in impotence—inability to gain an erection.

If the above conservative regimen fails, prompt surgical intervention is mandatory. A bilateral saphenous vein-corpora cavernosa shunt should be performed. If successful and done early, potency may be maintained. More recently, anastomosis of one corpus cavernosum to the corpus spongeosum has been suggested; the results are equivocal.

Becker, L. E., & A. D. Mitchell: Priapism. S Clin North America 45:1523-34, 1965.

Garrett, R. A., & D. E. Rhamy: Priapism: Management with corpus-saphenous shunt. J Urol 95:65-7, 1966.

Grace, D. A., & C. C. Winter: Priapism: An appraisal of management of 23 patients. J Urol 99:301-10, 1968.

Harrow, B. R.: Simple technique for treating priapism. J Urol 101:71-3, 1969.

Howe, G. E., & others: Priapism: A surgical emergency. J Urol 101:576-9, 1969.

Martin, D. C., Schapiro, A., & G. V. Burkholder: Corpus cavernosum-saphenous vein anastomosis for priapism. J Urol 102:221-3, 1969.

Rothfeld, S. H., & D. Mazor: Priapism in children: A complication of sickle cell disease. J Urol 105:307-8, 1971.

Rubin, S. O.: Priapism as a probable sequel to medication. Scandinav J Urol Nephrol 2:81-5, 1968.

Seeler, R. A.: Priapism in children with sickle cell anemia. Successful management with liberal red cell transfusions. Clin Pediat 10:418-9, 1971.

PLASTIC INDURATION OF THE PENIS
(Peyronie's Disease)

Fibrosis of the covering sheaths of the corpora cavernosa occurs without known cause, usually in men over 45 years of age. This fibrotic area will not permit lengthening of the involved surface with erection, so that the penis bends toward the involved area (chordee). In the early stages, erection is accompanied by pain. The degree of curvature may finally preclude coitus. Apparently the process begins as vasculitis in the connective tissue beneath the tunica albuginea of the penis and then extends to adjacent structures. This leads to fibrosis and at times calcification or even ossification.

Palpation of the shaft reveals a well-demarcated, raised plaque of fibrosis which is usually in the midline of the dorsum near the base of the organ, although it may be placed more laterally or distally. X-ray may reveal areas of calcification within the indurated area.

Treatment is unsatisfactory. Low-dosage x-ray therapy has some value. Injection of the plaque with hydrocortisone has been advocated, but its efficacy is questionable. Potassium para-aminobenzoate (Potaba®), 12 gm/day in divided doses, may decrease the chordee. It should be continued for 6 months to 2 years. Surgical resection of the plaque has been advocated, but there appears to be little enthusiasm for this mode of therapy.

DeSanctis, P. N., & C. A. Furey, Jr.: Steroid injection therapy for Peyronie's disease: A 10 year summary and review of 38 cases. J Urol 97:114, 1967.

Griff, L. C.: Peyronie's disease. The role of radiation therapy and a general review. Am J Roentgenol 100:916-9, 1967.

McRoberts, J. W.: Peyronie's disease. Surg Gynec Obst 129:1291-4, 1969.

Smith, B. H.: Subclinical Peyronie's disease. Am J Clin Path 52:385-90, 1969.

Williams, J. L., & G. G. Thomas: The natural history of Peyronie's disease. J Urol 103: 75-6, 1970.

Zarafonetis, C. J. D.: Antifibrotic therapy with Potaba. Am J M Sc 248:550-61, 1964.

PHIMOSIS

Phimosis is a disease in which it is impossible to retract the foreskin over the glans. It is usually secondary to infection beneath a redundant foreskin. Poor hygiene frequently contributes to the infection. Such a reaction causes tissue injury, and healing is by fibrosis. The preputial opening thereby becomes contracted, so that the foreskin cannot be retracted. This further facilitates the infectious process, usually by mixed organisms, including anaerobes, vibrios, and spirochetes. Such chronic irritation of many years' standing may be the cause of squamous epithelioma. Stones may form in the preputial sac.

The patient may merely complain of inability to retract the foreskin, but more commonly he is disturbed by symptoms and signs of infection (eg, redness and swelling of foreskin, purulent discharge, local pain).

Treatment consists of measures to control the infection (hot soaks, antibiotics). A dorsal slit of the foreskin is necessary if infection is marked. Circumcision should be performed when the inflammatory reaction has subsided.

PARAPHIMOSIS

Paraphimosis is a condition in which the foreskin, once retracted behind the glans, cannot be replaced in its normal position. This is due to chronic inflammation under the redundant foreskin, which leads to contracture of the preputial skin ring.

This tight ring of skin, caught behind the glans, causes venous occlusion which leads to edema of the glans and further disproportion between the size of the glans and the caliber of the preputial opening. If neglected, arterial occlusion may supervene and gangrene of the glans may develop.

Paraphimosis can usually be treated by squeezing the glans firmly for at least 5 minutes, thus reducing its size. The edema may also be reduced by subcutaneous injections of hyaluronidase into the edematous penile skin. The glans is then pushed proximally as the prepuce is moved distally. If manual reduction fails, incision of the constricting tissue is indicated. Once the inflammation and edema have subsided, circumcision should be performed.

Øster, J.: Further fate of the foreskin. Incidence of preputial adhesions, phimosis, and smegma among Danish boys. Arch Dis Childhood **43**:200-3, 1968.

Skoglund, R.W., Jr., & W.H. Chapman: Reduction of paraphimosis. J Urol **104**:137, 1970.

URETHRAL STRICTURE

Acquired urethral stricture is a rare complication of severe gonococcal urethritis and a common sequel of urethral injury. In either case the urethra heals by the proliferation of fibroblasts, producing contraction.

Pathogenesis and Pathology

A severe degree of stenosis causes changes typical of obstruction. These include (1) dilatation of the urethra proximal to the stricture, (2) compensatory changes in the bladder musculature, and (3) hydroureteronephrosis secondary to hypertrophy of the ureterotrigonal complex or vesicoureteral reflux. Because of stasis, infection occurs which may cause periurethral abscess, prostatitis, cystitis, and pyelonephritis. If the organisms split urea, renal calculi may form. Urethral stricture, then, may cause severe damage to the urinary tract.

Clinical Findings

A. Symptoms: The most common symptom is gradual diminution of the force and caliber of the urinary stream. Sudden urinary retention may occur if an infection at the site of stricture is exacerbated. A history of urethral injury or severe untreated gonorrhea can usually be obtained. Symptoms of cystitis may be noted. There may be fever secondary to prostatitis or pyelonephritis.

B. Signs: Periurethral induration may be found at the site of the stricture. A tender mass may be present if periurethral abscess has developed. Perineal urinary fistulas may be noted. A visible or palpable bladder may be found if urinary retention has supervened.

C. Laboratory Findings: If infection is present the white blood count may be elevated and pus and bacteria will be found in the urine. PSP excretion may be diminished if there is renal damage or residual urine.

D. X-Ray Findings: A urethrogram and voiding cystourethrogram will reveal the site and degree of the stricture. Fistulas may be demonstrated (Fig 24-4). A cystogram may show a thickened, trabeculated bladder and, possibly, ureteral reflux. Excretory or retrograde urograms may reveal urinary calculi or changes compatible with chronic pyelonephritis.

E. Instrumental Examination: A catheter or sound of average size (22 F) will be arrested at the site of stricture. Panendoscopy may visualize it. Cystoscopy (done after urethral dilatation) will show hypertrophy of the vesical muscle and, often, inflammation.

Differential Diagnosis

Prostatic or bladder neck obstruction may cause similar symptoms, but in this instance a catheter passes through the urethra with ease. An enlarged (or cancerous) gland is usually found on rectal examination.

Carcinoma of the urethra can mimic urethral stricture, but panendoscopy and biopsy
of the visualized tumor will establish the
proper diagnosis.

Complications

Prostatitis, cystitis, and pyelonephritis
are common complications of urethral stricture. Periurethral abscess may develop at the
stricture site; it may resolve or rupture
through the skin, causing a urethrocutaneous
fistula. Urinary stones may form secondary
to stasis and infection.

Treatment

A. Specific Measures:

1. Dilatation - After local urethral or
general anesthesia has been obtained and the
urethra lubricated, a 22 F sound should be
gently passed (Fig 9-4). If this is arrested,
a 20 F should be tried. Smaller sounds
should not be used, for their tips may perforate the friable urethra at the site of the
stricture.

Next, passage of a filiform should be attempted (Figs 9-5 and 9-6). If one passes to
the bladder, an appropriate follower can be
screwed onto its end. If the smallest follower
will not penetrate the stricture, the filiform
should be taped in place; the patient will be
able to void around it. This maneuver will
allow subsidence of the inflammatory reaction,
so that after a day or so dilation will be possible. If a filiform cannot be passed and the
patient is in urinary retention, suprapubic
cystostomy must be done.

Once an instrument has been passed

through the stricture, 2 methods for urethral
dilatation are available:

a. The stricture should be dilated to 18-20
F. A 14-16 F catheter should then be passed
into the bladder and left indwelling. After 48
hours, the next size can usually be easily
passed; this procedure can be repeated every
2 days until a 24-26 F catheter has been
placed. This method is relatively painless.

b. Sounds of increasing sizes should be
passed to the point of urethral tolerance. This
procedure can then be repeated, using larger
sounds at weekly intervals until a 24-26 F
sound can be passed. This method achieves
results more quickly but is more painful.

Dilatation of a urethral stricture is a palliative treatment; it is not curative. Sounds
should be passed at increasing intervals (eg,
2 weeks, 1 month, 3 months, 6 months). Periodic sounding must be done indefinitely.

2. Surgery - If the stricture contracts
rapidly so that the use of sounds is not feasible,
instrumental or surgical incision, excision, or
urethroplasty may be necessary.

B. General Measures: Hot sitz baths may
help combat local infection and decrease pain
after instrumentation.

C. Treatment of Complications: Infection
of the kidneys or bladder requires antimicrobial therapy, particularly at the time of urethral dilatation (which may exacerbate preexisting infection). Periurethral abscess may
resolve with medical treatment. If it does not,
surgical drainage will be necessary. Urethrocutaneous fistulas may close spontaneously

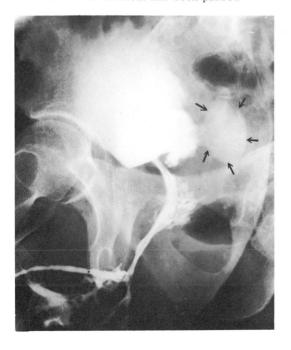

Fig 24-4. **Urethral stricture with multiple
perineal fistulas.** Voiding cystourethrogram showing stricture of perineal urethra,
multiple fistulas, dilated prostatic ducts,
and vesical diverticulum outlined by arrows.

once the stricture is dilated. If they do not, surgical correction must be done.

Prognosis

Most urethral strictures can be kept open by periodic dilatations; a few will require surgical treatment. Their deleterious effects on renal function must always be kept in mind.

Anderson, J.C., & W. Hynes: By-pass operation for strictures of the deep urethra. Brit J Urol **37**:148-56, 1965.

Colapinto, V.: Two-stage urethroplasty for stricture: Results and technical considerations. Brit J Urol **41**:494-504, 1969.

Devereux, M.H., & G.D. Burfield: Prolonged follow-up of urethral strictures treated by intermittent dilatation. Brit J Urol **42**:321-9, 1970.

Devine, P.C., & others: One-stage urethroplasty: Repair of urethral strictures with a free full thickness patch of skin. J Urol **9**:191-3, 1968.

Helmstein, K.: Internal urethrotomy - modifications in the operative technique. Acta chir scandinav. Suppl **340**, 1965.

Jessen, C.: Resection of urethral stricture and end-to-end anastomosis. Scand J Urol Nephrol **4**:87-91, 1970.

Katz, A.S., & K. Waterhouse: Treatment of urethral strictures in man by internal urethrotomy: A study of 61 patients. J Urol **105**:807-9, 1971.

Turner-Warwick, R.: The repair of urethral strictures in the region of the membranous urethra. J Urol **100**:303-14, 1968.

FISTULA

Fistulas between the urethra and penile skin usually follow an exacerbation of infection just proximal to a stricture. A fistula may develop secondary to a carcinoma of the urethra or to a foreign body which has been inserted into the channel (eg, bobby pin). Periurethritis and abscess formation may then develop. Spontaneous drainage may occur. Urethroscopy (panendoscopy) and urethrography will reveal the site and cause of the fistulous opening. Biopsy may be indicated. When all evidence of inflammation has disappeared, surgical closure can be performed.

THROMBOPHLEBITIS OF THE SUPERFICIAL PENILE VEINS

Not infrequently, thrombophlebitis of the circumferential veins just proximal to the corona develops. The patient notes a firm ridge of tender tissue, and redness of the overlying skin. Examination reveals thrombosis of the vein; this may also involve the longitudinal superficial dorsal vein. No treatment is required. Recanalization takes place in a few months.

Harrow, B.R., & J.A. Sloane: Thrombophlebitis of superficial penile and scrotal veins. J Urol **89**:841-2, 1963.

•   •   •

25...

Disorders of the Female Urethra

CONGENITAL ANOMALIES OF THE FEMALE URETHRA

DISTAL URETHRAL STENOSIS IN INFANCY AND CHILDHOOD

There has been considerable confusion about the site of lower tract obstruction in small girls who suffer from enuresis, slow, interrupted stream, recurrent cystitis, and pyelonephritis and who, on thorough examination, often exhibit ureterovesical reflux. Treatment has largely been directed to the bladder neck on rather empirical grounds. Most of these children, however, have congenital distal urethral stenosis with secondary spasm of the striated external sphincter rather than bladder neck contracture.

At birth, calibration of the urethra with bougies á boule reveals no evidence of a distal ring of urethral stenosis (Fisher & others). Within a few months, however, such a ring develops as a normal anatomic structure (Immergut & others). After puberty, the ring disappears. The inference is that the absence of estrogens leads to the development of this lesion. Lyon and Tanagho found that the ring calibrates at 14 F at age 2 and at 16 F between the ages of 4 and 10. They recognized, however, that from the hydrodynamic standpoint such a stenotic area should not be obstructive. Nonetheless, almost all observers recognize that destruction of the ring is successful in relieving symptoms and persistent infection or vesical dysfunction in 80% of these children. Lyon and Tanagho postulated that the basic cause of these urinary difficulties could be reflex spasm of the periurethral striated sphincter and noted that voiding cystourethrograms suggest this possibility (Fig 25-1).

Tanagho & others, measuring pressures in the bladder and in the proximal and mid urethra simultaneously in symptomatic girls, found resting pressures in the midurethral segment as high as 200 cm of water. Attempts at voiding caused intravesical pressures as high as 225 cm of water to develop. Under curare, the urethral closing pressures dropped to normal (40-50 cm of water), proving that these obstructing pressures were caused by spasm of the striated sphincter muscle. If the distal urethral ring was treated and symptoms abated, repeat pressure studies showed normal midurethral and intravesical voiding pressures. If, on the other hand, symptoms persisted, pressures were found to remain at their inordinately high levels.

It now seems clear, therefore, that the major cause of urinary problems in little girls is spasm of the external sphincter and not vesical neck stenosis.

In addition to recurrent urinary tract infection, these patients have hesitancy in initiating micturition and a slow, hesitant, or interrupted urinary stream. Enuresis and involuntary loss of urine during the day are common complaints. Abdominal straining may be required. Small amounts of residual urine are found, thus impairing the vesical defense mechanism. A voiding cystourethrogram may reveal an open bladder neck and ballooning of the mid urethra secondary to the spastic external sphincter (Fig 25-1).

While the voiding cystourethrogram may reveal evidence of the distal ring, the typical findings are not always seen, particularly if flow rate is slow. The definitive diagnosis is made by bougienage.

The simplest and least harmful treatment is overdilatation with sounds up to 32-36 F or with the Kollmann dilator. In either instance, the ring "cracks" anteriorly, with some bleeding. Recurrence of the lesion is rare. Internal urethrotomy has its proponents. In 80% of these children, a successful outcome is obtained: cessation of enuresis, normal free voiding pattern, cure of recurrent cystitis or persistent bacteriuria, and, at times, disappearance of vesicoureteral reflux. The latter is only to be expected of the "borderline" valve embarrassed by increased intravesical voiding pressure and infection. Since the ring disappears at puberty, it is probably this improvement in hydrodynamics that has caused spontaneous improvement in these girls.

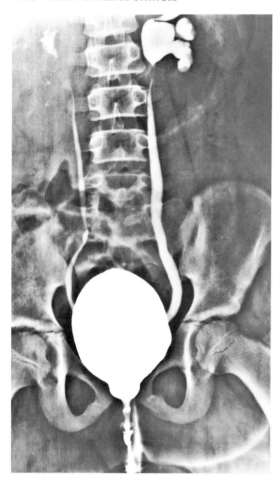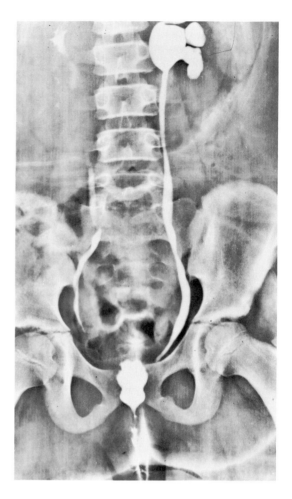

Fig 25-1. Distal urethral stenosis with reflux spasm of voluntary urethral sphincter. Left: Voiding cystourethrogram showing bilateral vesicoureteral reflux, a slightly trabeculated bladder, a wide-open vesical neck, and severe spasm of the striated urethral sphincter in the midportion of the urethra, secondary to distal urethral stenosis. **Right:** Postvoiding film. Bladder empty, vesical neck open, but dilated urethra contains radiopaque fluid proximal to the stenotic zone. Urethral bacteria thus can flow back into the bladder. (Courtesy of A. D. Amar, MD.)

It follows, therefore, that all little girls with enuresis, pants wetting, recurrent or persistent cystitis, or pyelonephritis must undergo bougienage and rupture of the ring as part of their diagnostic work-up and treatment.

Arnold, S. J.: Consequences of childhood urethral disease. Postgrad Med **43**:191-8, 1968.

Brannan, W., & others: Significance of distal urethral stenosis in young girls: experience with 241 cases. J Urol **101**:570-5, 1969.

Fisher, R. E., & others: Urethral calibration in newborn girls. J Urol **102**:67-9, 1969.

Graham, J. B., & others: The significance of distal urethral narrowing in young girls. J Urol **97**:1045-9, 1967.

Harvard, B. M.: Revision of the external urinary meatus in girls: A clinical appraisal. J Urol **103**:236-42, 1970.

Hinman, F., Jr.: Mechanisms for the entry of bacteria and the establishment of urinary infection in female children. J Urol **96**:546-50, 1966.

Kedar, S. S.: The urethra in the female child. Brit J Urol **40**:441-4, 1968.

Lyon, R. P., & S. Marshall: Urinary tract infections and difficult urination in girls: Long-term followup. J Urol **105**:314-7, 1971.

Shopfner, C. E.: Roentgen evaluation of distal urethral obstruction. Radiology **88**:222-31, 1967.

Smith, D. R.: Critique on the concept of vesical obstruction in children. JAMA **207**: 1686-92, 1969.

Tanagho, E. A., & R. P. Lyon: Urethral dilatation versus internal urethrotomy. J Urol **105**:242-4, 1971.

Tanagho, E. A., Meyers, F. H., & D. R. Smith: Urethral resistance: Its components and implications. I. Smooth muscle component. II. Striated muscle component. Invest Urol **7**:136-49 and 195-205, 1969.

Tanagho, E. A., & others: Spastic external sphincter and urinary tract infection in girls. Brit J Urol **43**:69-82, 1971.

Vermillion, C. D., Halverstadt, D. B., & G. W. Leadbetter, Jr.: Internal urethrotomy and recurrent urinary tract infection in female children. II. Long-term results in the management of infection. J Urol **106**:154-7. 1971.

ACQUIRED DISEASES OF THE FEMALE URETHRA

ACUTE URETHRITIS

Acute urethritis frequently occurs with gonorrheal infection in women. Urinary symptoms are often present at the onset of the disease. Cultures and smears establish the diagnosis. Cure is quickly effected by antibiotics. The detergents in bubble bath or certain spermatocidal jellies may lead to vaginitis and urethritis. Symptoms of vesical irritability may occur.

Bass, H. N.: ''Bubble bath'' as an irritant to the urinary tract of children. Clin Pediat **7**:174, 1968.

Marshall, S.: The effect of bubble bath on the urinary tract. J Urol **93**:112, 1965.

CHRONIC URETHRITIS

Because the distal portion of the channel normally harbors bacteria, chronic urethritis is one of the common urologic difficulties affecting women. Chronic urethral inflammation may occur (1) because of increase in the urethral flora from contaminated diapers; (2) from the trauma of coitus or childbirth, particularly if urethral stenosis, either congenital or following childbirth, is present; (3) because of the need for an indwelling urethral catheter following surgical or cystoscopic operations; or (4) from neighborhood cervicitis or vaginitis.

Clinical Findings

The urethral mucosa is reddened and quite sensitive. Granular areas are often seen, and polypoid masses may be noted just distal to the bladder neck. The urethra is often found to be stenosed.

A. Symptoms: The symptoms resemble those of cystitis, although the urine may be clear. Complaints include burning on urination, frequency, and nocturia. Discomfort in the urethra may be felt, particularly when walking.

B. Signs: Examination may disclose redness of the meatus, hypersensitivity of the meatus and of the urethra on vaginal palpation, and evidence of cervicitis or vaginitis. There is no urethral discharge.

C. Laboratory Findings: Collection of the initial and midstream urine in separate containers reveals pus in the first glass and none in the second. T-strain mycoplasmas are often identifiable in the first glass. These findings are similar to those observed in nonspecific urethritis in the male. Clinically, the presence of white blood cells in the absence of bacteria on a routine stain suggests this etiology.

D. Instrumental Examination: A catheter, bougie à boule, or sound may meet resistance because of urethral stenosis. Panendoscopy reveals redness and a granular appearance of the mucosa. Inflammatory polyps may be seen in the proximal portion of the urethra. Cystoscopy may show increased injection of the trigone (trigonitis), which often accompanies urethritis.

Differential Diagnosis

Differentiation from cystitis depends upon bacteriologic study of the urine; panendoscopy demonstrates the urethral lesion. Both diseases may be present.

Psychologic disorders may cause symptoms which are identical with those associated with chronic urethritis. A history of short bouts of frequency without nocturia is suggestive of functional illness. The neurotic make-up of the patient usually becomes obvious.

Treatment and Prognosis

Successful treatment requires removal of the cause of the urethritis. Gradual urethral dilatations (up to 36 F in the adult) should be given if there is urethral stenosis; this allows for some inevitable contracture. T-strain mycoplasmas are fairly sensitive to both tetra-cycline and erythromycin.

Essenhigh, D. M. , Ardran, G. M. , & V. Cope: A study of the bladder outlet in lower uri-nary tract infections in women. Brit J Urol **40**:268-77, 1968.

Marshall, S. , Lyon, R. P. , & J. Schieble: Nonspecific urethritis in females. Cali-fornia Med **112**:9-10, June 1970.

Moore, T. , Hira, N. R. , & R. M. Stirland: Differential urethrovesical urinary cell-count. Lancet **1**:626-7, 1965.

Zufall, R. : Treatment of the urethral syn-drome in women. JAMA **184**:894-5, 1963.

SENILE URETHRITIS

After physiologic (or surgical) menopause, hypoestrogenism occurs and retrogressive (senile) changes take place in the vaginal epi-thelium; it becomes rather dry and pale. Since the urethra arises from the same embryologic tissues as the female generative organs, sim-ilar degenerative changes develop in the lower urinary tract. Some eversion of the mucosa about the urethral orifice, from foreshorten-ing of the vaginal canal, is usually seen. This is commonly misdiagnosed as caruncle.

Clinical Findings

A. Symptoms: Many postmenopausal women have symptoms of vesical irritability (burning, frequency, urgency) and stress in-continence. They may complain of vaginal and vulval itching and some discharge.

B. Signs: The vaginal epithelium is dry and pale. The mucosa at the urethral orifice is often reddened and hypersensitive; eversion of its posterior lip due to foreshortening of the urethrovaginal wall is commonly seen.

C. Laboratory Findings: The urine is usually free of organisms. The diagnosis can be made by the following procedure: A dry smear of vaginal epithelial cells is stained with Lugol's solution. The slide is then washed with water and immediately examined micro-scopically while wet. In hypoestrogenism, the cells take up the iodine poorly and are there-fore yellow. When the mucosa is normal, these cells stain deep brown because of their glycogen content.

D. Instrumental Examination: Panendos-copy usually demonstrates a reddened and granular urethral mucosa. Some urethral stenosis may be noted.

Differential Diagnosis

Senile urethritis is often mistaken for ure-thral caruncle. Although there is eversion of the posterior lip of the urinary meatus in senile urethritis, a hypersensitive vascular tumor is lacking.

Before operations to relieve stress incon-tinence are performed, estrogenic (or andro-genic) vaginal therapy should be given. It may preclude the need for surgery.

Treatment

Senile urethritis responds well to diethyl-stilbestrol vaginal suppositories, 0.1 mg night-ly for 3 weeks. Estrogen creams applied lo-cally are also effective. Estrogen urethral suppositories have been recommended, but they offer no advantages and patients have dif-ficulty inserting them. After 3 weeks of treat-ment, the drug is withheld for 1 week and then the course is repeated. More than 2 courses are occasionally indicated, depending upon the symptoms and the appearance of the vaginal smear stained as outlined above.

Estrogen suppositories may cause con-siderable vaginal irritation or vaginal bleeding after withdrawal of the drug. If so, methyl-testosterone linguets (5 mg) can be used as vaginal suppositories with equally good results. They should be inserted daily for 5 to 8 weeks. Diethylstilbestrol, 0.1 mg/day by mouth, is also effective.

Prognosis

Senile urethritis usually responds prompt-ly to estrogen or androgen therapy.

Quinlivan, L. G. : The treatment of senile vag-initis with low doses of synthetic estrogens. Am J Obst Gynec **92**:172-4, 1965.

CARUNCLE

Urethral caruncle is a benign, red, rasp-berry-like, friable vascular tumor involving the posterior lip of the external urinary meatus. It is rare before the menopause. Microscopi-cally it consists of connective tissue containing many inflammatory cells and blood vessels, and is covered by an epithelial layer.

Clinical Findings

Symptoms include pain on urination, pain with intercourse, bloody spotting even from mild trauma, and the presence of a mass at the meatal orifice. A sessile or pedunculated red, friable, tender mass is seen at the posterior lip of the meatus.

Differential Diagnosis

Carcinoma of the urethra may involve the urethral meatus. Palpation reveals definite induration. Biopsy will establish the true diagnosis.

Senile urethritis is often associated with a polypoid reaction of the urinary meatus. In fact, it is the most common cause of masses in this region. The differentiation can be made by establishing the presence of hypoestrogen-ism and its response to replacement therapy. Biopsy should be done if doubt exists.

Thrombosis of the urethral vein presents as a bluish, swollen, tender lesion involving the posterior lip of the urinary meatus. It has the appearance of a thrombosed hemorrhoid. It subsides without treatment.

Treatment

Only if the lesion produces troublesome symptoms should local excision be done.

Prognosis

True caruncle is usually cured by excision, but in a few instances it does recur.

Marshall, F. C., Uson, A. C., & M. M. Meli-cow: Neoplasms and caruncles of the female urethra. Surg Gynec Obst 110:723-33, 1960.

THROMBOSIS OF THE URETHRAL VEIN

Spontaneous thrombosis of the urethral vein which occupies the floor of the distal ure-thra occurs in older women. The patient is conscious of sudden local pain and, shortly thereafter, a mass at the urethral orifice. Examination reveals a purple mass protruding from the posterior lip of the urethra; at the onset it is quite tender. Its abrupt onset tends to rule out caruncle or malignancy. Should doubt exist as to its nature, biopsy should be done.

No treatment is required in most instances; gradual resolution occurs. Evacuation of the clot has been recommended.

Falk, H. C.: Treatment of urethral vein thrombosis. Obst Gynec 23:85-8, 1964.
Harrow, B. R.: The thrombosed urethral hemorrhoid: 3 case reports. J Urol 98: 482, 1967.

PROLAPSE

Prolapse of the urethra is not common. It usually occurs only in children or in para-plegics suffering from a lower motor neuron lesion. The protruding urethral mucosa pre-sents itself externally as an angry red mass which, if not reduced promptly, may become gangrenous. Such a protruding mass in a little girl must be differentiated from prolapse of a ureterocele.

After reduction, cystoscopy should be done. Recurrences are rare once reduction has been accomplished; the accompanying in-flammation probably "fixes" the tissue in place as healing progresses. If the prolapsed urethra cannot be reduced, or if it recurs, an indwelling catheter should be inserted, traction placed upon it, and a heavy piece of suture material tightly tied over the tissue and cathe-ter just proximal to the mass. The tissue later sloughs off. Using this same technic, the tissue can be resected, preferably with an electrosurgical unit.

Capraro, V. J., Bayonet-Rivera, N. P., & I. Magoss: Vulvar tumor in children due to prolapse of urethral mucosa. Am J Obst Gynec 108:572-5, 1970.
Kamat, M. H., Del Gaizo, A., & J. J. Seebode: Urethral prolapse in female children. Am J Dis Child 118:691-3, 1969.
Potter, B. M.: Urethral prolapse in girls. Radiology 98:287-9, 1971.

URETHROVAGINAL FISTULA

Urethrovaginal fistulas may follow local injury secondary to fracture of the pelvis, or obstetric or surgical injury. Probably the most common cause is accidental trauma to the urethra or its blood supply in the course of surgical repair of a cystocele. Vaginal ure-throplasty is indicated.

Gray, L.: Urethrovaginal fistulas. Am J Obst Gynec 101:28-35, 1968.

DIVERTICULUM

Diverticulation of the urethral wall is not common, and its cause is obscure. Diverticula are at times multiple. Most cases are probably secondary to obstetric urethral trauma or severe urethral infection. A few cases of carcinoma in such diverticula have been reported. This disease is usually asso-ciated with recurrent attacks of cystitis. Puru-lent urethral discharge is sometimes noted as the infected diverticulum empties. On occa-sion the diverticulum may be large enough to be discovered by the patient.

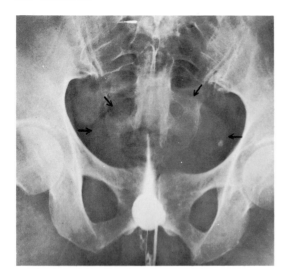 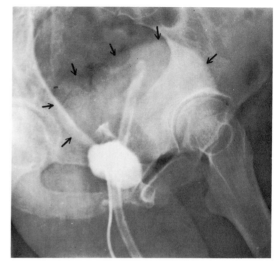

Fig 25-2. **Urethral diverticulum containing stone. Left:** Plain film showing stone. Arrows outline bladder. **Right:** Diverticulum filled with radiopaque fluid instilled through ureteral catheter. Bladder outlined by arrows.

The diagnosis is usually made on feeling a rounded cystic mass in the anterior wall of the vagina which, upon pressure, leaks pus from the urethral orifice. Endoscopy may reveal its urethral opening. It may be possible to introduce a small catheter through which radiopaque fluid can be instilled. Appropriate x-ray films are then exposed (Fig 25-2). The plain film may show the presence of a stone in the diverticulum. Should these methods fail, the following procedures can be used:

(1) Empty the diverticulum manually. Catheterize, and instill 5 ml of indigo carmine and 60 ml of contrast medium into the bladder. Remove the catheter and have the patient begin to void. Occlude the meatus with a finger. This maneuver usually causes filling of the diverticulum with the test solution. Take appropriate x-rays and do panendoscopy, seeking leakage of blue dye from the mouth of the diverticulum.

(2) Insert a Davis-TeLinde catheter. This looks like a Foley catheter, but it is surrounded by a second movable balloon. Pass the catheter to the bladder; inflate the proximal balloon. With tension on the catheter, slide the second balloon against the urinary meatus and inflate it. In the catheter, between the balloons, is a hole through which injected radiopaque fluid will escape, thus filling the urethra and diverticulum. X-rays are then exposed.

Treatment consists of removal of the sac through an incision in the anterior vaginal wall. The defect in the urethra must be repaired. An indwelling urethral catheter should be left in place for 10 days.

Prognosis is usually good unless the diverticulum is so situated that its excision injures the external urinary sphincter mechanism.

Borski, A. A., & R. E. Stutzman: Diverticulum of female urethra: A simplified diagnostic aid. J Urol **93**:60-1, 1965.

Presman, D., Rolnick, D., & J. Zumerchek: Calculus formation within a diverticulum of the female urethra. J Urol **91**:376-9, 1964.

Spence, H. M., & J. W. Duckett, Jr.: Diverticulum of the female urethra: Clinical aspects and presentation of a simple operative technique for cure. J Urol **104**:432-7, 1970.

Ward, J. N., Draper, J. W., & H. M. M. Tovell: Diagnosis and treatment of urethral diverticula in the female. Surg Gynec Obst **125**: 1293-300, 1967.

Widholm, O., & V. A. Ryynänen: Diverticulum of the female urethra. Acta obst gynec scandinav **46**:107-17, 1967.

Wishard, W. N., Jr., Nourse, M. H., & J. H. O. Mertz. Carcinoma in diverticulum of female urethra. J Urol **83**:409-13, 1960.

STRICTURE

Stricture of the adult female urethra is quite common and is often found to be the primary cause of nonspecific urethritis or cystitis. It may be congenital or acquired. The trauma of intercourse and especially that associated with childbirth may lead to periurethral fibrosis with contracture, or the stricture may be caused by the surgeon during vaginal repair. It may develop secondary to acute or chronic urethritis.

Hesitancy in initiating urination and a slow urinary stream are the principal symptoms of stricture. Burning, frequency, nocturia, and urethral pain may occur from secondary urethritis or cystitis. Pyelonephritis is uncommon. If secondary infection of the bladder is present, pus and bacteria will be found in the urine. A fairly large catheter (22 F) may pass to the bladder only with difficulty. Panendoscopy may visualize the point of narrowness and disclose evidence of urethritis. Cystoscopy often reveals trabeculation (hypertrophy) of the bladder wall.

Chronic cystitis may cause similar symptoms, but urinalysis will reveal evidence of infection. Cancer of the urethra causes progressive narrowing of the urethra, but indura-tion and infiltration of the urethra will be found on vaginal examination. Panendoscopy with biopsy establishes the diagnosis. Vesical tumor involving the bladder neck will cause hesitancy and impairment of the urinary stream. Cystoscopy is definitive. Chronic urethritis commonly accompanies urethral stenosis; either may be primary. Recurrent or chronic cystitis is often secondary to stenosis.

Treatment consists of gradual urethral dilatation (up to 36 F) at weekly intervals. Slight overstretching is necessary inasmuch as some contracture will occur after therapy is discontinued. Measures to combat urethritis and cystitis must also be employed.

With proper overdilatation of the urethra and specific therapy of the urethritis which is usually present, the prognosis is good.

Essenhigh, D. M., Ardran, G. M., & V. Cope: A study of the bladder outlet in lower urinary tract infections in women. Brit J Urol **40**:268-77, 1968.

26...

Disorders of the Testis, Scrotum, and Spermatic Cord

DISORDERS OF THE SCROTUM

Hypoplasia of the scrotum accompanies cryptorchism. Bifid scrotum is present with midscrotal or perineal hypospadias and in certain cases of intersexuality. In both instances the 2 scrotal sacs simulate labia majora.

Idiopathic edema of the scrotum is occasionally seen in children. It may be unilateral or may involve both sacs. The edema may involve the penis or may spread into the perineum or the inguinal region. The exact etiology is not known; it may represent an allergic response. The possibility of torsion of the spermatic cord must, however, be kept in mind. Antihistamines may be of value in treatment, though the process does resolve spontaneously.

In association with healed meconium peritonitis, masses may develop in the scrotum. At birth, examination may lead to the diagnosis of hydrocele, but 1 month later the scrotal masses have become firm. A plain film of the abdomen will reveal calcification in the masses as well as in the abdomen. This will differentiate the masses from teratoma.

Berdon, W. E., & others: Scrotal masses in healed meconium peritonitis. New England J Med **277**:585-7, 1967.

Nicholas, J. L., Morgan, A., & R. B. Zachary: Idiopathic edema of scrotum in young boys. Surgery **67**:847-50, 1970.

CONGENITAL ANOMALIES OF THE TESTIS

ANOMALIES OF NUMBER

Absence of one or both testes is very rare and can only be proved at autopsy. Polyorchi-

dism is very rare. A spermatocele or tumor of the spermatic cord is often mistaken for a third gonad.

Tibbs, D. J.: Unilateral absence of the testis. Eight cases of true monorchism. Brit J Surg **48**:601-8, 1961.

HYPOGONADISM

Males suffering from either congenital or prepuberal primary testicular eunuchoidism or pituitary hypogonadism (congenital or secondary to a brain lesion) are tall and have disproportionately long extremities because of delay in fusion of the epiphyses. The testes are small. There is lack of development of secondary sexual characteristics associated with some deficiency in libido and potency. These men are sterile. A somewhat feminine fat distribution may be noted and there are wrinkles about the eyes. The primary gonadal defect is often associated with color blindness and mental retardation.

X-ray studies of the bones reveal delay in closure of the epiphyses. The differential diagnosis of these 2 disorders often depends upon determination of FSH and 17-ketosteroid excretion in the urine. The pituitary type will excrete no FSH; the androgen level is very low. The gonadal eunuch excretes high levels of FSH (above 80 mouse units/24 hours) but only moderately decreased amounts of 17-ketosteroids. The pituitary eunuchoid male may have an enlarged sella turcica or visual field defects secondary to tumor.

Both types are treated with testosterone. Give long-acting esters of testosterone, 200 mg/month IM, or a comparable preparation by mouth daily.

For a discussion of Klinefelter's syndrome, see chapter 28.

Bryson, M. F., & S. Reichlin: Neuroendocrine regulation of sexual function and growth. P Clin North America **13**:423-36, 1966.

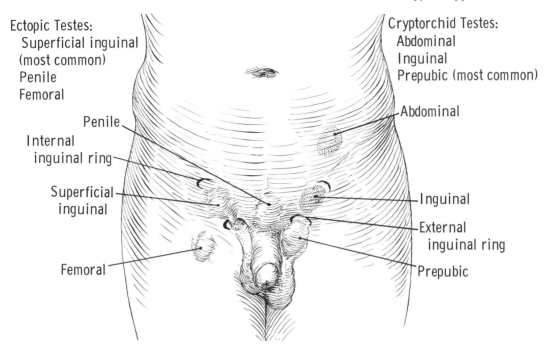

Ectopic Testes:
  Superficial inguinal
  (most common)
  Penile
  Femoral

Cryptorchid Testes:
  Abdominal
  Inguinal
  Prepubic (most common)

Penile
Internal inguinal ring
Superficial inguinal
Femoral

Abdominal
Inguinal
External inguinal ring
Prepubic

Fig 26-1. Undescended testes. Position of testes in various types of ectopy and cryptorchism.

Federman, D. D.: The assessment of organ function—the testis. New England J Med **285**:901-2, 1971.
Landau, R. L.: Tests of testicular function. JAMA **207**:353-5, 1969.

ECTOPY AND CRYPTORCHISM

In ectopy the testicle has strayed from the path of normal descent; in cryptorchism it is arrested in the normal path of descent. Ectopy may be due to an abnormal connection of the distal end of the gubernaculum testis which leads the gonad to an abnormal position. The ectopic sites are as follows (Fig 26-1):

(1) Superficial inguinal (most common site): After passing through the external inguinal ring, the testis proceeds superolaterally to a position superficial to the aponeurosis of the external oblique muscle.

(2) Perineal (rare): The testis is found just in front of the anus and to one side of the midline.

(3) Femoral or crural (rare): The testis is found in Scarpa's triangle superficial to the femoral vessels. The cord passes under the inguinal ligament.

(4) Penile (rare): The testis is placed under the skin at the root of the dorsum of the penis.

(5) Transverse or paradoxical descent (rare): Both testes descend the same inguinal canal. This condition is accompanied by findings compatible with pseudohermaphrodism.

(6) Pelvic (rare): The testis is found in the true pelvis (discovered only by surgical exploration).

Cryptorchism is a condition in which a testicle is arrested at some point in its normal descent. Thus it may be found anywhere between the renal and scrotal areas. Possibly 5% of newborn males will exhibit maldescent, but most of these testes will have assumed their normal positions within a few weeks. About 3% of boys are cryptorchid at puberty, but spontaneous descent may even then occur from the increased hormonal levels which develop at that time.

Etiology

The cause of maldescent is not clear. The following possibilities must be considered.

A. Abnormality of the Gubernaculum Testis: The gubernaculum is a cordlike structure which extends from the lower pole of the testis to the scrotum. In the embryo, of course, it is exceedingly short; differential growth of the body of the embryo appears to cause "descent" of the gonad from its lumbar origin. Absence or abnormality of the gubernaculum testis could lead to maldescent.

B. Intrinsic Testicular Defect: It may be that maldescent is due to a congenital gonadal defect which causes the testicle to be insensitive to gonadotropins. This theory best accounts for unilateral cryptorchism. It also would explain why many patients with bilateral cryptorchism, given definitive therapy at the optimum age, are sterile.

C. Deficient Gonadotropic Hormonal Stimulation: Lack of adequate maternal gonadotropins could account for incomplete descent. This seems to be the obvious explanation for bilateral cryptorchism in the premature infant, since the elaboration of maternal gonadotropins remains at a low level until the last 2 weeks of gestation. It is difficult, however, to apply this theory to unilateral cryptorchism, which is more common than bilateral arrest.

Pathogenesis and Pathology

Moore has clearly shown the efficacy of the scrotum as a temperature regulator for the testes. The spermatogenic cells are quite sensitive to body temperature. Cooper has demonstrated microscopic changes in the retained organ in boys at the age of 2. Robinson and Engle and others have reported definite diminution in the size of spermatogenic tubules and the number of spermatogonia in undescended testes in boys as young as 6 years of age.

After 6 years of age, the changes become more obvious. The diameter of the tubules is smaller than normal. The number of spermatogonia decreases, and fibrosis between the tubules becomes marked. The cryptorchid testis after puberty may be fairly normal in size, but it is markedly deficient in spermatogenic components; infertility is the rule.

It must be borne in mind, however, that about 10% of these testes are congenitally defective (primary hypogonadism, hypogonadism secondary to hypopituitarism). These gonads will show subnormal spermatogenic activity in spite of proper treatment.

Fortunately the Leydig cells are resistant to body temperature; they are therefore usually found in normal numbers in the cryptorchid organ. Impotence on an endocrinologic basis is therefore rare in this group.

Clinical Findings

A. Symptoms: The cardinal symptom of ectopy or cryptorchism is absence of one or both testes from the scrotum. The patient may complain of pain in the testis due to trauma to the organ which is situated in a vulnerable position (eg, over the pubic bone). The adult patient with bilateral cryptorchism may seek advice for infertility.

B. Signs: In true maldescent, the scrotum on the affected side is atrophic. The testis is either impalpable (lying within or even proximal to the inguinal canal) or can be felt external to the inguinal ring. It cannot be manipulated into the scrotum. A common position for such a testis is in the region of the inguinal canal. If one is felt in this area, it must be a superficial inguinal ectopic testis (lying subcutaneously) for it would be impossible to feel a small testis through the heavy external oblique aponeurosis. Inguinal hernia may be demonstrated on the affected side.

C. Laboratory Findings: Studies of the urinary 17-ketosteroids and gonadotropins may help in tracing the cause of cryptorchism. In primary hypogonadism, the urinary gonadotropins (FSH) are markedly elevated, whereas the 17-ketosteroids are moderately reduced. In primary hypopituitarism, the 17-ketosteroids and pituitary gonadotropins are definitely depressed. In "primary" cryptorchids, the 17-ketosteroids and pituitary gonadotropins are often moderately diminished.

Differential Diagnosis

Physiologic cryptorchism (retractile or migratory testis) is a common phenomenon which requires no treatment. Because of the small mass of the prepuberal testis and the strength of the cremaster muscle, which inserts upon the spermatic cord, the testes are apt to be involuntarily retracted out of the scrotum in cold weather or with excitement or physical activity. The diagnosis is made by noting that the scrotum on the suspected side is normally developed and that the "inguinal" testis can be pushed into and to the bottom of the scrotum. It may be necessary to place the child in a warm tub to afford maximum muscular relaxation.

Complications

Associated inguinal hernia is found in 25% of patients with maldescent. At the time of surgery, 95% prove to have a patent processus vaginalis.

Torsion of the spermatic cord is occasionally seen as a complication of cryptorchism. This must also be differentiated from strangulated hernia.

Most authorities agree that the danger of malignancy in a misplaced testis is significantly higher than in the organ which is normally descended. This further substantiates the theory that many of these testes are congenitally abnormal.

Treatment

Since definite histologic change can be demonstrated in the cryptorchid testis by the age of 6 years, placement of the testis in the scrotum should be accomplished by the age of 5. Scorer feels that surgical correction should be accomplished at about the age of 1 year. In association, he found that 83% had an inguinal hernia. However, a successful operation will not ensure fertility if the testis is congenitally defective.

A. Hormone Therapy: Chorionic gonadotropin should be administered in doses of 5000 IU intramuscularly daily for 3-5 days, depending upon the size of the child. Methyltestosterone, 5 mg/day, may be given by mouth for 1 month if the child refuses to accept the injections.

If physiologic cryptorchism has been carefully ruled out, hormone therapy will cause descent in not more than 10-20% of cases. It is more successful in bilateral than in unilateral cryptorchism. It is probably safe to say that if this treatment is successful, the testis would have descended spontaneously at puberty.

B. Surgical Treatment: If hormone therapy fails, or if inguinal hernia can be demonstrated, orchiopexy (and hernioplasty) should be done immediately. The testis must be placed at the bottom of the scrotum without tension; the blood supply to the organ must be meticulously preserved, though Fowler and Stephens and others believe that the spermatic artery can be sacrificed without harm to the testes.

Prognosis

Success of treatment is measured by fertility. The man with one untreated cryptorchid testis produces fewer sperm than the man with normally descended testes. Untreated, bilateral cryptorchism almost always causes infertility. If treated at the optimal age, 60% of these males will be fertile.

Altman, B. L., & M. Malament: Carcinoma of the testis following orchiopexy. J Urol **97**: 498-504, 1967.

Dajani, A. M.: Transverse ectopia of the testes. Brit J Urol **41**:80-2, 1969.

Ehrlich, R. M., & others: Effect of gonadotropin in cryptorchism. J Urol **102**:793-5, 1969.

Firor, H. V.: Two-stage orchiopexy. Arch Surg **102**:598-9, 1971.

Flinn, R. A., & L. R. King: Experiences with the midline transabdominal approach in orchiopexy. Surg Gynec Obst **133**:285-9, 1971.

Hortling, H., & others: An endocrinologic follow-up study of operated cases of cryptorchism. J Clin Endocrinol **27**:120-9, 1967.

Jacobson, C. E., Jr.: Midline approach to orchiopexy. J Urol **95**:74-6, 1966.

Kiesewetter, W. B., Shull, W. R., & G. H. Fetterman: Histologic changes in the testes following anatomically successful orchidopexy. J Pediat Surg **4**:59-65, 1969.

Lemek, C. N.: A study of the development and structural relationships of the testis and gubernaculum. Surg Gynec Obst **110**:164-72, 1960.

Miller, H. C.: Transseptal orchiopexy for cryptorchism. J Urol **98**:503-5, 1967.

Persky, L., & D. J. Albert: Staged orchiopexy. Surg Gynec Obst **132**:43-5, 1971.

Scorer, C. G.: Early operation for the undescended testis. Brit J Surg **54**:694-8, 1967.

Scorer, C. G.: The descent of the testis. Arch Dis Childhood **39**:605-9, 1964.

CONGENITAL ANOMALIES OF THE EPIDIDYMIS

Congenital absence of the epididymis is rare. At times the epididymis may be anterior rather than posterior to the testis. Lack of fusion of the epididymis and testis has been reported.

DISORDERS OF THE SPERMATIC CORD*

SPERMATOCELE

A spermatocele is a painless cystic mass containing sperm. It lies just above and posterior to the testis but is separate from it (Fig 26-2). Most spermatoceles are less than 1 cm in diameter, although they are occasionally quite large and may be mistaken for hydroceles. They may be firm, simulating solid tumor. The etiology is not entirely clear, although they probably arise from the tubules that connect the rete testis to the head of the epididymides (vasa efferentia) or from cystic structures on the upper pole of the testis or epididymis.

Since they are relatively small, spermatoceles are usually discovered by the physician during routine examination of the genitalia; at times they may be large enough to come to the attention of the patient. Examination reveals

---

*The only congenital anomaly which affects the spermatic cord is absence of the vas deferens. If bilateral, infertility is the result.

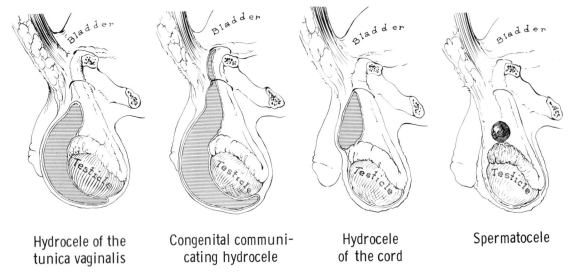

| Hydrocele of the tunica vaginalis | Congenital communicating hydrocele | Hydrocele of the cord | Spermatocele |

Fig 26-2. Hydrocele of the tunica vaginalis and cord; spermatocele.

a freely movable transilluminating cystic mass lying above the testicle. Microscopic examination of aspirated contents reveals sperm, usually dead. Grossly, the fluid is thin, white, and cloudy.

Spermatocele is differentiated from hydrocele of the tunica vaginalis in that the latter covers the entire anterior surface of the testicle. Aspiration of hydrocele recovers yellow but clear fluid. A tumor of the coverings of the spermatic cord (eg, mesothelioma, fibroma) may feel like a tense spermatocele. It does not, however, contain fluid, and will not transilluminate.

Spermatocele requires no therapy unless it is large enough to annoy the patient, in which case it should be excised.

Clarke, B. G., Bamford, S. B., & G. J. Gherardi: Spermatocele: Pathologic and surgical anatomy. Arch Surg 86:351-5, 1963.
Lord, P. H.: A bloodless operation for spermatocele or cyst of the epididymis. Brit J Surg 57:641-4, 1970.
Schoenberg, H. W., & J. J. Murphy: The differential diagnosis of intrascrotal masses. GP 25:82-8, March 1962.

VARICOCELE*

Varicocele is common in young men and consists of dilatation of the pampiniform plexus about the testis. The left side is most commonly affected. These veins drain into the internal spermatic vein in the region of the internal inguinal ring. This vein passes lateral to the vas deferens at the internal inguinal ring and, on the left side, drains into the renal vein. On the right it empties into the vena cava.

The left internal spermatic vein is particularly liable to have incompetent valves. This fact, plus gravity, may lead to poor drainage of the pampiniform plexus, the veins of which gradually undergo dilatation and elongation. At times they are painful, particularly in sexually continent men. Marriage in this instance may relieve symptoms.

The sudden development of a varicocele in an older man is sometimes seen as a late sign of renal tumor when tumor cells have invaded the renal vein, thereby occluding the spermatic vein.

Examination of a man with varicocele reveals a mass of dilated, tortuous veins lying posterior to and above the testis. It may extend up to the external inguinal ring and is often tender. Testicular atrophy from impaired circulation may be present.

No treatment is required unless the varicocele is thought to contribute to infertility or is painful or so large as to disturb the patient. A scrotal support will often relieve discomfort; otherwise, ligation of the internal spermatic vein at the internal inguinal ring is indicated. The results from this operation are uniformly excellent.

*See also chapter 30.

Ahlberg, N. E., & others: Phlebography in varicocele scroti. Acta radiol (diag) 4:517-8, 1966.

Clarke, B. G.: Incidence of varicocele in normal men and among men of different age groups. JAMA 198:1121-2, 1966.

Kiska, E. F., & G. T. Cowart: Treatment of varicocele by high ligation. J Urol 83:713-5, 1960.

HYDROCELE

A hydrocele consists of a collection of fluid within the tunica or processus vaginalis. Although it may occur within the spermatic cord, it is most often seen surrounding the testicle. A hydrocele may develop rapidly secondary to local injury, acute nonspecific or tuberculous epididymitis, or orchitis. It may complicate testicular neoplasm. Chronic hydrocele is more common. Its cause is usually unknown and usually afflicts men past the age of 40 years. Fluid collects about the testis, and the mass grows gradually. It may be soft and cystic or quite tense. The fluid is clear and yellow (Fig 26-2).

Hydrocele of the tunica vaginalis is common in the newborn, probably due to late closure of the processus vaginalis, which is continuous with the peritoneum. Most of these fluid collections subside spontaneously during the first few weeks of life.

Clinical Findings

Young boys with hydrocele commonly have a history of a cystic mass which is small and soft in the morning but larger and more tense at night. One can only conclude, in these instances, that a small communication exists in the processus vaginalis between the peritoneal cavity and the tunica vaginalis (Fig 26-2). Hernia or communicating hydrocele is therefore the proper diagnosis. Hydrocele is painless unless it is accompanied by acute epididymal infection. The patient may, however, complain of its bulk or weight.

The diagnosis is made by finding a rounded cystic intrascrotal mass which is not tender unless underlying inflammatory disease is present. The tumor transilluminates. If the hydrocele is enclosed within the spermatic cord, a cystic fusiform swelling is noted in the groin or in the upper scrotum.

A tense hydrocele must be differentiated from tumor of the testis, which does not transilluminate. However, if hydrocele develops in a young man without apparent cause, it should be aspirated so that careful palpation of the testicle and epididymis can be done in order to rule out cancer or tuberculosis.

Complications include compression of the blood supply of the testicle, which leads to atrophy; hemorrhage into the hydrocele sac following trauma (hematocele); or, rarely, infection complicating aspiration.

Treatment

Unless complications are present, active therapy is not required. The indications for treatment are a very tense hydrocele which might embarrass circulation to the testicle, or a large, bulky mass which is cosmetically unsightly and perhaps uncomfortable for the patient.

One aspiration of a hydrocele which is present during the first few months of life is often curative. Periodic aspiration is usually the treatment of choice in chronic hydrocele. Most chronic hydroceles refill slowly over a period of 6-20 weeks, at which time aspiration can be repeated. If the sac refills rapidly, or if the patient requests definitive therapy, the parietal tunica vaginalis should be resected. Secondary infection may require incision and drainage. Hematocele should be treated by resection of the hydrocele sac.

McGowan, A. J., & T. F. Howley: Experiences with the extrusion operation for hydrocele. J Urol 101:366-7, 1969.

Jordan, W. P., Jr.: Hydroceles and varicoceles. S Clin North America 45:1535-46, 1965.

Ross, J. G.: Treatment of primary hydroceles in infancy and childhood. Brit J Surg 49: 415-8, 1962.

Wallace, A. F.: Aetiology of the idiopathic hydrocele. Brit J Urol 32:79-96, 1960.

TORSION OF THE SPERMATIC CORD

Torsion of the spermatic cord (torsion of the testicle) is an uncommon affliction which is almost completely limited to prepubertal boys. It has been observed in the newborn. It causes strangulation of the blood supply to the testis. Unless treatment is prompt (within 3 or 4 hours), testicular atrophy may occur.

The cryptorchid testis is prone to undergo torsion. In most instances, congenital abnormality of the tunica vaginalis or spermatic cord is present. Torsion seems to be most often due to a voluminous tunica vaginalis which inserts well up on the cord. This allows the testis to rotate within the tunica. The initiating factor seems to be spasm of the cremaster muscle, which inserts obliquely on the cord. Its contraction causes the patient's left testis to rotate counterclockwise and his right testis clockwise (as the physician observes the patient from the foot of the bed). With vascular occlusion there is edema of the testis and the cord up to the point of occlusion. This leads to gangrene of the testis and epididymis.

Clinical Findings

The diagnosis should suggest itself when a young boy suddenly develops severe pain in one testicle, followed by swelling of the organ, reddening of the scrotal skin, lower abdominal pain, and nausea and vomiting. However, as Lyon has pointed out, torsion of the cord may be accompanied by little or no pain; only some scrotal swelling is observed.

Examination usually reveals a swollen, tender organ which is retracted upward as a result of shortening of the cord by volvulus. Pain may be increased by lifting the testicle up over the symphysis. (The pain from epididymitis, rare in children, is usually alleviated by this maneuver.) Within a few hours after onset, moderate fever and leukocytosis may develop.

The diagnosis may be made in the early stages if the epididymis can be felt in an abnormal position (eg, anterior). After a few hours, however, the entire gonad becomes so swollen that the epididymis cannot be distinguished from the testis by palpation.

Differential Diagnosis

The differential diagnosis includes acute epididymitis, acute mumps orchitis, and trauma. Epididymitis is rare before puberty. It is often accompanied by pyuria. Mumps orchitis is usually accompanied by parotitis; it is rare before puberty. Without history or findings of injury, traumatic orchitis may be misdiagnosed as torsion of the cord.

Treatment

If seen within a few hours of onset, manual detorsion may be attempted. Knowing that torsion causes the left testis to rotate counterclockwise and the right clockwise, one may twist a testis in the opposite direction. This maneuver is facilitated by infiltration of the spermatic cord, near the external inguinal ring, with 10-20 ml of 1% procaine hydrochloride. If this fails, immediate surgical detorsion must be performed, although after 4-6 hours infarction usually will have occurred in those testes subjected to a 720° twist of the cord. Whether the testis appears to be viable or not, it should be sutured down to preclude a subsequent torsion. Even though the seminiferous tubules may become necrotic, the more hardy interstitial cells may remain viable. Excision of the parietal tunica vaginalis will cause agglutination of the testicle to the scrotal wall. Since the opposite testicle usually is affected by the same abnormal attachments, prophylactic fixation of that organ must also be done.

Prognosis

Unfortunately, the diagnosis is usually made and treatment instituted too late, and atrophy is to be expected in most instances.

Frederick, P. L., Dushku, N., & A. J. Eraklis: Simultaneous bilateral torsion of the testes in a newborn infant. Arch Surg **94**:299-300, 1967.

Gelband, H., & M. A. Wulfsohn: Torsion of the spermatic cord in utero: Case report. J Urol **98**:506-7, 1967.

Hyams, B. B.: Torsion of the testis in the newborn. J Urol **101**:192-5, 1969.

Kaplan, G. W., & L. R. King: Acute scrotal swelling in children. J Urol **104**:219-23, 1970.

Lyon, R. P.: Torsion of the testicle in childhood. A painless emergency requiring contralateral orchiopexy. JAMA **178**:702-5, 1961.

Moharib, N. H., & H. P. Krahn: Acute scrotum in children with emphasis on torsion of spermatic cord. J Urol **104**:601-3, 1970.

Parker, R. M., & J. R. Robison: Anatomy and diagnosis of torsion of the testicle. J Urol **106**:243-7, 1971.

Skoglund, R. W., McRoberts, J. W., & H. Ragde: Torsion of the spermatic cord: A review of the literature and an analysis of 70 new cases. J Urol **104**:604-7, 1970.

TORSION OF THE APPENDICES OF THE TESTIS AND EPIDIDYMIS

On the upper poles of both the testis and epididymis there are small vestigial appendages which may be sessile or pedunculated (Fig 1-8). The latter type may spontaneously undergo torsion, which leads to an inflammatory reaction followed by ischemic necrosis and absorption.

This phenomenon usually affects prepuberal boys. Sudden onset of testicular pain is noted. Should the physician have the opportunity to examine the boy shortly after onset, a small tender lump may be felt at the upper pole of the testis or epididymis; this sign is pathognomonic.

If seen later, the entire testicle is swollen and tender. The differential diagnosis is then between torsion of these appendages and of the spermatic cord. Immediate surgical exploration is indicated, for time is a critical factor in treatment of torsion of the cord. If an appendix is twisted, it should be excised.

Bender, L., Prinz, L., & D. Presman: Torsion of the hydatid testis: A review of thirteen cases. Pediatrics **42**:531-4, 1968.

Rolnick, D., & others: Anatomical incidence of testicular appendages. J Urol **100**:755-6, 1968.

Skoglund, R. W., McRoberts, J. W., & H. Ragde: Torsion of testicular appendages: Presentation of 43 new cases are a collective review. J Urol **104**:598-600, 1970.

•   •   •

27...

Skin Diseases of the External Genitalia

Rees B. Rees, Jr., MD*†

SKIN DISEASES OF THE EXTERNAL GENITALIA

Almost any skin condition, including psoriasis, seborrheic dermatitis, lichen planus, eczema, etc, can affect the region of the external genitalia and perineum. The patient should be questioned and examined for other possible areas of involvement. In any case of itching or infected dermatitis in this area, it is important to rule out diabetes and pediculosis or scabies.

Associated vaginal and other urologic conditions should be corrected. Self-treatment and overtreatment may alter and complicate genital lesions. Emotional factors associated with repeated scratching and rubbing tend to prolong and complicate many genital conditions.

Many individuals with involvement in this area have a fear of venereal disease; if there is no question of this, the fear should be dispelled.

ECZEMATOID DERMATITIS

Eczematoid dermatitis is a broad descriptive term which denotes changes such as redness, vesiculation, scaling, weeping, lichenification (accentuation and thickening of skin markings), and excoriation. This type of eruption may become secondarily infected through scratching. Included in this group are such conditions as contact dermatitis, localized neurodermatitis, pruritus vulvae and scroti, atopic dermatitis, and intertriginous dermatitis. These conditions usually overlap in producing an eczematoid dermatitis, and treatment must take this into consideration.

Contact Dermatitis

Contact dermatitis includes changes produced both by primary irritants and true allergic sensitizers. Possible causes are cosmetics, feminine deodorant sprays, douches, contraceptives, soaps, local medications ("overtreatment dermatitis"), wearing apparel, plants (poison oak and ivy), etc.

Treatment must include removal of the suspected agent, if possible. Cool wet dressings constitute excellent treatment, and corticosteroid creams may be used topically if infection is not present. The fluorinated corticosteroid creams such as fluocinolone, triamcinolone, betamethasone, and fluocinonide are more likely to produce atrophic striae in the groin than is 0.25-1% hydrocortisone.

Fisher, A.A.: Contact Dermatitis. Lea & Febiger, 1967.

Circumscribed Neurodermatitis (Lichen Simplex Chronicus)

These thickened lesions are of great importance in the persistence of any vulval or scrotal skin condition regardless of the original cause. Rubbing and scratching can prolong any eruption indefinitely, and it is usually this problem that causes the patient to seek medical care. This may be done almost subconsciously. A continuing itch-scratch cycle is established which must be broken before healing can occur.

Treatment is as for contact dermatitis (above) plus counseling about the dangers of persistent trauma.

Obermayer, M.E.: Psychocutaneous Medicine. Thomas, 1965.
Verbov, J.L.: Pruritus ani. Practitioner **205**: 67-69, 1970.

Itching of Vulva and Scrotum

These are merely nonspecific terms used to classify some cases of marked pruritus of these areas with little or no skin changes. Treatment is as for contact dermatitis (above).

---

*Clinical Professor of Dermatology & Radiology, University of California School of Medicine, San Francisco.
†Venereal disease is discussed in Chapter 14; tumors in Chapter 17.

Atopic Dermatitis

This lesion presents as dry lichenified dermatitis on the penis, scrotum, in the groins, and on the vulva. Similar changes are usually present also on the face and neck and in the antecubital and popliteal spaces. Generalized dryness is present. There is usually a personal or family history of asthma or hay fever.

A high-potency corticosteroid cream (0.2% fluocinolone or 0.5% triamcinolone) rubbed in thinly 4 or 5 times daily is effective, although striae may supervene.

Baer, R.L.: Atopic Dermatitis. Lippincott, 1955.

Intertrigo

Intertrigo (sodden, macerated dermatitis) is due to chafing and friction of contiguous surfaces. It occurs in the groins, inframammary areas, skin folds, etc, usually in obese individuals, and is more common during hot, humid weather. Treatment must be directed toward drying the area and reducing chafing.

COMMON SUPERFICIAL INFECTIONS OF THE EXTERNAL GENITALIA

Pyodermas

Staphylococci are present in most of the infections discussed below, but streptococci may be found in as many as 40% of cases. A smear stained with Giemsa's stain will usually show many cocci. Systemic antibiotic treatment is mandatory to prevent nephritis and other serious complications. Pediculosis and scabies should be ruled out.

Sodium cloxacillin is the drug of choice since it is not destroyed by penicillinase. If the patient is allergic to penicillin, the drug of second choice is erythromycin. A polymyxin-bacitracin ointment such as Polysporin® may be used topically.

Pyodermas frequently complicate some other primary condition, such as pediculosis and scabies.

A. Folliculitis and Furunculosis: Infection of a hair follicle is usually acute but may be chronic and recurrent. Sharply pointed, extremely tender and hot swellings with central pustulation may be found.

B. Impetigo: Impetiginous involvement is more superficial and is characterized by "stuck-on crusts" and weeping. The mons pubis may be the sole site of involvement, but other areas are usually involved also.

C. Infectious Eczematoid Dermatitis: This is an acute reddened, weeping, spreading eruption. It is often associated with a draining process such as a furuncle or abscess or with vaginal discharge.

D. Hidradenitis Suppurativa: This is a deep chronic inflammatory infection of the apocrine sweat glands, characterized by cystic involvement and interconnecting sinus tracts. It usually involves the axillas and groins and may be an accompaniment of severe cystic acne. In addition to giving antibiotics, it may be necessary to unroof ("saucerize") or actually excise the lesions with or without grafting.

Maibach, H.I., & G. Hildick-Smith: Skin Bacteria and Their Role in Infection. McGraw-Hill, 1965.

Fungal Infections

Heat, moisture, and darkness favor these infections. They are frequently aggravated by overtreatment.

A. Tinea Cruris: Tinea cruris is characterized by marginated, slightly elevated, scaling patches on the inner thighs and in the groins. There may be an active vesicular border. Pruritus may be intense. Direct microscopic examination of skin scrapings in 15% potassium or sodium hydroxide solution will reveal hyphae or spores. The differential diagnosis includes seborrheic dermatitis, psoriasis, intertrigo, and localized neurodermatitis. Tinea cruris usually responds to treatment with 3% precipitated sulfur and 1% salicylic acid in an emulsion base. Griseofulvin (micronized), 500 mg orally, may be given daily after supper.

B. Anogenital Candidiasis: Infection with Candida albicans is characterized by erythematous, weeping, circumscribed lesions with peripheral epidermal undermining and satellite vesiculopustules. "Ping-pong" infections between sexual partners may occur. Pregnancy, diabetes, obesity, and hyperhidrosis are predisposing factors. Broad-spectrum antibiotic therapy or estrogen therapy may be followed by an overgrowth of candidal organisms. The skin involvement may be secondary to vaginal involvement. Lesions occur under the prepuce. High-power microscopic examination of skin scrapings in 15% potassium or sodium hydroxide solution shows clusters of tiny spores and fine mycelial filaments. Nystatin appears to be effective in most instances. It is available as dusting powder, cream, vaginal inserts, and oral tablets.

Conant, M.F., & others: Manual of Clinical Mycology. Saunders, 1971.

Virus Infections

A. Warts: Warts are common in the vulvar region, under the prepuce, and on the shaft of the penis. If present on the mucous or mucocutaneous surfaces, they are called condylomata acuminata. They are usually moist and macerated. They frequently respond to topical treatment with podophyllin resin, 25%, in compound tincture of benzoin. If this fails, 25% in mineral oil should be tried. Severe discomfort may follow application of podophyllin. Fulguration may be necessary if podophyllin is not successful. Liquid nitrogen can be used either with a cotton-tipped applicator or a copper disk on a long steel wand. Each lesion may be frozen for 10-30 seconds.

B. Herpes Simplex (Cold Sore, Fever Blister): Genital herpes is usually due to recurrent herpesvirus type 2 and is characterized by grouped vesiculopustular lesions. There may be secondary adenopathy. This can be a painful recurrent condition and has been implicated in the genesis of cervical carcinoma. Rarely, a primary herpes simplex infection is seen, with severe vulvovaginitis and systemic manifestations. Uncomplicated herpes simplex may be treated with 0.5% neutral red dye scrubbed into the lesion followed by exposure to a 15 watt fluorescent white light at 6 inches' distance for 15 minutes. A simple dusting powder such as BFI (bismuth formic iodide) may be useful.

Shelley, W. B.: Consultations in Dermatology With W. B. Shelley. Saunders, 1972.

OTHER INFLAMMATORY DISORDERS

Drug Eruptions

Drug eruptions may involve the genitals. A fixed drug eruption, due usually to phenolphthalein, broad-spectrum antibiotics, or barbiturates may cause a perfectly round, bright-red to purplish macular lesion which comes and goes with each reexposure to the drug. Other drug eruptions usually have manifestations elsewhere as well as on the circumscribed area.

Rees, R. B.: Cutaneous drug reactions. Texas Med **66**:92-3, 1970.

Urticaria and Angioneurotic Edema

These lesions ("hives" and "giant hives") may present on the vulva or male genitalia as a sole sign, at least initially. They may be confused with acute contact dermatitis, which can have an urticarial component. There may be a history of ingestion of an urticariogenic food such as shellfish, pork and pork products, strawberries, or yeast-containing foods. Penicillin is the most common drug cause. Treatment consists of removal of the cause plus cool wet dressings and antihistamines by mouth.

Zamm, A. V.: Chronic urticaria: A practical approach. Cutis 9:27-37, 1972.

Erythema Multiforme

Erythema multiforme may present as an acute inflammatory erosive process on the genitalia, although signs are usually present elsewhere, eg, the lips, tongue, and mouth, possibly with conjunctivitis. Erythema multiforme and its more severe variant, Stevens-Johnson disease, may be idiopathic or may be caused by drug reaction, herpes simplex, or other infection. Finding a typical "target" herpes-iris or "bulls-eye" lesion may make the diagnosis. Severe forms must be managed symptomatically with supportive treatment and hospitalization. Systemic corticosteroids may be necessary (unless contraindicated), and broad-spectrum antibiotics may be helpful as well.

Yaffee, H. S.: Erythema multiforme. In: Newer Views of Skin Diseases. Yaffee, H. S. (editor). Little, Brown, 1966.

PAPULOSQUAMOUS ERUPTIONS

Psoriasis

Psoriasis may involve flexural surfaces (inverse psoriasis) such as the groin and the perianal, internatal cleft, and intermammary areas. It tends to be bright red and moist, and usually free of scales. Itching may be intense. Occasionally the only involvement may be in the anogenital area. A solitary plaque may present on the penis, leading to confusion with Bowen's disease or some other more serious disorder. The diagnosis usually can be made by inspection and by noting other areas of involvement such as in the scalp and on the elbows and knees. Pitting of the nails, when present, is almost pathognomonic of psoriasis. Treatment is with 0.1% anthralin ointment rubbed in sparingly morning and night for intertriginous lesions.

Sidi, E., & others: Psoriasis. Thomas, 1968.

Seborrheic Dermatitis

Seborrheic dermatitis may appear as scurfy, scaly, erythematous patches and is easily confused with candidiasis, intertrigo, and psoriasis. Typical areas of involvement are usually present elsewhere, eg, the scalp, brows, creases of the cheeks and chin, in and around the ears, on the presternum, and in the axillas. Corticosteroid creams are very useful. Sulfur (3%) and salicylic acid (1%) in an emulsion base is also effective.

Derbes, V. J.: Seborrheic dermatitis. Cutis 4:553-8, 1968.

Lichen Planus

Lichen planus may appear on the glans penis or on the labia and introitus. The lesions are small polygonal violet-hued papules about 2-3 cm in diameter which have milky striations over their shiny surfaces. They may become clustered together to form plaques. Itching is usually a problem. There may be generalized involvement or typical lesions in the buccal mucosa which look like spilled milk.

Corticosteroid creams may be helpful in relieving the pruritus. The disease usually disappears after a course of several months.

Irgang, S.: Lichen planus. Cutis 6:887-97, 1970.

LICHEN SCLEROSUS ET ATROPHICUS

This is a distinct entity characterized by flat-topped white papules which coalesce to form white patches without infiltration. The surface shows comedone-like plugs or dells. The end stages may resemble very thin parchment or tissue paper. It occurs most frequently in patches on the upper back, chest, and breasts, mostly in women. It almost inevitably involves the anogenital regions, where painful fissures may develop and severe itching may be a distressing symptom. On the penis this condition occurs as balanitis xerotica obliterans, which may lead to urethral stenosis and atrophy with telangiectasia about the meatus and on the glans, with some shrinkage of the prepuce. There is a direct relationship between these conditions and carcinoma. Anogenital lichen sclerosus et atrophicus may be misdiagnosed as kraurosis vulvae with or without leukoplakia. At present, kraurosis is regarded as a descriptive term for the manifestation in a number of diseases.

Lichen sclerosus et atrophicus may involute spontaneously, especially in young girls.

Vitamin A ointment may be tried. For severe itching, one may use intralesional corticosteroids such as triamcinolone (Kenalog®) suspension injected into the skin with the dermajet apparatus or by syringe. Topical corticosteroids may give relief.

Circumcision for balanitis xerotica obliterans which is lichen sclerosus is not particularly helpful.

Barker, L. P., & P. Gross: Lichen sclerosus et atrophicus of the female genitalia. Arch Dermat 85:362-73, 1962.

•   •   •

General References

Domonkos, A. N.: Andrews' Disease of the Skin: Clinical Dermatology, 6th ed. Saunders, 1971.

Shelley, W. B.: Consultations in Dermatology With Walter B. Shelley. Saunders, 1972.

28 . . .

Intersexuality

The sex of an infant, judged by the appearance of the external genitalia, is in doubt in about one out of every 1000 births. The phallus may be small, and the question may arise whether the child has a micropenis or an enlarged clitoris. The phallus is often incurved ventrally (as in hypospadias), and the urethra may open in the perineum (as in penoscrotal or midscrotal hypospadias). In male pseudohermaphrodism the scrotum is often bifid, resembling labia majora; the testes are usually absent from the scrotum. At first glance, then, the appearance is usually that of advanced hypospadias, although the genitalia may be ambiguous.

Some of these infants have testes; others have ovaries. Many, despite the presence of testes, have well-developed structures of müllerian duct origin (uterus, fallopian tubes, upper vagina).

The evaluation of nuclear sex is of help in establishing the type of intersexuality. This can be ascertained by microscopic study of the cells in a buccal or vaginal smear. The percentage of cells containing the Barr chromatin mass of the female is determined. If 40% or more of the cells contain this body, the chromatin sex is positive. If less than 10% are positive (and these are artifacts), the chromatin sex is negative. Further information can be gained from cytogenetic studies. Chromosome number or morphology may be abnormal.

In most cases treatment is fairly satisfactory; in others it is not. Therapy in the infant depends largely upon the appearance of the external genitalia (except in the instance of congenital adrenal virilism); the child should usually be reared in the sex which surgical repair can best simulate.

Two types of intersexuality, Turner's syndrome (gonadal dysgenesis) and Klinefelter's syndrome, usually become apparent only at the time of puberty.

Barr, M. L. : The sex chromosomes in evolution and in medicine. Canad MAJ **95**:1137-48, 1966.

Bishop, P. M. F. : Intersexual states and allied conditions. Brit MJ **1**:1255-62, 1966.

Money, J. : Problems in sexual development. Endocrinologic and psychologic aspects. New York J Med **63**:2348-54, 1963.

Moore, K. L. : Sex determination, sexual differentiation and intersex development. Canad MAJ **97**:292-5, 1967.

Ross, G. T., & J. H. Tijo: Cytogenetics in clinical endocrinology. JAMA **192**:977-86, 1965.

Series of articles on genetics. Am J Med **34**: 583-720, 1963.

Wakefield, A. R. : Intersex and related problems. S Clin North America **47**:505-14, 1967.

Williams, D. L., & J. W. Runyan: Sex chromatin and chromosome analysis in the diagnosis of sex abnormalities. Ann Int Med **64**: 422-59, 1966.

INTERSEXUALITY NOTICEABLE AT BIRTH

FEMALE PSEUDOHERMAPHRODISM
(Female Intersex)

Congenital Virilizing Cortical Hyperplasia

This syndrome develops because of an inborn error of metabolism. The biosynthesis of cortisol is defective; this leads to increased secretion of ACTH, which causes adrenal hyperplasia and excessive secretion of androgens. The newborn female with anatomic changes caused by prenatal adrenocortical hyperplasia has normal ovaries, uterus, fallopian tubes, and vagina. However, the excess androgen has a masculinizing effect on the urogenital sinus and genital tubercle, so that the vagina is usually connected to the urethra, which in turn opens at the base of an enlarged clitoris. The labia are often hypertrophied. Externally, then, the appearance is that of severe hypospadias with cryptorchism. This is one of the common types of pseudohermaphrodism. It is

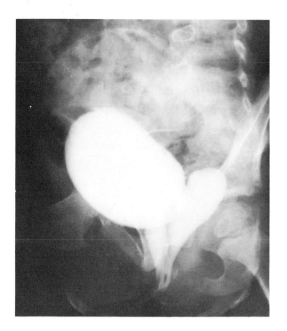

Fig 28-1. Urogenital sinus in congenital virilizing cortical hyperplasia. Oblique urethrogram showing connection of vagina with distal urethra. (Courtesy of Frank Hinman, Jr., MD.)

often familial and at times is accompanied by adrenal insufficiency.

Urethroscopy may permit visualization of the point at which the vagina opens into the posterior wall of the urethra. The vaginal tract can often be entered by the urethroscope and the cervix seen. A lateral urethrogram may visualize the vagina as well as the bladder (Fig 28-1).

Because hyperactivity of the adrenal cortex persists, the infant grows rapidly, and a definite increase in urinary 17-ketosteroids can often be demonstrated by the age of 2-4 months. Bone age is accelerated, as shown by radiograms. Nuclear sex is positive (female). Chromosome studies are normal. The other types of intersexuals, although similar in external appearance, demonstrate no abnormal hormonal reactions; acceleration of growth and maturation does not occur.

By giving corticosteroids, pituitary (ACTH) hyperactivity is suppressed, thereby decreasing the elaboration of adrenal androgen. In the infant, cortisone acetate, 25-50 mg IM, should be administered every day or every other day. It may also be given by mouth every 6 hours. Optimum dosage should cause the urinary 17-ketosteroids to drop to about 3 mg/day and the bone growth to approach normal.

Female pseudohermaphrodites usually adjust best toward the feminine side and should

be allowed to do so. If frequent erections of the hypertrophied clitoris occur, clitoridectomy should be considered. After the age of puberty it may be feasible to separate the urethra from the vaginal tract so that both empty on the perineum. A normal sexual and reproductive life may then be possible.

Nonadrenal Type

This rare disorder results from gestational virilization of the mother by administration of synthetic androgen or progestational compounds of the 19-nortestosterone type.

The gonadal and nuclear sex is female, and cytogenetically the child is a normal female. The uterus is present though often bifid. The vagina and urethra empty into a urogenital sinus whose opening on the perineal surface is often stenosed. This may lead to urinary obstruction and progressive renal damage. The vagina may become enlarged as a result of the hydrostatic pressure caused by the retained urine. Externally there is a hypertrophied clitoris which may contain a rudimentary urethra. The labia are normal.

This type of intersex is differentiated from female adrenal intersex by the fact that progressive masculinization does not occur, the 17-ketosteroids remain normal, and bone age is not advanced. Female intersex of this type may simulate true hermaphrodism, in which case exploratory laparotomy and gonadal biopsy are indicated.

Treatment consists of enlarging the vaginourethral opening in the perineum. If the vagina is enlarged, it should be resected. Partial clitoridectomy is often necessary.

Gross, R. E., Randolph, J., & J. F. Crigler, Jr.: Clitoridectomy for sexual abnormalities: Indications and technique. Surgery **59**:300-8, 1966.

Grumbach, M. M., & J. R. Ducharme: The effects of androgens on fetal sexual development. Fertil Steril **11**:157-80, 1960.

Jeffcoate, T. N. A., & others: Diagnosis of the adrenogenital syndrome before birth. Lancet **2**:553-5, 1965.

Kurlander, G. J.: Roentgenology of the congenital adrenogenital syndrome. Am J Roentgenol **95**:189-99, 1965.

New, M. I.: Congenital adrenal hyperplasia. P Clin North America **15**:395-407, 1968.

Seymour, R. J., & R. A. H. Kinch: Recession and relocation of the enlarged clitoris in congenital adrenogenital syndrome. Canad J Surg **9**:365-9, 1966.

Weldon, V. V., Blizzard, R. M., & C. J. Migeon: Newborn girls misdiagnosed as bilaterally cryptorchid males. New England J Med **274**:829-33, 1966.

MALE PSEUDOHERMAPHRODISM
(Male Intersex)

Some male intersex patients have perfectly normal external genitalia, except for cryptorchism, although a rudimentary uterus and fallopian tubes may be present. Others have a feminine psyche and body habitus, although the "clitoris" is enlarged. Breast development is normal (syndrome of testicular feminization). Most commonly, however, the male intersex patient has a markedly hypospadiac penis (often smaller than normal), a perineal urethral orifice, and, frequently, abdominal or inguinal cryptorchism. The scrotum is bifid, resembling labia majora. The prostatic utricle (a remnant of the müllerian duct) is enlarged, and a complete uterus and fallopian tubes may be found with the vagina opening into the posterior urethra. The testes may be suspended from the tubes in the position usually occupied by ovaries or found in femoral hernia sacs. They produce mostly estrogen. This is one of the most common forms of intersexuality.

Urethroscopy may or may not reveal the vaginal canal opening into the urethra; urethrograms may show this connection. By the age of 1 or 2 months and certainly by 6 months, determinations of urinary 17-ketosteroids will be normal. Bone age is also normal. The cells in a buccal smear lack the nuclear mass. These tests differentiate male intersexuality from the female congenital adrenogenital syndrome. The chromosome pattern is XY. If doubt still exists, exploratory laparotomy with biopsy of the gonads should be done.

If the phallus is of adequate size, treatment consists of repair of the hypospadiac penis. Cryptorchism should also be treated. If the testis cannot be brought down into the scrotum where it can be observed, orchiectomy should be done for, in association with this syndrome, about 15% of these testes will undergo malignant degeneration. The presence of the uterus and vagina can be ignored, for these organs will not develop.

If the phallus is very small, stimulation of its growth should be attempted by the administration of methyltestosterone, 5 mg/day orally. Often, unfortunately, no response is obtained, in which case the child is best raised as a girl. Appropriate plastic surgical repair can then be performed.

Alexander, D. S., & M. A. Ferguson-Smith: Chromosomal studies in some variants of male pseudohermaphroditism. Pediatrics **28**:758-63, 1961.

Schneider, K. M., Becker, J. M., & I. H. Krasna: Surgical management of intersexuality in infancy and childhood. Ann Surg **168**:255-61, 1968.

Weisberg, M. G., Malkasian, G. D., Jr., & J. H. Pratt: Testicular feminization syndrome. A review and report of 6 cases. Am J Obst Gynec **107**:1181-7, 1970.

TRUE HERMAPHRODISM
(Gonadal Intersex)

True hermaphrodites may have one ovary and one testis, although more often 2 ovotestes are present. At birth the external genitalia may resemble normal male or female genitalia, but they are usually similar to those seen in the male intersex (see above). These patients usually adjust well to the sex in which they are reared, and most cases tend to be feminine. Nuclear sex is positive in 75% of cases. The chromosomal pattern is usually XX, but a number of mosaics have been reported.

If psychic sex seems well established in a patient with one testis and one ovary, the antagonistic gonad should be removed and the external genitalia repaired if necessary. If bilateral ovotestes are present they should be removed and replacement therapy instituted.

Jones, H. W., Ferguson-Smith, M. A., & R. H. Heller: Pathologic and cytogenic findings in true hermaphroditism. Obst Gynec **25**:435-7, 1965.

MacMahon, R. A.: Hermaphroditism in infancy and childhood. Surgery **59**:290-9, 1966.

McDaniel, E. C., Nadel, M., & W. C. Woolverton: True hermaphrodite with bilaterally descended ovotestes. J Urol **100**:77-81, 1968.

Olsson, C. A., & others: True hermaphroditism. J Urol **105**:586-90, 1971.

INTERSEXUALITY WHICH BECOMES APPARENT PRIOR TO OR AFTER PUBERTY

GYNECOID EXTERNAL AND INTERNAL GENITALIA WITH RUDIMENTARY GONADS
(Turner's Syndrome, "Ovarian Dysgenesis")

If the gonads of a genetic male embryo fail to develop, the internal and external genitalia tend to be gynecoid. These children, then, appear to be girls at birth and are therefore reared as such. This very act establishes their psychic femininity. Such children are usually short and often exhibit congenital abnormalities such as web neck, increased carrying angle of the forearms, coarctation of the aorta, and congenital heart disease. The urine contains an increased amount of pituitary gonadotropins. The first sign of abnormality may be the absence of menses and breast development at the time of expected puberty.

The vagina leads to a hypoplastic uterus and fallopian tubes. The gonads at their extremities are mere "streaks" composed of stroma but without germinal cells. Sohval recommends their removal, because of the high incidence of malignant degeneration. Chromatin sex is negative in about 80% of cases, and corresponds to an XO or XO/XX mosaic.

Treatment consists of cyclic administration of estrogens, which causes withdrawal bleeding simulating menses, breast development, and assurance of a female sexual and social pattern. Growth stimulation may be obtained from fluoxymesterone, 5 mg/day orally.

A few cases of male Turner's syndrome have also been reported. These patients have small penises and small undescended testes. Sex chromatin is negative; analysis usually shows an XY sex chromosome.

Engel, E., & A. P. Forbes: Cytogenic and clinical findings in 48 patients with congenitally defective or absent ovaries. Medicine **44**:135-64, 1965.

Goldberg, M. B., & others: Gonadal dysgenesis in phenotypic female subjects. A review of eighty-seven cases, with cytogenic studies in fifty-three. Am J Med **45**:529-43, 1968.

Gordon, R. R., & E. M. O'Neill: Turner's infantile phenotype. Brit MJ **1**:483-5, 1969.

Greenblatt, R. B., & others: The spectrum of gonadal dysgenesis. A clinical, cytogenetic, and pathologic study. Am J Obst Gynec **98**:151-72, 1967.

Johanson, A. J., Brasel, J. A., & R. M. Blizzard: Growth in patients with gonadal dysgenesis receiving fluoxymesterone. J Pediat **75**:1015-21, 1969.

Meyerson, L., & G. Gwinup: Turner's syndrome in the male. Arch Int Med **116**:125-30, 1965.

Persky, L., & R. Owens: Genitourinary tract abnormalities in Turner's syndrome (gonadal dysgenesis). J Urol **105**:309-13, 1971.

Preger, L., & others: Roentgenographic abnormalities in phenotypic females with gonadal dysgenesis. Am J Roentgenol **104**:899-910, 1968.

Reveno, J. S., & A. J. Palubinskas: Congenital renal abnormalities in gonadal dysgenesis. Radiology **86**:49-51, 1966.

ANDROID EXTERNAL AND INTERNAL GENITALIA WITH SMALL TESTES
(Klinefelter's Syndrome, Seminiferous Tubular Dysgenesis)

At birth these children have an unequivocal male appearance; they are reared as boys and therefore feel like boys. With growth, some develop a eunuchoid appearance and many are obese. At the time of puberty, gynecomastia may develop. Mental retardation is common. Renal anomalies are occasionally seen.

Examination in all cases reveals small testes which, on biopsy, show degeneration of the seminiferous tubules but clumped though otherwise normal Leydig cells. The penis is usually normally developed. Study of urinary hormonal excretion shows a marked increase in pituitary gonadotropins but normal or only slightly subnormal 17-ketosteroids. Chromatin sex is positive in 50% of patients. Those that have positive chromatin masses (XXY, XXXY, or XXY/XX mosaic) have true Klinefelter's syndrome; those with negative genetic sex merely represent males with dysgenesis of the seminiferous tubules who suffer from no endocrine abnormality although they are infertile. The patients with true Klinefelter's syndrome are sterile and at times have a eunuchoid body habitus and gynecomastia; otherwise they are physically, psychically, and sexually male. Treatment consists of androgenic substitution to prevent eunuchoid symptoms and osteoporosis. Mastectomy is occasionally necessary. It has been observed that the incidence of breast cancer in Klinefelter's syndrome is the same as in the normal female.

Barr, M. L.: The natural history of Klinefelter's syndrome. Fertil Steril **17**:429-41, 1966.

Becker, K. L., & others: Klinefelter's syndrome. Arch Int Med **118**:314-21, 1966.

Cuenca, C. R., & K. L. Becker: Klinefelter's syndrome and cancer of the breast. Arch Int Med **121**:159-62, 1968.

Edlow, J. B., & others: Neonatal Klinefelter's syndrome. Am J Dis Child **118**:788-91, 1969.

Lubs, H. A., Jr.: Testicular size in Klinefelter's syndrome in men over fifty. New England J Med **267**:326-31, 1962.

Taylor, H., Barter, R. H., & C. B. Jacobson: Neoplasms of dysgenetic gonads. Am J Obst Gynec **96**:816-21, 1966.

•   •   •

29 ...

Renovascular Hypertension

Urologic renal disease is a not uncommon cause of hypertension. However, most cases of high blood pressure (ie, essential hypertension) are of unknown etiology. Coarctation of the aorta, polycystic kidneys, glomerulonephritis, and polyarteritis nodosa are often accompanied by hypertension.

Etiology

More than 35 years have passed since Goldblatt demonstrated in experimental animals that protracted renal ischemia could produce hypertension. In dogs unilateral renal ischemia can cause transient hypertension, or it can cause no change at all if the other kidney is not removed or rendered ischemic. In man, however, there is unequivocal evidence that unilateral renal ischemia causes hypertension which can be cured by nephrectomy or reconstruction of the renal artery.

Pathogenesis

Why the ischemic kidney causes elevation of blood pressure is not yet known. The most attractive theory has been the following: Decreased blood flow through the afferent glomerular arteries leads to an increased number of secretory granules in the juxtamedullary bodies which are thought to elaborate renin. This enzyme reacts with an alpha$_2$ globulin to produce angiotensin I, a rather inert substance. This is converted to angiotensin II, a potent vasoconstrictor which also acts to increase aldosterone secretion by the adrenal cortex. Thus, hypertension is established.

It is true that in severe hypertension caused by stenosis of the renal artery, renin has been recovered in increased amounts from the renal vein of the ischemic organ, and evidence of hyperaldosteronism (hypokalemic alkalosis) has been observed. However, in milder hypertensives such increased humoral activity may not be found.

Pathology

The common causes of stenosis of the renal artery are arteriosclerotic plaques, fibromuscular hyperplasia of the media (which usually affects relatively young females), and embolism or thrombosis. Stenosis in a renal artery may protect that kidney from the deleterious effects of hypertension while the other kidney remains hypertensive. Thus, the ischemic kidney is ultimately the better of the two; it should be preserved unless considerable atrophy has occurred.

In autopsy material, poor correlation between the presence of hypertension and stenosis of the renal artery has been observed. A lesion producing at least a 50% (and probably even a 70%) reduction in luminal diameter appears to be necessary in order to reduce renal plasma flow to the point where clinically significant ischemia is produced. Thus, the significance of a stenosis shown on aortography can only be estimated by tests of differential renal function.

The changes observed in the pyelonephritic kidney have already been described. From the standpoint of the genesis of hypertension the most striking lesion is the marked thickening of the arteriolar walls. There is considerable variation in the arteriolar changes in the renal parenchyma involved by other renal lesions, such as tumor and hydronephrosis. Correlation of these changes with high blood pressure is poor, but postoperative return to normotension has been reported as a result of nephrectomy in many instances.

Clinical Findings

The clinical features of those renal diseases that may cause hypertension have already been discussed (see chronic pyelonephritis, thrombosis of the renal artery, aneurysm of the renal artery, hydronephrosis, renal tumors, and renal tuberculosis).

A. Symptoms: Hypertension caused by renal ischemia should be considered (1) if there is a recent onset of hypertension in the absence of a family history of hypertension, particularly if the patient is under 30 or over 50 years of age; (2) if the patient has had severe flank or abdominal pain or trauma (suggesting embolism or thrombosis of a renal artery), with or without hematuria; (3) if there is abrupt acceleration of a preexisting hypertension, especially in an older person; or (4) in the presence of severe hypertension at any age.

B. Signs: In addition to a relatively sustained diastolic hypertension, changes typical of malignant hypertension may be found in the retinas. A systolic bruit should be sought anteriorly and posteriorly over the renal areas. The presence of an aortic aneurysm or vascular insufficiency of the extremities is suggestive.

C. Laboratory Findings: Bacteria and pus cells in the urine may indicate chronic pyelonephritis. In the malignant phase of hypertension, proteinuria, casts, and red cells will be seen. Unless malignant hypertension, polycystic disease, bilateral atrophic pyelonephritis, or bilateral renal artery stenosis is present, total renal function (as measured by PSP test and creatinine clearance) is usually normal. Hypokalemic alkalosis suggestive of aldosteronism may be found. Lactic acid dehydrogenase may be elevated in the presence of bilateral chronic pyelonephritis or malignant hypertension.

The angiotensin infusion test has been recommended to differentiate between renovascular and other causes of hypertension. Renovascular hypertension has been shown to be more resistant to angiotensin II; more than 6.5 ng/kg/minute are necessary to raise the systolic pressure 20 mm Hg. Other types of hypertension will respond similarly to less than 5 ng/kg/minute. It has therefore been suggested that 4 ng/kg/minute be given over a period of 5 minutes. A significant rise in blood pressure is presumptive evidence against renal ischemia.

D. X-Ray Findings: Excretory urography is the best generally available screening test for the presence of renal ischemia (Figs 29-1 and 29-2). It makes the presumptive diagnosis in 70-80% of cases. The bowel should be well prepared. Since delay in appearance of the radiopaque medium is an important sign, exposures should be made at 2, 3, and 5 minutes after rapid injection. The following findings are suggestive of renal ischemia: (1) a kidney at least 1 cm shorter than its mate (normally, the right kidney is 0.5 cm shorter than its mate); (2) lack of function of one kidney (with a normal pyelocalyceal architecture as shown by retrograde urography); (3) delayed appearance of visualization on the early films; (4) the occurrence, at times, of hyperconcentration of the radiopaque medium due to marked overreabsorption of water (a phenomenon which may be accentuated by making urograms with the patient hydrated); (5) narrow, delicate renal calyces, renal pelvis, and ureter because of diminution in the volume of urine excreted; (6) partial atrophy (contraction) of one pole; (7) normal, but small, calyceal pattern in a small kidney; and (8) scalloping or notching of the upper ureter caused by secondary arterial collaterals.

The urographic changes of chronic pyelonephritis, hydronephrosis, and polycystic kidneys should be obvious.

Although hyperconcentration of the radiopaque material typically occurs in the ischemic kidney because of overreabsorption of water, excretory urograms usually fail to reveal it. The urea washout test will more often reflect this phenomenon. Osmotic diuresis is initiated with urea; the radiopaque material is "washed out" of the normal kidney on late films but will be visible in the ischemic organ because of the relative concentration of the iodide.

Aortography (renal angiography) will demonstrate stenosis of the renal artery or its branches (Fig 29-3). The ischemic renal tissue will show less increase in density than normally vascularized tissue. Collateral vessels in the region of the upper ureter and renal pelvis may be seen (Fig 29-2).

E. Relative Renal Function Tests: If the history, physical examination, urinalysis, tests of total renal function, and excretory urograms suggest the possibility of renal hypertension, split-function studies of the kidneys should be performed. In the presence of heart failure or shock (diminished renal blood flow) normal kidneys modify their function and respond in the following manner: Urine volume, urine sodium, chloride, and BUN concentrations, total PSP excretion (test of renal blood flow), and urinary pH are reduced; and responses to clearance tests, such as creatinine, iodopyracet (Diodrast®), and PAH, are lowered. In addition, there is an increase in osmolality as well as increased concentration of creatinine, nitrogen, and potassium in the urine.

The ischemic kidney reacts in similar fashion. Its basic functional characteristic is marked reabsorption of water by the renal tubules; to an even greater extent, salt (both sodium and chloride) is absorbed. On the other hand, potassium and creatinine—though excreted in amounts smaller than those excreted by the normal kidney—are poorly reabsorbed, thus leading to an increase in their concentrations per unit volume.

In the presence of renal ischemia, urea—in contradistinction to creatinine—is significantly reabsorbed because of the slow flow of urine through the tubules. Thus, the urea nitrogen/creatinine ratio in the urine will be low compared to that of the normally vascularized organ. There is also a decrease in total PSP excretion but an increase in PSP

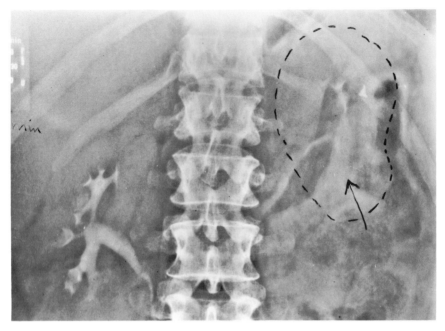

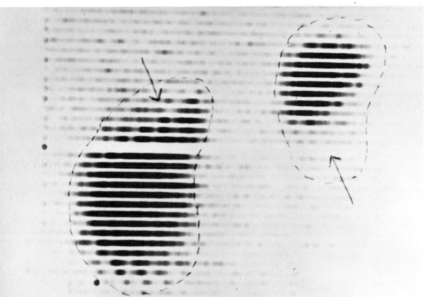

Fig 29-1. Renovascular hypertension. Above: Excretory urogram shows contraction of lower half of left kidney and failure of visualization of lower pole calyces. Right urogram normal. **Below:** Rectilinear scan, same patient, demonstrating ischemia of lower half of left kidney. Small area of upper pole of right kidney also ischemic. Renal angiogram showed stenosis of artery to lower pole of left kidney.

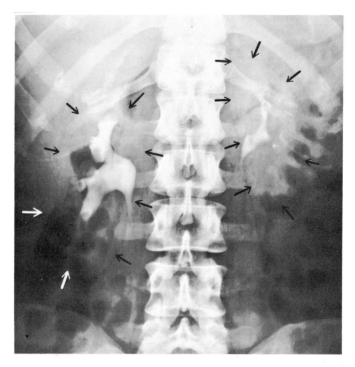

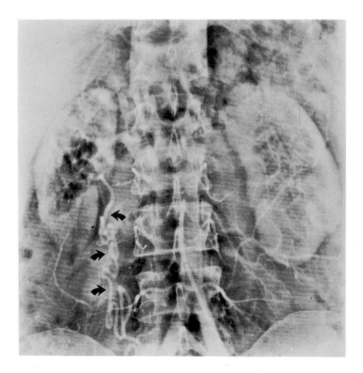

Fig 29-2. Hypertension caused by stenosis of left renal artery. Above: Ten-minute excretory urogram showing small left kidney with delayed and impaired excretion of radiopaque fluid. Because of diminution of urine volume, calyces and pelvis are smaller than in the contralateral kidney. **Below:** Angiogram in patient with complete occlusion of right main renal artery. Marked secondary periureteral collateral circulation allows persistence of some renal function.

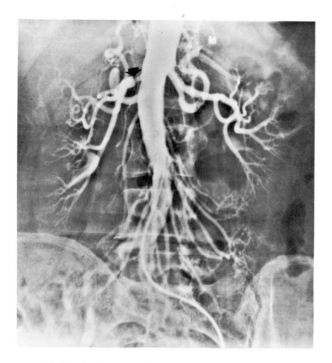
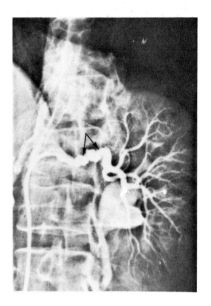

Fig 29-3. **Left:** Renal angiogram, "midstream" type, showing significant arteriosclerotic plaque at take-off of right renal artery. **Right:** Selective angiogram of left kidney, right posterior oblique position. Fibromuscular hyperplasia of renal artery.

concentration per milliliter of urine (because of overreabsorption of water) and an increase in osmolality of at least 15%.

1. Excretion of water, salt, and creatinine (Howard-Rapoport test) -

a. Technic -

(1) Normal salt diet for 3 days; no antihypertensive drugs for 5 days; good hydration. If performed under anesthesia, 1 L of 10% glucose should be administered to ensure adequate urine flow.

(2) Ureteral catheters are properly placed in the renal pelves or ureters. Urine specimens are collected for bacteriologic study. Three specimens of urine are then collected from each kidney after urine flow has become stabilized. The volume of one of the specimens should be 40-60 ml. The volume of each is measured and sodium and creatinine concentrations determined.

b. Interpretation of Howard-Rapoport test - The combinations of "positive" results shown in Table 29-1 suggest that nephrectomy or vascular reconstruction will tend to reduce hypertension.

Most cases of unilateral chronic pyelonephritis will yield a "negative" test (sodium concentration not decreased, or increased up

to 40%; creatinine concentration decreased 33-66%). Nephrectomy, in this group, will not affect the hypertension. Bilateral renal lesions, particularly if they are of equal degree, may give a negative or equivocal test; such lesions are obviously more difficult to diagnose.

2. Sodium chloride-urea-ADH-PAH test (Stamey test) - This test is also based upon the demonstration of abnormal reabsorption of water by the ischemic kidney; it is designed to exaggerate the evidence of this phenomenon. A normal saline infusion containing 8% urea, vasopressin (Pitressin®), and PAH is given after the placement of 8 F plastic catheters in the midureters. (Stamey prefers to leave these catheters in place for 12-24 hours. This appears to lessen the incidence of post-instrumental ureteral obstruction.) Three collections of urine taken at 10-minute intervals from each kidney are analyzed for volume and PAH concentration. The latter is significantly increased by the kidney affected by renovascular disease. (The reader is referred to Stamey's monograph for a detailed description of the test technic.)

The ischemic kidney is revealed by its diminished urine volume and its increased concentration of PAH as compared to its mate (Table 29-2).

Table 29-1. Interpretation of Howard-Rapoport Test.

Lesion	The ischemic kidney (in relation to the normal kidney) shows:		
	Urine Volume	Sodium Concentration	Creatinine Concentration
Stenosis of main renal artery	Decreased 60% or more	Decreased 15% or more	Increased 50-100%
Stenosis of branch of renal artery; chronic pyelo-nephritis with distal small artery disease	Decreased 33-50%	Decreased 0-20%	Increased 20-50%

Table 29-2. Interpretation of Stamey Test.

Lesion	Urine Volume	PAH Concentration
Stenosis of main artery, unilateral	Decreased 67% or more	Increased 100% or more
Stenosis of main artery, bilateral	Decreased 40% or more	Increased 36% or more
Stenosis of segmental artery, unilateral. Also essential hypertension, glomerulo-nephritis, chronic pyelonephritis (rare).	Decreased 50% or more	Increased 16% or more

3. Estimation of renal vein renin levels - Since it is believed that the ischemic kidney elaborates increased amounts of renin (thus causing hypertension), the expectation would be that measurements of the renin levels from both renal veins (when compared to peripheral venous levels) would be definitive in the diagnosis of renovascular hypertension. The correlation is good, but both false-positive and false-negative results have been reported. This test should be employed along with split function studies; the combination is superior to either one alone.

4. Measurement of urographic dye density with TS (total solids) meter - Because of over-reabsorption of water by the ischemic kidney, hyperconcentration of radiopaque contrast media occurs; it is surprising, however, how seldom this is portrayed on excretory urography. Hyperconcentration can be accurately estimated at the conclusion of the above differential function tests by injecting one of the urographic preparations intravenously. The specific gravity of the urine dripping from each catheter is measured every minute for 20 minutes using a TS (total solids) meter. Five to 10 minutes after the injection, the urine from the ischemic kidney shows hyperconcentration in comparison to that of its mate. When correlated with the Howard-Rapoport and Stamey studies, this technic has proved to be quite accurate.

The combination of the Howard-Rapoport and Stamey tests increases the accuracy of diagnosis. A "positive" test is an indication for renal aortography. Even when these tests are normal or equivocal, angiograms should still be made if the history, physical findings, and excretory urograms or isotope renograms suggest the presence of renal ischemia.

5. Renal isotope studies -

a. The ^{131}I-hippurate isotope renogram has proved to be a good screening test for evidence of renovascular hypertension. Because of the over-reabsorption of water by the tubules in the ischemic kidney, transport of the isotope to the pelvis is slow; its escape down the ureter is slowed. Furthermore, diminished renal blood flow decreases the amount of the iodide that reaches the kidney. Hence, the vascular spike from such a kidney is lower than that of its mate; its secretory phase is prolonged. Instead of the counts beginning to drop 3-5 minutes after injection, they tend to persist because of lack of "washout" (Fig 8-8).

b. The ^{203}Hg-Neohydrin® rectilinear scan measures renal tubular function and renal blood flow. It depicts the size and shape of the kidney. Thus, it may reveal polar atrophy (Fig 29-1) but it does not differentiate chronic pyelonephritis or renal infarct from ischemia.

c. Anger camera triple scan (Fig 8-5) - The ^{131}I-hippurate photos will show slow uptake of the isotope in the ischemic kidney. Because of the over-reabsorption of water, there is slow transport of the iodide to the pelvis. Therefore, by 8-10 minutes there is apt to be hyperconcentration of the isotope in the parenchyma as compared to the normal kidney. At 15 minutes, the normal kidney may have cleared the isotope, yet it still lingers in the renal pelvis of the ischemic kidney. An isotope renogram can be constructed from the counts that are recorded.

The iodide scan, made with the scintillation camera, may prove to be the best of all screening tests for renovascular hypertension.

Differential Diagnosis

Essential hypertension usually develops between ages 30-50 in a person with a family history of hypertension. Intravenous urograms are normal. The tests for ischemia are negative.

Coarctation of the aorta is characterized by relatively low blood pressure in the legs, a bruit over the vascular lesion, and evidence of collateral circulation.

Pheochromocytoma may be considered, especially if hypertension occurs in paroxysms associated with sweating and palpitation. The histamine or phentolamine (Regitine®) test is usually positive. Urinary VMA or serum or urinary catechols are elevated during hypertensive seizures. Excretory urograms may reveal displacement of a kidney by the tumor. Retroperitoneal gas insufflation (Fig 20-1) will delineate the suprarenal mass.

Secondary aldosteronism may accompany renovascular hypertension. In both primary and secondary aldosteronism, hypokalemic alkalosis is present; it responds to the administration of spironolactone (Aldactone®). Differentiation requires estimation of blood volume and serum sodium. In primary aldosteronism, both tend to be elevated. In secondary aldosteronism, they may be below normal.

Cushing's disease usually causes hypertension. Physical examination and hormonal assays establish the diagnosis.

Treatment

In the treatment of high blood pressure, nephrectomy is indicated for patients who have hypertension associated with serious unilateral renal lesions. The kidney should only be removed if its function is markedly deficient (eg, atrophic pyelonephritis, stenosis of the renal artery with marked atrophy, advanced hydronephrosis) or in order to save life (eg, cancer or tuberculosis of the kidney).

Endarterectomy, homograft, sleeve resection of the involved arterial segment, or arterial shunt or graft is indicated in a case of unilateral renal artery stenosis in which the involved kidney is of fairly good size. This is potentially the best kidney since it has been protected from the adverse effects of hypertension. Postoperatively, a "reversal" of the Howard test occurs; the repaired kidney excretes more PSP, water, and salt than its mate.

Bilateral stenosis of the renal arteries, found in 50% of cases, should be treated in a similar manner.

Prognosis

If split function studies are positive and the pressure gradient between the aorta and a point distal to the renal artery lesion is at least 50 mm Hg, successful arterial repair or nephrectomy will cure the hypertension in about 40% of cases. In another 40% of cases, the hypertension will show significant improvement.

•   •   •

Selected References

Ashken, M. H., & M. Chapman: A study of renal vascular patterns in hypertension and chronic pyelonephritis. J Urol **101:** 661-7, 1969.

Biglieri, E. G.: Evaluation of renal vascular hypertension and primary hyperaldosteronism. California Med **115:**40-7, Dec. 1971.

Bookstein, J. J.: Segmental renal artery stenosis in renovascular hypertension. Morphologic and hemodynamic considerations. Radiology **90:**1073-83, 1968.

Bourgoignie, J., & others: Renal venous renin in hypertension. Am J Med **48:** 332-42, 1970.

Brolin, I., & I. Stener: Collaterals in obstruction of the renal artery. Acta radiol (diag) **4:**447-62, 1966.

Catanzaro, F., & others: Angiotensin-infusion test. Arch Int Med **122:**10-7, 1968.

Chapman, W. H., & others: Diagnosis of renal hypertension using renal activity and renal vein pressor assay. J Urol **103:**549-53, 1970.

Clark, M. D., & others: The renogram in hypertension. Radiology **89:**667-75, 1967.

Clunie, G. J., & others: Autotransplantation of the kidney in the treatment of renovascular hypertension. Surgery **69:**326-31, 1971.

Conn, J. W., Rovner, D. R., & E. L. Cohen: Normal and altered function of the renin-angiotensin-aldosterone system in man. Ann Int Med **63:**266-84, 1965.

Coran, A. G., & S. R. Schuster: Renovascular hypertension in children. Surgery **64:**672-7, 1968.

Crocker, D. W., Newton, R. A., & J. H. Harrison: Results of surgical management of unilateral pyelonephritis with hypertension. Am J Surg **110**:405-10, 1965.

Fair, W. R., & T. A. Stamey: Differential renal function studies in segmental renal ischemia. JAMA **217**:790-3, 1971.

Fein, R. L., Norcott, E. A., & K. E. Van Buskirk: Utilization of the pyelogram—urea washout test in evaluating renal hypertension. J Urol **101**:12-5, 1969.

Foster, J. H., & others: Malignant hypertension secondary to renal artery stenosis in children. Ann Surg **164**:700-12, 1966.

Halpern, M., & J. A. Evans: Coarctation of the renal artery with "notching" of the ureter. Am J Roentgenol **88**:159-64, 1962.

Hamby, W. M., & others: Kidney function after surgery for renal hypertension. M Clin North America **51**:39-46, 1967.

Harrison, E. G., Jr., Hunt, J. C., & P. E. Bernatz: Morphology of fibromuscular dysplasia of the renal artery in renovascular hypertension. Am J Med **43**: 97-112, 1967.

Harwood-Nash, D. C. F., & E. L. Lansdown: Evaluation of the urea washout pyelogram and urography in the assessment of renovascular hypertension. Canad MAJ **96**:245-56, 1967.

Hollenberg, N. K., & others: "No man's land" of the renal vasculature. An arteriographic and hemodynamic assessment of the interlobular and arcuate arteries in essential and accelerated hypertension. Am J Med **47**:845-54, 1969.

Howard, J. E., & T. B. Connor: Use of differential renal function studies in the diagnosis of renovascular hypertension. Am J Surg **107**:58-66, 1964.

Hunter, J. A., Wilcox, H. G., & R. M. Kark: Problems in the management of renovascular hypertension. S Clin North America **47**:91-107, 1967.

Kaufman, J. J., & A. N. Lupu: Treatment of renal artery stenosis using hypogastric artery autografts. J Urol **106**:9-14, 1971.

Kaufman, J. J., & others: Diagnostic and predicative value of renal vein renin activity in renovascular hypertension. J Urol **103**:702-11, 1970.

Kincaid, O. W., & others: Fibromuscular dysplasia of the renal arteries. Am J Roentgenol **104**:271-82, 1968.

Loggie, J. M. H.: Hypertension in children and adolescents. I. Causes and diagnostic studies. J Pediat **74**:331-55, 1969.

Luke, R. G., & others: Results of nephrectomy in hypertension associated with unilateral renal disease. Brit MJ **3**: 764-8, 1968.

Luke, R. G., & others: Results of surgery in hypertension due to renal artery stenosis. Brit MJ **2**:76-80, 1968.

Lyon, R. P.: Urographic dye density as a measure of renal function and blood flow. J Urol **91**:444-50, 1964.

Marshall, S.: Urea-creatinine ratio in obstructive uropathy and renal hypertension. JAMA **190**:719-20, 1964.

Marshall, S., & R. P. Lyon: Differential renal function study. California Med **103**:9-12, 1965.

Maxwell, M. H., & A. N. Lupu: Excretory urogram in renal arterial hypertension. J Urol **100**:395-406, 1968.

Maxwell, M. H., Lupu, A. N., & J. J. Kaufman: Individual kidney function tests in renal arterial hypertension. J Urol **100**: 384-94, 1968.

O'Conor, V. J., Jr., & N. M. Simon: Are divided function studies necessary in the treatment of renovascular hypertension? J Urol **103**:119-25, 1970.

Palmer, J. M.: Prognostic value of contralateral renal plasma flow in renovascular hypertension. JAMA **217**:794-802, 1971.

Robertson, P. W., & others: Hypertension due to a renin-secretory renal tumor. Am J Med **43**:963-76, 1967.

Schacht, R. A., Conway, J., & B. H. Stewart: Split renal function studies in hypertension. Arch Int Med **119**:588-92, 1967.

Schreiber, M. H., & others: The normal pyelogram urea washout test. Am J Roentgenol **98**:88-95, 1966.

Stamey, T. A.: Renovascular hypertension— 1965. Editorial. Am J Med **38**:829-31, 1965.

Stamey, T. A.: Renovascular Hypertension. Williams & Wilkins, 1963.

Stewart, B. H., & others: Correlation of angiography and natural history in evaluation of patients with renovascular hypertension. J Urol **104**:231-8, 1970.

Strong, C. G., Boucher, R., & J. Genest: Renin, angiotensin and aldosterone in renovascular disorders. Postgrad Med **40**:337-43, 1966.

Turman, A. E., & others: Renal function studies in the detection of renal hypertension. J Urol **103**:115-8, 1970.

Vaughan, T. J., & others: Renal artery aneurisms and hypertension. Radiology **99**:287-93, 1971.

30...
Infertility

A couple can be judged infertile if conception does not occur after 12 months of adequate cohabitation. About 10% of marriages are barren; spermatogenic deficiencies in the male are responsible in at least 40% of these. Joël observes that 6% of habitual abortions are noted in association with highly abnormal semen.

From the clinical standpoint, the fertility of the male is judged through study of his sperm, including number, the percentage of motile sperm, their viability, and morphology. If sperm are absent from the ejaculate, testicular biopsy is indicated to differentiate between intrinsic deficiency of the germ cells (common) and obstruction of the conduction system (rare).

Pathogenesis

The common causes of male infertility are as follows:

A. Deficiencies in Maturation of Germ Cells: At least 85% of infertile men have intrinsic spermatogenic defects. The germ cells of the seminiferous tubules may be congenitally imperfect (aplastic), or incomplete maturation (spermatogenic arrest) may be observed secondary to hypogonadism or hypopituitarism.

Frequently orchitis due to mumps or trauma and exposure to x-ray radiation exert a deleterious effect upon spermatogenesis. In the cryptorchid testis, the temperature of the body causes injury to the germ cells.

B. Obstruction of the Conduction System: Bilateral epididymitis may cause occlusion of the ducts. Absence of connection between the vas deferens and the epididymis may be congenital or acquired (eg, vasoligation).

C. Hypothyroidism: Hypothyroidism is often associated with infertility and may have etiologic significance. A scientific explanation of this is lacking, but the administration of thyroid substance to hypothyroid infertile men with normal sperm may be followed by conception.

D. Hyperadrenalism: Hyperadrenalism causes an increase in volume of the ejaculate, diminished sperm count and motility, and an increased percentage of abnormal forms with evidence of desquamation.

E. Sperm Antibodies: There is increasing evidence that some men produce antibodies to their own sperm. This leads to (1) decrease in their power to penetrate cervical mucus, (2) spontaneous agglutination, and (3) decreased motility of the spermatozoa. Women may elaborate antibodies to sperm. To treat this phenomenon, a condom should be used for a year, during which time her titer gradually falls. This has led to a number of pregnancies in previously infertile couples.

F. Tight Clothing: The use of shorts or supporters that hold the testes close to the body leads to increase in testicular temperature which is deleterious to spermatogenesis.

G. Varicocele: The presence of varicocele causes (1) an increase in the percentage of immature forms, (2) a decrease in sperm count, and (3) a decrease in the percentage of motile sperm. The cause is not known. It has been shown that it is not due to increased scrotal heat from the pooled blood. It has been postulated that adrenal corticosteroids might move in a retrograde manner down the spermatic vein to the testes.

Testicular Histology and Pathology

A. Normal Development: Up to the age of 4 or 5 years, the testes are in a relatively quiescent state. The spermatogenic tubules are small. Adjacent to the basement membrane a number of ovoid or round cells are seen. Few spermatogonia are present. The interstitial tissue contains a few clumps of Leydig cells.

Between the ages of 5 and 10 years, the germinal tubules become more tortuous and their lumens increase in diameter. More spermatogonia are present. The interstitial tissues show a decrease in the number of fibroblasts.

At puberty, probably stimulated by increasing amounts of pituitary gonadotropins (FSH, LH), active spermatogenesis begins and mature spermatozoa make their appearance. Hyperplasia of the interstitial (Leydig) cells develops (Fig 1-8).

B. Abnormal Development: The pathologic changes found in the infertile testis have been carefully studied by gonadal biopsy. Many degrees of damage may be noted.

1. Germinal aplasia - The seminiferous tubules show a complete or almost complete lack of germ cells. Normal numbers of Sertoli cells are present, however. The cause of this change may be either congenital or secondary to lack of FSH (follicle-stimulating hormone) from the pituitary gland. If pituitary function is normal increased amounts of FSH may be found in the urine (Klinefelter's syndrome).

2. Spermatogenic arrest - The tubule and its cells are normal in appearance, but maturation fails to reach the adult stage.

3. Peritubular fibrosis - Normally the basement membrane of the tubule is quite thin. For some unknown reason, progressive peritubular fibrosis may occur. In all probability this impairs cellular nutrition and the sperm cells gradually disappear. At this stage the FSH excretion in the urine is increased.

4. Incomplete spermatogenesis - Some tubules may be quite normal, whereas others show lack of complete maturation. Both mature and immature sperm may be found in the tubular lumens. Men suffering from this defect have lowered sperm counts and an increase in the number of abnormal forms.

C. Spermatology: Clinically, there are 3 important criteria for normal semen.

1. Number - Most authorities state that "normal" semen contains at least 50 million sperm/ml in 2 ml of fluid. MacLeod found that 25% of fertile men have counts below 50 million/ml. He considers that true oligospermia consists of less than 20 million/ml, but he observes that, with excellent motility, conception may occur when the sperm count is as low as 10 million/ml.

2. Percentage of motile sperm and degree of motility - In most fertile men, at least 70% of the sperm are actively motile when the specimen is fresh. The fewer the motile forms, the greater the impairment of fertility. The degree of motility is also quite significant. The more sluggish the sperm, the greater the degree of infertility.

Generally speaking, the greater the percentage of motile forms the more vigorous is their motility.

3. Morphology - A differential count of normal and abnormal sperm affords considerable information. At least 70% of the sperm in most fertile men are normal.

Clinical Findings

A. History: The chief complaint of the patient is the inability to cause conception. Other information of importance includes childhood and adult illnesses (eg, mumps orchitis, cryptorchism, tuberculosis); operations, especially those which might cause injury to the testes or their ducts (eg, repair of inguinal hernia, orchiopexy); trauma to the external genitalia; genital infections, particularly epididymitis; pregnancy in present or previous wife, frequency of intercourse, and exposure to toxins (eg, x-rays).

B. Signs: A complete physical examination should never be neglected. Evidence of endocrinologic abnormality should be sought, including weight, height, body build, amount and distribution of hair, and gynecomastia. The degree of development of the penis should be noted and the scrotal contents carefully examined. (The testes of infertile men are usually normal in size and consistency.) Unilateral or bilateral changes may be noted. Small, flabby testes or the hard, pea-sized testes of Klinefelter's syndrome are usually azoospermic. Other testicular abnormalities may include cryptorchism and thickening of the epididymides (old epididymitis). The vas deferens should be carefully felt, for it may be absent or may fail to join the epididymis. Varicocele should be noted, for its presence offers the most hope when it comes to the point of treatment.

Rectal examination should include prostatic massage, although the significance of prostatitis in infertility is not clear. Fjällbrant believes that there is an increased incidence of sperm antibodies in some men who harbor this infection.

C. Laboratory Findings: Proteinuria or pyuria may be clues to chronic renal disease, which may depress spermatogenesis.

1. Examination of the semen - This is the most important step in the investigation of suspected infertility.

a. Method of collection - The ejaculate should be obtained after at least 4 days of abstinence from intercourse. It is best produced by masturbation in the physician's office. This ensures that the entire specimen is collected in a clean, dry glass. Condoms must not be used, for the sperm are quickly killed on contact with them. The specimen must be examined within 2 hours of its collection. Normally, the semen is quite gelatinous and ropy. Within a few minutes, at room temperature, the fluid becomes thin and homogeneous. Failure to liquefy is abnormal.

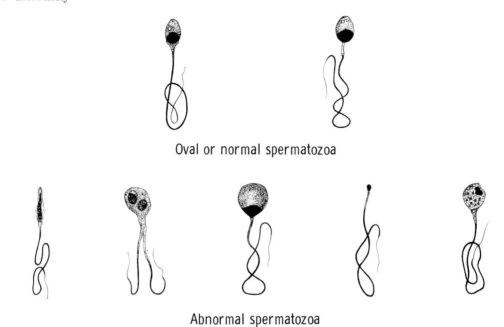

Oval or normal spermatozoa

Abnormal spermatozoa

Fig 30-1. Normal and abnormal spermatozoa. (Redrawn and reproduced, with permission, from Hotchkiss, R.S.: Fertility in Men. Lippincott, 1944.)

b. Sperm count - The technic is simple, requiring only a Neubauer blood cell counting chamber and a white cell pipet. Semen is drawn up to the 0.5 mark, and the rest of the chamber is filled with a saturated solution of sodium bicarbonate containing 1% phenol, which immobilizes the sperm. This mixture is then flooded over the counting chamber and covered with a coverslip. The number of sperm in the 5 blocks (80 small squares) is determined. To this number are added 6 ciphers. This equals the number of sperm per milliliter.

Most fertile men have at least 50 million sperm/ml. The absence of sperm means a severe defect of the seminiferous tubules or obstruction of the conducting system. The finding of a few dead sperm rules out obstruction.

Oligospermia is almost always due to disease of the germ cells. The lower the count, the poorer the prognosis.

c. Percentage of motile sperm and degree of motility - Semen is placed on a slide and covered with a coverslip sealed with Vaseline®. An estimate should be made of the percentage of motile forms, the degree of motility, and the duration of life of the sperm.

d. Morphology - Morphology may be judged by counting the normal and abnormal forms in a smear stained as follows:

(1) Dry a thin smear of semen in air.
(2) Flood with 10% formalin for 1 minute.
(3) Wash.
(4) Stain with Meyer's hematoxylin for 1 1/2 minutes.
(5) Wash in lukewarm water.

2. A basal metabolic rate or estimation of protein-bound iodine should be obtained in all men presenting themselves as possibly infertile, whether the ejaculate is normal or not. The hypothyroid male with normal semen may become fertile only after thyroid has been administered.

3. Testicular biopsy is usually indicated only if azoospermia is present. Study of the seminiferous tubules will permit differentiation between severe intrinsic gonadal disease and blockage of the conducting system. In the latter case, spermatogenesis is normal. There is, however, evidence to suggest that sperm counts are apt to be temporarily depressed after biopsy.

4. A buccal smear should receive nuclear chromatin analysis. If chromatin sex is positive (female), the diagnosis of Klinefelter's syndrome should be entertained. These patients are irreversibly sterile.

5. Pituitary gonadotropins (FSH) in the urine should be measured. An increase means primary gonadal deficiency; if FSH is decreased, hypopituitarism is present.

6. The estimation of 17-ketosteroids in the urine is the most important endocrinologic test. Hyperadrenocorticism is an indication that the excretion of adrenal androgens should

be suppressed. This is accomplished by prescribing cortisone or prednisone, which leads to an increase in the number of sperm and a greater percentage of normal forms.

Treatment

The results of treatment of infertility in the male are unsatisfactory except when a varicocele is found. Morphologic changes in the various components of the seminiferous tubules are largely irreversible.

A. Hormone Therapy:

1. If hypothyroidism can be demonstrated, thyroid or liothyronine (Cytomel®) should be given to the point of tolerance. The indication for the use of these drugs in the patient with euthyroidism is questionable; their effect may be psychotherapeutic.

2. Gonadotropins - The value of pituitary gonadotropins in therapy is equivocal, despite their stimulating effect on the development of the seminiferous tubules. Recently, however, it has been shown that the administration of human gonadotropins will maintain normal spermatology in hypophysectomized men. Glass and Holland have reported significant success (an increase to more than 10 million sperm/ml) in the treatment of oligospermia by the administration of human chorionic gonadotropin, 5000 IU intramuscularly 3 times a week for 4-8 weeks. This course can be repeated every 2-4 months.

3. Androgens - Small doses of androgen (eg, fluoxymesterone, 2-5 mg/day by mouth) may improve poor motility if the sperm count is high. This mode of therapy may also be helpful when the count is normal but the volume of ejaculate is low.

Heller and Heckel have recommended administering large doses of testosterone (50 mg 3 times a week) for 3 months in men whose sperm are markedly inadequate in quality and quantity. This causes complete azoospermia, but after cessation of treatment a "rebound" phenomenon may occur and the semen may show improvement over its pretreatment level in 15% of patients. Ten percent may be made worse, however.

B. General Measures: Sexual technic should be discussed with the couple. They should be apprised of the "fertile" period in the menstrual cycle. Intercourse should be avoided for 3 or 4 days before this time in order that the male can then deliver the best quantity and quality of semen. This is particularly important if the sperm count is deficient. Psychic factors should be sought. Should the volume of ejaculate be abnormally large, only the first portion should be instilled into the vagina, since the second part contains relatively few sperm.

If nonliquefaction of the semen is observed, Bunge has recommended that the woman insert a cocoa butter suppository containing 5 mg of alpha amylase powder into the vagina immediately after intercourse enacted during the time of ovulation.

The general health of the patient should be improved by regulating his diet and eradicating infections, particularly of the prostate gland. A reducing diet should be utilized if the man is overweight. The administration of thyroid substance may contribute to this goal. Alcoholic excesses should be curbed.

Vitamin B complex should be prescribed to ensure the normal inactivation of estrogens by the liver.

If treatment fails to improve the number, form, and motility of sperm, and if conception does not occur, a cap containing the inadequate semen can be placed over the cervix. This may improve the chances for conception.

If the man wears a supporter or shorts that hold the scrotal contents close to the body, he should be instructed not to do so.

If the temperature of the testis is increased for a few months by hot soaks or by an insulated jockstrap, the sperm count is significantly decreased. Cessation of this treatment may result in a rebound of spermatogenic activity and a consequent increase in the sperm count that may culminate in pregnancy.

C. Surgical Measures: The surgical procedures available for the correction of specific abnormalities are:

1. Vasovasostomy - If vasoligation has been performed, repair may be successful in 25-40% of cases.

2. Epididymovasostomy - If azoospermia is present but the testicular biopsy shows normal spermatogenesis and there is evidence of epididymal occlusion, epididymovasostomy should be considered. It may make conception possible in 10-20% of otherwise sterile matings.

3. Ligation of the spermatic vein at the internal inguinal ring as a cure for varicocele will usually improve the quality of the semen by improving motility of the sperm and their concentration. Pregnancy will occur in about one-half of this group.

4. Orchiopexy for undescended testes is of no value in the treatment of infertility after puberty.

Prognosis

The poorer the quality of the semen, the poorer the outlook for success in treatment. When the count is under 1 million/ml, there is little room for optimism. Azoospermia, unless caused by obstruction of the tubules of the of the epididymis, cannot be treated successfully.

• • •

General References

Agger, P.: Scrotal and testicular temperature: Its relation to sperm count before and after operation for varicocele. Fertil Steril 22:286-97, 1971.

Amelar, R. D., & R. S. Hotchkiss: The split ejaculate. Its use in the management of male infertility. Fertil Steril 16:46-60, 1965.

Ansbacher, R., Manarang-Pangan, S., & S. Srivannaboon: Sperm antibodies in infertile couples. Fertil Steril 22:298-302, 1971.

Behrman, S. J., & Y. Sawada: Heterologous and homologous inseminations with human semen frozen and stored in a liquid-nitrogen refrigerator. Fertil Steril 17:457-66, 1966.

Bourne, R. B., Kretzschmar, W. A., & J. H. Esser: Successful artificial insemination in a diabetic with retrograde ejaculation. Fertil Steril 22:275-7, 1971.

Brown, J. S., & others: Venography in the subfertile man with varicocele. J Urol 89:388-92, 1967.

Bruce, W. R., & others: Physical and chemical studies of sperm production. Canad MAJ 103:885-8, 1970.

Bunge, R. G.: Alpha amylase suppositories and non-liquefaction of human semen. J Urol 99:350, 1968.

Charny, C. W., & J. Y. Gillenwater: Congenital absence of the vas deferens. J Urol 93:399-401, 1965.

Dubin, L., & R. D. Amelar: Etiologic factors in 1294 consecutive cases of male infertility. Fertil Steril 22:469-74, 1971.

Dubin, L., & R. D. Amelar: Varicocele size and results of varicocelectomy in selected sub-fertile men with varicocele. Fertil Steril 21:606-9, 1970.

Fernandes, M., Shah, K. N., & J. W. Draper: Vasovasostomy: Improved microsurgical technique. J Urol 100: 763-6, 1968.

Fjällbrant, B.: Localization of human male antibodies on spermatozoa. Am J Obst Gynec 108:550-6, 1970.

Garduno, A., & D. J. Mehan: Testicular biopsy findings in patients with impaired fertility. J Urol 104:871-7, 1970.

Glass, R. H., & R. A. Vaidya: Sperm-agglutinating antibodies in infertile women. Fertil Steril 21:657-61, 1970.

Glass, S. J., & H. M. Holland: Treatment of oligospermia with large doses of human chorionic gonadotropin. Fertil Steril 14:500-6, 1963.

Joël, C. A.: Male factor in habitual abortion. Fertil Steril 17:374-80, 1966.

Kolodny, R. C., & others: Sperm-agglutinating antibodies and infertility. Obst Gynec 38:576-82, 1971.

Kom, C., Mulholland, S. G., & M. Edson: Etiology of infertility after retroperitoneal lymphadenectomy. J Urol 105:528-30, 1971.

Lehfeldt, H., & H. Guze: Psychologic factors in contraceptive failure. Fertil Steril 17:110-5, 1966.

Li, T. S., & S. J. Behrman: The sperm—and seminal plasma—specific antigens of human semen. Fertil Steril 21:565-73, 1970.

MacLeod, J.: Further observations on the role of varicocele in human male infertility. Fertil Steril 20:545-63, 1969.

MacLeod, J.: Semen analysis for infertility. Clin Obst Gynec 8:115-27, 1965.

Matheson, G. W., Carlborg, L., & C. Gemzell: Frozen human semen for artificial insemination. Am J Obst Gynec 104: 495-501, 1969.

Raboch, J., & L. Stárka: Hormonal testicular activity in men with a varicocele. Fertil Steril 22:152-5, 1971.

Robinson, D., & J. Rock: Intrascrotal hyperthermia induced by scrotal insulation: Effect of spermatogenesis. Obst Gynec 29:217-23, 1967.

Rowley, M. J., & C. G. Heller: The testicular biopsy: Surgical procedure, fixation, and staining technics. Fertil Steril 17: 177-86, 1966.

Rowley, M. J., O'Keefe, K. B., & C. G. Heller: Decreases in sperm concentration due to testicular biopsy procedure in men. J Urol 101:347-9, 1969.

Sandeman, T. F.: The effects of x irradiation on male human fertility. Brit J Radiol 39:901-7, 1966.

Schmidt, S. S.: Technics and complications of elective vasectomy. Fertil Steril 17: 467-82, 1966.

Schmidt, S. S.: Vasectomy: Indications, technic, and reversibility. Fertil Steril 19:192-6, 1968.

Scott, L. S.: Mumps and male fertility. Brit J Urol 32:183-7, 1960.

Sohval, A. R.: Sex chromatin, chromosomes, and male infertility. Fertil Steril 14: 180-207, 1963.

Wallace, D. M.: Vasectomy. Brit MJ 4: 100-2, 1971.

Wingate, M. B.: Recent advances in investigation and treatment of infertility. Canad MAJ 101:43-9, 1969.

31...
Psychosomatic Urologic Syndromes

Psychologic disturbances not uncommonly are reflected in disorders of the genitourinary organs. These include vesical irritability, urinary retention, enuresis, and impotence.

There are few references to these phenomena in the literature despite the fact that the effects of the emotions upon the cardiovascular, gastrointestinal, and respiratory systems are well documented and generally accepted. What is recorded in this chapter are the convictions of the author based upon his clinical experience.

PSYCHOSOMATIC CYSTITIS SYNDROME

Possibly 10% of women who suffer from "chronic cystitis" have urine specimens that are free of pus cells and bacteria. Cystoscopic examination may reveal nonspecific urethritis, urethral or vesical neck polyps, or senile urethritis. In half of this group, however, no organic changes are present and symptoms result entirely from emotional tension. Men seem to suffer from this syndrome less commonly than women.

Physiology and Psychodynamics

A. Anatomic Relationships: Embryologically and physiologically, the urethra and the trigone arise from the same embryologic fundament as the female generative organs and therefore have the same nerve and blood supply and are under the same hormonal influences. As a result of local hyperemia, many women have some symptoms of vesical irritability with their menstrual periods. Others experience similar symptoms after incomplete sexual gratification (ie, from unrelieved pelvic congestion). Suffering chronically from pelvic congestion, they develop chronic vesical irritability.

B. Preexisting Tension and Anxiety Patterns: A vesical pathway for the release of nervous tension seems to develop early in life. Many had prolonged enuresis as children; most

admit that with acute attacks of anxiety, urinary frequency occurs. Chronic anxiety may thus cause chronic frequency of urination.

C. Nerve Supply: Various hollow viscera (eg, stomach, intestine) have been shown to react to emotional tension. Since the bladder is likewise made up of smooth muscle and innervated by the autonomic nervous system, it too may be subject to abnormalities of function on an emotional basis.

An abnormal cystometrogram suggesting an uninhibited neurogenic bladder (Fig 19-7) may be obtained if the patient is tense. If the patient is mentally depressed, however, a curve similar to that found with the flaccid neurogenic bladder (Fig 19-8) may be seen. These changes demonstrate that bladder function may portray the state of the psyche (Straub).

D. Hormonal Factors: Some of these patients have short bouts of frequency because they suddenly excrete unusually large amounts of urine. This may follow temporary retention of salt and water during an acute "stress situation" or may be caused by a temporary decrease in the amount of antidiuretic hormone elaborated by the pituitary. Schottstaedt has pointed out that tension in a patient with congestive failure may lead to further retention of water and salt. Wakim reviewed the mode of action of antidiuretic hormone and recognized the effect of the emotions on its secretion. Anxiety or stress will cause changes in a radioisotope renogram similar to those obtained with epinephrine and norepinephrine. Under hypnosis, diuresis can be induced in a subject who has not ingested water.

E. Fluid Intake: Some nervous and tense people have a compulsion to drink large amounts of fluids. This will cause physiologic frequency. These persons may finally lose their renal concentrating power.

F. Threshold Variations: Emotionally unstable individuals seem to have low thresholds to painful and other stimuli. They may perceive minimal increase in bladder wall tension as a strong urge.

Clinical Findings

A. Symptoms: An anxious patient complains of periodic frequency, mostly in the morning. It may be noticed for a few days and then spontaneously subside for no obvious reason. Comparable nocturia is absent. With an attack, urgency may be severe even to the point of incontinence. Frequency is initiated or increased following emotional upsets (eg, "scenes" with husband or children) and after sexual intercourse, which is, almost without exception, unsatisfactory. The common denominator seems to be unrelieved pelvic congestion precipitated by sexual frustration.

Careful questioning reveals that the tense woman develops a tense small-capacity bladder so that she voids small amounts, whereas the woman suffering from frequency secondary to acute diuresis voids normal volumes. In the latter group, during the antidiuretic phase, the patient notes edema and a gain in weight which may amount to 10 lb over a period of 2-3 days. Following the diuresis, body weight promptly returns to normal.

Many of these women complain of hesitancy and a slow urinary stream, but questioning will reveal that, although some voidings are slow, others are normal. This rules out organic outlet obstruction and implies periodic spasm of the periurethral striated musculature. Sudden urinary retention may occur precipitated by acute depression.

These patients often volunteer the belief that their symptoms are due to "nerves." It is wise to accept this confession.

B. Signs: Careful evaluation and observation of the patient usually suggests anxiety and tension or depression. Vaginal examination may show tenderness of the urethra and pain on movement of the cervix, although no gynecologic pathology can be demonstrated.

Clues to the possibility of antidiuresis-diuresis or polydipsia can be obtained by having the patient record the time and volume of fluid intake and fluid loss through voiding over a period of a few days. Body weight should be checked morning and evening. If weight changes of 5-10 lb occur in 2 or 3 days, fluid is being retained. The inevitable diuresis must follow; weight then returns to normal.

C. Laboratory Findings: Urinalysis, stained smear of sediment, and culture are normal.

D. Instrumental Examination: The passage of even a small catheter is painful, apparently causing spasm of the urethral sphincters and simulating urethral stenosis. Cystoscopy may disclose trabeculation of the bladder wall (evidence of hypertrophy) secondary to increased urethral spasm. The urethra and trigone, which are normally redder than the rest of the bladder, are usually more hyperemic because of general pelvic congestion. This may lead to the erroneous diagnosis of trigonitis and urethritis. Bladder capacity may be diminished if the patient is anxious, or increased if she is depressed.

Differential Diagnosis

In true cystitis, both acute and chronic, the urine will show pus cells, bacteria, or both. Frequency is consistent both day and night.

Nonspecific urethritis may be difficult to differentiate from the psychosomatic cystitis syndrome. True urethral stenosis should be sought, but it must be differentiated from spasm, which is usually obvious from the history. Evidence of emotional difficulties will prove helpful in establishing the diagnosis.

Senile urethritis is always associated with local evidence of senile vaginitis and failure of the vaginal epithelial cells to take up iodine.

Multiple sclerosis often causes aberrations in bladder function typified by urgency, frequency, and nocturia. These symptoms, however, are not periodic as are those caused by psychic stimuli.

Fecal impaction in women or children can cause urinary retention; upper tract dilatation may also be found on urograms.

Complications

Some cases of interstitial cystitis may actually be the end stage of the psychogenic bladder. The contracture and fibrosis may be caused by chronic ischemia mediated through the sympathetic nervous system. Emotional "stress" of long standing may be the cause. It may be for this reason that corticotropin (ACTH) or corticosteroids often alleviate the symptoms and improves vesical capacity.

Treatment

It is often helpful to explain to the patient the ways in which "nerves" can affect the bladder.

Mistaken organic diagnoses are apt to lead to various treatments, including urethral instrumentation, or even transurethral resection of the vesical neck. Not only may these procedures be harmful; they further convince the patient that she has some serious disease. Although bladder sedatives may afford some relief, psychotherapy is the treatment of choice.

Prognosis

The bladder symptoms caused by psychogenic stimuli are not easy to relieve. Emphasis upon local therapy is detrimental in the long run, since it only serves to confirm the patient's belief that local disease exists. Patients do, however, accept the symptoms with equanimity after the mechanisms responsible for their troubles are explained.

Barnes, R., & W. W. Schottstaedt: The relation of emotional state to renal excretion of water and electrolytes in patients with congestive heart failure. Am. J. Med. 29:217-27, 1960.

Blomstrand R., & F. Löfgren: Influence of emotional stress on the renal circulation. Psychosom Med 18:420-6, 1956.

Bowers, J. E., Schwarz, B., & M. J. Leon: Masochism and interstitial cystitis: Report of case. Psychosom Med 20:296-302, 1958.

DeMaria, W. J. A., & others: Renal conditioning. Psychosom Med 25:538-42, 1963.

Dykman, R. A., & others: Inhibition of urine flow as a component of the conditional defense reaction. Psychosom Med 24:177-86, 1962.

Gerbner, M., Altman, K., & I. Mészáros: The mechanism of the increase in diuresis induced by hypnotic suggestion. J Psychosom Res 3:282-90, 1959.

Jeffcoate, T. N. A., & W. J. A. Francis: Urgency incontinence in the female. Am J Obst Gynec 94:604-18, 1966.

Khan, A. U.: Psychogenic urinary retention in a boy. J Urol 106:432-4, 1971.

Larson, J. W., & others: Psychogenic urinary retention in women. J. A. M. A. 184:697-700, 1963.

Ravich, L., Lerman, P. H., & N. B. Schell: Urinary retention due to fecal impaction. New York J Med 63:3289-91, 1963.

Schottstaedt, W. W., Grace, W. J., & H. G. Wolff: Life situations, behavior, attitudes, emotions and renal excretion of fluid and electrolytes. J Psychosom Res 1:75-83, 147-59, 203-11, 287-91, 292-8, 1956.

Shenken, L. I.: Psychogenic urinary retention. New Zealand MJ 64:153-5, 1965.

Smith, D. R., & A. Auerback: Pages 1-20 in: Encyclopedia of Urology, vol. 12. Springer, 1960.

Stevko, R. M., Balsley, M., & W. E. Segar: Primary polydipsic–compulsive water drinking. J Pediat 73:845-51, 1968.

Straub, L. R., Ripley, H. S., & S. Wolf: Disturbances of bladder function associated with emotional states. JAMA 141:1139-43, 1949.

Turner, R. D., & E. Bors: Some interesting observations in neurological urology. Urologia Internat 16:30-45, 1963.

Wahl, C. M., & J. S. Golden: Psychogenic urinary retention. Psychosom Med 25:543-55, 1963.

Wakim, K. G.: Reassessment of the source, mode and locus of action of antidiuretic hormone. Am J Med 42:394-411, 1967.

Zufall, R.: Treatment of the urethral syndrome in women. JAMA 184:894-5, 1963.

Enuresis originally meant "incontinence of urine," but usage has caused the term to be restricted to bedwetting after the age of 3 years. Most children have achieved normal bladder control by the age of $2^1/2$ years. Girls gain this control earlier than boys. At least 50% of cases are of psychic origin; 30% seem to be caused by delayed maturation of the nervous system or an intrinsic myoneurogenic bladder dysfunction; and perhaps 20% are secondary to more obvious organic disease. Most children with functional enuresis gain spontaneous nocturnal control by the age of 10 years.

Psychodynamics

Training in bladder control should begin after the age of $1^1/2$ years; attempts made before this are usually fruitless and may be harmful. If the parents fail in this teaching, the child may not develop cerebral inhibitory control over the infantile uninhibited bladder until much later in childhood. If the parents are emotionally unstable, their anxieties may be transmitted to the child, who may express his tensions through enuresis.

The birth of a sibling may cause a child to lose his paramount position in the family. He may then regress to an infancy pattern in order to recapture his parents' affection. An acute illness may be accompanied or followed by recurrence of incomplete nocturnal control. Physiologic or psychologic stress (fear and anxiety) may reestablish an uninhibited bladder.

Possibly 50% of enuretic children have electroencephalograms which are borderline or compatible with epilepsy. Many of these children have been shown to have bladders of small capacity.

Clinical Findings

A. Symptoms: The child may wet his bed occasionally or regularly. Careful questioning of the parents or observation by the physician reveals that the patient voids a free stream of normal caliber. This tends to rule out obstruction of the lower tract as a cause of the enuresis. Children with daytime incontinence usually have more than psychogenic enuresis.

There is no burning, although frequency and urgency are common. The urine is clear.

Careful observation of the parents usually reveals that they are anxious and tense; these traits are only increased by the bedwetting of their child.

B. Signs: General physical and urologic examinations are normal.

C. Laboratory Findings: In the emotional group, all tests, including urinalysis, are normal. An electroencephalogram may be abnormal, however.

D. X-Ray Findings: Excretory urograms show no abnormality. The accompanying cystogram reveals no trabeculation; a film of the bladder taken immediately after voiding shows no residual urine.

E. Instrumental Examination: A catheter of suitable size passes readily to the bladder, thereby ruling out stricture. If passed after urination, no residual urine is found. Urethrocystoscopy is normal. Cystometric studies are usually normal, but a curve typical of the "uninhibited" (hyperirritable) neurogenic bladder (Fig 19-7) is often obtained.

Differential Diagnosis

A. Obstruction: Lower tract obstruction (eg, posterior urethral valves, meatal stenosis) causes a urinary stream of decreased caliber. Painful, frequent urination during the day and night, pyuria, and fever (eg, pyelonephritis) are often present, and the bladder may be distended. Urinalysis almost always reveals evidence of infection. Anemia and impairment of renal function may be demonstrated.

Excretory urograms may show dilatation of the bladder and the upper urinary tract. Incomplete vesical emptying may be seen on the post-voiding film. Cystography may demonstrate distal urethral stenosis or reflux. Urethrocystoscopy will reveal the organic cause.

B. Infection: Chronic urinary tract infection not due to obstruction usually produces frequency both day and night and pain on urination, although such infections may occur without symptoms of vesical irritability. Recurrent fever with exacerbations is common.

General examination may be normal. Anemia may be noted. Urinalysis will show pus cells or bacteria, or both. Renal function may be deficient. Excretory urograms may be essentially normal, although changes compatible with healed pyelonephritis are often seen. Cystoscopy will show the changes caused by infection. Urine specimens obtained by ureteral catheter may reveal renal infection. Cystography may show vesicoureteral reflux.

C. Neurogenic Disease: Children suffering from sacral cord or root abnormality (eg, myelodysplasia) may have incomplete urinary control both day and night. Since they ordinarily have significant amounts of residual urine, infection is usually found on urinalysis.

The passage of a catheter, or the post-voiding film taken in conjunction with excretory urograms, will demonstrate the presence of residual urine. A plain film of the abdomen may reveal spina bifida.

The cystometrogram is usually typical of a flaccid neurogenic bladder. Cystoscopy demonstrates an atonic bladder, with moderate trabeculation and evidence of infection.

D. Distal Urethral Stenosis: This congenital anomaly is the cause of enuresis in many young girls, even in the absence of cystitis. Urethral calibration will establish this diagnosis.

Complications

The complications of functional enuresis are psychic, not organic. These children are particularly disturbed when they begin to attend school. Even more pressure is brought to bear by their parents; the child finds it impossible to stay overnight at the homes of his playmates. Unhealthy introversion may be his lot. Enuresis may be prolonged because of undue emphasis or as a result of punitive or shaming measures.

Late Sequelae

Occasionally an adult is seen who, under stress, develops nocturnal frequency without comparable diurnal frequency. Thorough urologic investigation proves to be negative. Many of these people will give histories of enuresis of long duration in childhood. It is suggested that their cerebrovesical pathways again break down under undue emotional tension; nocturnal frequency may be the adult expression of enuresis.

Treatment

Treatment should be considered if enuresis persists after the age of 3 years.

A. General Measures: Fluids should be limited after supper. The child should empty his bladder at bedtime and should be completely awakened a little before the usual time of bedwetting and allowed to void.

Drug therapy has its proponents.

1. Imipramine (Tofranil®) has been reported to cure 50-70% of patients. Start with 25 mg at bedtime. Increase the dose as needed to 50 mg. Twenty-five mg usually suffice.

2. Parasympatholytic drugs - Atropine (or belladonna), by decreasing the tone of the detrusor, has at times helped. Methantheline bromide (Banthine®), 25-75 mg at bedtime, is more potent.

3. Sympathomimetic drugs - Dextroamphetamine sulfate, 5-10 mg at bedtime, may cause enough wakefulness so that the child perceives the urge to void.

4. Diphenylhydantoin (Dilantin®) has been found to control some of those children whose electroencephalograms are abnormal.

5. The use of mechanical devices such as metal-covered pads which when wet cause an alarm to ring may be of benefit in cases of delayed maturation by setting up a conditioned reflex.

6. Urologic treatments (eg, urethral dilatation, urethral instillations of silver nitrate), though often recommended, should be condemned in the absence of demonstrable local disease. They are physically and psychically traumatic and can only cause further apprehension and fear in an already disturbed child.

B. Psychotherapy: Analytic evaluation and treatment may be indicated for the child and his parents. Responsibility for correction of the patient's feelings of insecurity rests with the parents, who must be cautioned not to punish the child nor in any way contribute further to his feelings of guilt and insecurity. The handling of the parents may prove difficult, in which case psychiatric referral may be necessary.

Prognosis

Retraining the enuretic child and, above all, reeducating the parents is difficult and time-consuming. Psychiatric referral for the parents and, at times, for the child may be necessary. Most patients conquer their enuresis by the age of 10 years. A few, however, do not, and may later develop vesical irritability of the psychogenic type under acute or chronic tension or anxiety.

Bakwin, H.: Enuresis in children. J Pediat 58:806-19, 1961.

Barbour, R. F., & others: Enuresis as a disorder of development. Lancet 2:787-90, 1963.

Campbell, E. W., Jr., & J. D. Young, Jr.: Enuresis and its relationship to electroencephalographic disturbances. J Urol 96:947-9, 1966.

Forsythe, W. I., & A. Redmond: Enuresis and the electric alarm: Study of 200 cases. Brit MJ 1:211-3, 1970.

Kunin, S. A., & others: The efficacy of imipramine in the management of enuresis. J Urol 104:612-5, 1970.

Linderholm, B. E.: The cystometric findings in enuresis. J Urol 96:718-22, 1966.

Martin, G. I.: Imipramine pamoate in the treatment of childhood enuresis. Am J Dis Child 122:42-7, 1971.

Oppel, W. C., Harper, P. A., & R. V. Rider: Social, psychological, and neurological factors associated with nocturnal enuresis. Pediatrics 42:627-41, 1968.

Oppel, W. C., Harper, P. A., & R. V. Rider: The age of attaining bladder control. Pediatrics 42:614-26, 1968.

Smith, D. R., & A. Auerback: Functional diseases. Pp 20-33, in: Encyclopedia of Urology, Vol 12. Springer-Verlag, 1960.

Starfield, B.: Functional bladder capacity in enuretic and nonenuretic children. J Pediat 70:777-81, 1967.

Werry, J. S., & J Cohrssen: Enuresis—an etiologic and therapeutic study. J Pediat 67:423-31, 1965.

IMPOTENCE

Various degrees of impotence in men are common, but it is rare to find definite organic cause for the complaints, which include inability to gain an erection, weak erections, premature ejaculation, loss of libido, or loss of normal sensation with ejaculation. The cause of almost all of these difficulties is psychogenic.

Most men are resistant to this concept, however. They are certain that the masturbation in which they indulged during adolescence or the gonorrhea they contracted later hurt their sexual organs. They have been taught that their symptoms are due to organic diseases, including prostatitis, verumontanitis, posterior urethritis, and decrease in androgen elaboration by the testes.

Physiology

The development of the male sexual attitude and power depends upon the presence of normal androgenic secretion at the time of puberty and the development of a male-oriented sexual attitude based on sociologic and psychogenic influences.

The ability to gain and maintain an erection that culminates in timed normal orgasm and ejaculation requires an intact nerve and blood supply to the lower genitourinary tract. The various aspects of potency are controlled by both autonomic and somatic nerves. Erection requires arteries of such caliber that an adequate flow of blood can be delivered to the penis.

A. Erection: This function is initiated by psychic or local influences. Sensory impulses reach the upper portion of the lumbar cord. Reflexes are set up through the sacral parasympathetic outflow (S2-4) which lead to relaxation of the arterioles to the corpora of the penis; the blood pressure within them approaches that of the carotid arteries. The cavernosus bodies are thus engorged under pressure. Lack of psychic stimulus, narrowed arterioles (atherosclerosis), or interruption of these nerves can impair the quality of erection.

B. Emission: Sensory nerve impulses from the glans penis reach the sacral cord and travel to the integrating center in the upper portion of the lumbar cord. These impulses set off a massive stimulus through the thoracolumbar sympathetic nerves which cause secretions from the prostate, seminal vesicles, and ejaculatory ducts to enter the prostatic urethra. Interruption of these nerves may preclude emission.

C. Ejaculation: Immediately after emission, spasmodic contractions of the muscles surrounding the urethra and those of the pelvic floor occur, thus forcing jets of semen down the urethra. The nerves involved are somatic S2-4. Accompanying the series of ejaculations is the rhythmic sensation of orgasm (S2-4). Hence, a lower motor neuron lesion in this zone could impair ejaculation and the sensation of orgasm.

D. Subsidence of Erection: The arterioles to the penis then contract and erection subsides.

Psychodynamics

With few exceptions, the causes of sexual difficulties in the male are psychic, ie, based on guilt, anxiety, jealousy, or frigidity on the part of the wife. Seldom is evidence of hypogonadism seen as an organic cause; androgen therapy as such is of little avail. Prostatitis may be an incidental finding; its treatment seldom improves sexual power unless the patient expects it to, in which case improvement is usually only temporary. After the age of 50 years, many men notice some diminution of desire and sexual power.

Clinical Findings

Partial or complete impotence is the only symptom. Complaints referable to the vascular system should be explored. Intermittant claudication might imply restriction of blood supply to the corpora. Vesical function will be abnormal if there is a neurologic defect causing impaired erection (S2-4). Survey, therefore, should include assay of peripheral pulses and neurologic examination with particular reference to S2-4. In most instances, however, no organic changes are found.

Many of these men are obviously tense and nervous. General and local examination of the external genitalia seldom shows any abnormality. The prostate may be hypersensitive and boggy due to lack of use of the organ. Cystoscopy may reveal increased sensitivity and redness of the trigone, posterior urethra, and the verumontanum. These changes are the effects, not the causes, of the sexual disability.

Differential Diagnosis

Primary or secondary hypogonadism is associated with small, often flabby testes; other endocrinologic changes are obvious. FSH may be elevated or low; urinary 17-ketosteroid or serum testosterone levels may be below normal. Thirty percent of diabetic men have evidence of hypogonadotropic hypogonadism and experience impotence and infertility or neurologic deficit.

Impotence may develop secondary to disease of, or surgical or traumatic injury to, the lumbar sympathetics, the spinal cord, or peripheral sacral nerves. Motor and sensory changes should be obvious.

In older men, poor erections may develop as a result of arteriosclerotic stenosis of the aorta or hypogastric arteries. Inability to maintain an erection is part of the Leriche syndrome, which leads to impaired blood flow through the hypogastric arteries, whose branches supply the corpora cavernosa. Arterial pulses in the legs are diminished, and a bruit may be heard over the femoral arteries. Angiography will reveal the vascular lesion. Gaskell finds low penile blood pressure in many impotent men despite lack of evidence of peripheral vascular disease. This may prove to be the main cause of impotence in men over the age of 60 years.

Certain drugs prescribed for the treatment of such diseases as peptic ulcer, hypertension, and hypersensitivity may adversely affect sexual power. These include estrogens (for prostatic carcinoma), parasympathetic and ganglionic blocking agents, antihistamines, and tranquilizers. Phenothiazine and phenoxybenzamine may interfere with the ejaculation and emission of semen.

Treatment

Psychiatric treatment is usually necessary. Sexual problems in the male are difficult to treat and usually require more time and skill than the physician without psychiatric training can give.

The placement of an intrapenile plastic prosthesis may be considered in the treatment of patients with neurologic defects. Lash utilizes this technic also in psychologic impotence. It seems to afford considerable satisfaction for these sexual cripples.

Organic treatment is contraindicated in the psychogenic group. It only further assures the patient that masturbation or an attack of gonorrhea has caused damage to his sexual organs. Painful (and expensive) treatment (eg, prostatic massage, urethral dilatations, fulguration of the verumontanum) at times appears successful because guilt and anxiety are thus relieved.

Prognosis

Unless the patient's difficulties are of short duration, he should be referred to a psychiatrist.

Bancroft, J.: Sexual inadequacy in the male. Postgrad MJ **47**:562-71, 1971.

Cooper, A.J., & others: Androgen function in "psychogenic" and "constitutional" types of impotence. Brit MJ **3**:17-20, 1970.

Ellenberg, M.: Impotence in diabetes: The neurologic factor. Ann Int Med **75**:213-9, 1971.

Finkle, A.L., & D.V. Prian: Sexual potency in elderly men before and after prostatectomy. JAMA **196**:139-3, 1966.

Finkle, A.L.: Sexual function during advancing age. In: Textbook of Geriatrics. I. Rossman (editor). Lippincott, 1969.

Gaskell, P.: The importance of penile blood pressure in cases of impotence. Canad MAJ **105**:1047-51, 1971.

Jakobvits, T.: The treatment of impotence with methyltestosterone thyroid (100 patients—double blind study). Fertil Steril **21**:32-5, 1970.

Lash, H.: Silicone implant for impotence. J Urol **100**:709-10, 1968.

Mudd, J.W., Jr., & R.J. Siegel: Sexuality— The experience and anxieties of medical students. New England J Med **281**:1397-402, 1969.

Newman, H.F., Northup, J.D., & J. Devlin: Mechanism of human penile erection. Invest Urol **1**:351-3, 1964.

Pearman, R.O.: Treatment of organic impotence by implantation of a penile prosthesis. J Urol **97**:716-9, 1967.

Shader, R.I.: Sexual dysfunction associated with thioridazine hydrochloride. JAMA **188**:1007-9, 1964.

Smith, D.R., & A. Auerback: Functional diseases. Pp 34-57, in: Encyclopedia of Urology, Vol 12. Springer-Verlag, 1960.

•   •   •

Index